User Manual for Minimally Invasive Surgical Equipment

Jasmeet Singh Ahluwalia
Editor

User Manual for Minimally Invasive Surgical Equipment

Description, Maintenance, Troubleshooting

Springer

Editor
Jasmeet Singh Ahluwalia
Director – Department of Bariatric & Minimal
Access Surgery
STAR Superspeciality Hospital
Jalandhar, Punjab, India

ISBN 978-981-95-9018-6 ISBN 978-981-95-9019-3 (eBook)
https://doi.org/10.1007/978-981-95-9019-3

This Springer imprint is published by the registered company Springer Nature Singapore Pte Ltd.
The registered company address is: 152 Beach Road, #21-01/04 Gateway East, Singapore 189721, Singapore

To my parents, the roots of my strength; to my wife, Mandeep, the heart of my journey; and to my children, Keerat and Amanat, the promise of every tomorrow.

Preface

> Instruments in hand, with a steady heart,
> Surgeon's touch makes science an art.
> The scalpel gleams, a trusted friend,
> Together they mend, together they tend.

The relationship between a surgeon and their instruments transcends mere technical necessity; it is a profound bond forged through trust, precision, and the shared objective of saving lives. For a surgeon, their instruments become extensions of their body, executing intricate movements that demand both control and sensitivity. With each incision and every stitch, these instruments become conduits for healing, yet also vessels for the surgeon's artistic expression.

Years of dedicated training and practice shape a surgeon's craft, and during this journey, their instruments become familiar companions. The weight of a scalpel, the tension of a suture, and the precision of a laparoscope become intuitively understood after countless hours of honing. This intimate connection allows surgeons to comprehend their instruments' capabilities, limitations, and nuances, akin to a musician's trust in their instrument.

> The true mark of excellence in Minimal Access Surgery lies not only in the surgeon's hands, but in the team's intimate understanding of their instruments—caring for them as extensions of their craft, preserving their integrity, and responding to every technical challenge with calm mastery.

Since the birth of laparoscopy in human medicine almost a century ago, the tools and technologies that define this field have evolved at an astonishing pace. What began with the ingenious use of reflected sunlight for illumination has advanced to an era where artificial intelligence and augmented reality are becoming integral to the operating room. The journey from crude optical systems to intelligent surgical platforms mirrors the broader evolution of surgery itself—one driven by innovation, precision, and the relentless pursuit of better outcomes.

While surgeons today are far more technologically adept than their predecessors, the intricate machinery that powers minimal access surgery—from laparoscopic towers to robotic and laser systems—often remains the domain of biomedical engineers. For many, the technical aspects of these systems can feel like navigating a foreign language. As a result, external assistance is frequently sought for procurement, setup, troubleshooting, and maintenance.

This dependence, though understandable, carries inherent disadvantages. In the high-stakes environment of the operating room, every moment counts. A limited understanding of technical systems can lead to delays or suboptimal use of equipment—outcomes that may directly affect patient safety.

This book was conceived to bridge that gap. It aims to provide a clear, practical understanding of the technology that drives minimal access surgery. Each chapter demystifies instruments and equipment, explaining their principles, maintenance, and troubleshooting in language accessible to medical professionals. The goal is not to replace the engineer, but to empower the surgeon—and by extension, the entire surgical team.

In minimal access surgery, precision and coordination are paramount. Most laparoscopic systems operate in a sequential and interdependent manner, where even a single point of failure can disrupt the entire process. From the assembly of equipment before surgery to its careful disassembly afterward, every step must follow established protocols to ensure efficiency, safety, and longevity of instruments. The clarity of the surgical image, the stability of pneumoperitoneum, the efficiency of hand instruments, and the safe operation of energy devices all rely on this delicate harmony.

When an intraoperative anomaly arises, the team must quickly diagnose and correct it without compromising patient safety or prolonging anesthesia. Without a structured understanding of the equipment, such moments can devolve into confusion and misplaced accountability. Knowledge of the intricate interplay between surgical devices and human expertise is therefore indispensable.

The primary objective of this book is to disseminate that knowledge to all members of the operating team, fostering confidence and preparedness. It encourages a culture where surgeons, trainees, and staff share a common technical language—one that strengthens teamwork and ensures patient safety. Ideally, each chapter should be studied alongside the corresponding equipment, allowing for hands-on familiarity that transforms theory into understanding.

The chapters have been carefully organized to cover each instrument's functional principles, practical usage, maintenance, and troubleshooting. Additional sections address the expanding domains of robotic surgery and laser technologies, which are increasingly integrated into laparoscopic practice. A dedicated chapter on sterilization techniques underscores the vital importance of proper sterilization in maintaining both safety and functionality.

We envision this book as a ready reference within the operating room—a companion for surgical teams striving for excellence in every procedure. Whether you are an experienced surgeon, a trainee, or an operating room technician, this resource is meant to support your journey toward mastering the art and science of minimal access surgery.

This book is a tribute to that sacred partnership—an exploration of the art and intimacy that define a surgeon's relationship with their tools. Yet, it is also something more. It is a celebration of global unity in the world of surgery, a tapestry woven from the experiences and wisdom of surgeons across continents.

From Asia, contributors hail from India, Singapore, Malaysia, Nepal, Bangladesh, the Philippines, and Taiwan—regions where ancient healing traditions meet modern innovation.

From Europe, voices from Portugal, Spain, and the United Kingdom lend depth, representing the precision and discipline honed in centuries of surgical evolution.

From the Middle East and Africa, surgeons from Jordan and Egypt bring insights shaped by resilience, dedication, and an enduring spirit of care.

From Latin America, contributors from Colombia, Brazil, and Mexico infuse the work with compassion, warmth, and the strength of communities that heal together.

From Central Asia, the inclusion of Kyrgyzstan reflects the growing global reach of surgical science and education.

And from North America, the presence of authors from the United States adds a voice of innovation, leadership, and academic excellence.

These instruments are not merely tools; they are silent partners in healing. They have witnessed triumphs, challenges, and countless moments of human resilience. When a surgeon grasps a familiar instrument, there is a quiet understanding—a rhythm between human hand and engineered precision. In the sterile theatre, where every second matters, these instruments offer assurance and stability, allowing surgeons to focus on the most unpredictable variable of all—the human body itself.

This book seeks to strengthen that bond—to bring the surgeon closer to their instruments, transforming familiarity into mastery and technology into trust.

> May this book offer some solace to the minimally invasive surgeon who valiantly undertakes the intricate and gratifying journey of this captivating surgical specialty.

Jalandhar, Punjab, India Jasmeet Singh Ahluwalia

Contents

Part I

Operating Room Setup

The Operating Room

1

Prasad Bhukebag and Roy Patankar

1.1 Introduction

The operating room (OR) is one of the most specialised and controlled environments within healthcare. Its design and organisation play a crucial role in determining surgical outcomes, efficiency, infection control, and team performance. For the surgeon, the configuration and functionality of the OR are directly relevant to safe and effective practice. Over time, the OR has evolved from basic surgical spaces to modern, high-precision environments that support advanced procedures. This chapter outlines the key principles of OR design, with a focus on practical considerations required for contemporary surgical practice. These include room dimensions, ergonomic layout, air handling systems, temperature and humidity control, door design, lighting, electrical infrastructure, and appropriate wall and flooring materials. Minimal access surgery places additional demands on the OR. Unlike open procedures, laparoscopic techniques rely on specialised instruments, video-assisted visualisation, and coordinated team workflow. This requires a well-planned environment that allows efficient equipment placement, clear visual access, and adequate working space. A thoughtfully designed OR improves operative efficiency, maintains patient safety, and supports the integration of evolving technologies, including robotic and energy-based systems. This chapter aims to provide a clear, practical overview of OR design principles, helping surgeons and institutions develop operating environments suited to current and future surgical needs.

P. Bhukebag (✉) · R. Patankar
Zen Multispeciality Hospital, Mumbai, Maharashtra, India

J. S. Ahluwalia (ed.), *User Manual for Minimally Invasive Surgical Equipment*,
https://doi.org/10.1007/978-981-95-9019-3_1

1.2 Historical Development

Surgery's earliest settings were far from ideal. Procedures took place wherever necessity dictated. In earlier times, surgeons travelled with their toolkits, conducting operations wherever needed—in patients' homes, makeshift camps, urban settings, or war zones. These non-specialised environments lacked dedicated facilities, proper anaesthesia, and infection control. Unsurprisingly, mortality rates remained high, with infection being the cause of death.

During the seventeenth and eighteenth centuries, amphitheatres became key venues for surgical practice, where surgeons performed operations, demonstrated techniques, and delivered lectures concurrently. Among these, the anatomy amphitheatre in Padua, Italy, gained particular fame [1]. In these settings, live patients underwent surgical procedures while an eager audience looked on. Little attention was paid to concerns about contamination, sepsis, or the considerable pain experienced by the patients during these public demonstrations. The term "operation theatre" originated from amphitheatre-style rooms where surgeries were performed before student audiences. The Old Operating Theatre at St. Thomas' Hospital in London (1822) is a fascinating preserved example of these early surgical spaces [2].

The surgical landscape transformed dramatically when Joseph Lister introduced antiseptic principles in 1867, using carbolic acid sprays and steam sterilisation [3] (Fig. 1.1). This marked the beginning of the aseptic era, emphasising contamination

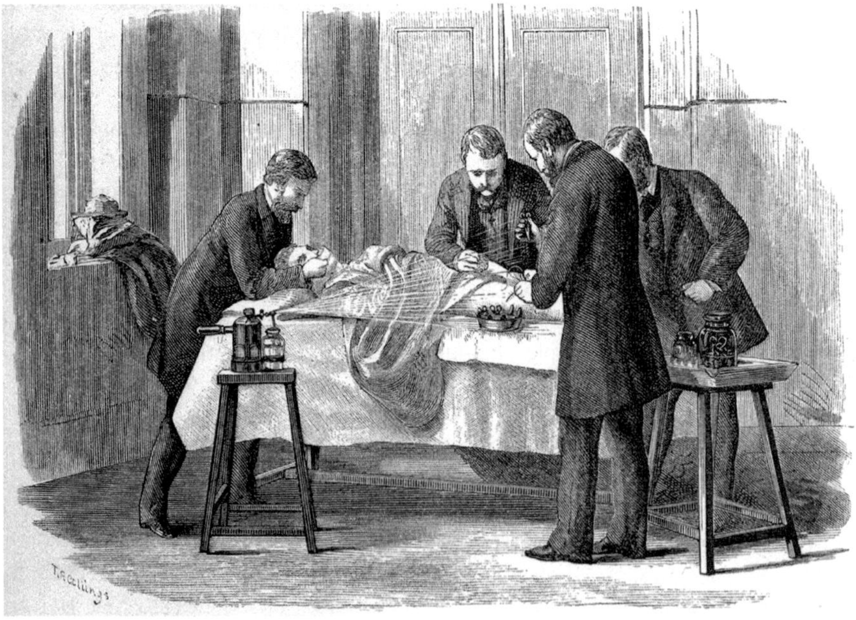

Fig. 1.1 Joseph Lister overseeing the use of carbolic acid spray during one of his early antiseptic surgical operations in 1865. (Source: https://wellcomecollection.org/works/c5yxmjue – Permission obtained from Wellcome Collection)

prevention through sterile environments and specialised equipment. Post-World War II advancements further revolutionised surgery, with purpose-built operating suites featuring overhead lighting, integrated anaesthesia systems, HEPA filtration, and laminar airflow [4]. Safety protocols and checklists also improved, reducing errors and enhancing outcomes [5].

Modern ORs now showcase technologies unimaginable to past surgeons: robotic systems for precision, real-time imaging, computer networks for patient data, and advanced ventilation to minimise infections. These innovations reflect two centuries of progress, prioritising infection control, efficiency, and patient safety—a remarkable journey from crude surgical spaces to today's high-tech facilities.

1.3 Spatial Design and Zonal Structure

ORs use a concentric zone design to maintain sterility and prevent infections during surgery. The innermost sterile zone includes the surgical field, used instruments, and scrubbed team members working under strict aseptic conditions. Surrounding this is the clean zone containing anaesthesia equipment and non-scrubbed personnel. Further out lies the semi-restricted zone with support areas like sub-sterile rooms and storage spaces. The outermost unrestricted zone includes pre-operative and post-operative areas where surgical attire isn't required. This arrangement protects sterility while allowing efficient patient movement [6].

1.3.1 Ideal Size of the Operating Room

The size of a laparoscopic OR must accommodate surgical personnel, essential equipment, and advanced technologies while ensuring sufficient manoeuvring space.

- Standard Laparoscopic OR: 400–600 square feet (37–56 square meters) is recommended [6].
- Robotic Surgery OR: A larger area of 600–800 square feet (56–74 square meters) is preferred to accommodate robotic arms, consoles, and additional monitors.
- Sufficient Clearance: The OR must allow free movement of the surgical team, anaesthesia workstation, and mobile equipment.

1.3.2 Special Flooring for the OR

The flooring of an OR plays a critical role in supporting hygiene, safety, and comfort.

- Seamless, Antimicrobial, and Non-Slip Flooring: Reduces bacterial growth and prevents accidents, particularly in a high-stakes surgical environment.

- Conductive Flooring: Designed to prevent static electricity, it is vital to avoid interference with sensitive surgical equipment, ensuring uninterrupted functionality during procedures.
- Easy-to-Clean Surfaces: Vinyl or epoxy flooring is preferred over traditional tile flooring to avoid grout lines where bacteria can accumulate.

1.3.3 Ideal Walls for the OR

Seamless, non-porous, and antimicrobial wall materials are ideal, as they prevent bacterial growth and can be cleaned efficiently.

Material Choices

- Stainless steel panels offer durability and sterility, while high-pressure laminate provides smooth, non-reflective surfaces that enhance the overall functionality of the space.
- Epoxy coatings can be applied to create a seamless finish, further reducing the risk of contamination.
- In cases where fluoroscopic procedures are performed, lead-lined walls are recommended to provide necessary radiation shielding.

1.3.4 Ideal Doors for the Operating Room

Doors are a critical component of the operating room, playing a vital role in infection control and facilitating ease of access.

- Hermetically sealed sliding doors are particularly advantageous as they prevent air leaks and significantly reduce the risk of contamination, ensuring a sterile environment.
- Automatic motion-sensor doors further enhance sterility by eliminating the need for physical contact, thereby minimising the transfer of pathogens.
- Doors with noise reduction features contribute to a quieter OR environment, helping maintain focus during delicate surgical procedures [7].

1.3.5 Layout and Design Considerations

A well-structured OR layout enhances workflow efficiency and minimises risks during surgical procedures.

- The operating table should be centrally positioned to allow 360-degree access for the surgical team, ensuring flexibility and ease of movement.

- Dedicated equipment zones are crucial, with laparoscopic towers, anaesthetic machines, and sterile trays assigned to specific areas to reduce clutter and streamline access.
- High-definition monitors must be strategically placed at ergonomic angles to provide optimal visualisation for the entire team, reducing strain and improving focus.
- Additionally, adequate storage solutions, such as built-in shelves or mobile units, should be incorporated to efficiently organise surgical instruments and supplies, maintaining a tidy and functional OT environment.

1.4 Essential Equipment and Infrastructure

1.4.1 Air Circulation, Temperature, and Humidity Control

A well-designed OR ventilation system is critical to maintaining a sterile environment and ensuring optimal conditions for surgery.

- Laminar Airflow System: HEPA-filtered laminar airflow systems should be installed to minimise airborne contamination, providing a continuous stream of purified air directed over the surgical field. However, evidence suggests that laminar airflow does not reduce surgical site infection rates [8].
- Positive Air Pressure: The OR must maintain positive air pressure relative to adjacent areas, acting as a barrier to prevent the ingress of contaminants.
- Temperature Control: The recommended OR temperature is 20–24 °C to ensure patient and staff comfort during procedures.
- Humidity Levels: Humidity levels should be carefully regulated between 40 and 60% to strike a balance that inhibits microbial growth while preserving the functionality of sensitive equipment [9].

1.4.2 Lighting Requirements for Laparoscopic Surgery

Proper lighting is a critical component for achieving precision in laparoscopic surgery, with both general and task-specific illumination playing vital roles.

- Ceiling-mounted LED-based general lighting provides uniform illumination across the operating room, with a recommended brightness level of 1000–1500 lux to ensure overall visibility.
- For direct illumination of the surgical site, shadow-free, adjustable surgical lights are essential, offering significantly higher brightness levels of 40,000–160,000 lux to create a well-lit surgical field. These surgical lights are equipped with adjustable arms, allowing surgeons to position them with precision to suit the specific requirements of the procedure [10].

1.4.3 Electrical Supply, Backup, and Cabinets

The OR should be equipped with dedicated power circuits, including isolated electrical systems, to prevent power fluctuations that could compromise sensitive equipment. In addition, a robust backup power system comprising an uninterruptible power supply (UPS) and a hospital-grade generator is essential to safeguard against unexpected disruptions. Adequate socket placement is equally critical, with multiple high-voltage outlets provided to accommodate laparoscopic equipment and other devices. Emergency shutoff switches should also be strategically located to enhance safety in case of an electrical hazard [11].

Glass-fronted storage cabinets are strategically integrated into the OR environment to organise instruments and supplies in a manner that ensures quick access while maintaining a sterile and clutter-free workspace. These transparent cabinets facilitate easy identification of essential tools and support infection control protocols by minimising unnecessary handling and exposure of sterile items.

1.4.4 Supporting Facilities for an Efficient OR Complex [6]

1.4.4.1 Scrubbing and Hand Hygiene Area

The design of an OR complex extends beyond the surgical suite itself, encompassing various supporting areas that contribute to seamless operations, patient safety, and staff efficiency. A dedicated scrubbing and hand hygiene area should be near the OR entrance to provide quick access for surgeons and staff. This area should feature automatic sensor-based faucets to minimise contamination risks, alongside wall-mounted scrub stations equipped with antimicrobial solutions. Adjacent to this, an instrument cleaning and sterilisation area is essential for the immediate processing of used instruments. This space should include cleaning, rinsing, and drying provisions, with sterilisation performed either within the OR complex or in a designated area. Separate entry and exit points for this zone help prevent cross-contamination, maintaining the sterility of the environment.

1.4.4.2 Patient Passage and Movement Areas

Patient movement and passage areas are equally critical in ensuring smooth workflows. Dedicated entry and exit routes should be established to prevent unnecessary contact with non-sterile zones. At the same time, wide corridors—a minimum of 2.5 m (8 feet) wide—are necessary to accommodate stretchers and allow easy movement of staff. Restricted access doors should be installed to prevent unauthorised personnel from entering the sterile field, safeguarding the integrity of the OR environment.

1.4.4.3 Pre-operative Patient Preparation Area

The pre-operative patient preparation area should include beds with privacy partitions to allow patients to be prepped for surgery in a dignified manner. Vital sign monitors should be available for pre-surgery assessments, and the area must have direct access to both the OR and the anaesthesia room to facilitate quick and efficient patient transfers.

1.4.4.4 Post-operative Recovery Room

The post-operative recovery room plays a vital role in patient care after surgery. Located near the OR, it ensures immediate attention can be provided during the critical recovery period. The recovery room should be equipped with cardiac monitors, oxygen supply systems, and comfortable beds with adjustable headrests to support patient comfort and monitoring during recovery.

1.4.4.5 Staff Working and Relaxation Area

For the surgical team, adequate provision of staff working and relaxation areas is essential to maintain morale and ensure optimal performance. A break room with lockers provides a space for rest, while a meeting room allows for case discussions and coordination among team members. Conveniently located toilets, pantry facilities, and changing rooms enable staff to change into scrub suits privately and access basic amenities, fostering a supportive and functional work environment.

1.5 Future Developments in OR Design

Rapid technological advancements, deeper digital integration, a stronger focus on sustainability, and greater attention to human factors shape the evolution of OR design. These emerging trends promise to enhance surgical precision, streamline operations, and improve patient outcomes and staff well-being.

Robotic systems are becoming smaller and increasingly precise, allowing for finer control during minimally invasive procedures, reducing tissue trauma and speeding recovery times. Future iterations may incorporate adaptive features, enabling robots to adjust to real-time changes in the operative field [12].

Artificial intelligence is poised to redefine theatre functionality by enhancing multiple aspects of surgical practice. It can refine scheduling by predicting procedure durations and resource needs, ensuring smoother transitions between cases [13].

Fifth-generation connectivity is set to expand the boundaries of surgery by enabling telesurgery, where experts can guide or perform procedures remotely with minimal delay. This could bring specialised care to distant locations, bridging gaps in surgical expertise. Meanwhile, Internet of Things devices are improving theatre efficiency by connecting equipment, monitors, and records into a cohesive network. These innovative systems track instrument usage, monitor patient vitals, and automate documentation, reducing manual tasks and freeing staff to concentrate on clinical priorities [14].

Sustainability and flexibility are paramount, reflecting both environmental considerations and the need for adaptability. Modular designs enable rapid reconfiguration of spaces to accommodate diverse procedures, maximising utility and future-proofing against regulatory changes or practice growth. Energy efficiency measures, such as LED lighting, smart climate controls, and heat recovery systems, reduce operational costs and environmental impact [15]. Waste reduction initiatives, including reprocessing programs and sustainable supply chains, align with global sustainability goals, while resource conservation efforts like water recycling and emission reductions contribute to greener healthcare facilities. Together, these strategies create surgical environments that are both environmentally responsible and highly adaptable to evolving clinical demands.

Digital integration is transforming theatres into highly coordinated environments. Centralised control systems allow staff to manage lighting, tables, and imaging from a single interface, reducing delays during surgery. Voice-activated documentation enables hands-free recording of notes, preserving sterility while capturing critical details. Data-driven enhancements analyse workflow patterns, identify bottlenecks, and suggest efficiency adjustments—such as repositioning equipment or streamlining staff movements.

Cloud connectivity is emerging as a powerful tool for real-time collaboration. By linking theatres to secure cloud platforms, surgical teams can share live data with colleagues for immediate input, whether for second opinions or multidisciplinary consultation. Post-procedure, cloud-stored records allow detailed analysis of outcomes, techniques, and complications, fostering continuous improvement across institutions [16].

Human factors are increasingly central to theatre design, addressing the physical and mental demands on surgical teams. Ergonomic improvements, such as adjustable tables and instrument layouts, reduce strain during lengthy procedures, preventing fatigue-related errors. Acoustic dampening materials lower ambient noise, creating a quieter environment that enhances concentration. Circadian-aligned lighting mimics natural daylight cycles, helping sustain alertness during extended shifts. Dedicated break areas offer respite between cases, while advanced communication systems improve coordination, ensuring clear instructions and reducing misunderstandings.

1.6 Conclusion

The modern OR integrates meticulous design with advanced technology to ensure procedural safety, efficiency, and optimal outcomes. Its zoned structure, robust environmental systems, and specialised equipment reflect a steadfast commitment to infection control and surgical precision. Future innovations, including artificial intelligence, robotics, and adaptable configurations, promise greater versatility and sustainability, meeting the evolving demands of surgical practice. These advancements enhance patient care whilst supporting the operational well-being of theatre teams, establishing the OR as a progressive, adaptable space.

References

1. Ferrari G. Public anatomy lessons and the carnival: the anatomy theatre of Bologna. Past Present. 1987;117:50–106. https://doi.org/10.1093/past/117.1.50.
2. The Old Operating Theatre Museum. Surgery and the Victorian operating theatre. London: The Old Operating Theatre Museum and Herb Garret. Available from: https://oldoperatingtheatre.com/surgery-and-the-victorian-operating-theatre
3. Lister BJ. The classic: on the antiseptic principle in the practice of surgery. 1867. Clin Orthop Relat Res. 2010;468(8):2012–6. https://doi.org/10.1007/s11999-010-1320-x. PMID: 20361283; PMCID: PMC2895849.
4. Memarzadeh F, Manning AP. Comparison of operating room ventilation systems in the protection of the surgical site. ASHRAE Trans. 2002;108(2):3–15.
5. Haynes AB, Weiser TG, Berry WR, Lipsitz SR, Breizat AH, Dellinger EP, Safe Surgery Saves Lives Study Group, et al. A surgical safety checklist to reduce morbidity and mortality in a global population. N Engl J Med. 2009;360(5):491–9. https://doi.org/10.1056/NEJMsa0810119.
6. Facility Guidelines Institute. Guidelines for design and construction of hospitals. St. Louis: FGI; 2018.
7. Chow TT, Yang X-Y. Performance of ventilation system in a non-standard operating room. Build Environ. 2003;38:1401–11. https://doi.org/10.1016/S0360-1323(03)00155-0.
8. Brandt C, Hott U, Sohr D, Daschner F, Gastmeier P, Rüden H. Operating room ventilation with laminar airflow shows no protective effect on surgical site infection rates in orthopaedic and abdominal surgery. Ann Surg. 2008;248(5):695–700. https://doi.org/10.1097/SLA.0b013e31818b757d.
9. Dharan S, Pittet D. Environmental controls in operating rooms. J Hosp Infect. 2002;51(2):79–84. https://doi.org/10.1053/jhin.2002.1217.
10. Knulst AJ, Mooijweer R, Jansen FW, Stassen LP, Dankelman J. Indicating shortcomings in surgical lighting systems. Minim Invasive Ther Allied Technol. 2011;20(5):267–75. https://doi.org/10.3109/13645706.2010.534169. Epub 2010 Nov 17.
11. Davey AJ, Diba A. Ward's anaesthetic equipment. 6th ed. London: Elsevier Health Sciences; 2012.
12. Marcus HJ, Ramirez PT, Khan DZ, Layard Horsfall H, Hanrahan JG, Williams SC, Beard DJ, Bhat R, Catchpole K, Cook A, Hutchison K, Martin J, Melvin T, Stoyanov D, Rovers M, Raison N, Dasgupta P, Noonan D, Stocken D, Sturt G, Vanhoestenberghe A, Vasey B, McCulloch P, IDEAL Robotics Colloquium. The IDEAL framework for surgical robotics: development, comparative evaluation and long-term monitoring. Nat Med. 2024;30(1):61–75. https://doi.org/10.1038/s41591-023-02732-7. Epub 2024 Jan 19. Erratum in: Nat Med. 2024 Apr;30(4):1213. https://doi.org/10.1038/s41591-024-02836-8
13. Loftus TJ, Tighe PJ, Filiberto AC, Efron PA, Brakenridge SC, Mohr AM, Rashidi P, Upchurch GR Jr, Bihorac A. Artificial intelligence and surgical decision-making. JAMA Surg. 2020;155(2):148–58. https://doi.org/10.1001/jamasurg.2019.4917. PMID: 31825465; PMCID: PMC7286802.
14. Elendu C, Elendu TC, Elendu ID. 5G-enabled smart hospitals: innovations in patient care and facility management. Medicine (Baltimore). 2024;103(20):e38239. https://doi.org/10.1097/MD.0000000000038239. PMID: 38758872; PMCID: PMC11098186.
15. McGain F, Naylor C. Environmental sustainability in hospitals – a systematic review and research agenda. J Health Serv Res Policy. 2014;19(4):245–52. https://doi.org/10.1177/1355819614534836. Epub 2014 May 9.
16. Levin M, McKechnie T, Kruse CC, Aldrich K, Grantcharov TP, Langerman A. Surgical data recording in the operating room: a systematic review of modalities and metrics. Br J Surg. 2021;108(6):613–21. https://doi.org/10.1093/bjs/znab016.

Operating Room Table

2

Raquel Rodrigues, Sónia Ribas, Nitin Choudhary, and Sankho Choudhury

2.1 Introduction

In recent decades, minimally invasive surgery continues to expand in several surgical areas. The operating room table is a crucial piece of equipment in surgical settings. It is designed to provide a stable and adjustable platform for patients during surgical procedures. Its versatility allows for various positions, ensuring optimal access for surgeons. For laparoscopic procedures, operating room tables need to facilitate patient positioning and access. They should have Trendelenburg and reverse Trendelenburg capabilities, as well as height and lateral tilt functionality to optimize for patient's comfort and optimal ergonomics. Additionally, the table must provide adequate space for the laparoscopic tower and instruments, ensuring seamless integration with the surgical team's workflow. Advanced models often feature electronic controls, enhancing precision and efficiency in the operating room.

R. Rodrigues
ULS Póvoa de Varzim – Vila do Conde, Porto, Portugal

S. Ribas
ULS Póvoa de Varzim – Vila do Conde, Porto, Portugal

Hospital Lusíadas Braga, Braga, Portugal

N. Choudhary (✉)
Department of Anaesthesiology, Pain Medicine & Critical Care, All India Institute of Medical Sciences (AIIMS), New Delhi, India

S. Choudhury
Department of Neuroanaesthesiology & Neurocritical Care, All India Institute of Medical Sciences (AIIMS), New Delhi, India

J. S. Ahluwalia (ed.), *User Manual for Minimally Invasive Surgical Equipment*,
https://doi.org/10.1007/978-981-95-9019-3_2

2.2 Mechanism of Function for Operating Tables

The operating room table operates through sophisticated mechanisms that involve components controlled by specialized handles, buttons, or panels. These mechanisms allow for precise adjustments and for ease of operating during surgery. The commonly used mechanisms are:

- *Motorized system*: Electronic controls for precise and smooth adjustments in height, tilt, and lateral movement. It is dependent on a power source and has potential for electronic malfunction.
- *Hydraulic system*: Use of hydraulic fluid to power adjustments in different sections of the table. It has a reliable and strong lifting capacity, but requires more maintenance, limited in adjustability compared to a motorized system.
- *Pneumatic system*: Air pressure-driven mechanism for smooth and controlled movement. It has quieter operation and is easy to control but may lack the fine-tuned adjustments of motorized tables.
- *Manual cranks or lever*: Hand-operated mechanism for adjusting the table's position, which makes it simple and reliable to use as it is not reliant on a power source. It is limited in terms of quick and precise adjustments and requires more physical effort to operate.

2.3 Parts

An operating room table typically consists of several essential parts (Fig. 2.1):

- *Tabletop*: The surface where the patient lies during the surgery. Preferably to have a radiolucent top to facilitate the use of fluoroscopy.

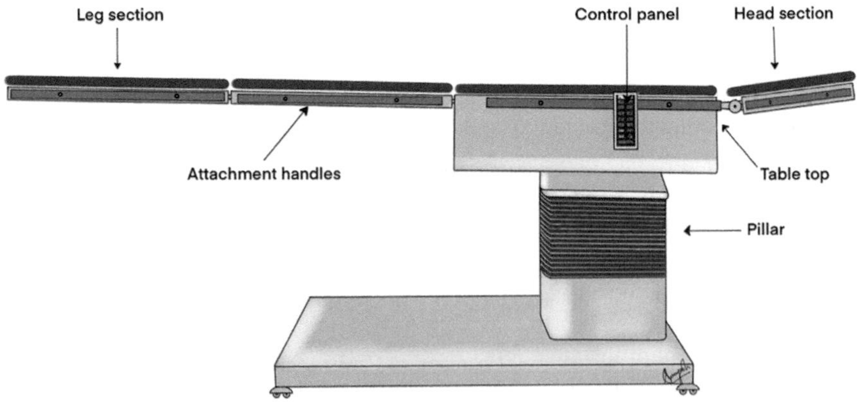

Fig. 2.1 Operating table components. (Courtesy Dr. Shreyash Agrawal)

- *Pillar*: The supportive structure providing stability to the table. It is usually placed off-center (as it allows for easy introduction of C-arm).
- *Adjustment mechanism*: Motor or manual control for height, tilt, and lateral movement.
- *Head section*: The upper part of the table, often removable with attachment points for headrests.
- *Leg section*: The lower part of the table, adjustable for procedures like lithotomy.
- *Control panel*: For regulating electronic adjustment and settings.
- *Accessory attachments*: Parts for adding specialized equipment or surgical tools as described below:

  1. *Attachment for patient positioning*: Such as arm boards, leg holders, or stirrups.
  2. *Safety straps and paddings*: It ensures patient stability during procedures.
  3. *Radiolucent tops*: Facilitates imaging during surgery.
  4. *Accessory rails*: Allows for additional equipment attachments.
  5. *Remote control*: For convenient adjustment of table setting.
  6. *Positioning aids*: Cushions and pads for patient comfort and stability.
  7. *Traction systems*: For orthopedic procedures.

2.4 Remote Control

Remote control functions for operating room tables allow surgeons or staff to make adjustments from a distance. The remotes usually have an LCD display to provide basic information on the operating table status with a backlit screen for viewing in darkened operating rooms. They are impact resistant to protect them from drops and damage, and the buttons may be colored to offer a quick identification for the most frequently used functions.

Some commonly used settings include (Fig. 2.2):

- *Height adjustment*: Raises or lower the table to the desired level.
- *Tilt control*: Adjusts the tilt of the table in Trendelenburg and reverse Trendelenburg positions.
- *Lateral movement*: Moves the table laterally to enhance access during surgery.
- *Head and leg section control*: Modifies the positioning of the head and leg sections as needed.
- *Level or "0" button*: It ensures that the table is positioned evenly and horizontally. Brings back the table to neutral position from any other position.
- *Memory setting*: Save and recall preferred table configurations for efficiency.
- *Emergency stop*: Quickly halt table movement in case of an emergency.
- *Lock*: It is crucial in securing the table's position. When locked, it prevents unintended movement of the table providing stability.
- *Unlock*: This allows medical staff to unlock the table to make adjustments and ensures precise and controlled positioning.

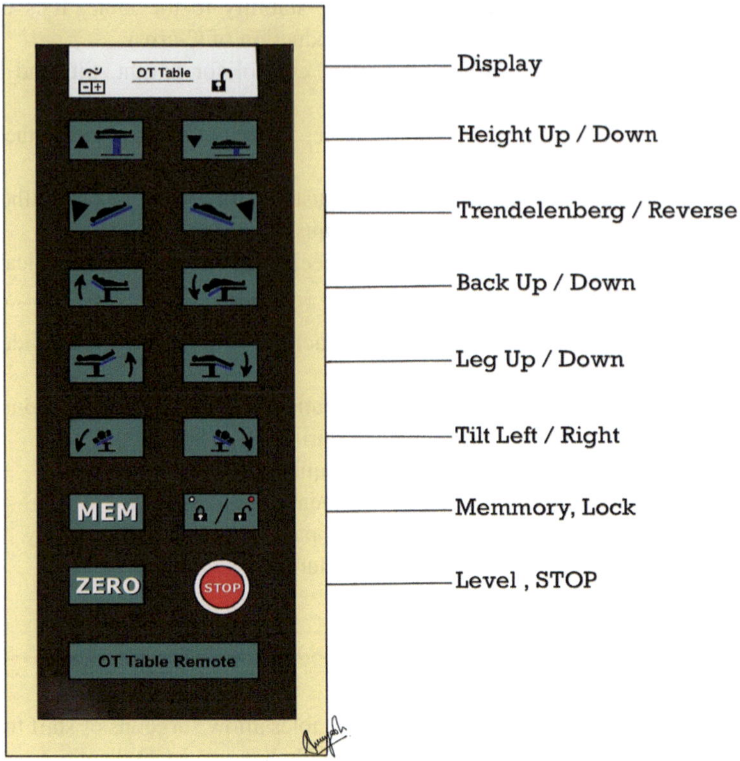

Fig. 2.2 Remote control. (Courtesy Dr. Shreyash Agrawal)

2.5 Dimensions of the Operating Table

2.5.1 Height

The maximum and minimum height of an operating room table depend on the specific model and its design. Typically, the minimum height allows for easy patient transfer and accessibility for surgical teams, while the maximum height provides flexibility for various procedures and surgeon preferences. Heights can vary, but common ranges might be around 28 inches (71 cm) minimum to 40 inches (102 cm) maximum or more. For laparoscopic surgery, the optimum height often falls within this range to align the instrument handles with the surgeon's elbow level. For bariatric surgery, lower height is recommended.

2.5.2 Length and Width

The dimensions of operating room tables can vary, but a standard table might have a length of approximately 75 to 80 inches (190 to 203 cm) and a width ranging from 20 to 30 inches (51 to 76 cm).

2.5.3 Weight

The maximum weight-bearing capacity of an operating room table typically ranges from 300 to 600 pounds (136 to 272 kilograms). It's crucial to adhere to the manufacturer's guidelines and specifications to ensure patient safety and the proper functioning of the table during a surgical procedure.

2.6 Bariatric Operating Room Table

Generally tailored for larger patients, these tables often exceed standard dimensions. Widths typically range from 26 inches (66 cm) to 32 inches (81 cm) or more, offering ample surface area for support. Length varies from approximately 78 inches (198 cm) to 84 inches (213 cm) or more. With a weight-bearing capacity ranging from 600 to over 1000 pounds (272 to 454 kilogram), these tables ensure a stable platform for bariatric surgeries. Specific dimensions may differ based on the model and manufacturer.

2.6.1 Positions

The most common surgical positions include (Fig. 2.3):

- *Supine*: Natural position of the body at rest. It is the most common position for surgery.
- *Trendelenburg*: The upper torso is lowered and the feet raised, aiding in pelvic organ visualization during laparoscopic and lower abdominal surgeries. To prevent the patient from slipping, padded straps or restraints should be used across the torso and legs to secure the patient. Ensure proper padding on the operating table to enhance friction and reduce slippage. Additionally, regularly check and adjust the straps to maintain a secure position throughout the procedure.
- *Reverse Trendelenburg*: Head-up and feet down position. It is suitable for head and neck procedures as well as upper abdominal laparoscopic surgeries. The feet should be supported to avoid the patient from slipping down.
- *Prone*: Patient lies flat on their stomach. It is commonly used for spine and rectal surgeries.
- *Lithotomy*: The patient lies supine with raised and abducted legs requiring stirrups.

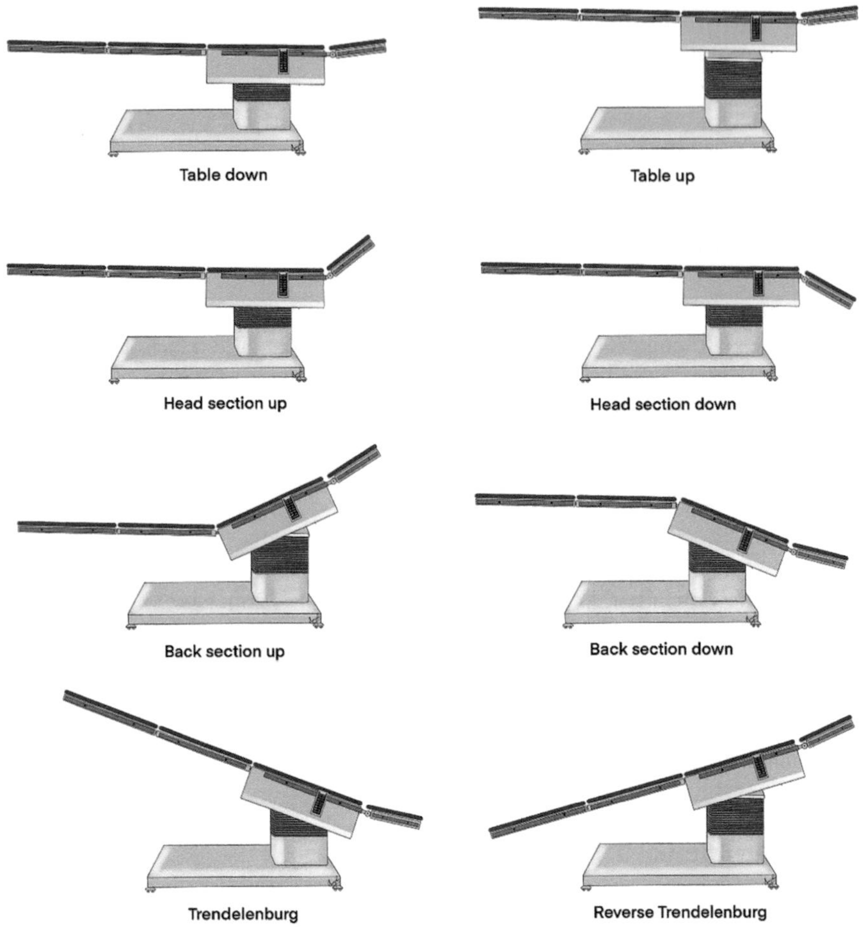

Fig. 2.3 Common operating table positions. (Courtesy Dr. Shreyash Agrawal)

- *Fowler's (sitting)*: Patient sits at a 90-degree angle, with knees slightly flexed and feet placed against a padded footboard. It is ideal for neurosurgery and facial operations.
- *Lateral*: Patient lies on the non-operative side for hip, chest, or renal surgeries. The patient should be secured by straps or restraints to avoid the risk of falling.

2.7 Maintenance

Regular maintenance of the operating room tables is crucial for their optimal performance. This includes cleaning surfaces after each use, checking hydraulic or electric components for any issues, inspecting moveable parts for wear and tear and ensuring that all adjustments function correctly. Following the manufacturer's guidelines for maintenance schedules and procedures is essential to keep the table in good working condition.

2.8 Troubleshooting

If an operating table is not functioning properly, it is imperative to address the issue as quickly as possible to avoid any disruption to patient care and prevent injuries.

Some commonly encountered problems and troubleshooting steps are (Table 2.1):

Table 2.1 Operating room table malfunction: tips, tricks, and troubleshooting

Issue	Possible cause	Solution
Table not powering on	Power cord unplugged or faulty connection	Check power cord, plug into a working outlet, and ensure secure connections.
	Blown fuse or tripped circuit breaker	Replace the fuse or reset the circuit breaker.
	Internal electrical fault	Contact biomedical engineering or manufacturer support.
Table movement is unresponsive	Low battery (for battery-operated models)	Charge or replace the battery.
	Faulty control panel or remote	Check for loose connections or replace the remote batteries.
	Hydraulic or motor failure	Inspect hydraulic fluid levels or call for service.
Unusual noise during movement	Lack of lubrication in moving parts	Apply appropriate lubricant to joints and moving mechanisms.
	Loose or worn-out components	Tighten or replace worn-out parts.
Table tilts unexpectedly or fails to lock in position	Faulty brake system	Engage the brakes properly or check for damage.
	Hydraulic or mechanical failure	Call for technical support or maintenance.
Leg or back section not adjusting	Obstruction or jammed mechanism	Inspect for debris or mechanical blockage and remove it.
	Motor or actuator failure	Contact technical support for repair or replacement.
Table height not adjusting	Low hydraulic fluid (for hydraulic models)	Refill hydraulic fluid if applicable.
	Electrical malfunction in motorized tables	Check wiring connections or call for service.
C-arm compatibility issues	Non-radiolucent table section in use	Ensure the correct radiolucent tabletop is being used.
Table remote or foot pedal not working	Battery drained or faulty connection	Replace remote batteries or check wired connections.
Unstable table movement	Uneven floor or broken wheels/casters	Adjust table levelling, inspect wheels, and replace if damaged.

2.9 Future

The future of operating room tables may involve advancements in smart technology, improved materials for enhanced infection control, and increased customization to accommodate various surgical techniques. Integration with artificial intelligence and robotics could further refine patient positioning and support surgical procedures. The focus may be on creating more ergonomic, efficient, and patient-friendly designs to elevate the overall surgical experience.

Lights Inside the OR

3

Darwin Salonga

3.1 Introduction

Surgical performance in the operating room (OR) relies heavily on effective illumination, as optimal lighting plays a critical role in ensuring precision, accuracy, and safety during procedures [1]. Adequate illumination helps mitigate the environmental, operational, and visual challenges inherent to surgery, including variable tissue reflectance, shadow formation, surgeon fatigue, and the need for continuous visual focus on complex anatomical structures. By enhancing visibility, reducing eye strain, and supporting consistent image perception, high-quality lighting contributes to improved surgical outcomes and overall workflow efficiency. OR lighting is one of the most important factors when setting up a minimally invasive surgery (MIS) OR. On the rise of state-of-the-art surgical suites where multiple monitors, advanced energy devices, ultrasound units, electro-cauteries, endoscopes, C-arms, and robots are positioned around the operating table, a well-lit MIS suite is a challenge as well as a must.

3.2 History

Before the advent of electricity and the introduction of lightbulbs into the operating room (OR), surgeons relied on candles as a primary source of illumination during procedures. Operations were also commonly scheduled during daylight hours to take advantage of natural sunlight, which offered more reliable visibility than artificial means available at the time. Over the more than century-long evolution that followed Thomas Edison's discovery of practical electric light in 1879, surgical lighting has undergone substantial transformation.

D. Salonga (✉)
Department of Surgery, De Los Santos Medical Center, Quezon City, Philippines

J. S. Ahluwalia (ed.), *User Manual for Minimally Invasive Surgical Equipment*,
https://doi.org/10.1007/978-981-95-9019-3_3

With the rise of advanced technologies and the development of hybrid operating rooms, one technical aspect that is often overlooked is the presence of natural sunlight. Beyond simply allowing individuals to perceive the time of day, exposure to natural light has been shown to enhance alertness, reduce fatigue, and alleviate stress among OR staff [2]. Historically, prior to the discovery of the light bulb, mankind made use of natural sunlight through strategically located windows with the addition of mirrors to reflect light appropriately.

Today, the challenge of allowing natural sunlight is limited due to the functional demands of other OR components. Limitations in spaces include wall, floor, and ceiling spaces that may be preferentially needed for monitors, equipment, or simply as general walking or standing areas to increase OR efficiency. Furthermore, opening a portion of the ceiling for a skylight or a wall window for natural sunlight may not be feasible at all times. For the past few years, there have been more discussions on the use of natural sunlight for operating rooms and hospital buildings more than ever.

3.3 The Ideal Modern OR Lighting

The OR lights of today should provide flexible adjustment capabilities, including customizable color temperature, intensity, and focus. These features allow surgical teams to adapt illumination to the specific requirements of a procedure. Equally important are comfortable and easily accessible controls that can be tailored to the surgeon's individual preferences and contribute to optimal performance during procedures. Such adaptability not only enhances visual clarity but also supports optimal ergonomic performance, contributing to improved efficiency and safety throughout the surgical workflow. An easy to control and adjust console panel, either attached to the OR table head or remotely in one of the walls of the OR, is preferable, so that the circulating nurse will be able to adjust and control the lights accordingly.

3.4 Factors to Consider

- *Luminance and Shadow Management:* OR lights should provide adequate luminance without causing eye strain. *Luminance* is measured in LUX, which is defined as the amount of light falling on a surface where one lux (1 lx) of light is equivalent to 1 lumen per square meter (lm/m^2). According to the International Electrotechnical Commission (IEC) [3, 4], the standard OR lights should provide a range of 40,000 lx to 160,000 lx in order to provide clear surgical visualization. Key features of modern OR lights should include power adjustments, intensity variations, shadow diffusion, and easy operability. Shadows and glare management can likewise pose a threat during operations. These lights should have multiple sources and easy adjustability that can be focused and directed in order to minimize shadows and glare. According to the American Academy of Ophthalmology (AAO), one of the primary contributors to eye strain (asthenopia) is exposure to excessive or improper illumination. This visual discomfort can be further exacerbated by the rapid and repetitive eye movements required for detailed visual tasks, a demand that is particularly pronounced in minimally invasive surgery [5, 6]. The risk of eye fatigue underscores the importance of appropriate OR lighting design and visual ergonomics.

- *Color Temperature and Color Rendering:* These are critical considerations when looking for the ideal OR lighting. To replicate natural daylight as closely as possible, the color temperature, measured in Kelvin (K), should generally fall between 3000 and 6700 K in contrast to a regular household bulb with 2700 to 3000 K. Achieving a daylight-like quality not only enhances visual comfort but also improves the accuracy of tissue visualization. Equally important is Color Rendering Index (CRI), ideally between 85 and 100, which ensures that colors are represented faithfully. A high CRI allows surgeons to distinguish subtle variations in body tissue and fluids, supporting precise assessment and decision-making throughout surgical procedures. The higher the CRI, the higher the precision. The International Electrotechnical Commission (IEC) criteria for chromaticity coordinates and correlated color temperature (CCT) demand a higher level of specificity. Although two light sources may share the same CCT and therefore be expected to exhibit a similar color appearance, such as yellowish-white, bluish-white, or something in between their actual visual characteristics can differ significantly. If the chromaticity coordinates of these light sources do not fall close to the *Planckian* locus, the emitted light may instead appear greenish or pinkish, despite having an equivalent CCT [7]. This is the importance of assessing both CCT and chromaticity when ensuring accurate and reliable illumination in the OR.
- *Heat Emission:* OR lights are a source of unwanted excessive heat that may cause discomfort not only to the surgeon and scrub nurse but also cause unwarranted tissue desiccation to the patient. There are various reports of burns cited in cases of overhead light use in varying severity due to ineffective heat shielding. Light-emitting diode (LED) technology can mitigate these untoward incidences by its reduced heat emission [1].
- *Surgical Ergonomics:* Accessibility and functionality should be highly considered in an ideal OR lights. Easy navigation and operability during the entire duration of surgery is vital to maximize its usage without causing strain and discomfort on the surgeon specially for long procedures. According to Stucky et al., comparing MIS versus open surgery, generalized pain was noted in 69% and 60% of MIS and open surgeons, respectively. Fatigue was likewise considerably more common in those performing MIS versus open procedures (83% vs. 37%). Many MIS surgeons have reported work-related injury such as cervical spinal stenosis, lumbar disc herniation, and carpal tunnel syndrome [5]. Therefore, it is mandatory to minimize such fatigue and maximize surgical ergonomics with properly equipped OR lights.
- *Integration and Compatibility:* Live surgery and virtual meetings are now part and parcel of continuing surgical education activities post COVID19 pandemic. The modern OR lights are now integrated with cameras to provide on-site video output as well as to record every procedure. They are likewise capable of audio output that can be disseminated to a broader audience inside and outside the operating theater. These features should then be compatible with other audio-visual set-ups for documentation, integration, and transmission to a local and international community.

3.5 Ambient OR Lights

With the advancement of LED technology, supplemental surgical lighting solutions are now available. OR can now be equipped with an optimal visual environment using GREEN and BLUE ambient light.

Green light interacts with a visual environment in ways that differ markedly from white light. Rather than producing distracting glare, creating hot spots, or washing out images on surgical displays, the use of ambient green lighting and its reflection from monitor surfaces has been shown to enhance image depth and contrast [8]. Because green light is more compatible with screen visibility, green luminaires can be remained illuminated throughout surgical procedures, providing essential light for support staff while allowing them to move safely and efficiently within the OR without compromising the surgeon's visual field.

In a study by Lembo et al. in 2015, blue light was also found to contribute to improved visual comfort in the OR. The researchers observed significant differences in illumination between surrounding areas and the visual task zones when blue lighting was used. Visual comfort was assessed through measurements of maintained illuminance (Em) and the luminance levels within the operating field, demonstrating that blue light can support visual ergonomics during procedures [9] (Fig. 3.1).

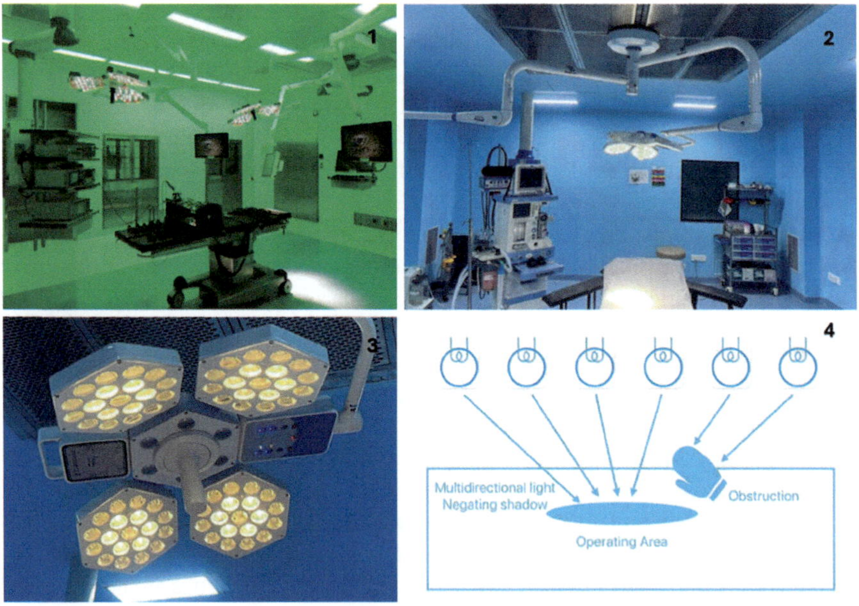

Fig. 3.1 (1) Modern OR with green ambient light. (2) Modern OR with integrated system. (3) Modern OR lights with and shadowless lighting. (4) Principle behind this feature

3.6 Conclusion

Selecting the ideal operating room (OR) lights is a critical decision that directly influences surgical outcomes, patient safety, and overall OR efficiency. Modern surgical lighting systems offer improved luminance, precise color rendering, reduced heat emission, and enhanced ergonomic features that collectively support greater surgical accuracy and comfort. These advancements have made today's OR lights more capable of delivering a safe, reliable, and efficient surgical environment. As technology continues to evolve, further innovations in surgical illumination are expected to emerge, shaping the operating theater of the future.

References

1. Curlin J, Herman CK. Current state of surgical lighting. Surg J (N Y). 2020;6(2):e87–97. https://doi.org/10.1055/s-0040-1710529. PMID: 32577527; PMCID: PMC7305019.
2. Golvani J, Roos L, Henricson M. Operating room nurses' experiences of limited access to daylight in the workplace – a qualitative interview study. BMC Nurs. 2021;20(1):227. https://doi.org/10.1186/s12912-021-00751-8. PMID: 34753467; PMCID: PMC8579627.
3. SIS Förlag AB. SS-EN 60601-2-41 medical electrical equipment—part 2:41: particular requirements for basic safety and essential performance of surgical luminaires and luminaires for diagnosis. Stockholm: SIS; 2010.
4. Illuminating Engineering Society of North America. RP-29-06. Lighting for health care facilities and hospitals. New York, NY: IESNA; 2006.
5. Stucky CH, Cromwell KD, Voss RK, et al. Surgeon symptoms, strain, and selections: systematic review and meta-analysis of surgical ergonomics. Ann Med Surg (Lond). 2018;27:1–8.
6. Toich, S. Surgical lighting to optimize and focus light intensity. https://www.lumitex.com/blog/surgical-lighting-ergonomics
7. Technical Guidance Document: LED Surgical Task Lighting. https://www1.eere.energy.gov/buildings/publications/pdfs/alliances/surgical_task_fs.pdf
8. Dana Porter, November 2022. https://www.architecturalssl.com/innovation/article/33001258/advantages-of-green-light-in-operating-rooms
9. Lembo M, Cannatà V, Militello A, Ritrovato M, Zaffina S, Derrico P, Borra M. Illuminazione artificiale e luce blu in sala operatoria: quali rischi per il chirurgo? [Artificial lighting and blue light in the operating room: what risks for the surgeon?]. Med Lav. 2015;106(5):342–50. Italian.

Suction Systems in the Operating Room

4

Wei-Liang Loh

A suction machine or system is a device that is used primarily used for removing fluid—like mucus, saliva, blood, or secretions—from a person's body cavity.

A cardiologist named Pierre Carl Edouard Potain was the first to introduce the first conventional aspirator in 1869 into medical practice. This was a simple machine that used a manual pump to drain excess fluid build-up in the chest, in an attempt to avert cardiac failure. As electricity supply became dependable and widespread, suction machines transitioned from manual pump devices to electric devices [1].

W.-L. Loh (✉)
Department of Hepatopancreatobiliary and Transplant Surgery, Singapore General Hospital, Singapore, Singapore

J. S. Ahluwalia (ed.), *User Manual for Minimally Invasive Surgical Equipment*,
https://doi.org/10.1007/978-981-95-9019-3_4

4.1 Types of Suction Systems—Central and Local Machines Inside OT

4.1.1 Central Suction Systems

Currently, most modern operating theatres are outfitted with central suction systems. These can be stationary, wall-mounted suction systems, or semi-movable towers that are mounted from the ceiling. A centralized suction system consists of one

Description of components of a central suction system (Fig. 4.1).

1. Pump(s): for generation of vacuum pressure; via various mechanisms such as rotary vane, etc.
2. Vacuum tank: stores the vacuum pressure created by the vacuum pump(s), for distribution on demand.
3. Vacuum control: allows a technician or engineer to control the vacuum pressure distribution and check on the status of the entire system.
4. Bacteria filter: traps bacteria and other micro-organisms that may have come through the distribution pipes, to prevent contamination of the vacuum tank and pump(s).
5. Secretion trap: prevents reflux of bodily fluids from the distribution pipes into the vacuum tank and pump(s).
6. Distribution system: piping system that distributes vacuum pressure from the vacuum tank to the rest of the hospital, where it is utilized on demand.

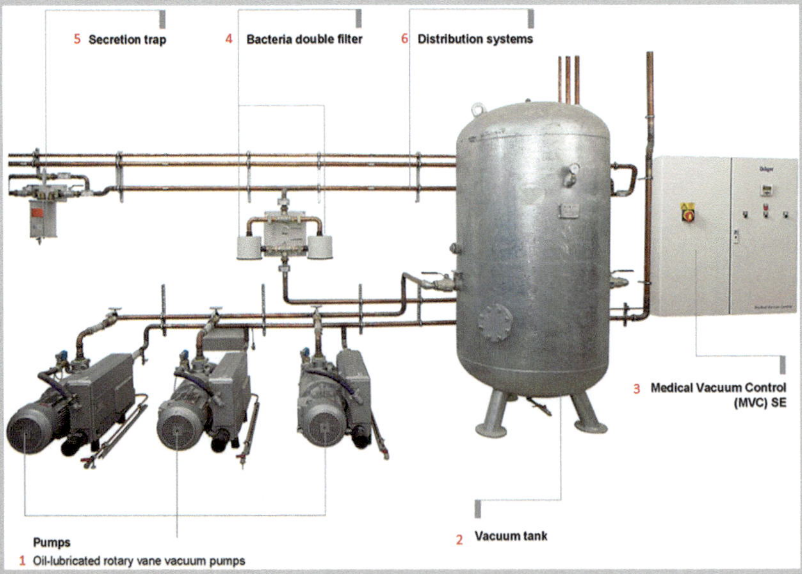

Fig. 4.1 Example of a centralized medical vacuum system. (© Drägerwerk AG & Co. KGaA, 2023)

or several pumps that can accommodate all the facility's equipment that requires suction.

Most centralized suction systems consist of vacuum pump(s), buffer tank(s), control panels, with bacteria filters and/or traps placed along the circuit (Fig. 4.1). The vacuum pumps generate vacuum, which is then transmitted to the buffer vacuum tank. Distribution pipes allow this vacuum to be transmitted to various points within the hospital (e.g., operating theatres, intensive-care, general ward, emergency room, etc.). The bacteria filters and secretion traps serve to prevent reflux of microorganisms and contaminated fluids back into the vacuum tank.

For the sake of redundancy and improved efficiency, systems have a minimum of two pumps and they are used alternately or additionally activated when more suction is required. Most pumps are single-stage rotary vane pumps with an ultimate pressure of around 1 mbar. The buffer vessels have volumes of 100 to 1000 liters, inlet filters, and a draining valve for condensed liquids and particles.

Distribution pipes provide vacuum pressure via ports in the operating theatre. These ports can be found either attached to the wall or ceiling-mounted towers (Fig. 4.2).

As centralized suction systems only generate vacuum, additional connection tubings, sterile patient tubings, and collection canisters are required in order to create a functional and seamless suction unit capable of providing suction capabilities during surgery (Figs. 4.2 and 4.3) [2].

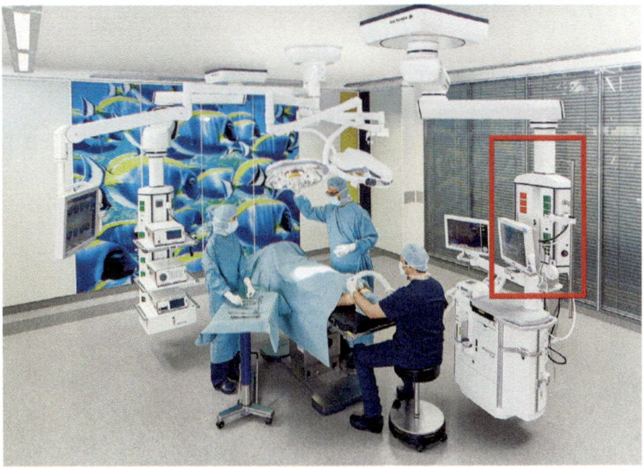

Fig. 4.2 Example of an operating theatre with a ceiling-mounted tower, capable of providing vacuum pressure via ports

Description: vacuum port-connecter tubing set-up (Fig. 4.3).

1. Vacuum port: distributes vacuum stored within vacuum tank to operating theatres; can be found attached to walls or on ceiling-mounted towers (as in this case).
2. Connection tubing: allows the vacuum pressure within the central system to be transmitted to canisters, and subsequently to the operative field.

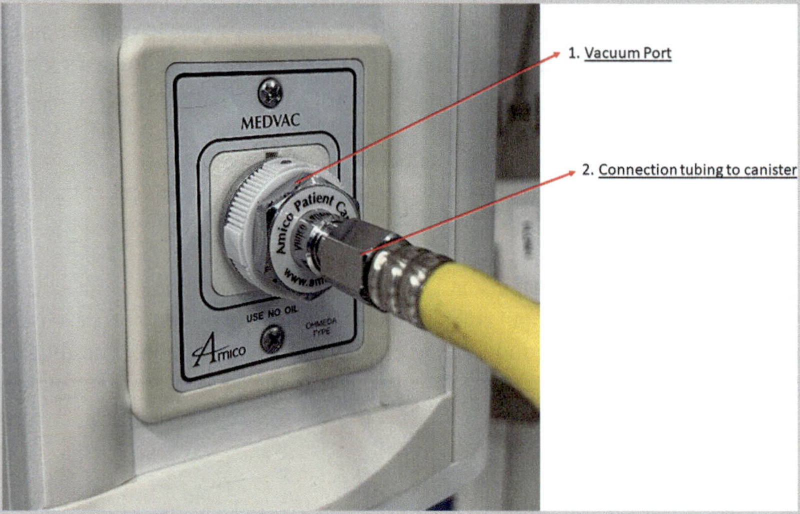

Fig. 4.3 Close-up of a connection tubing from a ceiling-mounted central suction system

Description: vacuum port connected to canister system set-up (Fig. 4.4)

1. Vacuum port: provides vacuum from central system.
2. Connection tubing: transmits vacuum from vacuum port to collection canister system.
3. Collection canister system: regulates the vacuum pressure and collects effluent from the surgical field.

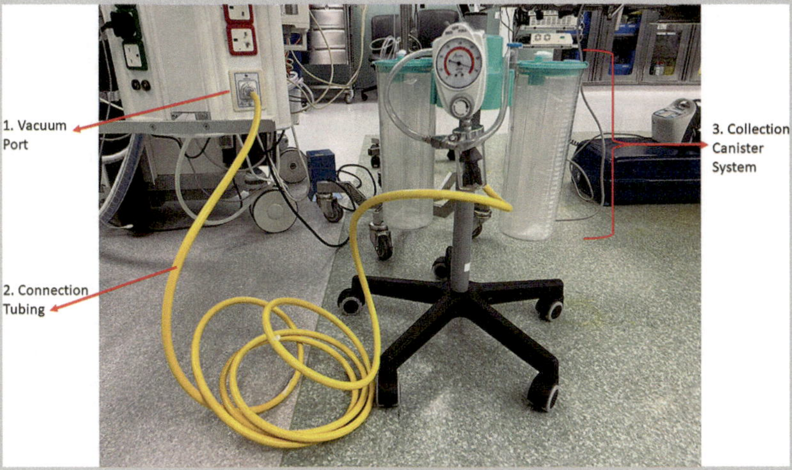

Fig. 4.4 Over-view of how a ceiling-mounted vacuum port is connected to canisters, which will then be connected to the surgical field

Description: how vacuum pressure is transmitted to collection canister system (Fig. 4.5)

1. Vacuum pressure regulator: contains switches and knobs to regulate the vacuum pressure that is transmitted to the collection canisters, and hence the surgical field.
2. Connection tubing: clear tubing that transmits vacuum pressure via (1) to collection canisters.
3. Connection tubing: yellow opaque tubing that transmits vacuum from vacuum port to (1).
4. Filter: connected between (1) and (2) to prevent contamination from the collection canisters into (1) and subsequently the vacuum port.

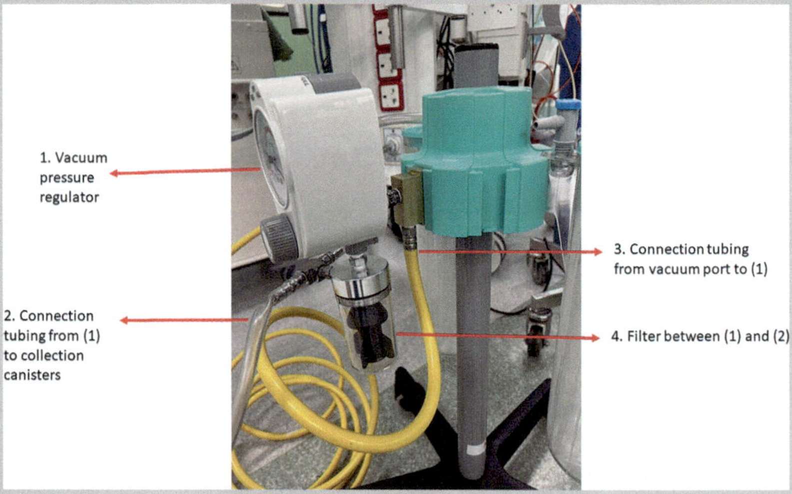

Fig. 4.5 Depiction of how vacuum pressure is transmitted to the collection canister system

Description: vacuum pressure regulator (Fig. 4.6)

1. Switch for vacuum pressure: in this particular example, it allows for vacuum pressure to be either "OFF," "REGULAR," or "FULL" power mode.
2. Vacuum pressure display: displays the vacuum pressure in units of mmHg that is being transmitted to the collection canisters and hence the surgical field.
3. Knob for vacuum pressure: in this particular example, this knob further regulates the vacuum pressure based on mmHg, after the power mode has been selected via (1).
4. T-connecter: this connects (1) to the clear connection tubings that lead to collection canisters (via the filter), and allows for up to 2 collection canisters to be in use at a time.

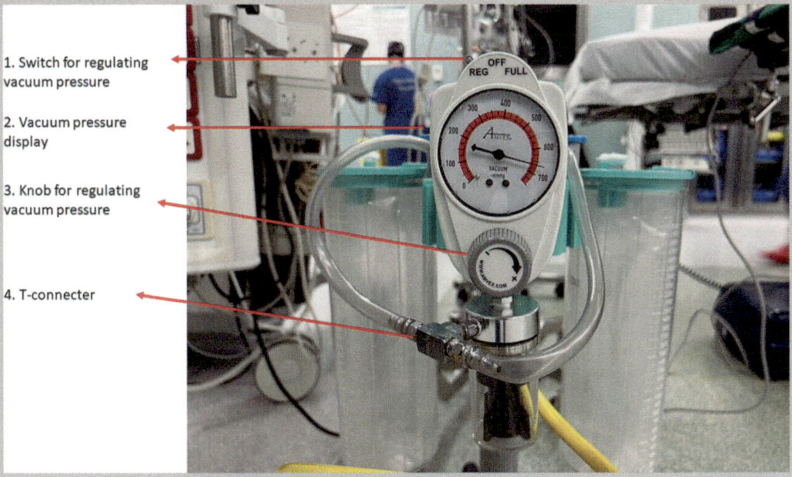

Fig. 4.6 Vacuum pressure regulator

Description: connections between canister stand and vacuum pressure regulator (Fig. 4.7)

1. Nozzle (white): In this model, the white nozzle is meant for the attachment of a connection tubing to the surgical field; this tubing evacuates effluent from the surgical field into the collection canister utilizing vacuum pressure.
2. Collection canister: collects effluent from the surgical field; this particular model has a capacity of 3 L.
3. Nozzle (grey): This nozzle connects the collection canister to the pressure regulator (via the filter and T-connector).
4. Connection tubing: This clear tubing connects the collection canister to the pressure regulator (via the filter and T-connector).
5. Canister stand: This model of canister stand allows for up to six canisters to be attached, and is equipped with a broad wheel base to allow for manoeuvrability in the operating room.
6. Attachment bracket: This allows for attachments of collection canisters and other compatible accessories (e.g., the pressure regulator).
7. T-connector: This allows for a pressure regulator to transmit vacuum pressure to up to two collection canisters.

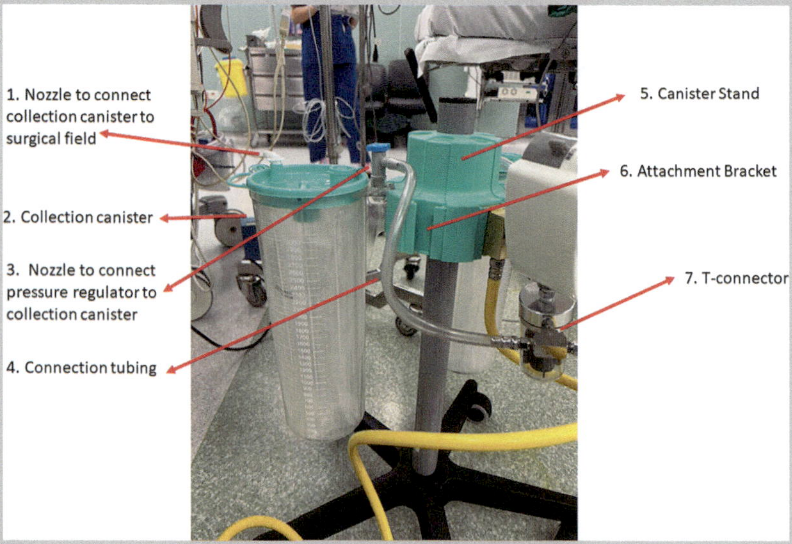

Fig. 4.7 Connections between canister stand and vacuum pressure regulator

Description: Depiction of collection canisters being serially connected (Fig. 4.8)

1. Canister stand: allows for multiple canisters to be mounted and connected, on a wheel base that allows for manoeuvrability in the operating room.
2. Connection tubing: connects the collection canister system to the surgical field for evacuation of effluent.
3. Connection tubing: these tubings allow effluent to flow from one canister to the next, hence increasing the capacity of the collection system.
4. Collection canisters: collects effluent from the surgical field.
5. Connection tubings: these tubins transmit vacuum pressure from the vacuum pressure source through to each of the collection canisters.
6. Connection tubing: connects vacuum pressure source to the entire collection canister system.

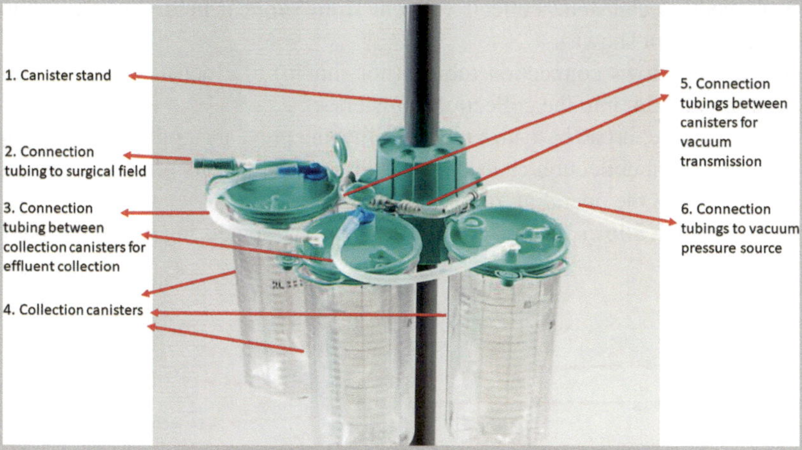

Fig. 4.8 Depiction of collection canisters being serially connected

4.1.2 Portable Suction Machines

However, some operating theatres still function mainly on local portable suction devices, and most hospitals will keep a few portable suction units in the rare event of a malfunctioning central suction system. They are otherwise known as point-of-use, or decentralized suction pumps. For operating theatres and in particular for the

Description: portable point-of-use pump (Fig. 4.9)

1. Pressure gauge: shows in mmHg or cmH_20 the vacuum pressure the machine is set to.
2. Pressure dial: enables user to increase or decrease the vacuum pressure as desired.
3. Power button: switches machine on or off.
4. Connection tubing with filter: transmits vacuum pressure from machine to collection canister, via a filter (prevents contamination of machine).
5. Collection canisters: collects effluent from surgical field via connection tubings (not shown).
6. Nozzle: allows connection tubing (not shown) to evacuate effluent from surgical field, into the collection canisters.
7. Wheel base: broad base provides stability and prevents toppling over, especially when collection canisters are full, and the wheels provide manoeuvrability in the operating room.
8. Foot pedal: allows for the foot-activation of suction during the operation if desired.

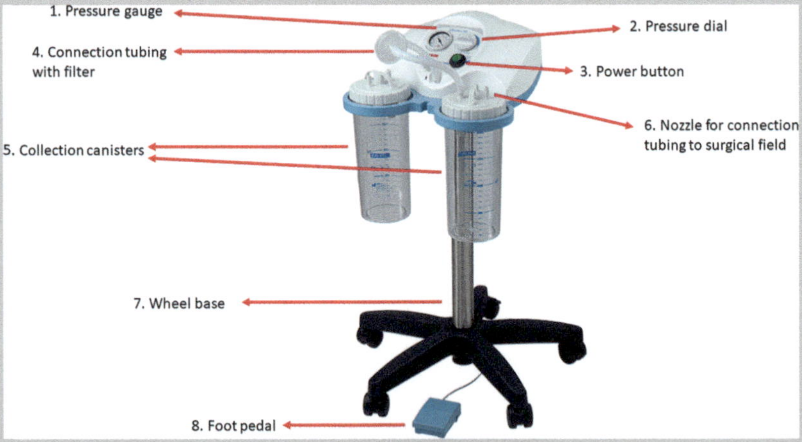

Fig. 4.9 Example of a point-of-use pump. Not shown is the connection tubings from the surgical field (© CA-MI)

Description: portable point-of-use pump (Fig. 4.10)

1. Control panel: contains switches and dials to turn machine on or off, adjust the vacuum pressure, and switch between collection canisters.
2. Collection system: contains connection tubings, collection bottles, collection canisters, filters.
3. Wheels: lockable wheels allow for manoeuvrability in the operating room.

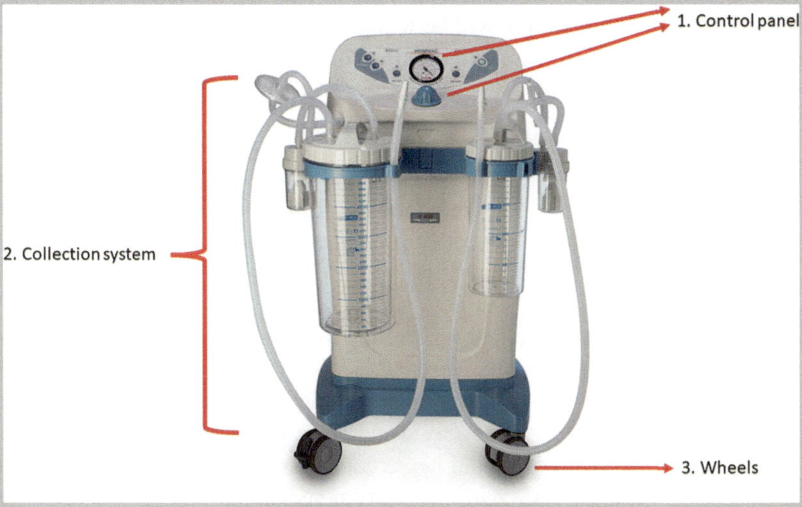

Fig. 4.10 Example of a point-of-use pump. Note in sequence the connection tubings from the surgical field to a canister, onto a sterilization filter, and into the machine itself (© CA-MI)

Description: detailed diagram of portable point-of-use pump (Fig. 4.11)

1. Power button: turns machine on or off.
2. Right and left output button: direct vacuum pressure to either right or left collection canisters, or both simultaneously.
3. Vacuum pressure gauge: allows user to see the amount of vacuum pressure being generated in mmHg or cmH2O.
4. Foot switch button: allows user to utilize foot pedal (not seen) for activation of suction.
5. Vacuum pressure dial: allows user to adjust vacuum pressure which will be reflected in (3).

(continued)

6. Filter with connection tubings: filter that prevents contamination of the machine from collection canister; it is the connection between the machine and the safetry trap bottle.
7. Safety trap bottle with connection tubings: additional barrier for safety against contamination, it is the connection between the filter and the collection canister.
8. Collection canister with connection tubings: collects effluent from the surgical field.
9. Connection tubing toward surgical field: this tubing is attached at its open end to a sterile tubing that will be within the surgical field; helps to collect effluent from the surgical field into the collection canister.

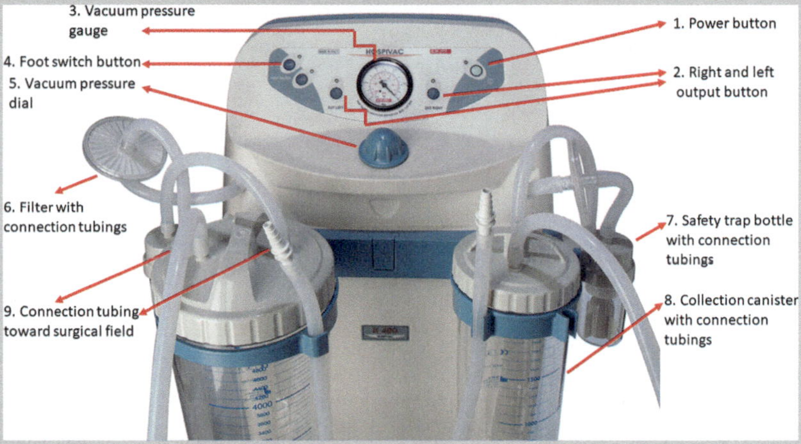

Fig. 4.11 A closer look at the control panel and gauges of a point-of-use suction pump (© CA-MI)

use during surgical procedures, these are pump machines that are dedicated to producing suction during the operation [3].

To generate negative pressure and remove secretions, portable suction machines depend on a few key technologies and components.

Suction/vacuum pump—This pump is often located inside the machine casing, and generates the negative pressure necessary for an operational suction machine.

Connection tubing—This connects the vacuum pump to the collection canister, and must not touch the contents within the collection canister.

Sterile patient tubing—This sterile tubing attaches to the sterile suctioning tip around the surgical field during the operation, and carries the patient's secretions into the collection canister. These are not re-usable and must be properly disposed of after a single use.

Disposable canister—This holds the fluid, secretions, and excrement from the surgical field, and usually provides overflow protection capabilities in circumstances where excess fluid content is suctioned from the surgical field. This canister should be disposable to ensure the rest of the suction machine remains sterile despite multiple usages.

Filters—Preferably, a disposable canister should allow the use of bacteria and/or viral filters to avoid contamination within the machine's inner components. There are special filters that may also be used to protect against dust and hazardous gases that can damage the machine.

Batteries—These ensure that the suction machines can provide suction capabilities even when a reliable power source is not readily available.

Power cord—It is used to charge up the machine's disposable batteries and/or provide electricity to the machine when close to a power outlet.

4.2 Benefits and Disadvantages of Both Systems

In the majority of modern hospitals, operating theatres now utilize central suction systems as their main source of suction capability during surgeries, given the various benefits that it provides over portable or decentralized machines [4] [5].

Energy Savings: A decentralized vacuum pump that is usually operating at full power while the process is running, although most machines allow for some degree of tailored power adjustment. Nonetheless, the machine needs to be switched on with inevitable power consumption even when vacuum is not required during the operation, resulting in unnecessary wastage of energy. Centralized vacuum systems, on the other hand, are controlled on a demand-driven basis. In contrast, central systems often allow for precise performance variations where the system only produces as much suction as is required, resulting in greater potential energy savings. In addition, central vacuum systems usually result in fewer vacuum pumps (albeit larger) than a decentralized vacuum system, where individual pumps are attached directly to each suction end-user interface.

The presence of point-of-use vacuum pumps also generates heat within the operating theatre; the extracted air is hot as it exits the pump, and the vacuum pump itself also radiates heat. This leads to increased air conditioning requirements in the operating theatres with raised costs.

Reduction in Maintenance Costs and Time-savings: Centralized systems use a single or usually multiple pumps located together in a designated area, allowing for easier accessibility, maintenance, and less disruptions to the operating theatre(s). The lesser number of machines required as opposed to having multiple individual suction machines in each operating theatre means that maintenance can be carried out more efficiently, with consequent time-savings. Furthermore, the centralized pumps are not at risk of being contaminated by bodily fluids, thus saving on machine maintenance.

Simple Expansion: Centralized systems offer flexibility when it comes to increasing operating theatre capacity by allowing extension of the existing central vacuum systems to the new operating theatre(s). This modular expansion allows for more efficient and less wasteful purchasing strategies.

Increased Productivity: Most centralized systems would incorporate backup pump(s) which would be activated automatically, hence allowing for uninterrupted operations in the event of failure of primary pumps. This built-in redundancy allows for continuous suction production while maintenance work is performed on the malfunctioning pump(s). In contrast, with point-of-use machines, a malfunction might lead to unnecessary delays in an operating theatre while the pump is fixed or replaced.

Increased Reliability and Lifetime: Due to ease of maintenance, the longevity of centralized vacuum pumps is increased as compared to point-of-use pumps. In addition, demand-driven centralized systems allow for less strain on the machines with consistent pressure generation, further increasing their lifespan and reliability.

Worker Safety and Comfort: As the vacuum pumps in a centralized system are in a dedicated area remote from the operating theatre, noise and heat emissions are drastically reduced during the operation, leading to increased comfort for healthcare workers. Additionally, the removal of oil-lubricated or water-cooled point-of-use pumps from the operating theatre, centralizing the system, eliminates potentially hazardous spills.

Heat Recovery: If space and planning allow for it, utilizing a central vacuum system with an oil-water heat exchanger might enable up to 50 to 70 percent of a motor's energy consumption to be recovered and used, consequently leading to increased energy and cost savings.

Point-of-use suction pumps, however, have several key traits that lend themselves to instances where they might be preferred over a central suction system.

Portability and Reliability: The ease of transport of point-of-use pumps allows for them to be utilized during surgical procedures, during patient transportation and evacuation, or in field hospitals. The advances in vacuum and battery technology have improved the reliability of such machines whilst allowing them to remain relatively lightweight.

Use in Disaster or Emergency Situations: A disruption to a hospital's centralized vacuum system due to unforeseen circumstances like a natural disaster may necessitate the use of individual point-of-use pumps as a stop-gap measure to allow essential operations from proceeding. In case of prolonged power outages, most portable suction pumps are able to run on alkaline batteries to ensure that surgeons can proceed with adequate suction during their operations during a critical time.

In a situation of a natural disaster or mass casualty scenario where there is an immediate surge of life-threatening injuries requiring surgical procedures, a hospital's operating theatre capacity may be overwhelmed. Portable suction machines would be one of the items necessary for the establishment of make-shift operating rooms.

In summary, proper usage of a central vacuum supply system in operating theatres can generate significant energy savings and allow for extra advantages to be appreciated. They are by far the most common system used in most modern hospitals. Nevertheless, portable suction machines remain an essential back-up to a hospital's centralized vacuum system. Hospitals should plan for a contingency cache of portable suction machines in the event of catastrophic loss of their central vacuum system or an unexpected surge in patients requiring surgical procedures, in order to provide uninterrupted suction capabilities in the operating rooms.

4.3 Pressure Settings

Here is a table with recommended suction machine pressure settings for various types of surgeries [4]:

Type of surgery	Recommended pressure setting (mmHg)
General surgery	120–150 mmHg
Abdominal surgery	120–150 mmHg
Neurosurgery	100–120 mmHg
ENT surgery (ear, nose, throat)	100–150 mmHg
Thoracic surgery	80–120 mmHg
Liposuction	200–600 mmHg (depending on technique)
Orthopedic surgery	150–200 mmHg
Gynecological surgery	120–150 mmHg
Urological surgery	120–150 mmHg
Dental/oral surgery	80–120 mmHg
Endoscopic procedures	80–120 mmHg
Pediatric surgery	50–100 mmHg (lower to avoid tissue damage)
Plastic & reconstructive surgery	100–150

Note:
Suction pressure should be adjusted based on patient condition, surgical field, and tissue sensitivity.
Higher pressures are used in procedures like liposuction where large amounts of fat are aspirated.
Lower pressures are preferred for delicate tissues, pediatrics, and neurosurgery to prevent damage.
Always refer to manufacturer guidelines and surgical team preferences for optimal settings.

4.4 Ideal Characteristics

An ideal suction pump meant for use in the operating theatre requires a combination of multiple important features, to ensure its safe, reliable, and frequent utilization [3].

Contamination-resistant: A medical grade vacuum pump must not allow any contaminants to pass through; hence, an oil-free compressor is preferable to reduce the risk of oil contamination. Pumps can be usually classified as rotary vane (dry or oil-sealed), scroll, or dry-claw pumps. A detailed technical understanding of the different categories of pumps is not required for a medical professional and is outside the scope of this chapter.

Low noise production or noise-free: It is ideal for a suction pump to be noise-free or emit low volume of noise so that patient monitoring systems are not drowned out, and the surgical team's concentration is not interfered with. Low noise production also facilitates timely and concise communication between healthcare professionals in the operating theatre.

Durability: It is desirable for a suction pump to be durable despite multiple and frequent usage; this cuts down on maintenance in a hospital or operating theatre, and decreases the down-time experience during these episodes.

Adjustability of pressure: Different types of surgeries or bodily cavities require different levels of vacuum suction during the operation for optimal surgical performance. An ideal suction machine would need to have its suction pressure adjustable in order to cater to the wide range of surgical procedures it will be used for.

Strong suction capacity: At times, certain procedures may require high volume rates of fluid to be suctioned or evacuated from a bodily cavity; it is essential that a suction pump is up to the task so that adequate visualization of the surgical field is maintained. A flow rate of 30 liters per minute is minimally required.

High vacuum power: A machine with a high level of maximal vacuum pressure is mandatory because there might be occasions where short bursts of high suction pressure are required to preserve a dry surgical field. A minimum of 300 mmHg is recommended.

Portability: This refers to portability within the operating theatre, as different operations require various theatre set-ups and the suction machinc has to compete with multiple other auxiliary medical machines for real estate during the operation. It is essential that the suction machine is readily and easily shifted to fit a variety of set-ups.

Compatibility: This refers to a point-of-use suction machine's ability to be compatible with the local electrical grid, as well as locally used sterile suction tubings and apparatus that are used in the surgical field. For a central suction system, this refers to the capability for its suction ports to be used with locally used bottle collection systems.

Battery life and rechargeability: This refers to point-of-use vacuum machines, where a long battery life is desirable in the case of disaster situations or catastrophic disruption of central suction and power supply. A unit that charges quickly provides greater flexibility and reliability too.

4.5 Troubleshooting If It Doesn't Work at All or Low Pressure or High Pressure

Medical vacuum pumps are intended to remove undesired gases and fluids, and their optimal running is essential in an operating theatre. Frequent protective maintenance of the vacuum systems maintains the efficiency and turn-around time of the operating theatre and reduces time and labor wastage during a malfunction.

If the malfunction is that no vacuum is being generated, it is wise to test the vacuum as close to the output of the device as possible. Remove all the accessory tubing, the collection jars, and the safety trap to determine if a vacuum is being generated at all and test all modes. If no vacuum is created, then either a power failure or internal faults are probable.

Thus, when the suction machine fails to generate any suction at all, the first thing to do would be check its power supply. This applies mainly to point-of-use machines which will be powered either by a power cable or batteries. The fault can be as simple as realizing the machine is not plugged into a power supply, or that the power supply is not switched on, otherwise the machine itself may not be switched on. If the machine is being battery-operated, the batteries may have gone flat and back-up batteries may need to be inserted and the machine may be attempted to switch on again.

Once the machine is switched on by way of either the power supply or batteries, then check if vacuum can be generated. It would be best to check for the presence of vacuum as close to the machine's output connection port as possible. If the unit's vacuum gauge is deflecting and yet no vacuum is felt directly from the machine, then an internal occlusion or mechanical issue with the machine is highly likely. Suction machines may be occasionally disassembled for cleaning. Incorrect reassembly or an inadvertent misplacement of a crucial part may cause an internal malfunction. Fluid interference within the machine can occur due to inadequate cleaning, condensation, or faulty filters. This can lead to internal filters being damaged, valves becoming occluded, and gauges being inoperable. Other common faults that can be found in any electrical appliance such as wiring, transformer, capacitor, or fuse issues can also cause a malfunction.

However, if there is adequate suction directly from the machine, and yet there is a lack of or inadequate suction at the distal end of the tubing near the operative site, then an occlusion or leak along the connection tubings or canister is the likely source.

For central vacuum systems which are ceiling or wall mounted, first attach the connection tubing to the vacuum port and test for suction generation either by feel or by the vacuum gauge. If there is no suction, then either the port is faulty or there is an occlusion or leak in the central system, or worse, a central failure of the vacuum generator pump. Similarly, if the vacuum port can generate vacuum and yet there is insufficient or absent vacuum at the operative side, then one has to investigate for a leak or blockage along the connection tubings or canister.

The cause of leakage or occlusion along the connection circuit can usually be attributed to a few key issues. Wrong accessories or incorrectly attached accessories can lead to either occlusion or leakage of vacuum suction. Tubings or canisters may have cracks that lead to leakages with subsequent unsatisfactory suction power. Occlusion or poor flow during the course of the operation can also be due to particulate debris.

If there is a suspected issue with the central vacuum system either at the vacuum port, pipes within the hospital infrastructure, or at the main pumps, engineers or technicians familiar with the system should be alerted to troubleshoot and rectify the issue [5].

4.6 Maintenance

Maintenance can range from daily protocols to yearly schedules. Every step goes a long way in ensuring optimal working of this crucial component in any operating room [6].

1. Daily Maintenance
   - Pre-use Functional Check: Ensure the machine is operational and suction pressure is adequate.
   - Inspection of Tubing and Connections: Check for leaks, cracks, or loose fittings; replace if necessary.
   - Collection Canister Management: Empty and dispose of collected fluids as per hospital protocol. Clean and disinfect the canister after each use.
   - Filter Inspection: Check bacterial and overflow filters for clogging or contamination; replace if required.
   - Surface Cleaning: Wipe down the machine with a hospital-grade disinfectant to maintain hygiene.
2. Weekly Maintenance
   - Suction Line Cleaning: Flush tubing with sterile saline or as recommended by the manufacturer to prevent blockages.
   - Vacuum Pump and Regulator Inspection: Ensure proper function and check for any unusual noises.
   - Electrical Component Check: Inspect power cables, plugs, and switches for any damage.
   - Lubrication of Moving Parts: Follow manufacturer guidelines for lubrication, if applicable.
3. Monthly Maintenance
   - Suction Pressure Calibration: Verify and adjust suction settings to ensure optimal performance.
   - Wear and Tear Assessment: Inspect canister seals, tubing, and regulator knobs for any deterioration.
   - Filter Replacement: Change bacterial and hydrophobic filters according to manufacturer recommendations.
   - Footswitch and Accessory Inspection: Test all controls for responsiveness and functionality.
4. Annual Maintenance and Servicing
   - Biomedical Engineering Evaluation: Schedule a complete inspection and servicing by technical staff.
   - Vacuum Pump Maintenance: Clean or replace the pump if necessary.
   - Performance Testing: Assess the machine's ability to maintain consistent suction pressure.
   - Component Replacement: Replace aging parts, including tubing, gaskets, and worn-out components.

4.7 Troubleshooting

Problem	Possible causes	Solutions
No suction at all	Machine not powered on Loose or disconnected tubing Collection canister lid not sealed properly Full canister Clogged filter	Check power supply and switch on Reconnect and secure tubing Ensure canister lid is tightly sealed Replace or empty canister Replace clogged filter
Weak or insufficient suction	Partial tubing blockage Canister almost full Suction pressure too low Worn-out or leaking tubing Clogged bacterial filter	Check and clear tubing Empty or replace canister Increase suction pressure as per need Replace damaged tubing Change bacterial filter
Intermittent suction loss	Loose tubing connections Leak in tubing or canister lid Vacuum pump issue	Secure all connections Replace leaking tubing/canister lid Call for biomedical technician support
Excessive noise or vibration	Faulty motor or vacuum pump Loose machine parts Obstruction in system	Inspect motor and vacuum pump Tighten loose parts Clear any blockages
Overflow of fluids into the pump	Overfilled canister Faulty overflow protection mechanism No bacterial filter installed	Empty canister before it reaches max level Check and repair overflow mechanism Install bacterial filter
Burning smell or overheating	Motor overload Clogged air vents Prolonged use without rest	Turn off and let the unit cool down Clean air vents Reduce usage duration and allow cooling
Alarm or warning light on machine	Machine malfunction Power supply issue Internal component failure	Refer to user manual for error codes Check power supply Contact biomedical engineering department
Blood or debris in tubing	Inadequate flushing Tubing not properly positioned No in-line filter	Flush tubing with sterile saline Ensure tubing placement is correct Use an in-line filter to trap debris
Unable to adjust suction pressure	Faulty regulator knob Blocked suction pathway Internal mechanical failure	Inspect and replace regulator knob if needed Check and clear blockages Service the machine if issue persists

4.8 Conclusion

Medical suction machines play a critical role in maintaining a clear surgical field, ensuring patient safety, and facilitating various procedures in the operating room. Proper selection, setup, and usage of these devices are essential for optimal performance. Regular maintenance, including daily checks, periodic servicing, and prompt troubleshooting, is crucial to prevent malfunctions and ensure reliability. A well-maintained suction system contributes significantly to the overall success of surgical interventions.

References

1. Joseph KC, Macaulay B, Hassan G, Khairat A, David O, Jamal Q, Richard S, Zulikhat L, Anuoluwapo A, Patience KG, Inioluwa T, Sekinat O, Bankole O, Sarah A, Comfort A, Martha O, Joyce T, bolaji A, Roqeebat N, Adekemi E. Design and construction of a low cost suction machine for Lagos state primary healthcare needs. Int J Res Publ Rev. 2024;5(8):4269–80.
2. Jacques S, Christe B. Chapter 2 – Healthcare technology basics. In: Jacques S, Christe B, editors. Introduction to clinical engineering. Academic; 2020. p. 21–50., ISBN 9780128181034. https://doi.org/10.1016/B978-0-12-818103-4.00002-8.
3. Peri SR, Akhter F, De Lorenzo RA, Hood RL. Portable medical suction and aspirator devices: are the design and performance standards relevant? Sensors (Basel). 2022;22(7):2515. https://doi.org/10.3390/s22072515.
4. Lamb W, Pursely D. The principles of vacuum and clinical application in the hospital environment. Ohio Medical Corporation; 2014.
5. International Standard Organization. Medical Suction Equipment ISO 10079-1, 10079-2, 10079-3. 2015.
6. Chun C, Zohdy M. Medical suction and fluid waste management: patient and workplace safety considerations for health care organizations. Joint Commission International; 2017.

C-Arm Fluoroscope

5

Mohammad Talal Abdallah Al-Zubi, Khayry Al-Shami, Manar Al-Shami, and Almu'atasim Khamees

The C-arm machine is a kind of advanced medical imaging device that functions based on the concept of X-rays. They are fluoroscopy machines, which are also referred to as image intensifiers. However, the picture intensifier is technically just an ingredient of the machine, which is referred to as a detector. The C-arm device is named after the C-shaped arm, which is used to link the X-ray source to the detector. Such C-arm machines find application in orthopedic, complicated surgery; pain treatments (anesthetics); urological procedures; and emergency surgeries. Its X-ray fluoroscopy technology allows the device to provide high-resolution images of the X-ray in real-time, enabling the surgeon to observe the treatment progress and make relevant decisions [1].

Fluoroscopy is a common practice in the majority of endourologic operations, including ureteroscopy, and contributes to the augmented radiation. The concern with radiation exposures in the long term is the higher possibility of cancer; thus, it is essential to measure the radiation exposure during such therapies. The timing of the fluoroscopy, the machine parameters, the distance between the source and the skin, and patient thickness have also been identified as some of the variables that are known to lead to the aggregate radiation dose during ureteroscopy. In order to

M. T. A. Al-Zubi (✉)
Department of General Surgery and Anesthesia, Faculty of Medicine, Yarmouk University, Irbid, Jordan
e-mail: Mzubi@yu.edu.jo

K. Al-Shami · M. Al-Shami
Department of Medical Science, Faculty of Medicine, Yarmouk University, Irbid, Jordan
e-mail: 2014899029@alumni.yu.edu.jo

A. Khamees
Department of Medical Science, Faculty of Medicine, Yarmouk University, Irbid, Jordan

Department of General Surgery, Princess Basma Teaching Hospital, Ministry of Health, Irbid, Jordan

J. S. Ahluwalia (ed.), *User Manual for Minimally Invasive Surgical Equipment*,
https://doi.org/10.1007/978-981-95-9019-3_5

overcome these effects, pulse fluoroscopy, collimation, and the proximity of the fluoroscope image intensifier to the patient are some of the strategies that have been developed to combat these effects [2]. There are numerous fluoroscopy technologies, such as fixed fluoroscopy tables and C-arm portable fluoroscopies, that are used in endourologic procedures. Some of the fixed table units have over-the-table radiation sources, with the majority of C-arm units having under-the-table energy sources. Due to the highest absorption of dose of radiation during proximity to the X-ray emitter, the placement of the radiation source will determine the location of the organs affected by the radiation beam [3].

Time of fluoroscopy is not a sufficient index of radiation dose and dose taken by patients, as it fails to capture the size of the patient, machine mode, and dispersal of the radiation beam [4]. Urologists should be conscious of the amount of radiation that they expose their patients to. The providers are also expected to know the availability of the fluoroscopy unit in their institution and make all efforts they can to restrict fluoroscopy, particularly when using an over-the-table fluoroscopy unit. There are those providers who opt to use fixed fluoroscopy equipment since it can easily be manipulated by the surgeon and does not need the services of a fluoroscopy technician. The X-ray emitter of the C-arm is mobile, which provides more flexibility in the organization of the operating room. Besides, the C-arm can be easily rotated, which can be easily accessed by the patient during percutaneous treatment. Moreover, with the C-arm, the table also creates some dispersion of the radiation, and therefore the total radiation that the patient absorbs as a whole is affected during the course of the fluoroscopy (Fig. 5.1) [5–7].

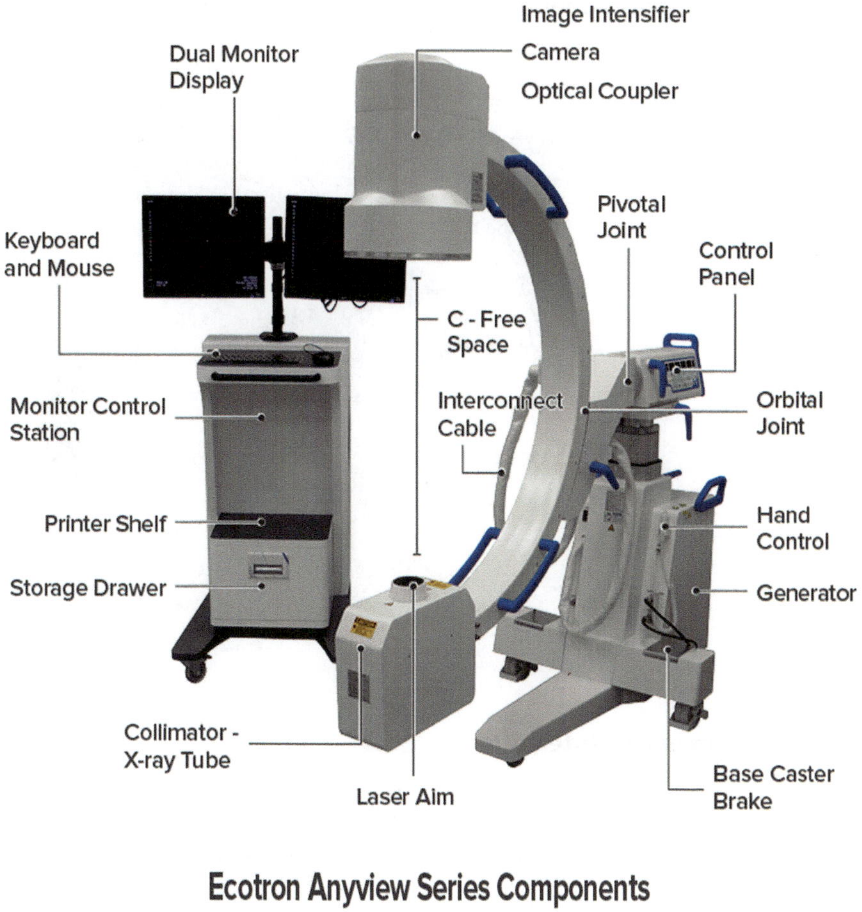

Fig. 5.1 Illustration of C-arm fluoroscope components [7]

5.1 Main C-Arm Parts

Knowing the essential components and parts of your C-arm machine is vital in maintaining its optimal operation. Identifying potential issues promptly and taking necessary measures to repair or prevent them is crucial to avoid downtime. Below, you will find the key constituents and elements that comprise your C-arm. While we have utilized images of OEC 9800, these parts are generally applicable to various other models and brands (Figs. from 5.2, 5.3, 5.4, 5.5, and 5.6) [8].

5.1.1 C-Arm X-ray Tubes

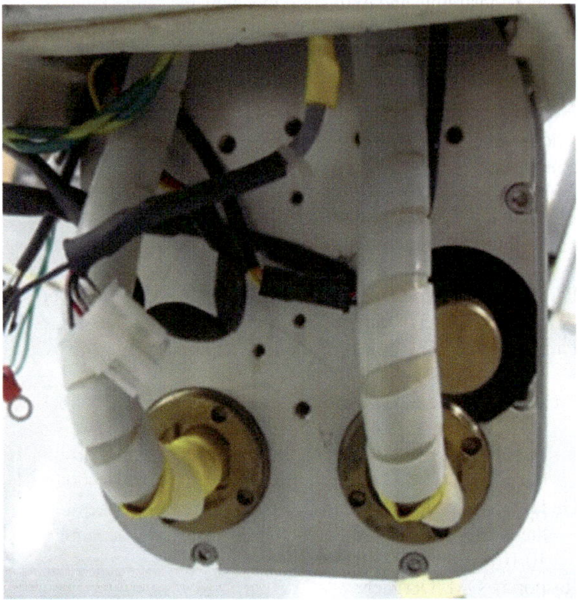

Fig. 5.2 The tube on the C-arm machine is used to generate X-rays on C-arm

5.1.2 C-Arm Image Intensifier

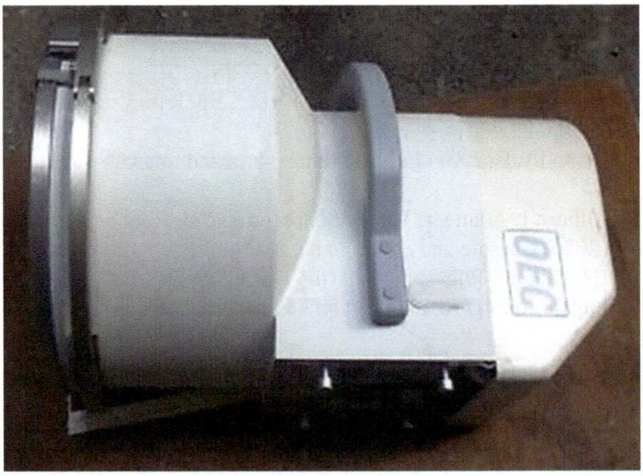

Fig. 5.3 The X-ray image intensifier is responsible for converting X-rays into visible light with significantly higher intensity compared to regular fluorescent screens

5.1.3 C-Arm CCD Camera

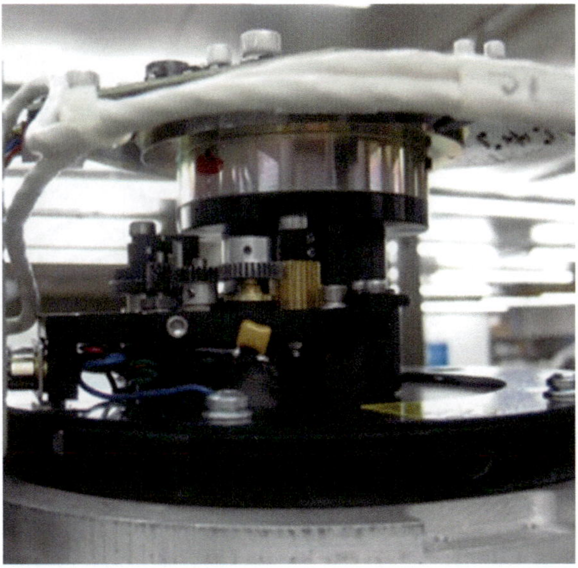

Fig. 5.4 The charge-coupled device (CCD) camera produces high-resolution images in different lighting conditions. When combined with the image intensifier, these two components work together to ensure the quality of images

5.1.4 C-Arm High-Voltage Cables

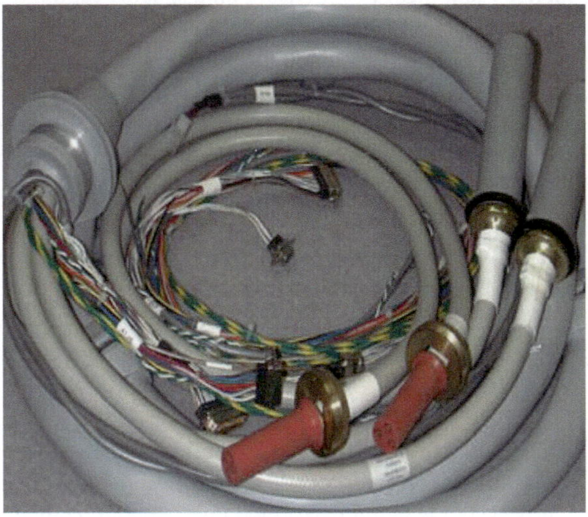

Fig. 5.5 High-voltage cables are installed to ensure reliable connections for the twisting and turning movements that occur within the C-arm

5.1.5 C-Arm CPU Board

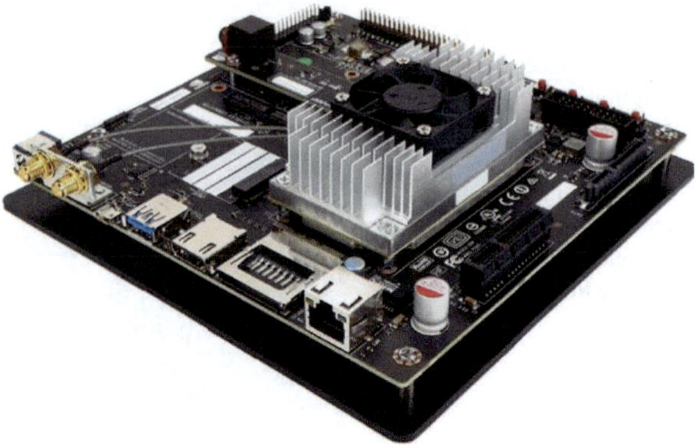

Fig. 5.6 The central processing unit (CPU) serves as the core component or "brain" of C-arm

5.2 Buttons of C-Arm Fluoroscope

Look at Fig. 5.7 *to see the illustration of C-arm buttons:*

A-Image Rotation & Image Orientation Keys: Rotates image.

B-Field Size: This is used to adjust the size of the X-ray beam field that reaches the patient and the detector. This helps in optimizing image quality while minimizing unnecessary radiation exposure.

Smaller Field Size: For focusing on a specific region (e.g., spine, joints) to improve contrast.

Larger Field Size: When a *wider anatomical view* is needed, like during vascular or orthopedic procedures.

C-Collimator Leaf Rotation: It is used to adjust the angle of the collimator blades (leaves). This helps in optimizing the X-ray beam shape and direction for better imaging and reduced radiation exposure.

It allows the collimator leaves to be adjusted diagonally or at different angles instead of just horizontally or vertically, helps match the X-ray beam shape to the specific anatomy being imaged, reducing unnecessary exposure, reduces scatter radiation, resulting in a sharper and clearer image, and minimizes patient and operator exposure.

D-Manual Contrast/Brightness: These are applied to enhance contrast and reduce brightness (or vice versa) when a live X-ray is being displayed or when post-processing is being performed on the previous image stored.

E-kVp Adjust: Controls the amount of voltage, overrides auto.

F-mA/mAs Adjust: Controls the amount of current, overrides auto.

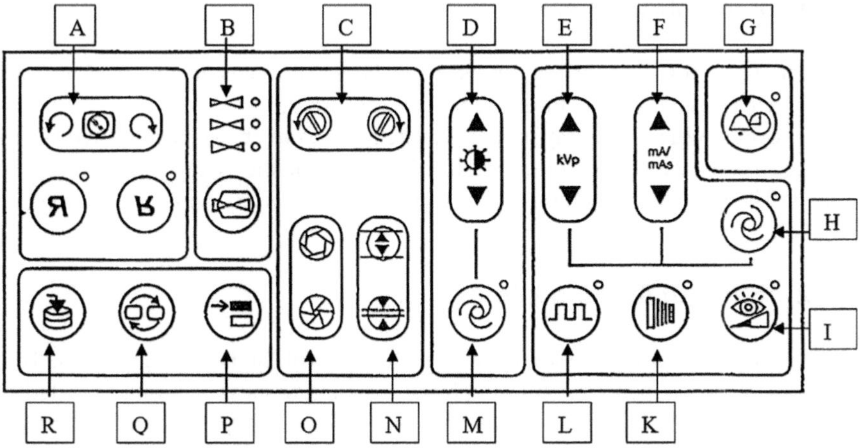

Fig. 5.7 Illustration of C-arm buttons

G-Alarm Reset: A clock is used to note X-ray time used when the X-ray switch is on (considering the quantity of time of the length of pulses and the quantity of pulses). An alarm will be raised at 5 min of registered fluoroscopy time. This button will reset it.

H-Auto Contrast/ Brightness: Auto selects optimal contrast/brightness.

I-Low Dose Mode: Reduces exposure dose to patient.

K-Film Image intensifier control: Enables film operation.

L-Pulse Mode: This is a preprogrammed number of X-ray pulses that are produced per second when the X-ray switch is pressed. Here, it is utilized in order to minimize the total radiation dose to the patient. It is not applicable in film or digital spot mode.

M-Auto Technique: Enables the system to produce optimal technique.

N-Collimator Leaf Open/Close: Opens/closes collimator leaves.

O-Iris Collimator Open/Close: Opens/closes collimator iris.

P-Mode: Switch between normal fluoroscopy mode and vascular imaging mode when the C-arm is attached to a vascular/cardiac workstation.

Q-Swap workstation: It is operated during the production of live X-rays, or when an X-ray is dead, swaps live to still image. Capturing a new image discards the old image.

R-Save workstation: Saved by pressing when there is a real-time X-ray or after saving the last image that was viewed on the left monitor [9].

5.3 The Settings of C-Arm Fluoroscope Depending on the Case of Patient

To optimize imaging outcomes while prioritizing patient safety, precise adjustments of kilovolt peak (kVp) and milliampere seconds (mAs) are paramount. Tailoring these settings for different patient groups—adults, pediatrics, geriatrics, trauma, and orthopedics—takes into account anatomical variations and radiation sensitivity.

5.3.1 kVp (Kilovolt Peak)

What it stands for: kVp stands for "Kilovolt Peak." It represents the peak voltage applied across the X-ray tube during the exposure.

How it works: When the X-ray tube is activated, electrons are accelerated across this voltage. These accelerated electrons hit the anode of the X-ray tube, producing X-rays. The kVp setting controls the energy level of the X-ray photons produced.

5.3.2 Effect of Altering kVp

Higher kVp: Increasing the kVp results in X-rays with higher energy levels. This leads to greater penetration through the patient's tissues, resulting in a darker image on the fluoroscopy monitor. It is useful for imaging denser body parts or larger patients.

Lower kVp: Reducing the kVp results in X-rays with lower energy levels. This leads to less penetration and a lighter image. Lower kVp is used for imaging less dense body parts or pediatric patients.

5.3.3 mAs (Milliampere-Seconds)

What it stands for: mAs stands for "Milliampere-Seconds." It represents the product of the X-ray tube current (in milliamperes, mA) and the exposure time (in seconds, s).

How it works: The mAs setting controls the quantity or amount of X-rays produced. It directly relates to the number of X-ray photons emitted during the exposure.

5.3.4 Effect of Altering mAs

Higher mAs: Increasing the mAs setting results in a higher quantity of X-ray photons being produced. This leads to a darker image with improved visibility of anatomical details. It's useful when a high level of image quality is required or when imaging thicker body parts.

Lower mAs: Reducing the mAs setting results in a lower quantity of X-ray photons. This leads to a lighter image with reduced visibility of details. Lower mAs may be used when lower radiation exposure is required or when imaging thinner body parts.

kVp and mAs are essential parameters in C-arm fluoroscopy. While kVp primarily controls the quality of X-ray images by adjusting the energy level of the X-ray photons, mAs controls the quantity of X-ray photons, directly affecting image brightness. Adjusting these settings appropriately based on the patient's characteristics and the specific procedure helps achieve optimal image quality while minimizing radiation exposure to the patient and medical staff.

For adult patients, a kVp range of 70–90 is generally effective. This range balances tissue penetration with radiation dose. Adjustments to the mAs setting, reflecting radiation quantity and exposure time, depend on body size and the specific procedure. Larger adults may necessitate higher mAs to attain sufficient image quality, particularly in regions with denser structures.

Pediatric patients require specialized settings due to their heightened radiation sensitivity. A kVp range of 60–80 is commonly used to reduce exposure while capturing the required details. Low mAs settings are preferred to mitigate radiation dose to their developing tissues. Because pediatric patients may struggle with staying still during imaging, shorter exposure times are crucial. Techniques such as distraction or immobilization help maintain image clarity.

Geriatric patients may have unique needs due to age-related anatomical changes. A kVp range of 70–85 strikes a balance between tissue penetration and radiation dose. Adjustments to mAs should consider factors like tissue density and patient size. Longer exposure times may be necessary if mobility is compromised, ensuring image acquisition without patient discomfort.

Trauma patients, often requiring swift and precise imaging, benefit from a kVp range of 80–100. This higher energy setting is essential for visualizing fractures or injuries. Due to potential obstructions from bandages or immobilization devices, adjusting mAs is necessary to achieve accurate image quality. Flexibility in settings allows adapting to the patient's specific condition and the procedure's demands.

Orthopedic procedures demand meticulous visualization of bones and joints. A kVp range of 80–90 is suitable to achieve high-resolution images. Tailoring mAs settings to the specific joint or orthopedic device enhances clarity. Larger joints might require higher mAs settings for optimal detail.

These guidelines serve as a foundation but must be tailored for each case. Close collaboration with a radiologist or medical professional ensures the best settings for patient needs. Factors such as patient history, clinical requirements, and equipment capabilities are pivotal. Patient safety remains the top priority when determining the appropriate kVp and mAs settings.

5.4 What Sets a C-Arm Apart from Radiography or Fixed Fluoroscopy Machines?

Radiography involves mainly the use of X-rays to take images, digital or on X-ray film. Fixed fluoroscopy procedures include barium meal studies, which are real-time fluoroscopy imaging procedures using X-rays to visualize body parts and the movement of fluid, such as blood or contrast agents, to identify blockages and other diseases. Diagnostic procedures are used both in radiography and fixed fluoroscopy. A C-arm, on the other hand, although it is also used as a fluoroscopy machine, is specifically used in surgical procedures [3].

5.5 Dimensions and Maneuverability of C-Arm Machine

Mobility of mobile C-arm units in hospital environments and flexibility in positioning are some of the key factors in this case. The size of the unit is thus an important factor. A rich depth of C-arm is preferable, as it should be able to fit patients of all sizes. Meanwhile, it is not supposed to be too huge and impede its mobility in the operating theater. Moreover, the C-arm must be low profile so that it can be installed under hospital beds and operating tables. The range of swivel and angulation that is appropriate and has the ability to carry out orbital, horizontal, vertical, and lateral motions is also another concern that a surgeon should take into account. The distance between the X-ray source and the image intensifier is also another important parameter, not to mention the isocentric rotation that has its center of rotation as the midpoint between the X-ray tube focal point and the image intensifier. All this makes the C-arm machine effective and maneuverable overall [10].

5.6 Maintenance

Proper maintenance of a C-arm fluoroscopy machine ensures optimal performance, image quality, and patient safety while extending the machine's lifespan. Regular preventive maintenance minimizes breakdowns, reduces downtime, and ensures compliance with radiation safety standards.

After each use:

- Wipe down the X-ray tube, image intensifier, and monitor with a soft, lint-free cloth.
- Use approved disinfectants to prevent contamination.
- Avoid liquid spills on control panels and screens.
- Tow with care and save machine in a place where there is no unusual traffic and moderate temperature.

Monthly:

- Remove dust buildup from ventilation areas to prevent overheating and replace air filters if required.
- Perform a full system check: Inspect cables, connectors, and control panels for wear and tear. Verify that *all software settings and presets* are functioning.
- Ensure software is up to date.

Annually:

- Perform a full calibration of the X-ray tube, detector, and fluoroscopy system and ensure the machine meets radiation safety standards.

5.7 Troubleshooting

Table below delineates some problems, their possible causes, and solutions:

Problem	Possible cause	Solution
No power/C-arm won't turn on	Power cable unplugged or loose	Check and securely plug in the power cable.
	Blown fuse or circuit breaker tripped	Replace fuse/reset breaker and check power supply.
	Emergency stop button engaged	Release the emergency stop and restart.
Poor or no image on screen	Low kVp or mA settings	Increase kVp/mA settings as needed.
	Detector or X-ray tube misaligned	Adjust positioning for optimal image capture.
	Detector dirty or obstructed	Clean detector with a soft cloth.
	Collimator shutters closed too much	Open collimator slightly to allow proper imaging.
Blurry or noisy image	Low mA setting causing insufficient exposure	Increase mA slightly to reduce noise.
	Motion blur due to patient or C-arm movement	Stabilize patient and use pulsed fluoroscopy.
	Scatter radiation affecting clarity	Use collimation and grid to reduce scatter.
Image too dark or too bright	Incorrect kVp/mA settings	Adjust kVp/mA to optimize contrast and brightness.
	Auto-exposure control (AEC) not working properly	Manually adjust exposure settings.
Fluoroscopy mode not working	Footswitch malfunctioning	Check footswitch connection and test with another.
	Software glitch	Restart system or call for technical support.
C-arm movement issues	Locking mechanism engaged	Disengage locks and check for obstructions.
	Hydraulic/electronic failure	Restart system; if unresolved, call for service.
Overheating warning	Continuous use causing tube overheating	Allow machine to cool down before resuming.
	Faulty cooling fan	Check fan function; if faulty, service is needed.
Radiation dose too high	High mA/kVp settings	Optimize exposure settings to minimize dose.
	Collimator not adjusted properly	Narrow field size to reduce unnecessary exposure.

Additionally, it is crucial to inform the biomedical team of any warning messages after a case to prevent further damage to the tube and electronics. Disregarding error messages on the C-arm can exacerbate issues, necessitating the removal of the machine from circulation to prevent further damage.

The C-arm constitutes a critical component of OR. With proper maintenance and adherence to the mentioned guidelines, the C-arm can provide years of reliable service [11, 12].

In conclusion, the diversity of patients and procedures demands adaptability in C-arm fluoroscopy settings. Balancing radiation dose, image quality, and patient comfort is paramount. As medical technology advances, continuous refinement of these settings, coupled with clinical expertise, contributes to improved diagnostic accuracy and patient outcomes [13].

References

1. Healthcare Trivitron: All you need to know about the C-arm X-ray machines. https://www.trivitron.com/blog/all-you-need-to-know-about-the-c-arm-x-ray-machines-2/?fbclid=IwAR2dEHIMX8iZbhxpUH3b6AiNJd9MwB8-EO3Hl5mnsB4WkfF5umq6E9NPqSY. 2018. Accessed.
2. Park S, Pearle MS. Imaging for percutaneous renal access and management of renal calculi. Urol Clin. 2006;33(3):353–64.
3. Lipkin ME, Mancini JG, Toncheva G, Wang AJ, Anderson-Evans C, Simmons WN, et al. Organ-specific radiation dose rates and effective dose rates during percutaneous nephrolithotomy. J Endourol. 2012;26(5):439–43.
4. Jaco JW, Miller DL. Measuring and monitoring radiation dose during fluoroscopically guided procedures. Tech Vasc Interv Radiol. 2010;13(3):188–93.
5. Violette PD, Szymanski KM, Anidjar M, Andonian S. Factors determining fluoroscopy time during ureteroscopy. J Endourol. 2011;25(12):1837–40.
6. Cabrera FJ, Shin RH, Waisanen KM, Nguyen G, Wang C, Scales CD, et al. Comparison of radiation exposure from fixed table fluoroscopy to a portable C-arm during ureteroscopy. J Endourol. 2017;31(9):835–40.
7. Medical aAHSc: C-Arm – fluoroscopy machines. https://www.dremed.com/catalog/index.php/cPath/603_1005. 2017. Accessed.
8. Imaging Primary Medical: C-Arm parts. https://www.primarymedicalimaging.com/c-arm-parts/. 2017. Accessed.
9. Quizlet: C-Arm Buttons. https://quizlet.com/367150822/c-arm-buttons-diagram/. 2023. Accessed.
10. Equipment Perlove Medical: What is a C-arm machine? What are C-arms used for? http://www.perlove.com.cn/about/detail.asp?Id=294. 2023. Accessed.
11. Corporation SHVE: Application notes – X-ray generators. https://www.spellmanhv.com/en/Technical-Resources/Application-Notes-X-Ray-Generators/AN-02#Inactivity. 2023. Accessed.
12. Electric Clover: What is electrical arcing and what are the warning signs?. https://www.clover-electric.com/what-is-electrical-arcing. 2023. Accessed.
13. American Association of Physicists in Medicine, Organizations AOFO, for medical physics, organisations EFO, physics FM: diagnostic radiology physics: a handbook for teachers and students. https://www-pub.iaea.org/MTCD/Publications/PDF/Pub1564webNew-74666420.pdf. 2014. Accessed.

Intermittent Pneumatic Compression Devices

6

Burgos Rueda Hugo Alejandro
and Arévalo Guerra Orlando Favio

Venous thromboembolism (VTE) is common in the postoperative setting with about half of the population at moderate risk. VTE, including deep vein thrombosis (DVT) and pulmonary embolism (PE), is a life-threatening complication. DVT, that is, the development of thrombi within the deep veins of the legs, can be complicated by PE, resulting from the movement of these thrombi from the veins of the legs to the pulmonary artery or its branches. This PE is known to be one of the most common preventable causes of in-hospital death after surgery, and clinicians should be aware that thromboprophylaxis reduces, but does not eliminate, the risk of VTE and VTE-related mortality [1, 2]. The high incidence of VTE and the current availability of effective prevention methods indicate that thromboprophylaxis should be considered for most surgical patients [3].

Guidelines recommend pharmacological (PP) or mechanical prophylaxis (MP). PP options include anticoagulation (low molecular weight heparins [LMWH], new oral anticoagulants, or warfarin) and aspirin, but these may increase the risk of bleeding. MP with IPCD is recommended, particularly in populations at elevated risk of bleeding, due to decreased risk of major bleeding and surgical site bleeding. The recommendation that patients should be mobilized quickly after surgery unless contraindicated should be seen as universally applicable, regardless of the type of prophylaxis chosen [4].

Compared with no prophylaxis, the use of IPCD reduces the risk of DVT (including asymptomatic and distal DVT) by 60%; and although IPCD may offer protection against VTE, adherence is usually suboptimal (53–78%), and efficacy may vary between devices [3, 5].

B. R. H. Alejandro · A. G. O. Favio (✉)
Cirugía general, universidad del Valle, Cali, Valle del Cauca, Colombia
e-mail: orlando.arevalo@correounivalle.edu.co

J. S. Ahluwalia (ed.), *User Manual for Minimally Invasive Surgical Equipment*,
https://doi.org/10.1007/978-981-95-9019-3_6

6.1 Intermittent Pneumatic Compression Devices

IPCD prevents thrombosis by two mechanisms. On the one hand, they stimulate the venous flow of the lower limbs, thus avoiding stasis. This effect is achieved by mechanical compression of the foot or calf only, or by sequential compression of the foot and calf, or calf and thigh. On the other hand, IPCD also reduces tissue plasminogen activator inhibitor (PAI-1), increasing endogenous fibrinolytic activity [3, 6].

Meta-analyses report that the use of IPCD is superior to non-prophylaxis and graduated compression stockings (GCS) and may offer additional benefits to surgical patients with LMWH. Adhesion, proper fit, and discomfort are major problems with IPCD [1, 3].

Although there are different contraindications for the use of these devices, most of them are relative and the decision is submitted to the clinician's discretion. In this sense, some authors recommend not using IPCD in patients with evidence of leg ischemia (e.g., severe or critical peripheral arterial disease) [5], although this contraindication is usually mainly for GCS and compression bands [7]. Other contraindications include patients with burns or extensive skin lesions; patients with neuropathies, and with hereditary predisposition to pressure paralysis; patients with massive edema of lower extremities; patients with congestive heart failure; deformity of the leg or foot; and suspected pre-existing DVT. On the other hand, IPCD can present adverse events ranging from quite common events, such as skin irritation, to rare but severe situations, such as cardiac decompensation [7–9].

There is a wide variety of devices available that differ in the anatomical location of the sleeve, the number and location of air bladders, compression cycle patterns, and the length of inflation and deflation time. In general, IPCD can be classified into (Table 6.1).

Single-chamber or multi-chamber devices, constant pressure or sequential pressure devices, gradual slow inflation or rapid inflation devices, and portable or non-portable devices. Portable ones offer the added advantage of continuous use during ambulation in the early postoperative period. Moreover, non-portable ones should be removed when the patient wanders [3].

6.2 Time and Duration of Thromboprophylaxis

The time to onset of MP or PP is unknown and should be individualized according to factors such as type of surgery (urgency or elective), duration, risk of bleeding, and baseline risk of VTE.

In patients with a low risk of bleeding, experts agree that mechanical methods can be started just before surgery or in the operating room and continued with few interruptions until discharge. Pharmacological agents can be started between 2 and 12 h preoperatively.

In terms of duration, in most cases, VTE prophylaxis is continued until the patient becomes fully ambulatory or until discharge from the hospital. Ten to

Table 6.1 Some IPCD devices available

Manufacturer	Device name	Sleeve location	Single vs multiple bladder	Average cycle duration (s)	Average compression duration (s)	Pressure pattern	Inflation rise	Portable	Hour meter
Aircast	VenaFlow	Calf	Multiple	60	6	Sequential	Rapid	No	Yes
Huntleigh	Flowtron	Calf	Single	60	12	Constant	Slow	No	No
Jobst	Anthrombic pump	Calf	Multiple	60	7–8	Sequential	Slow	No	No
NuTech	PlexiPulse	Foot, foot-calf	Multiple	20–60	2.5	Constant	Rapid	No	No
Kendall	Kendall SCD	Calf, calf-thigh	Multiple	20–60	11	Sequential	Slow	No	No
Medical compression systems	ActiveCare DVT	Calf	Multiple	30–60	10	Sequential	Slow	Yes	Yes
	WizAir DVT	Calf	Multiple	60	8	Sequential	Slow	Yes	Yes
Novamedix	A-V impulse system	Foot	Single	20–50	3	Constant	Rapid	No	Yes

fourteen days of thromboprophylaxis may be indicated in patients at high surgical risk, including those with cancer. It is worth mentioning that some guidelines (ACCP, AHS) indicate extended therapy, in certain scenarios, for up to 4 weeks [5, 10].

6.3 Device

The system consists of the controller, hoses or tubes, and garments/sleeves for a single patient (Fig. 6.1).

6.3.1 Details of the Machine

A typical IPCD has following controls/features:

- *Power Button*: Turns the device on or off.
- *Mode Selection Button*: Allows the user to choose from different compression modes.
- *Pressure Adjustment Buttons*: Adjust the pressure levels based on patient requirements.
- *Timer Button:* Sets the duration of the therapy session.
- *Start/Pause Button***:** Starts or pauses the compression cycle.
- *LCD Display*: Shows real-time information, including pressure settings, mode, and time remaining.
- *Indicator Lights*: Signals the device's operational status, errors, or malfunctions.

6.3.2 Inflatable Cuffs/Sleeves

These wrap around the limb and inflate with air to apply compression. Different types of cuffs are available based on the medical needs and limb size.

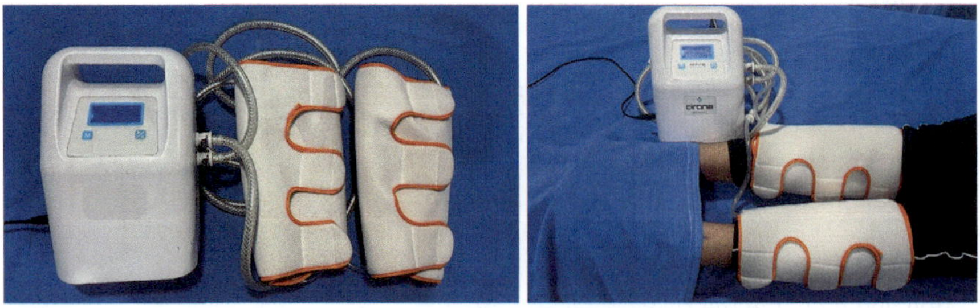

Fig. 6.1 Device images. Personal archive from the author

- *Standard Leg Cuffs:* Designed for lower limb therapy, covering the foot and calf.
- *Full-Length Cuffs:* Extend from foot to thigh for comprehensive compression.
- *Segmented or Multi-Chamber Cuffs:* Have multiple chambers that inflate sequentially to provide gradient compression.
- *Adjustable-Size Cuffs:* Equipped with Velcro or elastic straps to fit different limb sizes.
- *Arm Cuffs:* Used for upper limb lymphedema and post-surgical swelling.
- *Boot-Style Cuffs:* Encase the entire foot and ankle, ideal for treating swelling in the lower extremities.
- *Torso or Abdominal Cuffs:* Used for specialized applications in reducing fluid build-up in the abdominal region.

6.3.3 How to Use IPCD Device

1. *Prepare the Patient:* Ensure the patient is in a comfortable position with the affected limb exposed.
2. *Wrap the Cuffs:* Secure the cuffs around the limb snugly but not too tight.
3. *Connect the Tubing:* Attach the tubing between the control unit and the cuffs.
4. *Power On the Device:* Press the power button to turn on the unit.
5. *Select Mode and Settings:* Adjust pressure levels, mode (detailed below), and duration as per the medical recommendation.
6. *Start Compression Therapy:* Press the start button to initiate the therapy.
7. *Monitor the Process:* Check for any discomfort, leaks, or irregular operation.
8. *End the Session:* Turn off the device, remove the cuffs, and store it properly.

6.3.4 Modes of Operation

Depending upon the make of the machine, some or all of the following modes may be available:

- *Sequential Compression Mode:* Inflates the cuffs in a sequence, starting from the lower end of the limb toward the heart. This mimics the natural flow of venous return and is useful for treating venous insufficiency and DVT prevention.
- *Gradient Compression Mode:* Applies higher pressure at the extremity and gradually decreases pressure as it moves toward the upper limb. This mode enhances lymphatic drainage and reduces swelling.
- *Continuous Compression Mode:* Maintains a constant level of compression throughout the treatment session. This mode is useful for post-surgical recovery and pain management.
- *Pulsatile Compression Mode:* Delivers rapid, rhythmic inflation and deflation cycles that simulate muscle contractions. It is beneficial for enhancing circulation and reducing the risk of blood clots.

- *Targeted Zone Compression Mode:* Allows the user to apply varying pressure levels to different segments of the limb. This is particularly useful for patients with localized edema or post-traumatic swelling.
- *Intermittent Compression Mode:* Cycles between inflation and deflation at regular intervals, promoting better blood flow and lymphatic drainage. This mode is widely used for reducing leg fatigue and managing chronic venous disorders.

6.3.5 Maintenance

- Regular Cleaning: Wipe the control unit and cuffs with a disinfectant cloth after each use.
- Inspect Tubing and Cuffs: Check for leaks, wear, or damage regularly.
- Store Properly: Keep the device in a clean, dry place when not in use.
- Replace Filters: If the unit has filters, replace them periodically.
- Battery Care (If applicable): Ensure the battery is fully charged and avoid overcharging.
- Check for Software Updates: Some modern devices may require firmware updates.

6.4 Troubleshooting

Issue	Possible cause	Solution
Device not turning on	Power cord unplugged; battery drained	Check power connection and charge battery
Weak or no compression	Tubing disconnected, leaks in the cuffs	Reconnect tubing, check for leaks
Uncomfortable high pressure	Pressure settings too high	Adjust pressure level accordingly
Cuffs not inflating properly	Kinked tubing, clogged air filter	Ensure tubing is straight, replace filter if necessary
Device overheating	Continuous use for long hours	Allow the device to cool before restarting
Error codes on display	System malfunction	Refer to the user manual for specific error codes

6.5 Conclusion

A pneumatic compression device is an essential tool for preventing circulatory complications and managing conditions like DVT and lymphedema. A proper understanding of its components, operation, and maintenance ensures effective and safe therapy. Regular troubleshooting and care can enhance its longevity and efficiency, providing optimal benefits to patients.

References

1. Kakkos S, Kirkilesis G, Caprini JA, et al. Combined intermittent pneumatic leg compression and pharmacological prophylaxis for prevention of venous thromboembolism. Cochrane Database Syst Rev. 2022;1(1):CD005258.
2. Urbankova J, et al. Intermittent pneumatic compression and deep vein thrombosis prevention: a meta-analysis in postoperative patients. Thromb Haemost. 2005;94(6):1181–5.
3. Williams JW, Pavon JM, Adam SS, et al. Effectiveness of intermittent pneumatic compression devices for venous thromboembolism prophylaxis in high-risk surgical and medical patients. Durham: Evidence-based Synthesis Program (ESP) Center Durham Veterans Affairs Healthcare System; 2015.
4. Johanson N, Lachiewicz P, Lieberman J, et al. Prevention of symptomatic pulmonary embolism in patients undergoing total hip or knee arthroplasty. J Am Acad Orthop Surg. 2009;17(3):183.
5. Gould MK, Garcia DA, Wren SM, et al. Prevention of VTE in nonorthopedic surgical patients. Antithrombotic therapy and prevention of thrombosis, 9th ed: American College of Chest Physicians evidence-based clinical practice guidelines. Chest. 2012;141(2 SUPPL):e227S–77S.
6. Venclauskas L, Maleckas A, Arcelus JI. European guidelines on perioperative venous thromboembolism prophylaxis. Eur J Anaesthesiol. 2018;35(2):147–53.
7. Rabe E, et al. Risks and contraindications of medical compression treatment—a critical reappraisal. An international consensus statement. Phlebology. 2020;35(7):447–60.
8. Operation and Service Manual. Kendall SCD. 700 sequential compression system. Covidien.
9. Lott N, et al. Intermittent pneumatic compression devices: time to reassess the evidence. ANZ J Surg. 2023;93:812–4.
10. Anderson DR, Morgano GP, Bennett C, et al. American Society of Hematology 2019 guidelines for management of venous thromboembolism: prevention of venous thromboembolism in surgical hospitalized patients. Blood Adv. 2019;3(23):3898–944.

Mesh

7

Paulo H. Fogaça de Barros, Rodrigo Galhego,
and Álvaro Cota Carvalho

7.1 Introduction

The use of meshes to repair abdominal wall hernias has been a standard practice in surgical treatment, as there is a lower degree of recurrence over time [1, 2]. The use of synthetic materials for repairing hernias began in the 1950s [3–5], and in 1989, Lichtenstein treatment became popular for treating inguinal hernias because of its low cost, low rate of complications, and recurrence [6, 7].

Since then, several meshes have been developed from various polymers, filament structures, mesh patterns, and collagen matrices, as they can be synthetic (absorbable or not) or biological. The interaction between the mesh and tissues is affected by several factors, such as mesh material, mesh structure, pore size, and implantation technique. This incorporation process can result in complications, such as adherence or granulomas. It is important to choose a surgical mesh that is compatible with the surrounding tissues and that can adequately integrate to provide long-lasting structural support.

The host response to the mesh in the reconstruction process can be described as a series of factor, as the incorporation of the mesh, when the graft is infiltrated by the host cells, allowing neovascularization and collagen deposition; encapsulation, when the collagen and connective tissue deposits at the periphery of the material; and resorption, when the full graft is replaced by host cells.

The implantation position, degree of local contamination, and characteristics of each polymer must be considered when selecting among the different types of

P. H. Fogaça de Barros (✉)
Einstein Hospital Israelita, São Paulo, Brazil

R. Galhego
Casa De Saúde São José, Rio de Janeiro, Brazil

Á. C. Carvalho
Hospital Felício Rocho, Belo Horizonte, Brazil

J. S. Ahluwalia (ed.), *User Manual for Minimally Invasive Surgical Equipment*,
https://doi.org/10.1007/978-981-95-9019-3_7

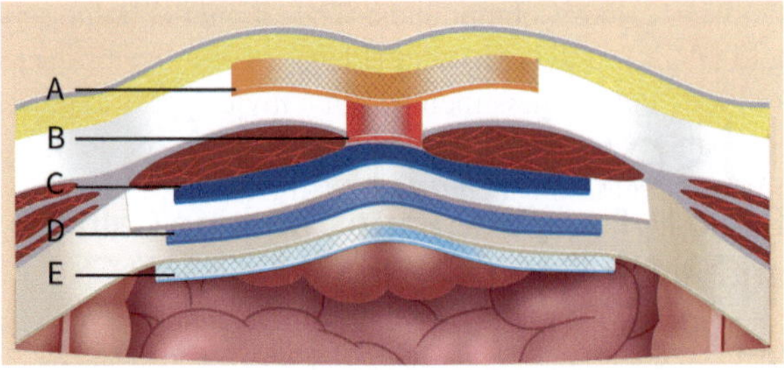

Fig. 7.1 Diagram of ventral hernia and mesh positioning. (**a**) Onlay mesh. (**b**) Inlay mesh. (**c**) Retrorectus sublay mesh. (**d**) Underlay preperitoneal. (**e**) Underlay intraperitoneal

meshes. Meshes can be implanted in onlay, retromuscular sublay, and underlay preperitoneal or intraperitoneal positions (Fig. 7.1). Polypropylene and polyester mesh can be implanted in the onlay, retromuscular, or preperitoneal underlay positions. These meshes can't be in direct contact with intra-abdominal organs due to the risk of organ erosions.

LeBlanc was the first to describe the minimally invasive ventral hernia repair in 1993. He used an intra-abdominal mesh made of polytetrafluoroethylene (PTFE), a hydrophobic polymer that decreases adherence to intestinal loops [8]. Biological meshes, PTFE, polyvinylidene fluoride (PVDF), and composite meshes can be used when they touch intestinal loops [9]. Retromuscular repairs gained importance when Abdalla described the use of a robotic platform for performing the minimally invasive Rives Stoppa technique [10]. In 2013, Ballecer introduced the use of a robotic platform to separate components. In 2015, Bx elyansky and Daes published a procedure for performing a total extraperitoneal access. [11, 12].

7.2 Non-absorbable Synthetic Meshes

7.2.1 Polymers

Polypropylene It is the most commonly used polymer because it is inert and extremely resistant to tissue degradation. However, it induces a highly intense inflammatory reaction even though it is hydrophobic. It forms foreign body granulomas that, when confluent, can encapsulate the mesh, decrease its size, and cause rigidity, and possibly lead to fractures [9, 13]. Nowadays, since it has become widely used, it's a useful resource of comparison between different meshes. The polypropylene mesh can be found in the market in different presentations, in relation to its weight (light, medium, or high) and porosity (microporous or macroporous).

Polyester Polyester is a polymer containing an ester functional group in every repeating unit of its main chain. Alcohol and carboxylic acid reactions were used to synthesize these compounds. The aliphatic homopolymers include polyglycolic acid (PGA), polylactic acid (PLA), and polycaprolactone (PCL), whilst the semi-aromatic copolymers include polyethylene terephthalate (PET). Polyesters are biocompatible and hydrophilic in nature. Polyester fibers are extremely strong, durable, and resistant to most chemical products. However, PET can be degraded after long-term implantation [9, 13].

A comparison between polypropylene and polyester is unavoidable. Some studies have questioned the efficacy of surgical polyester mesh, especially the multifilament type. However, there is no evidence of significant clinical differences in infection or recurrence between polyester and polypropylene [14, 15].

Expanded Polytetrafluoroethylene (ePTFE) The polytetrafluoroethylene is a common polymer used in kitchenware, and the expanded form is marketed as an unabsorbable mesh, once its pores allow cellular ingrowth through the mesh. The e-PTFE is chemically stable and is produced by free polymerization of polytetrafluoroethylene. These meshes are highly hydrophobic and microporous and can be utilized to touch the intestinal loops due to their laminar microporous nature. It can create a well-structured "neo-peritoneum" surface with thin mesothelial cells, allowing bridging reconstruction and sublay placement of the mesh [9, 13]. Nowadays, it is proposed to use a composite mesh with PTFE/polypropylene that, in animal models, suggests a continuous gain of strength compared with the ePTFE plateau strength. However, they face complications due to infection after implantation, such as fragmentation, fractures, and superficial detachment [16]. No PTFE mesh exhibited physiological elasticity [13].

Polyvinylidene Fluoride (PVDF) PVDF is a type of thermoplastic fluoropolymer that is highly inert and pure and is produced by the polymerization of vinylidene difluoride. PVDF surgical meshes are more resistant to hydrolysis and degradation than PET surgical meshes and display improved biocompatibility and durability. In addition, the structure of the polymer can arrange a higher surface with a lower grammage when compared with a polypropylene mesh. No increase in retraction of the graft over time is seen when compared to polypropylene mesh. The mechanical properties of PVDF were highly stable, maintaining 92.5% of its initial resistance after implantation for 9 years [9, 13]. A novel clinical trial published in 2022 showed that PVDF has similar surgical site occurrence in the first 30 days after surgery when used in contaminated environments compared to clean wounds, although the study has limitations concerning the number of patients involved, its results demonstrate the stability of the material even in complex hernia surgery [30].

7.2.2 Mesh Structure

Porosity Porosity is important for reducing any reaction from foreign bodies in the polypropylene structures. Pores larger than 1 mm allow inflammatory proteins to permeate macrophages and form new surrounding vessels, fostering mesh integration and collagen deposition [9, 13]. This way, the meshes can be classified as macroporous, when their pores are larger than 1 mm, and microporous, when their size is narrower.

Grammage Surgical meshes can be classified according to their weight as lightweight (LW) or heavyweight (HW) meshes. The mesh weight classification was unrelated to the molecular weight of the polymer, but the mesh density was measured in grams per square meter (g/m^2). The lightweight meshes were less than 50 g/m^2, whereas the heavyweight density was greater than 80 g/m^2. Mesh densities ranging from 50 to 80 g/m^2 are frequently specified as medium weight (MW). The difference between these meshes is mainly related to their mechanical resistance and capability to bear tension (tensile strength). Heavier meshes are generally stronger and longer lasting, but are stiffer and less flexible. The lighter meshes are generally more flexible and easier to handle but can be less resistant to tension [9] (Table 7.1).

The high grammage meshes can be a risk factor for chronic pain when used for inguinal hernia reconstruction, mainly when placed on anterior reconstruction due to nerve entrapment between the mesh encapsulation. The HerniaSurge data base

Table 7.1 Polypropylene mesh classified according to weight

Mesh	Weight	Manufacturer
Bard™ Soft Mesh	Light	Bard
3DMax™ Light Mesh*	Light	Bard
Optilene® Mesh LP	Light	Bbraun
Optilene® Mesh Elastic	Light	Bbraun
Prolene® Soft Mesh	Light	Ethicon
Parietene Light™	Light	Medtronic
Parietene™	Light	Medtronic
Optilene® Mesh	Medium	Bbraun
Prolene® Mesh	Medium	Ethicon
Parietene Standard™	Medium	Medtronic
Bard™ Mesh	Heavy	Bard
3DMax™ Mesh *	Heavy	Bard
Premilene® Mesh	Heavy	Bbraun
Dextile™	Heavy	Medtronic

Table 7.2 Composite meshes classified as grammage and composite materials

Mesh	Weight	Composite formation	Manufacturer
Symbotex™	Light	Polyester + collagen biofilm	Medtronic
Composix™ L/P Mesh	Light	PET + ePTFE	Bard
Ventralight™ ST	Light	PGE + PET + hydrogel	Bard
Proceed® Surgical Mesh	Light	PET + oxidized cellulose	Ethicon
Sepramesh™ IP composite	Medium	PGA + PET + hydrogel	Bard

suggests large pore monofilament synthetic flat meshes with a burst strength of $16N/m^2$ [31].

Elasticity The elasticity of the abdominal wall at 32 N/cm is approximately 38%. Most porous meshes present approximately 20–35% to 16 N/cm, whereas smaller pore meshes range from 4 to 16% at 16 N/cm. This suggests that the meshes generate restricted flexibility of the abdominal wall at an increased rate in the small-pore meshes [2, 17].

Filament Structure Multifilaments increase the surface by at least 1.57x compared with monofilaments, as said earlier, meshes with higher surface favor the tissue growth, hence increasing mesh incorporation with lower grammage. On the other hand, it also can favor bacterial persistence at the implantation site. However, this is not sufficient to create a clinically apparent infection, which can explain why infections can develop sequentially in the mesh [9, 13, 18].

Composite Meshes Composite synthetic meshes contain one coated side to avoid adherence inside the abdominal cavity, whereas the other surface is integrated into the abdominal wall. This layer gets absorbed after 30 days, providing sufficient time to regenerate the peritoneum from days 5 to 7 [19, 20]. Omega-3 fatty acids, oxidized cellulose, and collagen are utilized to form this layer (Table 7.2).

7.3 Absorbable Synthetic Meshes

Absorbable synthetic meshes made from polyglycolic acid, polyglactin 910, or carbon cellulose can be degraded by hydrolysis. They have been utilized for a long time in bridge treatment of abdominal walls in cases of contamination and infection. They are not associated with long-term repairs, because they degrade rapidly [9, 21].

Materials that reabsorb more slowly are used in abdominal wall reconstruction and have shown good initial results. Three meshes adhere to this principle: GORE BIO-A (Gore), Phasix (Bard), and TIGR Matrix (Novus Scientific). GORE BIO-A consists of a poly-copolymer (glycolyl: trimethylene carbonate), a synthetic bioabsorbable. Therefore, the mesh must not be used as a bridge. Phasix is a

Table 7.3 Absorbable synthetic meshes classified as composite materials and resorption time

Mesh	Fiber	Complete resorption	Material structure	Manufacturer
ETHICON VICRYL® Woven Mesh	92% PGA 8% PLLA	2–3 months	Multifilament 2-D knit	Ethicon
GORE® BIO-A® Tissue Reinforcement	67% PGA 33% TMC	6 months	Laminar 3-D web	Gore
BARD® DAVOL PHASIX Mesh	P4HB	12–18 months	Monofilament 2-D knit	Bard
NOVUS SCIENTIFIC TIGR® Resorbable Matrix	1) Primary matrix: PGA:PLA:TMC	3 years	Dual-filament 2-D knit	Novus scientific
	2) Secondary matrix: PLLA:TMC			

monofilament mesh with fibers composed of poly-4-hydroxybutyrate (P4HB), which is reabsorbed from 12 to 18 months. TIGR Matrix is a multifilament mesh consisting of two types of fiber: a fiber that is reabsorbed rapidly (40% lighter in weight) and a reabsorption fiber absorbed slowly [22] (Table 7.3).

A clinical trial demonstrated infrequent complications and 22% recurrence in the following 60 months in patients submitted to abdominal wall reconstruction utilizing the Phasix mesh [21]. The slower absorptive synthetic meshes seem less expensive than biological meshes, although further studies are necessary.

7.4 Biological Meshes

Most biological meshes comprise porcine acellular dermal matrix, although there are biological matrix meshes based on bovine, equine, and human compounds used in complex hernias of the abdominal wall with contamination and fistulas [23–25]. Collagen reticulation is performed during the mesh manufacturing process to strengthen the matrix structure and prevent degradation by collagenase [26]. The balance between collagen matrix deposition and mesh degradation is critical for successful repair. Immunological and inflammatory factors can also affect this process. It is postulated that the collagen framework of the biological matrix favors neoangiogenesis, making the mesh more resistant to infection than the synthetic meshes, which are associated with biofilm formation.

There is a great deal of heterogeneity in publications on the utilization of biological meshes; however, repairs using biological meshes from contamination defects have displayed considerably high rates of complications at surgical sites [27], and in meta-analysis studies, the occurrence of surgical wounds can vary 40–37%, related to surgical wound infections 27–18% [23]. Recurrence (36%) was the most

Table 7.4 Biological meshes matrix, thickness, and manufacturer

Biological mesh	Matrix	Thickness (mm)	Manufacturer
FlexHD	Human dermal tissue	0.4–4.0	MedTronic, Minneapolis, KS
Biodesign Hernia Graft	Porcine small intestine submucosa	NA	Cook medical, Bloomington, IN
XenMatrix	Porcine dermal tissue	1.8–2.5	Bard, Warwick, RI
XCM BIOLOGIC	Porcine dermal tissue	1.5	DePuy Synthes, West Chester, PA
Strattice	Porcine dermal tissue	2.5	Acelity, San Antonio, TX
Permacol	Porcine dermal tissue	0.5–1.5	MedTronic, Minneapolis, KS

consistent postoperative complication when compared with reconstruction of the abdominal wall with PET, particularly when used in bridged reconstruction [23, 27, 28].

In a randomized clinical study comparing the use of biological and synthetic meshes on contaminated ventral hernias, the findings were more favorable in the long-term follow-up using synthetic meshes, as there were fewer recurrences and no significant differences in the risk of surgical wound occurrences that require intervention in both groups or re-operation [29]. The biological meshes represent a cost 200 times higher than that of synthetic meshes.

Even though there is still uncertainty about the real benefits of near-biological mesh, the currently published guidelines recommend the use of biological mesh for contaminated sites. For abdominal wall reconstruction, whilst there is The Center for Disease Control (CDC) classification for surgical site infection, contaminated (class III) and dirty (class IV) wounds should be treated with biological matrix mesh.

The great challenge upon infected sites is the need for mesh explant whilst there is an active infection on the surgical site. Meanwhile there is debate if we have a benefit between synthetic mesh reconstruction when compared to biological mesh implant in complex hernia surgery [29, 32] (Table 7.4).

References

1. Luijendijk RW, Hop WC, van den Tol MP, de Lange DC, Braaksma MM, IJzermans JN, Boelhouwer RU, de Vries BC, Salu MK, Wereldsma JC, Bruijninckx CM, Jeekel J. A comparison of suture repair with mesh repair for incisional hernia. N Engl J Med. 2000;343(6):392–8. https://doi.org/10.1056/NEJM200008103430603.
2. EU Hernia Trialists Collaboration. Repair of groin hernia with synthetic mesh: meta-analysis of randomized controlled trials. Ann Surg. 2002;235(3):322–32. https://doi.org/10.1097/00000658-200203000-00003. PMID: 11882753; PMCID: PMC1422456.
3. Usher FC. Use of lyophilized homografts of dura mater in repair of incisional hernias. AMA Arch Surg. 1958;76(1):58–61.
4. Usher FC, Wallace SA. Tissue reaction to plastics; a comparison of nylon, orlon, dacron, teflon, and marlex. AMA Arch Surg. 1958;76(6):997–9.

5. Usher FC, Ochsner J, Tuttle LL Jr. Use of marlex mesh in the repair of incisional hernias. Am Surg. 1958;24(12):969–74.
6. Lichtenstein IL, Shulman AG, Amid PK, Montllor MM. The tension-free hernioplasty. Am J Surg. 1989;157(2):188–93. https://doi.org/10.1016/0002-9610(89)90526-6.
7. Amid PK. The Lichtenstein repair in 2002: an overview of causes of recurrence after Lichtenstein tension-free hernioplasty. Hernia. 2003;7(1):13–6. https://doi.org/10.1007/s10029-002-0088-7. Epub 2002 Oct 5.
8. LeBlanc KA, Booth WV. Laparoscopic repair of incisional abdominal hernias using expanded polytetrafluoroethylene: preliminary findings. Surg Laparosc Endosc. 1993;3(1):39–41.
9. Todros S, Pavan PG, Natali AN. Synthetic surgical meshes used in abdominal wall surgery: part I-materials and structural conformation. J Biomed Mater Res B Appl Biomater. 2017;105(3):689–99. https://doi.org/10.1002/jbm.b.33586. Epub 2015 Dec 16.
10. Abdalla RZ, et al. Procedimento de Rives/Stoppa modificado robô-assistido para correção de hérnias ventrais da linha média. ABCD. Arquivos Brasileiros de Cirurgia Digestiva (São Paulo). 2012;25:129–32.
11. Belyansky I, Zahiri HR, Park A. Laparoscopic Transversus abdominis release, a novel minimally invasive approach to complex abdominal wall reconstruction. Surg Innov. 2016;23(2):134–41. https://doi.org/10.1177/1553350615618290. Epub 2015 Nov 24.
12. Belyansky I, Daes J, Radu VG, Balasubramanian R, Reza Zahiri H, Weltz AS, Sibia US, Park A, Novitsky Y. A novel approach using the enhanced-view totally extraperitoneal (eTEP) technique for laparoscopic retromuscular hernia repair. Surg Endosc. 2018;32(3):1525–32. https://doi.org/10.1007/s00464-017-5840-2. Epub 2017 Sep 15.
13. Binnebösel M, von Trotha KT, Jansen PL, Conze J, Neumann UP, Junge K. Biocompatibility of prosthetic meshes in abdominal surgery. Semin Immunopathol. 2011;33(3):235–43. https://doi.org/10.1007/s00281-010-0237-5. Epub 2011 Jan 12.
14. Rosen MJ. Polyester-based mesh for ventral hernia repair: is it safe? Am J Surg. 2009;197(3):353–9. https://doi.org/10.1016/j.amjsurg.2008.11.003.
15. Totten C, Becker P, Lourd M, Roth JS. Polyester vs polypropylene, do mesh materials matter? A meta-analysis and systematic review. Med Devices (Auckl). 2019;12:369–78. https://doi.org/10.2147/MDER.S198988. PMID: 31572024; PMCID: PMC6747676.
16. Bellon JM, Contreras LA, Bujan J. Ultrastructural alterations of polytetrafluoroethylene prostheses implanted in abdominal wall provoked by infection: clinical and experimental study. World J Surg. 2000;24:528–31.
17. Junge K, Klinge U, Prescher A, Giboni P, Niewiera M, Schumpelick V. Elasticity of the anterior abdominal wall and impact for reparation of incisional hernias using mesh implants. Hernia. 2001 Sep;5(3):113–8. https://doi.org/10.1007/s100290100019.
18. Klinge U, Junge K, Spellerberg B, Piroth C, Klosterhalfen B, Schumpelick V. Do multifilament alloplastic meshes increase the infection rate? Analysis of the polymeric surface, the bacteria adherence, and the in vivo consequences in a rat model. J Biomed Mater Res. 2002;63(6):765–71. https://doi.org/10.1002/jbm.10449.
19. van 't Riet M, de Vos van Steenwijk PJ, Bonthuis F, Marquet RL, Steyerberg EW, Jeekel J, Bonjer HJ. Prevention of adhesion to prosthetic mesh: comparison of different barriers using an incisional hernia model. Ann Surg. 2003;237(1):123–8. https://doi.org/10.1097/00000658-200301000-00017. PMID: 12496539; PMCID: PMC1513975.
20. Schreinemacher MH, Emans PJ, Gijbels MJ, Greve JW, Beets GL, Bouvy ND. Degradation of mesh coatings and intraperitoneal adhesion formation in an experimental model. Br J Surg. 2009;96(3):305–13. https://doi.org/10.1002/bjs.6446.
21. Roth JS, Anthone GJ, Selzer DJ, Poulose BK, Pierce RA, Bittner JG, Hope WW, Dunn RM, Martindale RG, Goldblatt MI, Earle DB, Romanelli JR, Mancini GJ, Greenberg JA, Linn JG, Parra-Davila E, Sandler BJ, Deeken CR, Badhwar A, Salluzzo JL, Voeller GR. Long-term, prospective, multicenter study of Poly-4-Hydroxybutyrate mesh (Phasix mesh) for hernia repair in cohort at risk for complication: 60-month follow-up. J Am Coll Surg. 2022;235(6):894–904. https://doi.org/10.1097/XCS.0000000000000363. Epub 2022 Nov 15. PMID: 36102523; PMCID: PMC9653100.

22. Miserez M, Jairam AP, Boersema GSA, Bayon Y, Jeekel J, Lange JF. Resorbable synthetic meshes for abdominal wall defects in preclinical setting: a literature review. J Surg Res. 2019;237:67–75. https://doi.org/10.1016/j.jss.2018.11.054. Epub 2019 Jan 30.
23. Samson DJ, Gachabayov M, Latifi R. Biologic mesh in surgery: a comprehensive review and meta-analysis of selected outcomes in 51 studies and 6079 patients. World J Surg. 2021;45(12):3524–40. https://doi.org/10.1007/s00268-020-05887-3. Epub 2021 Jan 8.
24. Latifi R. Practical approaches to definitive reconstruction of complex abdominal wall defects. World J Surg. 2016;40(4):836–48.
25. Slater NJ, Montgomery A, Berrevoet F, Carbonell AM, Chang A, Franklin M, et al. Criteria for definition of a complex abdominal wall hernia. Hernia J Hernias Abdom Wall Surg. 2014;18(1):7–17.
26. Novitsky YW. Biology of biological meshes used in hernia repair. Surg Clin North Am. 2013;93(5):1211–5. https://doi.org/10.1016/j.suc.2013.06.014. Epub 2013 Aug 12.
27. Atema JJ, de Vries FE, Boermeester MA. Systematic review and meta-analysis of the repair of potentially contaminated and contaminated abdominal wall defects. Am J Surg. 2016;212(5):982–995.e1. https://doi.org/10.1016/j.amjsurg.2016.05.003. Epub 2016 Jun 12.
28. Köckerling F, Alam NN, Antoniou SA, Daniels IR, Famiglietti F, Fortelny RH, Heiss MM, Kallinowski F, Kyle-Leinhase I, Mayer F, Miserez M, Montgomery A, Morales-Conde S, Muysoms F, Narang SK, Petter-Puchner A, Reinpold W, Scheuerlein H, Smietanski M, Stechemesser B, Strey C, Woeste G, Smart NJ. What is the evidence for the use of biologic or biosynthetic meshes in abdominal wall reconstruction? Hernia. 2018;22(2):249–69. https://doi.org/10.1007/s10029-018-1735-y. Epub 2018 Jan 31. PMID: 29388080; PMCID: PMC5978919.
29. Rosen MJ, Krpata DM, Petro CC, Carbonell A, Warren J, Poulose BK, Costanzo A, Tu C, Blatnik J, Prabhu AS. Biologic vs synthetic mesh for single-stage repair of contaminated ventral hernias: a randomized clinical trial. JAMA Surg. 2022;157(4):293–301. https://doi.org/10.1001/jamasurg.2021.6902. PMID: 35044431; PMCID: PMC8771431.
30. Birolini C, Tanaka EY, de Miranda JS, Murakami AH, Damous SHB, Utiyama EM. The early outcomes of complex abdominal wall reconstruction with polyvinylidene (PVDF) mesh in the setting of active infection: a prospective series. Langenbeck's Arch Surg. 2022;407(7):3089–99. https://doi.org/10.1007/s00423-022-02625-2. Epub 2022 Jul 29.
31. HerniaSurge Group. International guidelines for groin hernia management. Hernia. 2018;22(1):1–165. https://doi.org/10.1007/s10029-017-1668-x. Epub 2018 Jan 12. PMID: 29330835; PMCID: PMC5809582.
32. Katzen M, Ayuso SA, Sacco J, Ku D, Scarola GT, Kercher KW, Colavita PD, Augenstein VA, Heniford BT. Outcomes of biologic versus synthetic mesh in CDC class 3 and 4 open abdominal wall reconstruction. Surg Endosc. 2023;37(4):3073–83. https://doi.org/10.1007/s00464-022-09486-2. Epub 2022 Aug 4.

Anaesthesia Workstation

8

Choro Athiphro Kayina and Saranlal Ajai Mokandasan

8.1 Introduction

We don't know where exactly in brain the anaesthetic agents precisely act. Yet what makes the practice of anaesthesia safer is that we know how exactly to control it so as to safely provide a mix of amnesia, ataxia, anaesthesia and areflexia which together enables surgical procedure. Modern anaesthesia machine is a comprehensive workstation that enables safe delivery of gas mixture at preset rates, adds inhalational agents as required, and includes an inbuilt attached mechanical ventilator to deliver positive pressure ventilation. It also has monitoring systems to enable continuous measurement of patient's vital parameters in cardiovascular, respiratory, thermo-regulatory and neuromonitoring domains.

8.2 Components

Anaesthesia workstation incorporates a complex system with multiple pipelines, connections, valves and flow-adjusting knobs that function to deliver a safe amount of gases in a controlled manner and to continuously monitor the patient's vitals. Anaesthesia workstation can be separated into multiple components to enable easy understanding (Fig. 8.1):

1. The gas delivery system
2. The vaporisers
3. Electronic flow meters
4. The ventilator

C. A. Kayina (✉) · S. A. Mokandasan
Anaesthesiology Pain Medicine and Critical Care, All India Institute of Medical Sciences, New Delhi, New Delhi, India

J. S. Ahluwalia (ed.), *User Manual for Minimally Invasive Surgical Equipment*,
https://doi.org/10.1007/978-981-95-9019-3_8

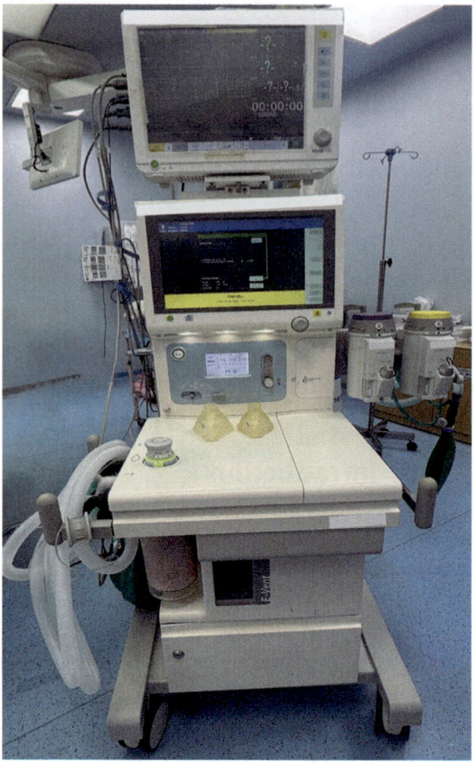

Fig. 8.1 Anaesthesia workstation

5. Sensors
6. Breathing systems
7. Carbon dioxide (CO_2) absorbers
8. Monitors
9. Scavenging system

There are two general systems comprising the anaesthesia workstation: the electrical system and the pneumatic system.

(a) *Electrical System*

   (i) *Master switch*: Turning the master switch activates both the electrical and pneumatic functions of the anaesthesia machine. When the master switch is in the OFF position, only the backup battery charger and electrical outlets are active (Fig. 8.2a).
   (ii) *Power failure indicator*: The workstations are equipped with a visual or audible indicator to alert the anaesthesia provider on loss of main electrical power (Fig. 8.2b).
   (iii) *Reserve power*: A backup source is usually provided with the modern anaesthesia workstation, as electricity is crucial for the functioning of the

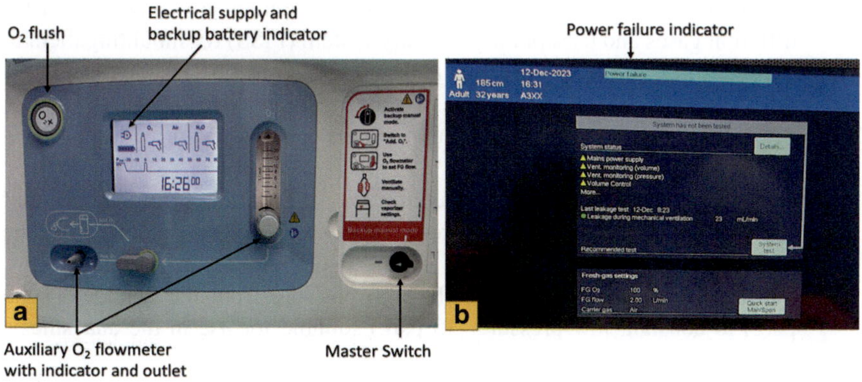

Fig. 8.2 (**a**) Anaesthesia workstation showing master switch, O_2 flush, auxiliary O_2 and power supply. (**b**): Visual indicator showing main electrical supply being cut-off

Table 8.1 Components of pressure system

High pressure system	Intermediate pressure system	Low pressure system
(a) Cylinder	(a) Pipeline inlet connections	(a) Flow indicators
(b) Hanger yolk system	(b) Pipeline pressure indicators	(b) Unidirectional check valve
(c) Check valve	(c) Oxygen pressure failure devices	(c) Pressure relief device
(d) Pressure regulator	(d) Oxygen supply failure alarm	(d) Vaporiser mounting device
(e) Cylinder pressure indicator	(e) Oxygen flush valve	(e) Common fresh gas outlet
	(f) Second stage pressure regulator	(f) Auxiliary O_2 flowmeter
	(g) Flow control valves	

machine. The status of the battery should be checked as part of the pre-use anaesthesia machine check (Fig. 8.2a).

(iv) *Electrical outlets*: To power the monitors and other anaesthesia devices, electrical outlets have been provided at the back of the machine. These outlets should not be used to power anything other than anaesthesia devices and cannot supply electricity if there is power failure.

(b) *Pneumatic System:*

The pneumatic part of the machine has been divided into three parts, namely, high, intermediate and low pressure system (Table 8.1)

1. *High Pressure System*: Part of the machine that is confined to the cylinders and their primary pressure regulators.

Cylinder: Reserve source of inspiratory gases. Cylinders are colour coded for different gases and uses pin index safety system (PISS) for mounting them to the anaesthesia workstation (Figs. 8.3a and 8.4). This PISS enables accidental misconnection of wrong cylinders to wrong gas input.

Hanger yolk assembly: Orients and supports the cylinder and provides gas tight seal (Fig. 8.3a).

Check valve: The check valve allows unidirectional flow of gas from the cylinder to the machine. This valve also prevents backfilling of the cylinder from the pipeline.

Pressure regulator: Converts variable high pressure from the cylinder (1900 psig) to constant low pressure (45 psig) suitable for use in the anaesthesia machine.

Cylinder pressure indicator/gauge: Bourbon-type gauges were used in older machines. Newer machines use electronic pressure transducers to continuously measure cylinder pressure (Fig. 8.5).

2. *Intermediate Pressure System*: Begins at the regulated cylinder supply sources downstream to the flow control valve.

   Pipeline inlet connection: Each gas pipeline is attached via a gas-specific connection. The pipeline attaches to the terminal wall unit (which carries gas from the hospital manifold) on one end and the machine end on the other (Figs. 8.3b and 8.4b).

   Pipeline pressure indicators: Present on the pipeline side of the check valve for measuring pipeline pressures continuously. Pressure is maintained between 50 and 55 psig (Fig. 8.5).

   Oxygen pressure failure devices: The function is to prevent delivering hypoxic gas mixture to patients if the oxygen pressure in the pipeline/cylinder falls or oxygen flow stops. (It will be great if we could mark all parts in the pictures.)

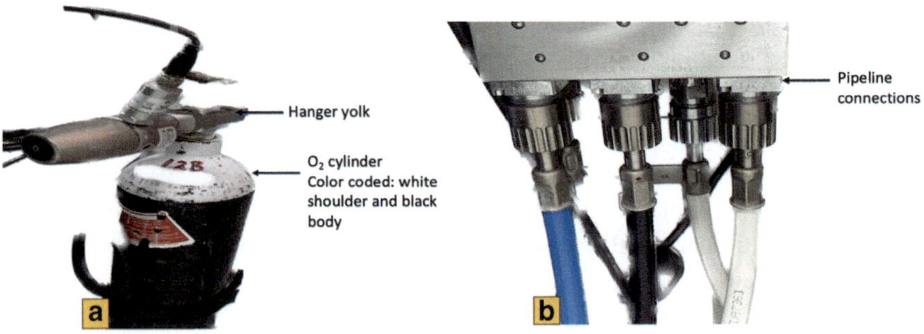

Fig. 8.3 (**a**): Oxygen cylinder with hanger yolk assembly. (**b**): Gas pipeline connections; colour coded: blue—nitrous oxide, black—air, white—oxygen

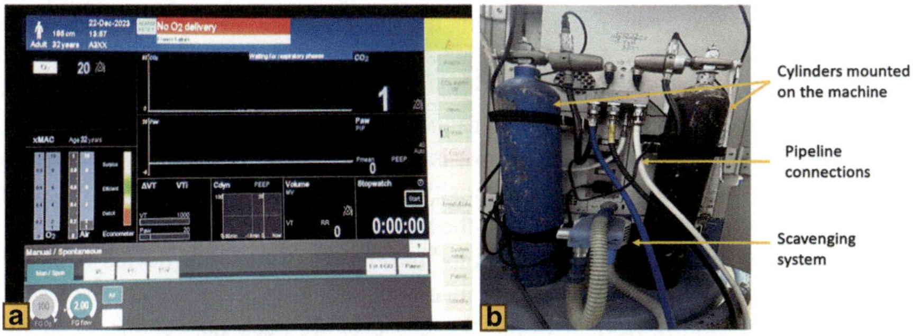

Fig. 8.4 (**a**): Oxygen failure alarm system activated due to oxygen supply failure. (**b**). Cylinder and pipeline connections mounted at the back of the anaesthesia workstation

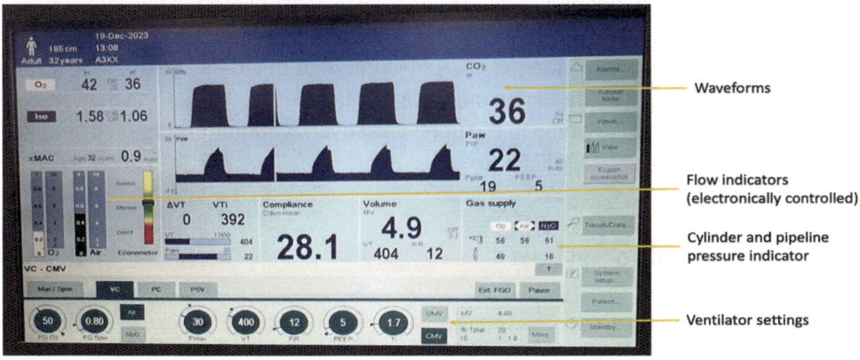

Fig. 8.5 Workstation interface showing ventilation waveform and graphics

Oxygen supply failure alarm: When oxygen supply pressure falls below a specific threshold (e.g. 38 psig), oxygen failure alarm opens and shows audible and visual indicators of the same (Fig. 8.4a).

Oxygen flush: Supply 100% oxygen at high flow rates (35-75 L/min) from pipeline or cylinder at 45–55 psig (Fig. 8.2a). A safety mechanism that can be activated even when the master power switch is turned off or when there is an electronic power failure that causes shut down of the workstation.

Second stage pressure regulator: Reduces pressure further to 14 psig for oxygen and 26 psig for nitrous oxide. The purpose is to eliminate fluctuations in pipeline pressure and ensure constant flow.

Flow control valves: Controls gas flow rate. Modern devices have electronic flow meters with an electronic display of the flow rates (Fig. 8.5). Flow control knobs are colour coded for easy identification of the associated gas (white for O_2, blue for N_2O).

3. *Low Pressure System*: Extends from the flow control valve to the common gas outlet.
   Flow indicators: Flowmeters may be mechanical or electronic. Modern workstations use electronic flow sensors to indicate flow rates. (Fig. 8.5).
   Unidirectional check valve: The valve is located between the vaporisers and the common gas outlet. It prevents positive pressure from the breathing system from being transmitted back into the machine.
   Pressure relief device: Some machines have a pressure relief device near the common gas outlet to protect the machine from high pressure.
   Vaporiser mounting device: Some devices provide back bars/connections for mounting two vaporisers. Push the button to be activated before the dial can be turned on.
   Common gas outlet: Receives all the gases and vapours from the machine and delivers them to the breathing circuit. Newer machines have internal connections to the breathing system. Pressure delivered at the end is 5–8 psig.
   Auxiliary oxygen flow meters: It is a self-contained flowmeter with its own flow control valve, flow indicator and outlet (Fig. 8.2a). Works independent of electrical/computer control. It can be used even without turning on the anaesthesia machine.

8.3 Scavenging System

Collects and removes waste anaesthetic gases from both the anaesthesia machine and anaesthesia location (Fig. 8.4b).

Types:

1. Active: has a central evacuation system to eliminate waste gases.
2. Passive: the pressure imposed by the venting of the breathing circuit drives flow.

8.4 The Vaporisers

An instrument designed to change a liquid anaesthetic agent into its vapour and to add a controlled amount of this vapour to fresh gas flow. These are portable equipment which can be fitted into the anaesthesia workstation interchangeably. Most modern devices use agent-specific vaporisers that are colour coded and can be fitted into the workstation in the backbars, which are located distal to the flowmeters (Fig. 8.6a). Part of the gas flows through the vaporiser and pickups the anaesthetic vapours to be delivered at the fresh gas outlet.

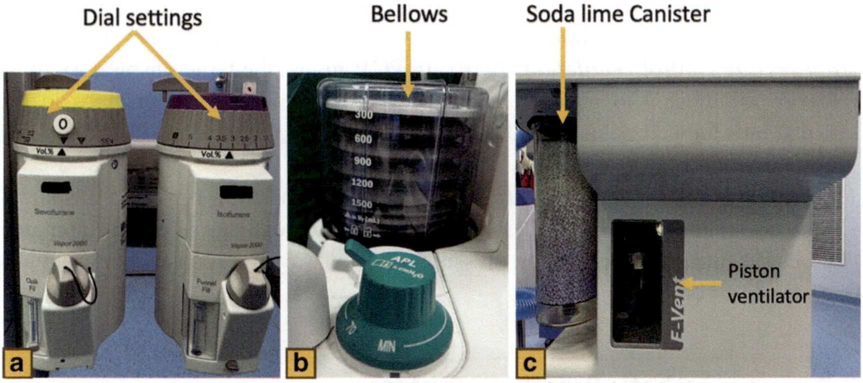

Fig. 8.6 (**a**): Sevoflurane and isoflurane vaporiser (colour coded). (**b**): Bellows type of ventilator; adjustable pressure limiting (APL) valve. (**c**): Piston type of ventilator; soda lime showing colour change indicating exhaustion

8.5 Ventilator

The ventilator is a device designed to provide positive pressure ventilation to the patient. The ventilators are attached between the expiratory valve and the CO_2 absorber with a manual/ventilator switch in between. In ventilator mode, the ventilator drives the gas mixture into the patient. In manual mode, ventilation can be assisted by compressing the reservoir bag with an adjustable pressure limiting (APL) valve set to the desired pressure level to enable manual ventilation (Fig. 8.6b). In a spontaneously breathing patient, the reservoir bag is kept free and the APL valve set to the desired PEEP pressure for assisting the patient's efforts. Ventilators can be bellows or piston type.

(a) *Bellows type*: The bellows are housed in a clear plastic cylinder, which allow bellow movement to be observed. In these ventilators, pressurised driving gas compresses the bellows and bellows in turn deliver the tidal volume. Example of bellows type ventilator (Fig. 8.6b).
(b) *Piston type*: Piston ventilator uses an electric motor to compress the gas in the breathing system to deliver the ventilation. The computer determines the amount the piston must move to deliver the required tidal volume. They do not have bellows nor require driving gas.

Example of piston-type ventilator (Fig. 8.6c).

Ventilation Modes in Anaesthesia Ventilators: The common modes of ventilation in modern anaesthesia workstations are as follows.

(a) *Volume control ventilation (VCV):* In this mode, preset volume is delivered with constant flow. Peak airway pressure varies with patient compliance and airway resistance. Typical ventilator settings in VCV are—tidal volume (TV): 6-10 ml/kg body weight; respiratory rate: 10–14/min; PEEP: 5 cm of water (Fig. 8.7a).

(b) *Pressure control ventilation (PCV):* In PCV mode, the target inspiratory pressure is adjusted to generate adequate TV. According to the changes in the patient's lung compliance and airway resistance, the delivered tidal volume varies (Fig. 8.7b).

(c) *Pressure support ventilation (PSV):* This mode is useful for patients in spontaneous respiration under general anaesthesia. The ventilator supports spontaneous breathing by augmenting pressure to the airway in response to the patient's supported breaths (Fig. 8.7c).

8.6 Anaesthetic Breathing Systems

Fresh gas departs from the gas supply system and enters the anaesthetic breathing circuit through the fresh gas line. The function of the breathing system is to deliver oxygen and anaesthetic gases and eliminate CO_2. The circle system is most commonly used in an anaesthesia workstation. The circle system is so named as it allows circular, unidirectional flow of gases which is facilitated by the unidirectional valves (Fig. 8.8).

8.7 CO_2 Absorbers

Circle systems require a means of CO_2 removal from the expired gases to avoid rebreathing and CO_2 retention. Hence, CO_2 absorbers are used to absorb the CO_2 from the expired air before adding it to the inspiratory limb. The canister houses the CO_2 absorbent which is a base, soda lime (NaOH + KOH) or lithium hydroxide (LOH) which absorbs CO_2, forming sodium bicarbonate or lithium carbonate

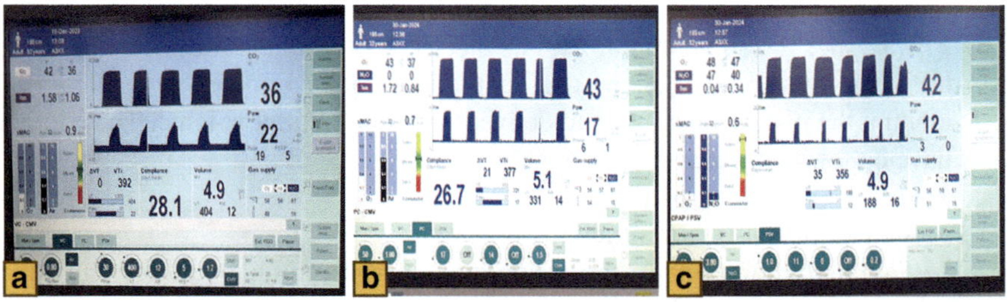

Fig. 8.7 Workstation interface showing ventilation waveform and different modes of ventilation. (**a**): *Volume control ventilation (VCV)*—TV set at 400 ml and patient's peak airway pressure is 22cmH_2O with respiratory rate (RR) set at 12/min. (**b**): *Pressure control ventilation (PCV)*—Inspiratory pressure set at 17 cmH_2O which generates TV of 377 ml and set RR of 14/min. (**c**): *Pressure support ventilation (PSV)*—with pressure support of 11 cmH_2O, TV generated is 356 ml

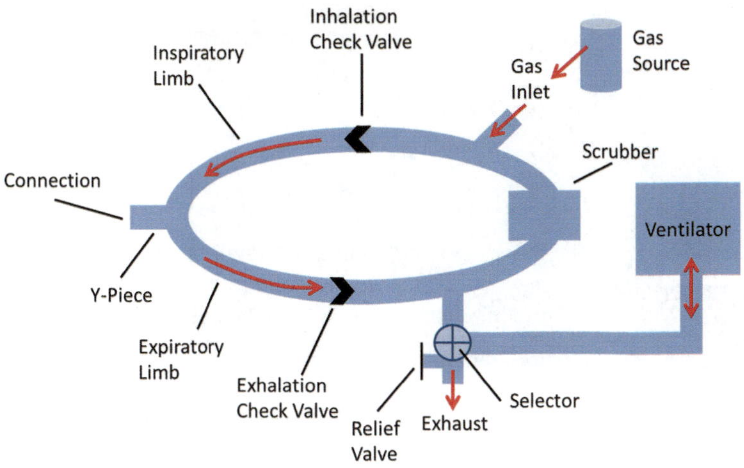

Fig. 8.8 Circle system—schematics (During inspiration, fresh gas flows through the inspiratory limb and inspiratory unidirectional valve to the patient. During expiration, the inspiratory valve closes and the expired gases flow through the expiratory unidirectional valve in the expiratory limb to soda lime canister (scrubber) and reservoir bag)

(Fig. 8.6c). This is an exothermic reaction and hence needs to be separated from the patient.

8.8 Monitors

American Society of Anaesthesiology (ASA) practice guidelines require all patients presenting for surgery need to be continuously monitored in the domains of temperature, oxygenation, ventilation and circulation. Anaesthesia workstation comes equipped with multiple monitoring sensors, which enable continuous monitoring of heart rate, electrocardiogram (ECG), oxygen saturation (SpO_2), capnography (expired CO_2), respiratory rate, blood pressure (BP), temperature, airway pressure, flow and volumes (Fig. 8.9). Advanced monitoring includes sophisticated devices for measuring unconsciousness (processed electroencephalogram like Entropy), degree of muscle relaxation (neuromuscular monitoring), invasive BP (beat-to-beat monitoring), volume responsiveness predictors such as systolic pressure variation (SPV) and pulse pressure variation (PPV) (Fig. 8.9). These vitals are constantly updated in colour display in real time with visual and audible alarms. They are also stored locally to enable data retrieval at a later point.

8.9 Trouble Shooting

The commonly encountered device failures and the troubleshooting are listed in the table below (Table 8.2).

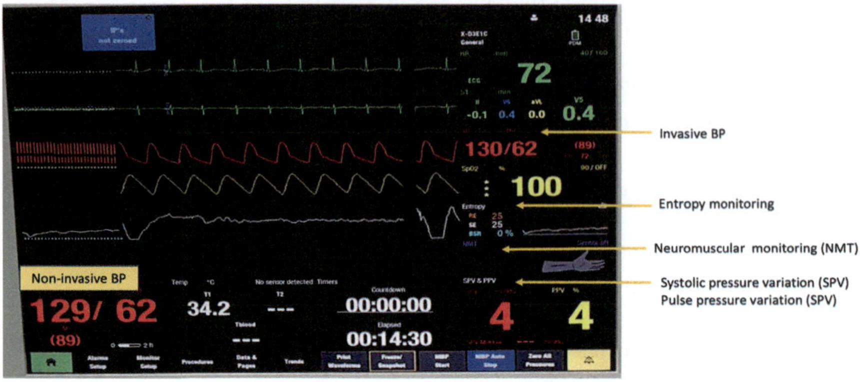

Fig. 8.9 Workstation interface showing patient vitals (basic as well as advanced monitoring)

Table 8.2 Troubleshoot of commonly encountered anaesthesia workstation failure

Feature failure	Display alarm	Cause	Device adjustments
Power failure	Power fail	Electrical supply failure	Workstation continues to work in UPS mode. If that fails, only manual ventilation would be possible.
Gas failure	No O_2/air/ N_2O supply	Central gas supply failure	Reserve cylinder should be opened; if the cylinder is exhausted, the machine automatically uses ambient air.
Ventilation failure	Ventilator fail	Ventilator failure	Manual ventilation is possible in manual/ spontaneous mode.
Fresh gas delivery failure	Gas mixer fail	Anaesthesia workstation gas mixer failure	Emergency O_2 safety control valve set to required flow. Can deliver controlled ventilation with a vaporiser.
Leak in system	Tidal volume not attained	Fresh gas flow is not adequate	Increase the flows and check for any leak in the system.
Oxygen failure	Oxygen supply failure alarm	Inadequate supply of oxygen	Check for the source of oxygen (cylinder and pipeline). Restoring oxygen pressure should restore other gases.
Increase airway pressure	High peak pressure	Increase resistance to the flow of gases	Check for any kind of endotracheal tube (ETT), or secretions inside the ETT. Also, can be due to intrinsic problem with the patient's lung.

8.9.1 Automatic Self-Test of Workstation

Modern anaesthesia machines have been equipped with fully automatic self-test features and calibration of all sensors to ensure proper functioning. The self-test result will be displayed on the monitor dashboard (Fig. 8.10).

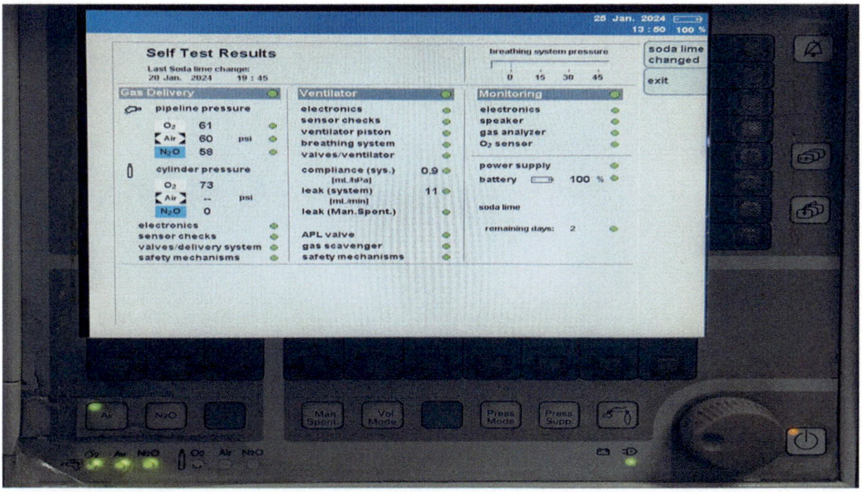

Fig. 8.10 Self-test result displayed on the dashboard of the anaesthesia workstation

8.9.2 Upcoming Technology in Anaesthesia Workstation

The modern practise of anaesthesia is inextricably dependent on technology. It is technology that made anaesthesia possible, then subsequently ensured its safety and will strive to enhance its scalability over time. As the twenty-first century dawns, advances in the anaesthesia workstation have been developed in the area of automation and monitoring.

1. *Automation*: Automation in the delivery of anaesthetics such as closed-loop anaesthesia delivery system (CLADS), which relies on the "closed" feedback loop system. The hallmark of this automation is the ability of the machine to alter its function without direct-user input but a pre-defined feed objective.
2. *Monitoring*: With innovation, monitoring has become less invasive. Cardiac output (CO) monitoring, which required invasive lines such as pulmonary artery catheter, now uses a BP cuff attached to a finger, such as the CNAP system (CNSystems Medizintechnik GmbH, Graz, Austria).

Lastly, artificial intelligence (AI) has been applied to all fields of medicine, not sparing anaesthesiology. Ongoing research is underway on the use of AI in the control of mechanical ventilation, monitoring the depths of anaesthesia and delivery of neuromuscular blockade.

Multiparameter Monitor

9

Nitin Choudhary and Sankho Choudhury

A multiparameter monitor is a state-of-the-art medical device designed to simultaneously measure and display multiple physiological parameters of a patient on one screen. Some of the most common parameters that can be measured include heart rate, blood pressure, respiratory rate, oxygen saturation, electrocardiogram, temperature and capnography. The monitor integrates all this essential information into a user-friendly interface, offering a comprehensive overview of the patient's health status, thus streamlining the monitoring process, saving time and enhancing healthcare providers' efficiency.

These devices are portable and come in various shapes and sizes and can be used in a variety of settings including intensive care units, emergency department, operation theatres, critical care transport units and long-term care facilities making them very versatile to use.

They offer continuous, real-time and extensive monitoring of vital signs with accurate and reliable measurements, thus useful for early detection of irregularities in a patient's condition. The early warning system incorporated in these monitors use multitude of alarms that can be customised by the healthcare professional based on individual needs, ensuring the monitor's alerts are tailored to the patient's condition, thus reducing risk of human errors and increasing patient safety. Other features include trend analysis, wherein the monitor can record and display trends in vital signs over time, assisting in treatment planning and assessing the effectiveness of intervention. These monitors often come with built-in data recording capabilities, helping in accurate documentation and analysis of patient's progress.

N. Choudhary (✉)
Department of Anaesthesiology, Pain Medicine & Critical Care, All India Institute of Medical Sciences (AIIMS), New Delhi, India

S. Choudhury
Department of Neuroanaesthesiology & Neurocritical Care, All India Institute of Medical Sciences (AIIMS), New Delhi, India

J. S. Ahluwalia (ed.), *User Manual for Minimally Invasive Surgical Equipment*,
https://doi.org/10.1007/978-981-95-9019-3_9

Some multiparameter monitors can transmit data wirelessly to central monitoring stations, enabling healthcare teams to monitor patients from a distance and allocate resources effectively.

Overall, multi-parameter monitors have significantly revolutionised patient care and monitoring in the healthcare industry. As technology continues to advance, multi-parameter monitors will remain at the forefront of improving patient outcomes and elevating the standard of healthcare worldwide.

9.1 Identify Controls/System Components

The specific buttons may vary depending on the monitor's make and model, but some common ones include:

9.1.1 Front View (Fig. 9.1a)

- *Power on/off button*: Used to turn the monitor off or on.
- *AC power LED status indicator*: Is lit when the monitor is receiving AC power.
- *Battery LED status indicator*: Indicates when the monitor is functioning on battery power.
- *Freeze/unfreeze*: Press to take a snapshot of data at a specific moment.
- *Alarm silence button*: Mutes the system alarm sound temporarily (usually for 2 min). Alarm may automatically reactivate after the specific time has ceased.
- *Alarm lamp*: Patient status alarm that changes colour based on alarm condition.
- *Technical alarm*: It is lit when there are system status alerts.
- *Manual NIBP button*: Press to start or stop non-invasive blood pressure measurement.
- *Navigation knob*: It can be used to confirm menu selection.
- *Display screen*: Can be a TFT/LED/LCD panel of different manufacturers' specifications.
- *Main screen button*: Press to return to the main screen from other screens.
- *Handle*: Used to transport the monitor.

9.1.2 Side and Bottom View (Fig. 9.1b)

- *Module racks*: The cable for different parameters connect to the module rack

  1. Invasive blood pressure (IBP)
  2. Temperature
  3. Pulse oximetry
  4. NIBP
  5. ECG and impedance respiration connector

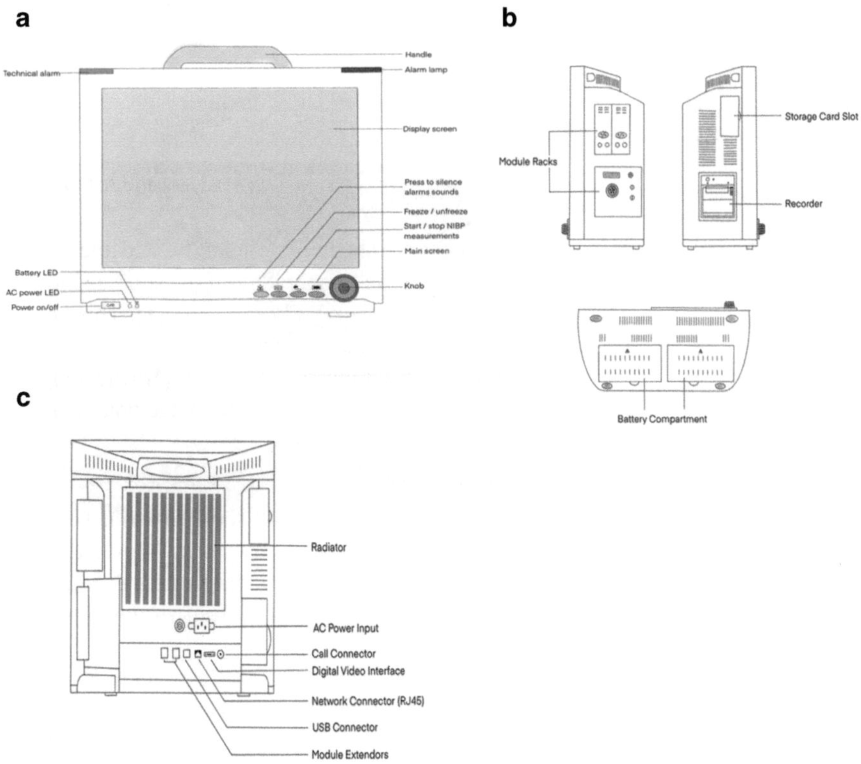

Fig. 9.1 (**a**) Multiparameter monitor front view; (**b**) side view and bottom view; (**c**) rear view. (Courtesy Dr Shreyash Agrawal)

- *Battery compartments*: contains battery to allow the monitor to run on battery power
- *Storage card slot*: slot for inserting a memory card
- *Recorder*: connect the recorder via this connector

9.1.3 Rear View (Fig. 9.1c)

- *AC power input*: connects the AC power to the monitor via a power cord
- *USB connector*: connects a USB storage device to save and download logs
- *Network connector*: connects the monitor to a network
- *Radiator*: grills/bars for ventilation, dissipating heat from the monitor
- *Call connector*: monitor communicates with the central monitoring station
- *Digital video interface*: HDMI port to connect to other devices

9.1.4 Display Screen (Fig. 9.2)

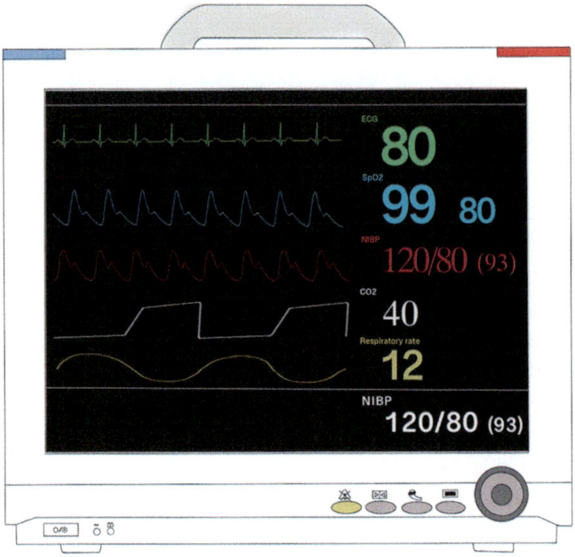

Fig. 9.2 Display screen of multiparameter monitor showing the various waveform tracings and values of monitored parameters. (Courtesy Dr. Shreyash Agrawal)

9.1.5 Waveform Area (Fig. 9.2)

1st trace: ECG waveform
2nd trace: Plethysmogram for SpO2 measurement
3rd trace: Arterial waveform from invasive blood pressure recording
4th trace: Capnography tracing
5th trace: Impedance respiration waveform

9.1.6 Parameter Area

It displays each parameter's value, unit and icon, etc. The navigation knob can be moved to the parameter panel (such as SpO2, ECG, etc.) to highlight it and then the knob can be pressed to enter into the parameter setting screen.

9.1.7 Alarms

Alarms in a multi-parameter monitor are critical safety features that alert the health-care provider when vital signs deviate from preset or acceptable ranges.

Table 9.1 Showing various physiological and technical alarms settings in the multiparameter monitor

Physiological alarms	Technical alarm
HR over limit, ST over limit, asystole SpO2 over limit RR over limit Temp over limit SYS over limit, DIA over limit, MAP over limit, PR over limit NIBP over range	Low battery, self-checking failure ECG leads off Temp probe off Unable to detect SpO2 Weak SpO2 signal Cuff error, air leakage, BP motion artifact, BP measuring timeout, BP reset

9.1.8 Categories (Table 9.1)

- *Physiological alarms*—also known as patient status alarm and are triggered when there is a deviation from set alarm limits
- *Technical alarm*—also known as system status alarm and are triggered by device malfunction or mechanical problems
- *Prompt messages*—are displayed in the prompt message category

9.1.9 Alarm Indicators (May Vary Among Manufacturers) (Table 9.2)

Table 9.2 The significance of colour coding of alarms based on their priority [1]

Alarm lamp colour	Alarm level
Red flashing	High priority alarm
Yellow flashing	Medium priority alarm
Yellow	Low priority alarm
Green	Normal

9.2 Electrocardiogram (ECG)

An electrocardiogram monitor is used in the operation theatre to record the electrical activity of the heart and to measure the heart rate, assess the rhythm and to diagnose abnormalities such as ischemia, arrythmias and detect pacemaker function.

- Lead II is ideal for detecting arrhythmias.
- Lead V is useful for detecting ischemia.

9.2.1 Components of ECG Monitor

- *Electrodes*: They are made up of foam pads with a conducting gel and silver chloride impregnated electrodes which are ideally placed on a clean, dry and hair-free bony prominence of the body for precise measurement without much electrical interference. They are connected to an ECG monitor via lead wires.
- *Lead wires*: These are colour coded cables with ends made in a snap or grabber design to attach to the electrodes for transmission of signals to the monitor. They are available in three and five lead version.
- *ECG module*: It is the main component responsible for processing the electrical signals received from the electrodes and converting them into ECG waveforms.
- *A display screen*: A monitor is present to display the real-time waveform of the ECG. The standard ECG display speed of 25 mm/second and sensitivity of 1 mV/cm is used.
- *A high-pass and low-pass filter*: It removes the 'unwanted noise' and produces a clear signal.
- *Visual and audible alarms* are present to alert the healthcare provider of any abnormality of rate, rhythm disturbance, ischemia, etc., helping them quickly respond to any potential issues.

9.2.2 Placement of Leads (AHA Standard) (Table 9.3)

Table 9.3 Colour coding of various ECG leads with their site of placement on the body [2]

Colour code	Label on lead	Electrode position
White	RA	Right arm: intersection between centreline of the right clavicle and 2nd rib
Black	LA	Left arm: intersection between the centreline of left clavicle and 2nd rib
Red	LL	Left leg: left part of the upper abdomen
Green	RL	Right leg: right part of the upper abdomen
Brown	V	Anywhere on the chest

9.2.3 ECG and Laparoscopic Surgery

- *Tachycardia*: It may be seen due to sympathetic stimulation of the patient during insufflation with carbon dioxide.
- *Bradyarrhythmia and asystole*: It may occur during insufflation of the abdomen due to stimulation of the vagus nerve. It is recommended to insufflate the abdomen slowly with a reduced pressure and flow rate. If bradyarrhythmia persists, remove gas from the abdomen and atropine may be used.

9.3 Non-invasive Blood Pressure (NIBP)

Principle of Measurement NIBP measurement in multi-parameter monitors utilises the oscillometric method. It is easy to use, accurate, provides reliable and consistent readings and can be utilised for continuous monitoring.

A cuff is used to occlude the artery by inflating it above the patient's systolic BP (generally 150 mm Hg for adults, 120 mm Hg for paediatric and 70 mm Hg in neonates) and then incrementally reduced while a transducer senses the pressure oscillations in the cuff. The point of maximum oscillations correlates to the mean blood pressure, whereas the systolic blood pressure can be detected as the point of initial rise of oscillation and diastolic blood pressure is calculated indirectly using algorithms set in the device according to the manufacturers.

9.3.1 Modes of Measurement

- *Manual*: measurement of BP on demand
- *Auto*: BP recordings continuously repeated at set time intervals
- *STAT*: continuous rapid series of BP measurements over a 5-min interval

9.3.2 Taking a BP Reading

- Check the patient information on the monitor. Select a correct patient type.
- Ideally neonate, paediatric and adult option can be selected on most monitors. The operator should select the patient type cautiously to avoid untoward injury to children and neonates due to high inflation pressures during BP measurement.
- Select a correct cuff size according to the patient. Generally, the cuff width should be 40% of the limb circumference and the length should encircle 50-80% of the limb.
- The residual air inside the cuff should be emptied before measurement is commenced.
- Place the cuff in such a way so that the arrow mark (↓) lies over the artery (brachial) for the detection of clearest pulsation.
- The BP cuff should be tightened such that one finger can be inserted comfortably.
- The air hose, which connects the cuff to the monitor, should be straight without any tangles.
- The lower end of the cuff should be 2 cm above the elbow joint.
- Start and stop the NIBP measurement by pressing the NIBP button on the monitor.
- The NIBP readings should be taken at appropriate intervals as required during surgery.
- American Society of Anaesthesiologists (ASA) recommends NIBP monitoring at least every 5 min for patients undergoing surgery under anaesthesia.

9.3.3 Limitations

- Improper calibration may produce unreliable reading.
- It may not be reliable in patients with arrhythmias, shock, etc.
- Cuff size should be selected appropriately. A cuff that is too small may lead to erroneously high BP, whereas a larger cuff may result in falsely low readings.
- Motion artefacts (e.g. shivering, movement) may give false or no readings at all.
- Nerve damage, limb ischemia and bruising may result due to frequent BP readings.

9.3.4 NIBP Setting and Panel Display

- *NIBP*—non-invasive blood pressure label
- *mm Hg*—unit of BP reading, other units can be selected
- *PR bpm*—pulse rate in beats per minute
- *Mode (Manual/STAT/Auto)*—modes of measurement. The auto mode displays a countdown timer which indicates the duration after which BP cycling occurs
- *Cycle*—it indicates the time interval between measurement when mode is set to Auto
- *Cuff size*—can select adult/paediatric or neonate from the options
- *Inflation pressure*—cuff pressure to be inflated initially (can be selected depending on the patient type, i.e. neonates 70 mm Hg, paediatric 120 mm Hg and adult 150 mm Hg)
- *SYS Hi/Lo*—high and low alarm limits for systolic blood pressure
- *DIA Hi/Lo*—high and low alarm limits for diastolic blood pressure
- *MAP Hi/Lo*—high and low alarm limits for mean arterial pressure
- *PR Hi/Lo*—high and low alarm limits for pulse rate

9.3.5 Blood Pressure and Laparoscopic Surgery

- *Pneumoperitoneum*: The creation of pneumoperitoneum causes an increase in abdominal pressure, which may lead to reduced venous return to the heart and subsequently lower cardiac output. As a result, there may be a decrease in blood pressure.
- *Anaesthetic drugs*: The use of intravenous and inhalational anaesthetics can lead to a drop in blood pressure due to vasodilation.
- *Positioning*: Trendelenburg position may lead to an increase in venous return to the heart, thereby causing an elevated blood pressure, whereas a reverse Trendelenburg position may lead to reduced blood pressure recordings.
- *Pre-existing conditions*: Patients with cardiovascular conditions, such as hypertension, may be more susceptible to blood pressure changes during laparoscopic surgery.

9.4 Invasive Blood Pressure (IBP)

It is a method of measuring the patient's blood pressure in real-time. It involves inserting a catheter with a pressure transducer into a blood vessel. It is considered the gold standard for accurate and continuous blood pressure measurement.

9.4.1 Principle of Measurement

The sensor for IBP measurement uses a transducer that consists of four strain gauges, which are thin semiconductor wafers bound to a membrane. This forms a Wheatstone bridge and can measure changes in pressure variation that are transmitted as electrical signals to the monitor and displayed as a pressure waveform.

9.4.2 Method of Measurement

- *Insertion and sites of insertion*: Arterial catheter is inserted into a suitable artery using proper aseptic techniques. The most common sites of insertion are the radial, brachial, dorsalis pedis, posterior tibial and femoral artery.
- *Pressure transducer*: It is a sensitive strain gauge device that converts the mechanical pressure exerted by the blood into an electrical signal. The transducer is connected to the catheter and measures the pressure changes in the artery (Fig. 9.3).
- *Position of the pressure transducer*: With the patient lying in the supine position, the transducer should be placed at the level of the heart along the mid axillary line in the 4th or 5th intercostal space.
- The catheter and transducer system are connected to a saline heparin solution which flows at a rate of 3–5 ml/h from a pressurised intravenous bag to the tubing, past the sensor and into the catheter to prevent clotting at the catheter tip (Fig. 9.3).
- A three-way stop cork is attached between the catheter and transducer allowing for flushing and sampling from the arterial system (Fig. 9.3).
- *Calibration and zeroing the sensor*: Before obtaining blood pressure recordings, the pressure transducer should be calibrated to atmospheric pressure (zero reference point on the monitor indicated as IBP reading 0/0 mm Hg) which ensures accurate and reliable pressure readings. This is done by turning the three-way stop cork in a manner so that heparinised saline exists between the transducer and atmospheric air.
- The three-way stop cork can then be turned 'in line' so that the transducer sensor and cannula along with saline bag system is open to the patient, thereby displaying the IBP reading.

Invasive blood pressure transducer showing (a) normal measurement mode and (b) pulling open of the flush to allow heparinised saline to be flushed into the system.

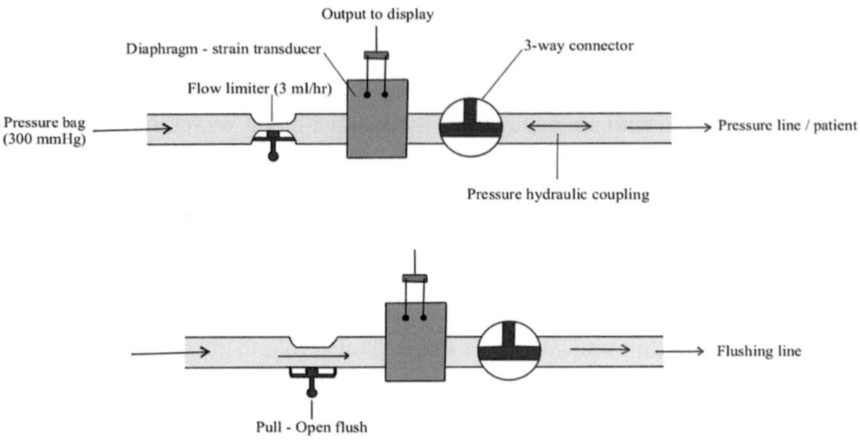

Fig. 9.3 Mechanism of functioning of arterial pressure transducer. (Courtesy Dr. Shreyash Agrawal)

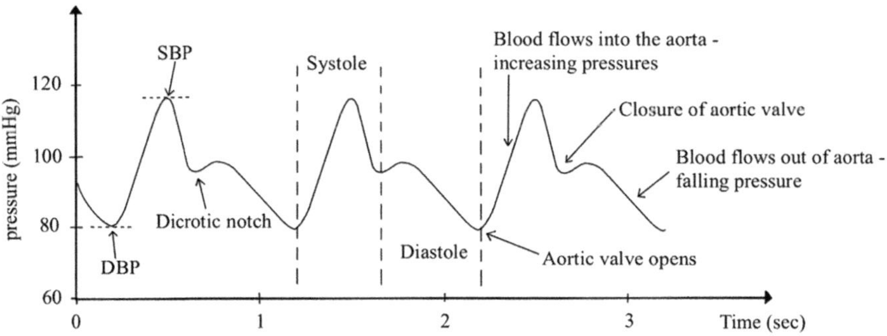

Fig. 9.4 Arterial pressure waveform: its parts and clinical relevance. (Courtesy Dr. Shreyash Agrawal)

- *Arterial waveform analysis*: By analysing the shape and characteristics of the pressure waveform generated by each heartbeat, the clinicians can assess the arterial compliance, vascular resistance, cardiac function, systolic, diastolic and mean arterial pressure (Fig. 9.4).

- *The systolic peak*: The highest point of the waveform represents the systolic blood pressure, i.e. the pressure generated by the contracting heart when it ejects blood into the aorta.
- *The diastolic downstroke*: It represents the decline in arterial pressure during ventricular relaxation.
- *Dicrotic notch*: It is caused by the closure of the aortic valve.
- *Diastolic pressure*: It is indicated by the lowest point of the waveform and reflects the minimum pressure in the arteries.

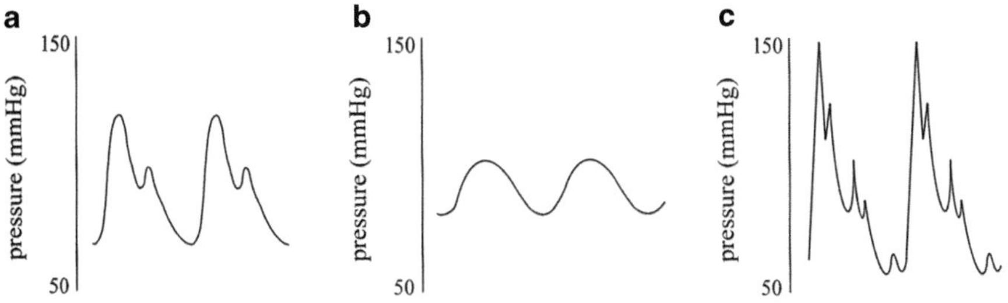

Fig. 9.5 Various types of arterial pressure waveforms: (**a**) normal; (**b**) over-damped; (**c**) under-damped. (Courtesy Dr. ShreyashAgrawal)

- *Normal arterial waveform* (Fig. 9.5a): Showing the systolic peak, the diastolic trough and the dicrotic notch, which is a small dip following the systolic peak
- *Over-damped system* (Fig. 9.5b): Seen as a flattened curve with reduced amplitude. It occurs when there is inadequate flushing of the catheter or when the arterial cannula becomes partially or completely occluded or due to ageing or arteriosclerosis (decreased arterial compliance).
- *Under-damped system* (Fig. 9.5c): It is characterised by exaggerated oscillations, rapid upstrokes and downstrokes and overshooting and undershooting resulting in higher systolic and diastolic values. It occurs due to increased compliance due to sepsis or anaemia or low vascular resistance such as in vasodilation or shock.

9.5 Temperature

Temperature monitoring of patients in the operation theatre is a critical aspect to ensure the safety and well-being of patients. Maintaining optimal temperature is essential for patient comfort, prevention of coagulopathy, surgical site infection and for smoother recovery after surgery.

9.5.1 Principle of Temperature Monitoring

The body temperature is measured using a thermistor, which are temperature-sensitive resistors. They are made up of semiconductors and exhibit a change in resistance with temperature variations. They are accurate, have a quick response and are popular due to their miniature size, inexpensiveness and convenience.

9.5.2 Monitoring Sites

- *Core body temperature*: Probes can be placed in the nasopharynx, oesophagus, rectum or bladder. It reflects a more accurate patient's overall body temperature.

- *Peripheral temperature monitoring*: Axillae and skin are used most commonly, but they are not as accurate as core temperature readings. The normal skin temperature is 36.5 to 37.5 °C.

9.5.3 Key Points Regarding Temperature Monitoring

- Body temperature should be ideally measured in all patients undergoing general anaesthesia for more than 30 min
- It should be monitored continuously
- Intra-operative temperature should be maintained >36 °C

9.6 Capnography

End tidal carbon dioxide ($EtCO_2$) monitoring provides continuous feedback on the patient's ventilation status during surgery. It helps determine if the patient is adequately ventilated and if there are any abnormalities in CO_2 elimination and also shows the perfusion status, as $EtCO_2$ levels are influenced by cardiac output and pulmonary blood flow. Thus, capnography monitoring ensures patient safety, helps in optimising ventilation and improving overall surgical outcomes.

9.6.1 Principle of Measurement

The collected sample gas is analysed using the principle of infrared absorption spectroscopy. Polyatomic gases like CO_2 absorb infrared radiation at a peak wavelength of 4.28 micrometres.

$$\text{The percentage of } CO_2 = \frac{\text{Partial pressure of } CO_2}{\text{Atmospheric pressure}} \times 100\%$$

The value and waveform are calculated as shown above once per breath on the capnograph, and units are calculated in volume percent or represented as partial pressure of CO_2 in mm Hg or kPa (normal range is 35–45 mm Hg).

9.6.2 Waveform Analysis (Fig. 9.6)

The capnometer generates a graphical waveform known as a capnogram which represents the concentration of CO_2 over time during the respiratory cycle.

- *Phase 0 (Inspiratory downstroke)*: The CO_2 concentration rapidly decreases during inhalation.
- *Phase I (Expiratory upstroke)*: As the patient begins to exhale, the concentration increases and is represented by a rapid rise in the capnogram. It reflects the CO_2 concentration in the anatomical airway (trachea and bronchi).

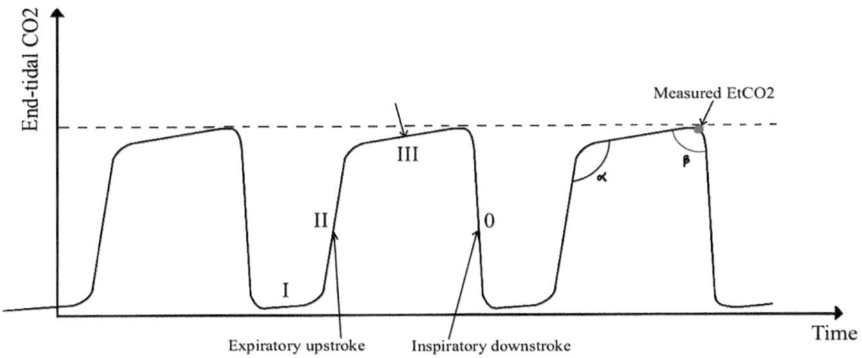

Fig. 9.6 Tracing of capnogram waveform showing the different parts of the waveform. (Courtesy Dr. Shreyash Agrawal)

- *Phase II (Expiratory upslope)*: It represents the mixing of alveolar gas with the dead space gas.
- *Phase III (Expiratory plateau)*: It represents the alveolar plateau where the concentration of CO_2 is maximum during expiration and reflects the CO_2 level in the alveoli.

9.6.3 Techniques of Capnography Measurement (Table 9.4)

- *Main-stream method*: It is the 'in line' method of capnography, i.e. the sensor is directly placed in the patient's airway tubing, thus responding immediately to changes in concentration of CO_2 (Fig. 9.7).
- *Side-stream sampling method*: It involves extracting a sample of the patient's exhaled gas using a small, flexible sampling tube and analysing it away from the patient's airway. This method has a lag time in representation of the waveform, and the sampling tube is vulnerable to occlusion (Fig. 9.7).

9.6.4 Anaesthetic Consideration of Capnography for Laparoscopic Surgery

- *Insufflation*: Insufflation during creation of pneumoperitoneum will cause an increase in CO_2 concentration and an increase in the $EtCO_2$ readings.
- *Pneumothorax*: Laparoscopic surgery involves creating pneumoperitoneum, which may lead to pneumothorax. This can be detected by showing an early abrupt increase in $EtCO_2$ levels as ventilation becomes compromised and CO_2 cannot be eliminated effectively as it builds up in the lung, which causes a higher concentration of CO_2 to be exhaled in each breath. Later, as the pneumothorax enlarges, it may decrease the cardiac output, which may cause less CO_2 to be delivered to the lung for exhalation.

Table 9.4 Comparison of the characteristics between mainstream and sidestream capnography

Characteristics	Main stream	Side stream
Response time	Fast	Slow
Waveform	Accurate	Distorted frequently
Sensor size	Large and heavy	Small and light
Amount of dead space	Large	Small

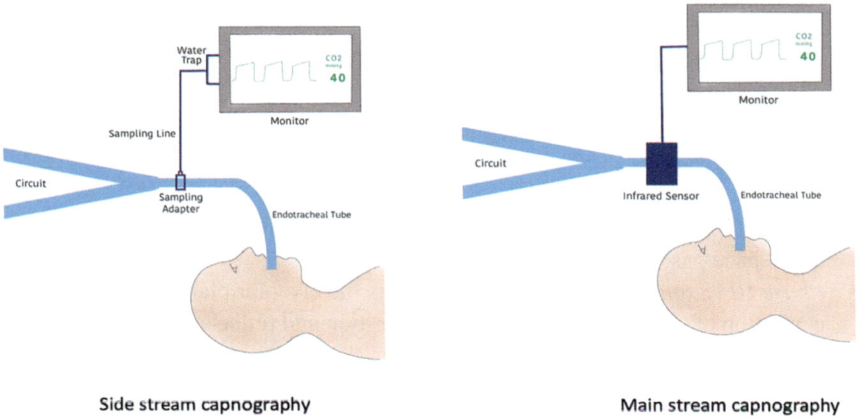

Fig. 9.7 Mainstream and sidestream sampling techniques of capnography. (Courtesy Dr. Shreyash Agrawal)

- *Monitoring perfusion*: $EtCO_2$ levels can indirectly reflect the patient's cardiac output and tissue perfusion. A decrease in $EtCO_2$ value can suggest inadequate tissue perfusion or reduced cardiac output, as less blood is reaching the lungs for gas exchange.
- *Assessing the effects of Trendelenburg position*: This position is widely used in laparoscopic surgeries to improve surgical exposure. This position can affect respiratory mechanics and gas exchange.
- *Detecting air/CO_2 embolism*: The insufflation of CO_2 during laparoscopic surgery can potentially cause embolism. A sudden decrease in $EtCO_2$ levels may indicate its presence as CO_2 emboli may cause obstruction to right ventricular blood flow resulting in reduced perfusion of lungs resulting in right and left ventricular failure, systemic hypotension and cardiovascular collapse.

9.7 Pulse Oximetry

Pulse oximetry is a non-invasive and highly effective method used in operation theatres to continuously monitor the oxygen saturation level in the patient's blood. The pulse oximeter offers real-time and continuous monitoring throughout surgery and helps in early detection of hypoxemia and to take corrective measures to maintain optimal oxygen levels. It helps determine the baseline oxygenation of a patient and monitor the heart rate which is crucial in detecting arrhythmia or other cardiac abnormalities during surgery. Thus, it plays a pivotal role in ensuring patient safety during surgical procedures.

9.7.1 Principle of Measurement (Fig. 9.8)

Pulse oximetry utilises the principle of spectrophotometry. The device emits light from two wavelengths, i.e. red and infrared, through a patient's tissue. Oxygenated and deoxygenated haemoglobin molecules absorb light differently, and the oximeter's photodetector measures the light absorption. The pulse oximeter calculates the ratio of light absorbed at the red (wavelength of 660 nm) and infrared wavelengths (wavelength of 940 nm) to determine the relative amounts of oxygenated and deoxygenated haemoglobin. This ratio is used to calculate the oxygen saturation level as a percentage.

9.7.2 Using a Pulse Oximeter

- Connect the pulse oximeter probe to the patient's finger and make sure that the nail covers the light window.
- The wire of the pulse oximeter and light emitting side should be towards the nail (backside of the hand).
- The multi-parameter monitor will display the patient's oxygen saturation along with heart rate.
- Normal oxygen saturation recording ranges from 97–100%.

9.7.3 Limitations of Pulse Oximetry

- *Haemoglobin variants*: Presence of carboxyhaemoglobin, methaemoglobin and foetal haemoglobin may lead to erroneous values.
- *Motion artefacts*: Frequent movement of the sensor (e.g. shivering) may result in erroneous readings.

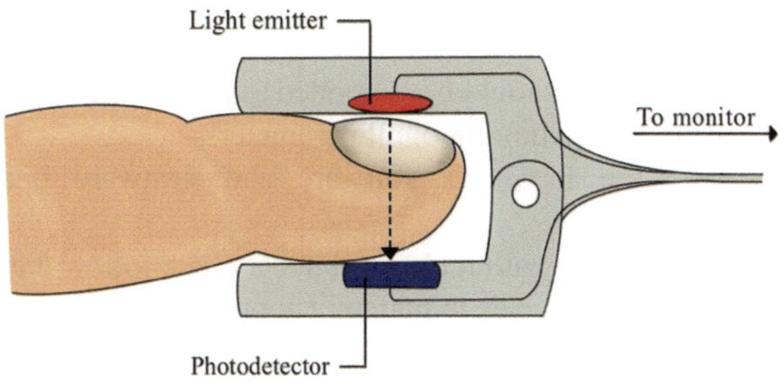

Fig. 9.8 Principle of pulse oximetry. (Courtesy Dr. Shreyash Agrawal)

- Avoid placing the pulse oximetry probe on the same extremity as an NIBP cuff, as it may cause a false alarm.
- *Low perfusion states*: Conditions such as shock and hypothermia can lead to unreliable readings or difficulty in obtaining a signal.
- *Dark skin pigmentation and nail polish*: It may lead to inaccuracy of readings.

9.7.4 Oxygen Saturation and Laparoscopic Surgery

- *Patient selection*: Preoperative assessment and patient selection are crucial. For example, a patient with a pre-existing respiratory condition or compromised lung function may require special attention and adjustments of oxygen flow rate during the procedure to optimise oxygenation.
- *Positioning*: The Trendelenburg position is commonly used during laparoscopic surgery which may lead to reduced lung volumes. The anaesthetist should monitor the patient's oxygen saturation and respiratory parameters closely during changes in position.
- *Positive pressure ventilation (PPV)*: Laparoscopic surgery requires PPV to overcome the increased intra-abdominal pressure during Trendelenburg position. However, excessive PPV may impair venous pressure and reduce cardiac output, potentially affecting oxygen delivery. Thus, balance should be maintained between ventilation pressure by use of positive end expiratory pressure (PEEP) to maintain adequate oxygenation while minimising adverse hemodynamic effects.

9.8 Maintenance

Proper maintenance of a multi-parameter monitor is essential to ensure its reliability, accuracy and longevity. Along with the specific device manufacturing guidelines which should be adhered to, some basic routine maintenance practices are as follows (Table 9.5):

- The monitor surface and display should be cleaned regularly according to the manufacturer's guidelines so as to avoid damage to sensitive equipment.
- Inspect sensors and cables regularly for signs of wear and tear. Any damage to the device component should be replaced promptly to maintain its proper functioning.
- The monitor should be calibrated as per the manufacturer's recommendations for accurate functioning of all parameters.
- Keep the monitor's software and firmware updated to maintain optimal performance.
- For monitors with rechargeable batteries, follow the recommended charging and discharging cycles to maintain appropriate health.

Table 9.5 Troubleshooting in multi-parameter monitor

Problem	Possible reason	Solution
No power or display issues	No power sources Power cable is damaged or has loose connections	Ensure the monitor has a charged battery or is properly plugged into a power source and verify that the power switch or button is turned on Inspect the power cable for any damage or loose connections If the display remains black, try restarting the monitor
Alarm not sounding or false alarm	Alarm may be muted or volume may not be set appropriately Alarm limits may not be configured appropriately for each parameter being monitored False alarms due to patient movement or other conditions	Ensure that the alarm volume is set appropriately and is not muted Verify alarm limits are correctly configured Decrease movement and treat the appropriate problem
Sensor or cable issues	Damaged or worn-out sensor or cable Wrong placement of sensor or incompatible attachments Loose sensor	Replace any damaged parts Ensure correct placement of sensors on the patient and compatibility with the monitor Verify sensor connections are secure
Data transmission or connectivity problems	Inspect the cables and attachments for loose or damaged connections For wireless monitors, check network connection	Ensure proper attachments of cables, or if any attachment damaged, replace them Restart the monitor or the network router if there are connectivity issues
Inaccurate reading	Calibration of monitor not up to date	Recalibrate the modules of the monitor following the manufacturer's guidelines
Software or firmware errors	Outdated software or firmware	Install updates if available
Overheating or ventilation issues	Monitor is covered or obstructed	Place the monitor in a well-ventilated and cool area

- Ensure the monitor is placed on a horizontal surface and kept in a well-ventilated room to prevent overheating.
- When not in use, the monitor should be stored in a cool, safe and dry place. Protect the monitor from extremes of heat, humidity and dust.
- Regular inspection and servicing by the company's service engineer should be performed to identify potential issues and perform any necessary adjustments.
- Ensure that healthcare staff is adequately trained to use the monitor to reduce misuse and damage to device.
- Maintain a detailed record of the monitor's maintenance history, including calibration dates, repairs and any software updates.

9.9 New Innovations/Future Directions

- *Miniaturisation and wearable device*: There is a growing trend towards miniaturising monitoring devices and incorporating them into wearable technologies. This allows continuous monitoring of various parameters like heart rate, blood pressure, oxygen saturation levels and provides real-time data for health tracking.
- *Internet of Things (Iot) integration*: Multi-parameter monitoring devices could be integrated into IoT networks, thus enabling seamless connectivity between devices and systems, thereby allowing data transmission, analysis and early detection of health issues.
- *Artificial intelligence (AI) and predictive analytics*: AI plays a crucial role in processing a vast amount of data collected from multiple monitoring devices. AI-powered analytics can help detect patterns, identify anomalies and predict potential health risks.
- *Non-invasive techniques*: Research is ongoing to develop non-invasive methods for monitoring multiple parameters so as to enhance convenience and reduce patient discomfort. For instance, advancements in optical and infrared technologies for non-invasive blood glucose monitoring are promising.
- *Integration of biomarkers*: Future technologies may integrate biomarkers from various body fluids like saliva, sweat, tears to provide a more comprehensive health monitoring.
- *Long-term health data tracking*: By incorporating multi-parameter monitoring into everyday wearable devices, long-term health data tracking becomes more accessible. This can help individuals and healthcare professionals make better-informed decisions about management plans of the patient.

9.10 Conclusion

Multipara monitors play a crucial role in modern healthcare by continuously tracking vital parameters such as heart rate, blood pressure, oxygen saturation and respiratory rate. These devices enhance patient safety, allowing healthcare professionals to detect abnormalities early and respond promptly. Advancements in technology have led to the development of more accurate, user-friendly and interconnected monitors, improving efficiency in patient care. As hospitals continue to adopt smart and AI-integrated monitoring systems, the future of patient monitoring promises even greater precision and proactive healthcare management.

References

1. Mindray Medical International. BeneVision CMS central monitoring system: operator's manual. Shenzhen: Mindray; 2021. Available from: https://www.mindray.com/content/dam/xpace/en_us/service-and-support/training-and-education/resource%2D%2Dlibrary/technical%2D%2Ddocuments/operators-manuals-1/centralized/H-046-007960-00-BeneVision-CMS-Ops-ManualFDA-4.0.pdf
2. Cooper DS, Pike R. ECG essentials: electrode placement, lead systems, and common pitfalls. J Electrocardiol. 2014;47(6):914–8.

Ergonomics in Minimal Access Surgery 10

Kalpesh Jani

10.1 Introduction

Work-related musculoskeletal disorders (WMSDs) are defined as 'musculoskeletal disorders (injuries or disorders of the muscles, nerves, tendons, joints, cartilage, and spinal discs) in which the work environment and performance of work contribute significantly to the condition; and/or the condition is made worse or persists longer due to work conditions' [1]. In industries, WMSDs are of special significance as they result in absenteeism and loss of workforce, which in turn impacts productivity and profit, ultimately causing a significant financial loss to the industry as a whole. WMSDs result in losses of over $20 billion annually in the USA. Moreover, changing the working environment to suit the workers has been demonstrated to reduce wastage of raw materials, allow optimum use of machinery and equipment, result in greater efficiency, decrease cost, result in better public perception of the industry implementing such measures and enhance employee satisfaction [2, 3]. As a result, major research is undertaken as to how to improve the working environment, in order to primarily reduce WMSDs and increase productivity. Thus, the science of ergonomics came into being.

The etymology of 'ergonomics' can be traced to two Greek words—*ergon* meaning labour or work and *nomia* meaning arrangement. The International Ergonomics Association Council defines it as 'the scientific discipline concerned with the understanding of interactions among humans and other elements of a system, and the profession that applies theory, principles, data and methods to design to optimize human well-being and overall system performance' [4]. In simpler terms, it can be described as designing of the working environment to fit the worker, rather than forcing the worker to fit the working environment [5]. While the interaction of

K. Jani (✉)
Department of GI, Laparoscopic and Bariatric Surgery, Sunshine Global Hospital, Vadodara, Gujarat, India

J. S. Ahluwalia (ed.), *User Manual for Minimally Invasive Surgical Equipment*,
https://doi.org/10.1007/978-981-95-9019-3_10

human labourers and their working environment has been a source of interest since ancient Greek times, it was only after the Second World War, that ergonomics became a formal field of study when the Human Factors Society was established in the USA in 1957. Their stated goal is 'to reduce human error, increase productivity, and enhance safety and comfort with a specific focus on the interaction between a human and the thing of interest', with the primary aim 'to promote the discovery and exchange of knowledge concerning the characteristics of human beings that are applicable to the design of systems and devices of all kinds' [6].

As is true for workers everywhere, surgeons are also susceptible to WMSD. However, since surgeons rarely report these injuries to their parent institutions, do not claim compensation from their employers for the same, and perhaps are not even aware of how they can be avoided, for a long time, not much data was available except empirical reports. We all know a surgical colleague who has an injured shoulder, or early onset cervical spondylitis, or chronic back pain, or knee pain. But we assume that this is a hazard of our profession, afflicting the unlucky few. In fact, the statistics are staggeringly frightening: the occurrence of WMSD ranges from 66% to 94% for open surgery [7–13], and is even higher for laparoscopic surgery (73–100%) [14–19].

Even robotic surgery, touted for being tailored for surgeon's comfort, is not truly immune from WMSD, with occurrences of the latter in the range of 23–80% for robotic-assisted laparoscopic surgery [20–25].

As in other industries, WMSDs in the field of minimal access surgery also has far reaching consequences. Once the operating surgeons realize that it is the poor ergonomics that is causing physical problems, they attempt to improve the ergonomic situation by either changing their position, altering the position of the monitor and resorting to exercises. To alleviate the pain caused by the WMSDs, surgeons have resorted to various forms of therapies apart from standard medical treatment, ranging from physical therapy, massage, intra-articular injections and services of a chiropractor. Some have shifted to robotic surgery. In severe cases, they may need surgery themselves to tackle their problem. When all else fails, they have no resort but to either decrease their work load or give up operating altogether [17].

10.2 Ergonomic Problems Associated with Laparoscopic Surgery

Before we discuss the ergonomics associated with laparoscopic surgery, it is necessary to define some terms.

The 'Elevation Angle' is the angle formed by drawing a straight line passing perpendicular to the surface of the lens tip of the laparoscope ('the visual axis or the optical axis') to the target organ and a horizontal line over the floor of the abdomen (Fig. 10.1). For a zero-degree laparoscope, the physical axis of the scope and the optical axis will coincide. However, for angled laparoscopes, the physical axis and the optical axis will diverge depending on the angulation of the scope (Fig. 10.2). This has clinical importance because to obtain the same elevation angle, angled

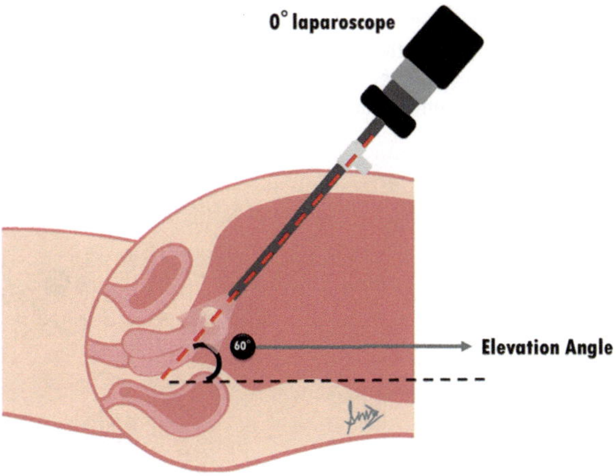

Fig. 10.1 The optical axis and the physical axis of a zero-degree laparoscope coincide. The elevation angle is the angle formed by the extension of the optical axis of the laparoscope to the target organ with the floor of the abdomen

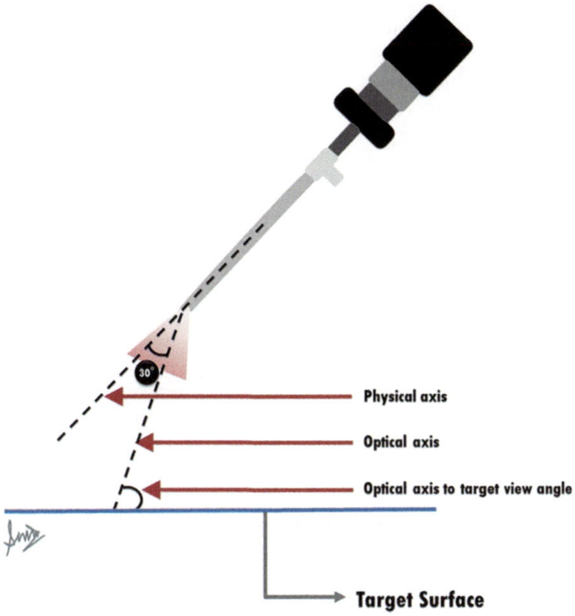

Fig. 10.2 With angled laparoscopes, the optical axis of the scope diverges from its physical axis depending on the angulation of the lens

laparoscopes have to be placed further away from the target organ than zero-degree laparoscopes and vice versa.

The 'Manipulation Angle' is the angle formed between two lines drawn from each of the working trocars such that they intersect at the target organ (Fig. 10.3).

The 'Azimuth Angle' is the angle formed between the line drawn from one working trocar and the visual axis, as they intersect at the target organ (Fig. 10.4).

Certain factors are unique to laparoscopic surgery, making it more difficult to adapt to than open conventional surgery:

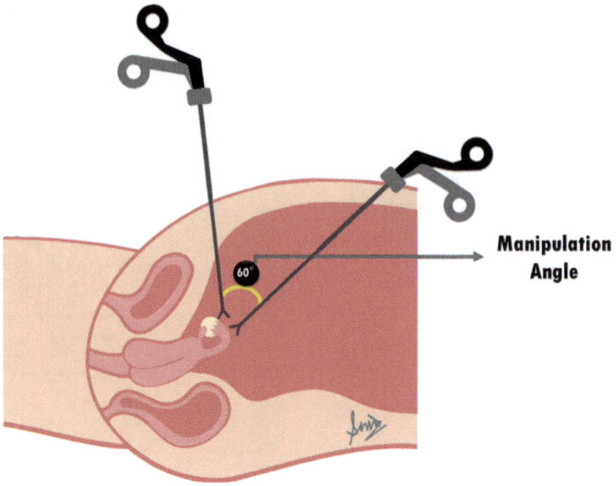

Fig. 10.3 The manipulation angle is the angle formed between the two working instruments at the target organ

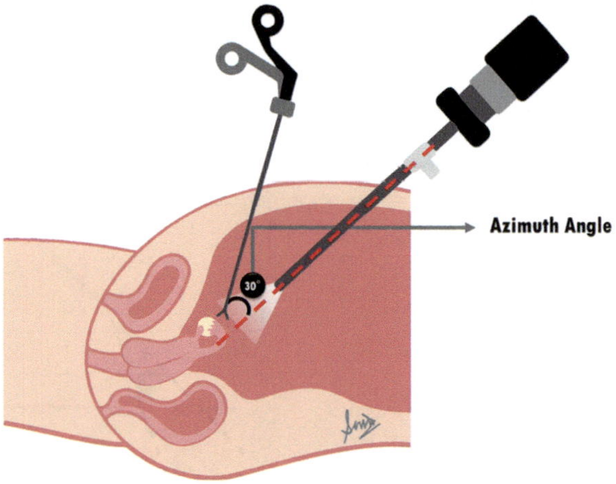

Fig. 10.4 The Azimuth angle is the angle formed between the optical axis and one working instrument at the target organ

1. In conventional surgery, the surgeon is looking directly at his/her hands which are operating on the target organ. In other words, the visual axis and the motor axis are congruous. However, in laparoscopic surgery, the surgeon is looking at a monitor placed in a different direction from the direction in which his working instruments are operating, i.e. there is de-coupling of the visual-motor axes.
2. There is a loss of tactile feedback to a large extent in laparoscopic surgery.
3. Since most laparoscopic surgeons use a two-dimensional camera, there is a loss of depth perception.
4. The laparoscopic surgeon sees a limited portion of the operating field, which narrows even further as the camera surgeon zooms in. Thus, there is a restricted field of vision.
5. The elevation, manipulation and azimuth angles may not be ideal and cannot be corrected as once the ports are placed, they become fixed. In open surgery, the surgeon simply changes his/her body position to obtain the optimum angles.

6. The 'fulcrum effect': The laparoscopic surgeon works through fixed ports which leads to a fulcrum effect on the instruments at their point of entry into the abdomen. This, in turn, results in two things:
   (i) If more of the instrument is inside than outside, minor side-to-side manipulation of the instrument handle outside will lead to magnified movements of the instrument tip inside. The converse also holds true, in that, if more of the instrument is outside than inside, to obtain the desired position of the instrument tip inside, the outside handle would need to be swung in a much larger arc, perhaps, clashing with other instruments, scope or light cable.
   (ii) Due to the fulcrum effect, there will be a paradoxical movement of the instrument tip vis-à-vis the instrument handle. For example, to move the tip to the left, the handle outside will have to be pushed to the right, and to move the tip upwards, the handle will have to be moved downwards.
7. Laparoscopic instruments are long and thin. As such they are difficult to handle as compared to their open counterparts. Involuntary tremors of the surgeon's hands are greatly magnified due to the length of the instruments.
8. The instrument and handle design have not changed practically from the inception of therapeutic laparoscopy in the late 1980s and early 1990s.
9. Loss of degrees of freedom: In open conventional surgery, the surgeon uses several body joints, right from the foot, ankle, knee, hip, vertebral column and pelvic rotation, vertebral flexion-extension and sideward bending, scapulo-thoracic joint, shoulder, elbow, wrist and finger joints to obtain the correct ergonomic position, enabling a total of more than 36 degrees of freedom. In contrast, a laparoscopic surgeon is reduced to 4 degrees of freedom through the use of rigid instruments passing through fixed ports of entry.

10.3 Mechanisms of Injury in Laparoscopic Surgery

In 1989, Kroemer published a monograph, identifying the mechanisms of WMSDs, which he termed as cumulative trauma disorders, their progression and their prevention [26]. He postulated the following mechanisms or their combinations as the source of injury, of which four are applicable to laparoscopic surgery:

A. Repetitive movements
B. Prolonged or repetitive exertion
C. Body parts held in awkward positions
D. Unmoving posture for a prolonged period of time

He described three stages of progression of the WMSD:

Stage 1: Symptoms of the injury appear during working, but relief is immediate on cessation.
Stage 2: Symptoms persist for at least 24 h beyond the activity.

Stage 3: Symptoms are persistent and affect the surgeon's other activities as well as sleep.

Various injuries have been described in surgeons in general, caused by various repetitive motions, prolonged positions or instrument design: [27–36]

1. Trigger finger—caused by flexion of the finger, especially distal phalanx alone, as seen during working the suction-irrigation cannula of a particular design.
2. 'Laparoscopist's thumb'—paraesthesia of part of the thumb surface due to digital nerve compression by the ring of the laparoscopic instrument handle.
3. Carpal tunnel syndrome—due to rapid flexion, extension and rotation of wrist.
4. Epicondylitis—pronation in extension position of wrist, as practised during intracorporeal suturing.
5. Pronator Teres syndrome, wrist tendinitis—as a result of forceful wrist flexion and extension.
6. Ulnar nerve entrapment—prolonged flexion/extension of wrist with pressure of instrument handle on the hypothenar aspect, as seen during retraction of viscera.
7. Shoulder tendinitis, rotator cuff injury, recurrent trapezitis—due to prolonged abduction of the shoulder.
8. Cervical spine disorders, neck tension syndrome—due to rotation and extension of the cervical spine.
9. Pectoral tendinitis—owing to prolonged strain, as in retracting viscera.
10. Thoracic outlet syndrome—shoulder flexion and hyperextension of the arm.
11. Low back pain—due to continuous standing with the trunk rotated or bent over.
12. Varicose veins—prolonged standing in a static posture also makes the surgeon prone to the development of varicosity of the lower limb veins.

All this leads to increased need of analgesic consumption among surgeons, resort to various alternative medicinal procedures to relieve chronic pain, physical and rehabilitative therapy. The surgeon also may need to take repeated sick leaves or, in the worst-case scenario, resign from his or her post [37–40].

In addition, surgeons are also exposed to various other hazards in their work environment like exposure to cautery smoke, ethylene oxide gas, formic acid fumes, inhalational agents, needle-prick and scalpel injuries, blood-transmitted viruses, cautery burns due to glove punctures and many more, but they do not fall within the purview of this chapter.

10.4 Tools to Study Ergonomics in Surgery

Various subjective and objective tools have been developed and used to study the ergonomics associated with surgery in general. The Body Part Discomfort (BPD) Scale is one of the most frequently used tools employed in several studies of ergonomics in surgery. It documents discomfort in 27 different body areas [41].

Another such tool is the NASA-Task Load Index, originally developed for the aircraft industry, but subsequently modified for the surgical fields. The surgical iteration of the same is also known as the Surgery Task Load Index [42, 43]. Apart from this, some have used the commonly used Likert scale (visual analogue scale), mental stress and local discomfort questionnaire, Dundee Stress State Questionnaire, Cornell Musculoskeletal Questionnaire, Dutch Musculoskeletal Questionnaire or an unvalidated technique of asking the participants to mark out the areas of discomfort on human diagrams [42, 44–53]. Yet another technique employs videos of surgeons taken while operating and subsequent analysis using tools like the Rapid Upper Limb Assessment (RULA) [54], Strain Index [55] or the Rapid Entire Body Assessment (REBA) [56].

However, these subjective techniques suffer from some common drawbacks, namely, recall bias, inter- and intra-observer variability and lack of correlation between the subject's perception of injury and actual injury at the tissue level. To overcome these subjective shortcomings, objective tools have been developed and used in various studies of surgical ergonomics. These include tracking joint markers based on reflective markers applied externally [50, 57, 58], measuring action potentials of various muscle groups using electromyography (EMG) [59]. Physiologic stress has been also measured during various steps of surgery using techniques like goniometry [49, 60], forceplate study [57, 61], workload measurements [45, 48, 52], computer software to measure stress during posture [62, 63] and accelerometry [45, 64].

These objective measures, while being free from inter- and intra-observer variability and more accurate, come with their own special problems. Tools like EMG and others, which require sensors applied to surgeon's body and hands, are not possible during actual surgery due to the issue of sterility, and hence, such studies are usually carried out on simulators and in the animal lab. Those that rely on capturing signals reflected from the surgeon's body parts, whether ultrasonic or infra-red, are hampered by the interference of other equipment and instruments inside the operation theatre. However, a new device that helps to measure inertia, through wearable sensors that can be covered by sterile surgical gowns, holds promise for future research in actual real-time surgery in this field [25].

10.5 Technical Aspects of Laparoscopic Ergonomics

In conventional open surgery (in fact, in any human activity), the surgeon is trained to use both his hands (operating appliances) which are placed on either side of the eyes (visual axis). This arrangement of the two operating appliances entering the visual field on either side of the visual axis is called 'triangulation'. In laparoscopic surgery, triangulation is obtained when the camera port is placed in the centre of two working ports which are placed more or less equidistant from it on either side. Since this mimics the arrangement of the operating appliances and visual axis of conventional open surgery, the hand-eye co-ordination of the surgeon is optimum with this arrangement. However, occasionally, it may be required to place both the working instruments through ports lying on the same one side of the camera port. This arrangement is called 'sectorization' [65].

10.6 Ergonomics of Laparoscopic Surgery and Their Effects on the Surgeon [42, 43, 63, 66–77]

1. Most laparoscopic surgeries take longer to perform than their open counterparts. Prolonged surgical stress leads to mental exhaustion, impaired judgement, irritability, which Cuschieri termed as surgical fatigue syndrome. He observed that such a state was likely to occur after more than 4 h of continuous laparoscopic performance.
2. By its very nature, laparoscopic surgery involves the surgeon having to continuously stare at a monitor, inducing greater eye strain as compared to open surgery.
3. The 'laparoscopist's thumb' or 'laparoscopic surgeon's thumb' is a well-described entity, entailing paraesthesia and sensation of pressure around the base of the thumb as a result of digital nerve compression caused by continuous and prolonged pressure of the ring of the instrument handle.
4. Poor instrument design can lead to unnatural stress on different parts of the upper limb of the surgeon, leading to WMSDs, especially due to prolonged abduction of the shoulder joints, flexion of the wrist joint and excessive ulnar deviation of the hand. Matern and colleagues studied normal functional anatomy of the human hand and the various grip and areas of the human hand involved in laparoscopic surgery. Based on this, they compared various designs of laparoscopic instrument handles and made several recommendations [78, 79].
5. The laparoscopic instruments have another inherent design flaw which is unavoidable—they enter the patient's body through fixed ports creating a fulcrum effect. Moreover, they are very long and a combination of these two factors results in the surgeon have to move the hands through fairly large arcs outside to enable smaller movements of the instrument tips inside the body at some stages of a laparoscopic surgery.
6. Most of the energy sources are activated and controlled using foot switches—monopolar coagulation electrosurgery, monopolar cutting electrosurgery, bipolar electrosurgery, vessel-sealing current, ultrasonic shears, etc. This leads to a large number of foot pedals surrounding the surgeon's feet. The surgeon has to place his entire weight on one foot while reaching around for different energy source pedals with the other foot.
7. Laparoscopic surgery requires the surgeon remain in a static position, with head and neck fixed in space, for a prolonged period of time, putting excessive stress on the neck, back and spine, which will be exacerbated by an ill-positioned monitor.

It is no wonder that the prevalence of WMSDs amongst laparoscopic surgeons has been reported in the range of 73–100%. The most vulnerable regions of the surgeon are the wrist, elbow, shoulder, neck and back. Several risk factors are associated with a higher prevalence of WMSDs. Younger surgeons were more prone to WMSDs as compared to older surgeons [15, 17]. While this finding seems counter-intuitive at first glance, the explanation may lie in the fact that younger surgeons take longer to perform the same operations than their more experienced older colleagues. Moreover, younger surgeons may also not be placing their equipment or holding their instruments in the most ergonomic way. This is also supported by the fact that as the surgeons become more experienced, the incidence of WMSDs seems to reduce [17]. However, another study reported that the incidence of chronic WMSDs was directly related to the number of years the surgeon had been performing laparoscopic surgeries [80].

Short stature is also associated with a higher incidence of WMSDs. This is probably due to the fact that short-statured surgeons would need to abduct their shoulders more to access the instruments placed through different ports. This is probably the reason why these injuries are more common with smaller glove sizes. However, female gender of the surgeon renders them more susceptible to injuries, irrespective of their height, age and glove size. Higher BMI of patients had a worse impact on the surgeons with a higher occurrence of WMSDs.

Increasing case loads are associated with a higher frequency of WMSDs [16, 80]. The same study also reported a higher occurrence of injuries in the surgeon's dominant hand. Female surgeons reported more problems in the upper extremity while males reported an increased incidence in their lower extremity.

10.7 Ergonomics of Robotic Surgery

Robotic surgery is the new 'kid on the block', touted to be designed to improve ergonomics and surgeon comfort. While the instrument ergonomics are undeniably greatly improved, yet for the surgeons, it is not totally exempt from the risk of WMSDs, with various studies reporting a prevalence ranging from 8–80% [20–25, 81].

Overall, surgeons report less pain in robotic surgery as compared to laparoscopic surgery, especially in the regions of foot, ankle, knee, hip, back, shoulder, elbow and wrist. However, certain other areas may be at a higher risk including fingers, hand, neck and may be more prone to eyestrain. Overall, robotic surgery does seem to place less strain on all muscle groups as compared to laparoscopic surgery, except for the trapezius muscle. This may lead to overall less musculoskeletal injuries in robotic surgeons vis-à-vis laparoscopic surgeons [82]. Surgeons reported less pain and discomfort associated with robotic surgery as compared to both laparoscopic and open surgery; however, eye strain, neck pain and thumb pain were more as compared to laparoscopic surgery. Though less, physical discomfort is still a significant issue in robotic surgery, and there is a major scope for improvement in the ergonomic aspects of robotic console designing [81].

10.8 Recommendations to Improve the Ergonomics of Laparoscopic Surgery

A large amount of interest has been generated in the field of ergonomics of minimal access surgery and the measures that can be undertaken to improve them. These measures can be broadly classified into three types:

(i) Personal protective equipment—These are the instruments, equipment, or tools that the surgical team members may employ to improve the ergonomic outcomes, e.g. use of support frame to rest the body during surgery.
(ii) Engineering controls—These are the alterations that can be done in the theatre setup and instrument arrangements, e.g. changing the height of the OT table, or using equipment mounted on pendants rather than on a trolley.
(iii) Administrative controls—These are the behavioural changes brought about by interventions in the theatre staff and surgical and anaesthetic team members, e.g. instituting stretching exercises at pre-determined intervals among the surgical team members during prolonged procedures [83].

Majority of the surgeons in practice have not received any formal training in ergonomics nor do they recollect being taught the proper ergonomics during their training in minimal access surgery [84].

The various measures can be summarized as under: [45, 65, 76, 85–102]

1. *Monitor*: Various sources agree that the best position is for the monitor to be below the eye level of the surgeon. However, there is no concurrence as to how much below it should be, with a recommended range of 10° to 45°. While keeping it lower improves the concurrence of the visual-motor axis and hence is believed to improve the hand-eye co-ordination, flexion of the neck beyond 30° places an excessive stress on the neck muscles as well as the cervical spine, and so, most authorities recommend placing the monitor such that the surgeon's neck is flexed between 10–30°. Also, axial rotation of the neck is to be avoided, keeping it less than 15°. Its distance from the surgeon is dependent on its size. Placing a large monitor too close to the surgeon causes excessive strain on the extraocular muscles of the eyes as they try to converge on the view and leads to over-accommodation of the eyeballs. Too far off and the surgeon would be straining and staring to make out the details which would be lost in delineation.
2. *Table height*: The table height should be adjusted as per the ergonomic comfort of the tallest surgical team member (operating surgeon, camera surgeon, assistant surgeon). The remaining members should stand on appropriately tall broad stools to match the tallest surgeon's height. Objectively, the height of the table should be such that the ventral surface of the patient lying on it is at a height equal to 0.7 or 0.8 times the distance of the surgeons' elbow from the ground.

3. *Support*: Static position of the laparoscopic surgeon places a lot of stress on the trunk muscles. This can be avoided by using a support to distribute the weight. Especially ergonomically designed seats for this purpose have also been developed. Intraoperatively, it is recommended to take a break during prolonged surgeries and perform periodic stretching, including squats.
4. *Foot pedals*: The foot pedals should be placed such that while operating them, the surgeon does not shift his/her entire weight to the other foot. Also, dorsal flexion of the foot greater than 5° should be avoided when operating the pedals. Some authorities even recommend placing the foot pedal in front of the patient, in line with the instrument, target organ and monitor.
5. *Arm rests*: To all the surgical team access and enable utilization of the entire side of the table, the patient's arms should be tucked as far as possible.
6. *Manipulation, azimuth and elevation angles*: The ports should be planned such that the manipulation angle is between the working instruments is between 45–75°, with equal azimuth angles for both the working instruments. The elevation angle should also be matched accordingly to the manipulation angle.

   Ideal manipulation angle would be 60° with equal azimuth angles of 30° on each side in a triangulation configuration.
7. *Fulcrum*: The ports should be planned and placed in such a way that while operating half of the operating instrument is intra-corporeal and half is extra-corporeal, i.e. the fulcrum lies at the centre of the instrument.
8. *OT flooring*: Anti-skid flooring should be installed so that the surgeon does not slip.
9. *Posture*: The surgeon should stand erect, comfortably, with shoulders and spine in neutral position. A 'head forward' position with shoulders rolled back should be avoided as this puts excessive stress on the cervical spine. Increasing bend of the head over a prolonged period should be avoided as it can cause tension and pain in the neck muscles.
10. *Lower limbs*:

    (a) For prolonged surgery, the surgeon should consider putting on elastic support for the lower limb as a prophylaxis towards development of lower limb varicose veins.
    (b) The surgeon should stand with the feet slightly apart and with equal distribution of body weight on both the feet.
    (c) Locking of the knees should be avoided.

11. *Upper limbs*:

    (a) The shoulders should be relaxed and adducted. Any abduction more than 30° has to be avoided by standing on a broad stool.
    (b) The upper arms should be near perpendicular to the floor. The neutral position of the arm would be with a minimal abduction and internal rotation. This position puts the least strain on the muscles involved.

(c) The height of the table is adjusted such that the angle of the elbow is in a range of 90–120°. The most ergonomic position of the arm would be if the elbow is at 90° with the lower arm parallel to the ground and held in a neutral position mid-way between complete pronation and complete supination.
(d) Wrist movements should remain in a range encompassing a maximum of 25° of ulnar deviation to 15° of radial deviation and 20° of flexion to 40° of extension.
(e) Instrument design should be such that excessive force (>15 N) is not required to close the instrument's tips.

12. *Intra-operative*: During prolonged surgeries, the surgeon should take short intermittent breaks during surgery to either rest or stretch the different body joints, especially the neck (flexion-extension and side-to-side rotation), upper limbs (hand raise), trunk (side-to-side twist, forward and backward bending) and lower limbs (squats, sitting knee and hip flexion). These so-called 'micro-breaks' may reduce errors, improving workflow and communications within a team performing major non-routine surgery.

    There is also a lack of consensus on what constitutes a micro-break, with opinions varying from 20 s every 20 min, 1–2 min break every 20–40 min or 5 min break every 25 min.
13. *Laparoscopic instruments*: The design of laparoscopic instrument handles is archaic and usually consists of ringed offset handles. Continuous pressure of the ring of the handles on the fingers leads to paraesthesia and related injuries. The surgeon may consider using the palm of his/her hand and the shaft of the thumb without inserting the latter into the ring to open/close the handle. Multifunctionality of instruments should be avoided with each instrument being designed to perform a specific task. Van Veelen (2004) had described in detail the ergonomically optimal design of laparoscopic surgical instruments. Similarly, Matern (2001) had described 22 criteria for designing the handles of laparoscopic instruments.
14. *Assistant surgeons*: Assistant surgeons should consider rotating places so that they would not be required to stand static in the same awkward posture for prolonged periods.
15. *Training in ergonomics*: 59–99% of minimally invasive surgeons in a meta-analysis reported that they had no formal ergonomic training during their residency nor could they remember any ergonomic recommendations from their training fellowships. Franasiak et al found that a bespoke ergonomic training program, i.e. training a surgical team in various ergonomic measures deemed most beneficial to their practice and the physical characteristics of the team members did benefit from them. Thus, teaching ergonomic principles and their applications in work situations is definitely a need of the hour. This has been confirmed in a study by Park et al where they found that among surgeons who are aware of various ergonomic recommendations, more than 93% applied them in their own practice [16].

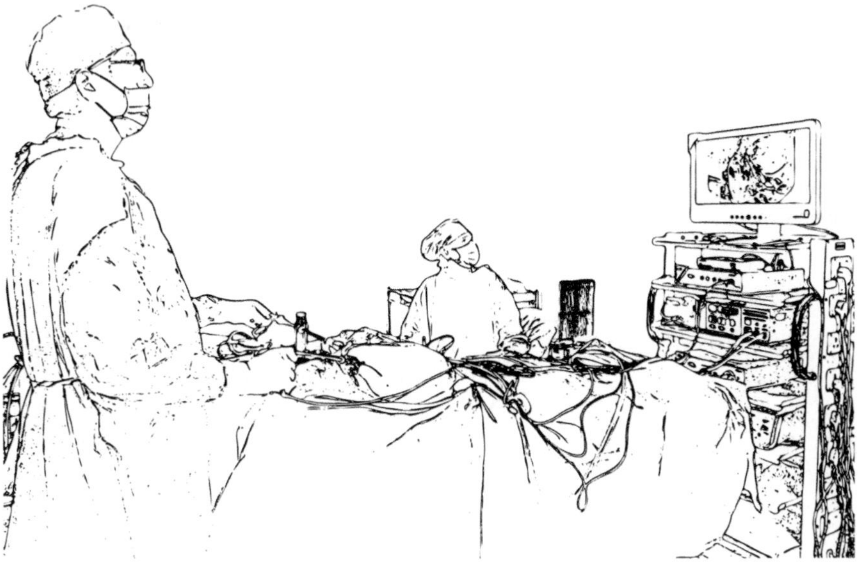

Fig. 10.5 This photograph encapsulates an ergonomically correct posture of the surgeon. The surgeon is standing erect with the head in a neutral position, shoulders relaxed, arms slightly abducted at the shoulders and body weight evenly distributed on both feet. The monitor is placed about 10° below the eye level. The operation table has been elevated to allow the elbows to maintain an angle of 90–100° flexion

The posture of the surgeon, placement of the monitor, height of the table and use of foot pedals have been depicted in Figs. 10.5 and 10.6. During prolonged surgeries, taking short breaks (even as small as 20-s breaks every 20 min) has been found to reduce the stress among surgeons, decrease errors and discomfort [94, 100].

Specialized exercise and posture training regimes like the Alexander Technique have also been shown to improve the ergonomics of minimal access surgery by improving posture [103]. Winters and colleagues have described an exercise regimen for surgeons to improve postural ergonomics. These involve workouts for the head and neck muscles, shoulder girdle, thoracic and lumbar spine, pelvic girdle and lower limbs [104].

10.9 Conclusion

Work-related musculoskeletal disorders are a common occurrence among laparoscopic surgeons, though they may be under-reported. These are primarily due to the poor ergonomics associated with laparoscopic surgery due to various factors that have been described above. Understanding these factors and adopting measures to counter them to improve the ergonomics of a laparoscopic surgeon enables him/her to reduce injuries, improve technique and enable pursuance of a career as a minimal access surgeon for a longer duration.

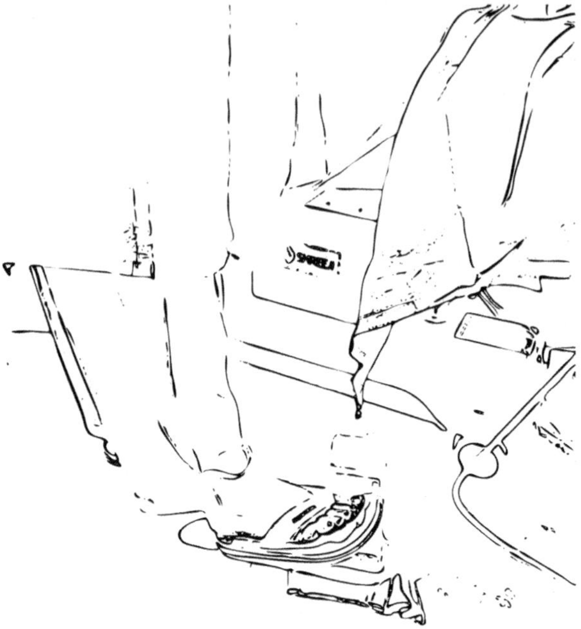

Fig. 10.6 When using foot pedals, the surgeon should distribute weight evenly between non-dominant foot and dominant heel. The arch of the dominant foot is placed over the pedal to be compressed

Acknowledgements Dr. Samir Contractor has created the figures depicting the various ergonomic angles (Figs. 10.1, 10.2, 10.3 and 10.4)

References

1. Bernard BP, editor. U.S. Department of Health and Human Services, Centers for Disease control and Prevention, National Institute of Occupational Safety and Health. Musculoskeletal disorders and workplace factors: a critical review of epidemiologic evidence for work-related musculoskeletal disorders of the neck, upper extremity, and lower back. 1997. DHHS (NIOSH) Publication No. 97-141. Available from: https://www.cdc.gov/niosh/docs/97-141/
2. Hendrick HW. Determining the cost-benefits of ergonomics projects and factors that lead to their success. Appl Ergon. 2003;34(5):419–27.
3. Beevis D. Ergonomics – costs and benefits revisited. Appl Ergon. 2003;34(5):491–6.
4. Catanzarite T, Tan-Kim J, Whitcomb EL, Menefee S. Ergonomics in surgery: a review. Female Pelvic Med Reconstr Surg. 2018;24(1):1–12. https://doi.org/10.1097/SPV.0000000000000456. PMID: 28914699.
5. Stylopoulos N, Rattner D. Robotics and ergonomics. Surg Clin North Am. 2003;83(6):1321–37.
6. https://www.hfes.org/About-HFES/What-is-Human-Factors-and-Ergonomics. Accessed on 31.1.23.
7. Babar-Craig H, Banfield G, Knight J. Prevalence of back and neck pain amongst ENT consultants: national survey. J Laryngol Otol. 2003;117(12):979–82.
8. Matern U, Koneczny S. Safety, hazards and ergonomics in the operating room. Surg Endosc. 2007;21(11):1965–9.
9. Szeto GP, Ho P, Ting AC, et al. Work-related musculoskeletal symptoms in surgeons. J Occup Rehabil. 2009;19(2):175–84.

10. Soueid A, Oudit D, Thiagarajah S, et al. The pain of surgery: pain experienced by surgeons while operating. Int J Surg. 2010;8(2):118–20.
11. Capone AC, Parikh PM, Gatti ME, et al. Occupational injury in plastic surgeons. Plast Reconstr Surg. 2010;125(5):1555–61.
12. Auerbach JD, Weidner ZD, Milby AH, et al. Musculoskeletal disorders among spine surgeons: results of a survey of the Scoliosis Research Society membership. Spine. 2011;36(26):E1715–21.
13. Sivak-Callcott JA, Diaz SR, Ducatman AM, et al. A survey study of occupational pain and injury in phthalmic plastic surgeons. Ophthal Plast Reconstr Surg. 2011;27(1):28–32.
14. Wauben LS, Van Veelen MA, Gossot D, et al. Application of ergonomic guidelines during minimally invasive surgery: a questionnaire survey of 284 surgeons. Surg Endosc. 2006;20(8):1268–74.
15. Sari V, Nieboer TE, Vierhout ME, et al. The operation room as a hostile environment for surgeons: physical complaints during and after laparoscopy. Minim Invasive Ther Allied Technol. 2010;19(2):105–9.
16. Park A, Lee G, Seagull FJ, et al. Patients benefit while surgeons suffer: an impending epidemic. J Am Coll Surg. 2010;210(3):306–13.
17. Franasiak J, Ko EM, Kidd J, et al. Physical strain and urgent need for ergonomic training among gynecologic oncologists who perform minimally invasive surgery. Gynecol Oncol. 2012;126(3):437–42.
18. Miller K, Benden M, Pickens A, et al. Ergonomics principles associated with laparoscopic surgeon injury/illness. Hum Factors. 2012;54(6):1087–92.
19. Esposito C, El Ghoneimi A, Yamataka A, et al. Work-related upper limb musculoskeletal disorders in paediatric laparoscopic surgery. A multicenter survey. J Pediatr Surg. 2013;48(8):1750–6.
20. Bagrodia A, Raman JD. Ergonomics considerations of radical prostatectomy: physician perspective of open, laparoscopic, and robot-assisted techniques. J Endourol. 2009;23(4):627–33.
21. Lee J, Kang SW, Jung JJ, et al. Multicenter study of robotic thyroidectomy: short-term postoperative outcomes and surgeon ergonomic considerations. Ann Surg Oncol. 2011;18(9):2538–47.
22. Santos-Carreras L, Hagen M, Gassert R, et al. Survey on surgical nstrument handle design: ergonomics and acceptance. Surg Innov. 2012;19(1):50–9.
23. Plerhoples TA, Hernandez-Boussard T, Wren SM. The aching surgeon: a survey of physical discomfort and symptoms following open, laparoscopic, and robotic surgery. J Robot Surg. 2012;6(1):65–72.
24. Franasiak J, Craven R, Mosaly P, et al. Feasibility and acceptance of a robotic surgery ergonomic training program. JSLS. 2014;18(4).
25. Yu D, Dural C, Morrow MM, et al. Intraoperative workload in robotic surgery assessed by wearable motion tracking sensors and questionnaires. Surg Endosc. 2016;31(2):1–10.
26. Kroemer KH. Cumulative trauma disorders: their recognition and ergonomics measures to avoid them. Appl Ergon. 1989;20(4):274–80.
27. Williams B. Some surgeons and their hand injuries. Practitioner. 1974;23:717.
28. Campbell-Semple J. Tenosynovitis, repetitive strain injury, cumulative trauma disorder and overuse syndrome et cetera. J Bone Joint Surg [Am]. 1991;73-A:536–8.
29. Campbell CS. Gamekeeper's thumb. J Bone Joint Surg [Br]. 1955;
30. Westreich M. Breast augmentor's arm. JAMA. 1978;239:401. (Letter)
31. Belsole RJ, Greeley JM. Surgeon's acute carpal tunnel syndrome: an occupational hazard? J Fla Med Assoc. 1988;75(6):369–70. PMID: 3397708.
32. Kano N, Yamakawa T, Ishikawa Y, Miyajima N, Ohtaki S, Kasugai H. Prevention of laparoscopic surgeon's thumb. Surg Endosc. 1995;9(6):738–9. https://doi.org/10.1007/BF00187955. PMID: 7482178.
33. Majeed AW, Jacob G, Reed MW, Johnson AG. Laparoscopist's thumb: an occupational hazard. Arch Surg. 1993;128(3):357. https://doi.org/10.1001/archsurg.1993.01420150117022. PMID: 8442697.

34. Sackier JM, Berci G. A laparoscopic hazard for the surgeon. Br J Surg. 1992;79(7):713. https://doi.org/10.1002/bjs.1800790751. PMID: 1386552.
35. Norheim EP, Black MH, Ngor EW, Shi JM, Safran MR, Navarro RA. Cervical spine disease in surgeons performing arthroscopy or laparoscopy. Arch Environ Occup Health. 2019;74(4):206–14. https://doi.org/10.1080/19338244.2017.1392277. Epub 2017 Nov 7. PMID: 29035681.
36. Kumar S. Trunk rotation: ergonomic and evolutionary perspective. Theor Issues Ergon Sci. 2002;3(3):235–56.
37. Esposito C, El Ghoneimi A, Yamataka A, Rothenberg S, Bailez M, Ferro M, Gamba P, Castagnetti M, Mattioli G, Delagausie P, Antoniou D, Montupet P, Marte A, Saxena A, Bertozzi M, Philippe P, Varlet F, Lardy H, Caldamone A, Settimi A, Pelizzo G, Becmeur F, Escolino M, De Pascale T, Najmaldin A, Schier F. Work-related upper limb musculoskeletal disorders in paediatric laparoscopic surgery. A multicenter survey. J Pediatr Surg. 2013;48:1750–6.
38. Mohseni-Bandpei MA, Ahmad-Shirvani M, Golbabaei N, Behtash H, Shahinfar Z, Fernandez-De-Las-Penas C. Prevalence and risk factors associated with low back pain in Iranian surgeons. J Manip Physiol Ther. 2011;34:362–70.
39. Davis WT, Fletcher SA, Guillamondegui OD. Musculoskeletal occupational injury among surgeons: effects for patients, providers, and institutions. J Surg Res. 2014;189:207–12.
40. Soueid A, Oudit D, Thiagarajah S, Laitung G. The pain of surgery: pain experienced by surgeons while operating. Int J Surg. 2010;8:118–20.
41. Olendorf MR, Drury CG. Postural discomfort and perceived exertion in standardized box-holding postures. Ergonomics. 2001;44(15):1341–67.
42. Nguyen NT, Ho HS, Smith WD, et al. An ergonomic evaluation of surgeons' axial skeletal and upper extremity movements during laparoscopic and open surgery. Am J Surg. 2001;182(6):720–4.
43. Wilson MR, Poolton JM, Malhotra N, et al. Development and validation of a surgical workload measure: the surgery task load index (SURG-TLX). World J Surg. 2011;35(9):1961–9.
44. van Veelen MA, Kazemier G, Koopman J, et al. Assessment of the ergonomically optimal operating surface height for laparoscopic surgery. J Laparoendosc Adv Surg Tech A. 2002;12(1):47–52.
45. Berquer R, Smith WD, Davis S. An ergonomic study of the optimum operating table height for laparoscopic surgery. Surg Endosc. 2002;16(3):416–21.
46. Veelen MA, Jakimowicz JJ, Goossens RH, et al. Evaluation of the usability of two types of image display systems, during laparoscopy. Surg Endosc. 2002;16(4):674–8.
47. Lee EC, Rafiq A, Merrell R, et al. Ergonomics and human factors in endoscopic surgery: a comparison of manual vs telerobotic simulation systems. Surg Endosc. 2005;19(8):1064–70.
48. Berquer R, Smith W. An ergonomic comparison of robotic and laparoscopic technique: the influence of surgeon experience and task complexity. J Surg Res. 2006;134(1):87–92.
49. Szeto GP, Ho P, Ting AC, et al. A study of surgeons' postural muscle activity during open, laparoscopic, and endovascular surgery. Surg Endosc. 2010;24(7):1712–21.
50. van der Schatte Olivier RH, Van't Hullenaar CD, Ruurda JP, et al. Ergonomics, user comfort, and performance in standard and robot-assisted laparoscopic surgery. Surg Endosc. 2009;23(6):1365–71.
51. Xiao DJ, Jakimowicz JJ, Albayrak A, et al. Ergonomic factors on task performance in laparoscopic surgery training. Appl Ergon. 2012;43(3):548–53.
52. Hubert N, Gilles M, Desbrosses K, et al. Ergonomic assessment of the surgeon's physical workload during standard and robotic assisted laparoscopic procedures. Int J Med Robot. 2013;9(2):142–7.
53. Alleblas CC, Formanoy MA, Könemann R, et al. Ergonomics in gynecologists' daily practice: anationwide survey in The Netherlands. Work. 2016;55(4):841–8.
54. McAtamney L, Corlett E. RULA: a survey method for the investigation of work-related upper limb disorders. Appl Ergon. 1993;24(2):91–9.

55. Stephens JP, Vos GA, Stevens EM, et al. Test-retest repeatability of the Strain Index. Appl Ergon. 2006;37(3):275–81.
56. Hignett S, McAtamney L. Rapid Entire Body Assessment (REBA). Appl Ergon. 2000;31(2):201–5.
57. Lee G, Lee T, Dexter D, et al. Ergonomic risk associated with assisting in minimally invasive surgery. Surg Endosc. 2009;23(1):182–8.
58. Kolwadkar YV, Brown SI, Abboud RJ, et al. Comparison of two actuation systems for laparoscopic surgical manipulators using motion analysis. Surg Endosc. 2011;25(3):964–74.
59. Koneczny S, Matern U. Instruments for the evaluation of ergonomics in surgery. Minim Invasive Ther Allied Technol. 2004;13(3):167–77.
60. Sancibrian R, Gutierrez-Diez MC, Torre-Ferrero C, et al. Design and evaluation of a new ergonomic handle for instruments in minimally invasive surgery. J Surg Res. 2014;188(1):88–99.
61. Berguer R, Remler M, Beckley D. Laparoscopic instruments cause increased forearm fatigue: a subjective and objective comparison of open and laparoscopic techniques. Minim Invasive Ther Allied Technol. 1997;6(1):36–40.
62. Vereczkei A, Feussner H, Negele T, et al. Ergonomic assessment of the static stress confronted by surgeons during laparoscopic cholecystectomy. Surg Endosc. 2004;18(7):1118–22.
63. Kant IJ, De Jong LC, Van Rijssen-Moll M, et al. A survey of static and dynamic work postures of operating room staff. Int Arch Occup Environ Health. 1992;63:423–8.
64. Collins SA, O'Sullivan DM, Tulikangas PK. Surgeon activity in robotic versus abdominal gynecologic surgery. J Robot Surg. 2012;6(4):333–6.
65. Supe AN, Kulkarni GV, Supe PA. Ergonomics in laparoscopic surgery. J Minim Access Surg. 2010;6(2):31–6. https://doi.org/10.4103/0972-9941.65161. PMID: 20814508; PMCID: PMC2924545.
66. Cuschieri A. Whither minimal access surgery: tribulations and expectations. Am J Surg. 1995;169(1):9–19.
67. Horgan LF, O'riordan DC, Doctor N. Neuropraxia following laparoscopic procedures: an occupational injury. Minim Invasive Ther Allied Technol. 1997;6(1):33–5.
68. Neuhaus SJ, Watson DI. Laparoscopic surgeons' thumb-is it a training phenomenon? Minim Invasive Ther Allied Technol. 1997;6(1):31–2.
69. Berguer R, Rab GT, Abu-Ghaida H, et al. A comparison of surgeons' posture during laparoscopic and open surgical procedures. Surg Endosc. 1997;11(2):139–42.
70. Gallagher AG, McClure N, McGuigan J, et al. An ergonomic analysis of the fulcrum effect in the acquisition of endoscopic skills. Endoscopy. 1998;30(7):617–20.
71. Hemal AK, Srinivas M, Charles AR. Ergonomic problems associated with laparoscopy. J Eleendourol. 2001;15(5):499–503.
72. Matern U, Giebmeyer C, Bergmann R, et al. Ergonomic aspects of four different types of laparoscopic instrument handles with respect to elbow angle. An electromyogram-based study. Surg Endosc. 2002;16(11):1528–32.
73. Berguer R, Chen J, Smith WD. A comparison of the physical effort required for laparoscopic and open surgical techniques. Arch Surg. 2003;138(9):967–70.
74. Reyes DA, Tang B, Cuschieri A. Minimal access surgery (MAS)-related surgeon morbidity syndromes. Surg Endosc. 2006;20(1):1–13.
75. Elhage O, Murphy D, Challacombe B, et al. Ergonomics in minimally invasive surgery. Int J Clin Pract. 2007;61(2):186–8.
76. Matern U. Ergonomic deficiencies in the operating room: examples from minimally invasive surgery. Work. 2009;33(2):165–8.
77. Tarr ME, Brancato SJ, Cunkelman JA, et al. Comparison of postural ergonomics between laparoscopic and robotic sacrocolpopexy: a pilot study. J Minim Invasive Gynecol. 2015;22(2):234–8.
78. Matern U, Waller P. Instruments for minimally invasive surgery: principles of ergonomic handles. Surg Endosc. 1999;13(2):174–82.
79. Matern U, Eichenlaub M, Waller P, Rückauer K. MIS instruments. An experimental comparison of various ergonomic handles and their design. Surg Endosc. 1999;13(8):756–62.

80. Gofrit ON, Mikahail AA, Zorn, et al. Surgeons' perceptions and injuries during and after urologic laparoscopic surgery. Urology. 2008;71(3):404–7.
81. Wee IJY, Kuo LJ, Ngu JC. A systematic review of the true benefit of robotic surgery: ergonomics. Int J Med Robot. 2020;16(4):e2113. https://doi.org/10.1002/rcs.2113. Epub 2020 May 6. PMID: 32304167.
82. Shugaba A, Lambert JE, Bampouras TM, Nuttall HE, Gaffney CJ, Subar DA. should all minimal access surgery be robot-assisted? A systematic review into the musculoskeletal and cognitive demands of laparoscopic and robot-assisted laparoscopic surgery. J Gastrointest Surg. 2022;26(7):1520–30.
83. Koshy K, Syed H, Luckiewicz A, Alsoof D, Koshy G, Harry L. Interventions to improve ergonomics in the operating theatre: a systematic review of ergonomics training and intra-operative microbreaks. Ann Med Surg (Lond). 2020;55:135–42.
84. Stucky CH, Cromwell KD, Voss RK, Chiang YJ, Woodman K, Lee JE, Cormier JN. Surgeon symptoms, strain, and selections: systematic review and meta-analysis of surgical ergonomics. Ann Med Surg (Lond). 2018;27:1–8.
85. van Veelen J, Kazemier. Improved physical ergonomics of laparoscopic surgery. Minim Invasive Ther Allied Technol. 2004;13(3):161–6. https://doi.org/10.1080/13645700410033193. PMID: 16754505.
86. Matern U, Faist M, Kehl K, et al. Monitor position in laparoscopic surgery. Surg Endosc. 2005;19(3):436–40.
87. Zehetner J, Kaltenbacher A, Wayand W, Shamiyeh A. Screen height as an ergonomic factor in laparoscopic surgery. Surg Endosc. 2006;20(1):139–41. https://doi.org/10.1007/s00464-005-0251-1.
88. van Det MJ, Meijerink WJ, Hoff C, van Veelen MA, Pierie JP. Ergonomic assessment of neck posture in the minimally invasive surgery suite during laparoscopic cholecystectomy. Surg Endosc. 2008;22(11):2421–7.
89. Manasnayakorn S, Cuschieri A, Hanna GB. Ideal manipulation angle and instrument length in hand-assisted laparoscopic surgery. Surg Endosc. 2008;22(4):924–9.
90. Zheng B, Martinec DV, Cassera MA, Swanström LL. A quantitative study of disruption in the operating room during laparoscopic antireflux surgery. Surg Endosc. 2008;22(10):2171–7.
91. van Det MJ, Meijerink WJ, Hoff C, Totté ER, Pierie JP. Optimal ergonomics for laparoscopic surgery in minimally invasive surgery suites: a review and guidelines. Surg Endosc. 2009;23(6):1279–85.
92. Hullfish KL, Trowbridge ER, Bodine G. Ergonomics and gynecologic surgery. J Pelvic Med Surg. 2009;15(6):435–9.
93. Nagpal K, Vats A, Ahmed K, Smith AB, Sevdalis N, Jonannsson H, Vincent C, Moorthy K. A systematic quantitative assessment of risks associated with poor communication in surgical care. Arch Surg. 2010;145(6):582–8.
94. Engelmann C, Schneider M, Kirschbaum C, et al. Effects of intraoperative breaks on mental and somatic operator fatigue: a randomized clinical trial. Surg Endosc. 2011;25(4):1245–50.
95. Xiao DJ, Jakimowicz JJ, Albayrak A, Goossens RH. Ergonomic factors on task performance in laparoscopic surgery training. Appl Ergon. 2012;43(3):548–53.
96. Seagull FJ. Disparities between industrial and surgical ergonomics. Work. 2012;41(Suppl 1):4669–72.
97. Szeto GP, Cheng SW, Poon JT, Ting AC, Tsang RC, Ho P. Surgeons' static posture and movement repetitions in open and laparoscopic surgery. J Surg Res. 2012;172(1):e19–31.
98. Rosenblatt PL, McKinney J, Adams SR. Ergonomics in the operating room: protecting the surgeon. J Minim Invasive Gynecol. 2013;20(6):744.
99. Craven R, Franasiak J, Mosaly P, et al. Ergonomic deficits in robotic gynecologic oncology surgery: a need for intervention. J Minim Invasive Gynecol. 2013;20(5):648–55.
100. Dorion D, Darveau S. Do micropauses prevent surgeon's fatigue and loss of accuracy associated with prolonged surgery? An experimental prospective study. Ann Surg. 2013;257(2):256–9.

101. Franasiak JM, Gehrig PA, Craven R. Feasibility and effectiveness of an ergonomics training program to address high rates of strain among robotic surgeons. J Minim Invasive Gynecol. 2013;20(6).
102. Park AE, Zahiri HR, Hallbeck MS, Augenstein V, Sutton E, Yu D, Lowndes BR, Bingener J. Intraoperative "micro breaks" with targeted stretching enhance surgeon physical function and mental focus: a multicenter cohort study. Ann Surg. 2017;265(2):340–6.
103. Reddy PP, Reddy TP, Roig-Francoli J, Cone L, Sivan B, DeFoor WR, Gaitonde K, Noh PH. The impact of the alexander technique on improving posture and surgical ergonomics during minimally invasive surgery: pilot study. J Urol. 2011;186(4 Suppl):1658–62. https://doi.org/10.1016/j.juro.2011.04.013. Epub 2011 Aug 19. PMID: 21855928.
104. Winters JN, Sommer NZ, Romanelli MR, Marschik C, Hulcher L, Cutler BJ. Stretching and strength training to improve postural ergonomics and endurance in the operating room. Plast Reconstr Surg Glob Open. 2020;8(5):e2810. https://doi.org/10.1097/GOX.0000000000002810. PMID: 33133890; PMCID: PMC7572150.

Part II

Laparoscopic Equipment

Cables Used in OR

11

C. Chandramaliteeswaran and Lokesh Arora

11.1 Introduction

As surgeons are getting familiar with laparoscopic and robotic procedures, the practical knowledge on electrical and electronic components of laparoscopic setup becomes indispensable. Often while operating, the surgeon relies on technicians whenever display issues occur, and if not corrected, the surgical team is left paralysed. A good working knowledge allows the operating surgeon to do the basic troubleshooting, especially when experienced technical personnel are not available. As a primer to subsequent chapters, this section focuses on the basics of various cables used in laparoscopic armamentarium.

11.2 Basic Laparoscopic Cable Outlay

Essential laparoscopic setup consists of image processor, light source, gas supply unit, energy source and monitor. All these components have their corresponding cables. They can be viewed as two types:

Front-end cables: All the cables from the components entering the surgical field in the surgeon's view. These can include:

1. Camera cable
2. Light cable
3. Gas tubing
4. Energy source cables

C. Chandramaliteeswaran (✉)
Department of Surgical Gastroenterology, SVIMS, Tirupati, India

L. Arora
Department of Surgical Gastroenterology, AIIMS, Rishikesh, Uttarakhand, India

J. S. Ahluwalia (ed.), *User Manual for Minimally Invasive Surgical Equipment*,
https://doi.org/10.1007/978-981-95-9019-3_11

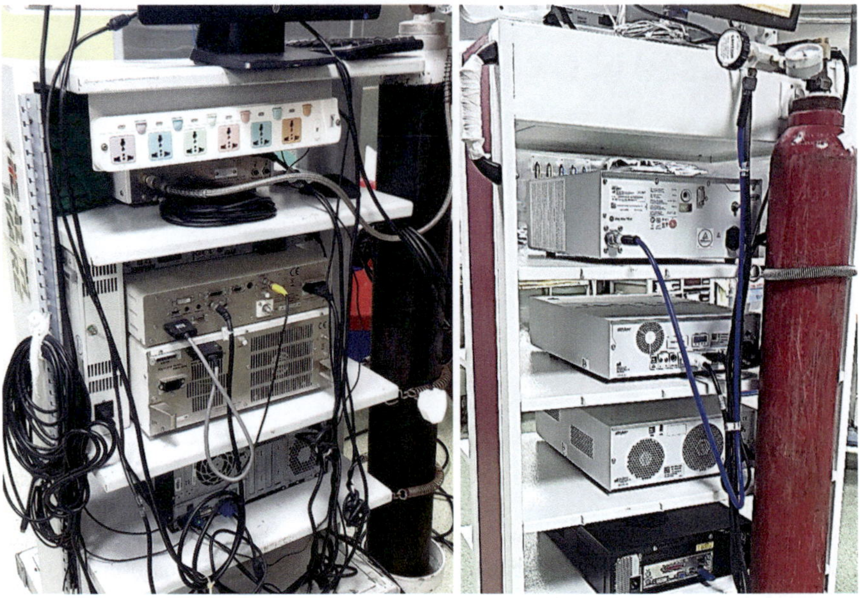

Fig. 11.1 Typical disorganised rear-end cables of laparoscopic trolley (left) and an organised minimalistic cable management system (right)

Rear-end cables: all the cables powering the units, shielded from the surgeon's view (Fig. 11.1). These may include:

1. Power cables
2. Video connectors

11.3 Power Cables

Laparoscopic trolleys are equipped with an inbuilt expansion board which is ideally connected to 15amp 3pin wall socket with UPS (uninterrupted power supply) backup. Three-pin socket ensures earthing of the sensitive components. If any equipment shows evidence of mild electric shock on touch, the circuit must be checked for proper earthing.

The output sockets should be at least six in number and preferably the 5/15amp hybrid 3-pin type (Fig. 11.2). This allows direct plugging without using adapters as some components come with 15 amps power adapter and others with 5amp adapter. The shape and electric load compatibility of plugs vary from region to region, and the user must ensure compatibility before plugging in. In case there is no inbuilt expansion board, an appropriate extension box with individual switches should be fixed to the trolley system.

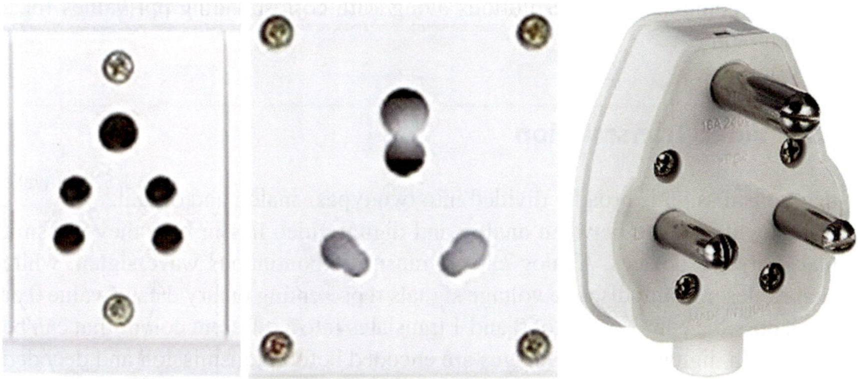

5amp socket Hybrid 5/15amp socket 3pin AC wall adapter

Fig. 11.2 Typical electric socket and adapter in India

Table 11.1 Various video resolutions with their pixel density and ppi values for 32-inch monitor

Common format	Pixel density	Vertical resolution	Pixel per inch (for 32-inch monitor)
Standard definition (SD)	640 × 480	480p	~30
High definition (HD)	1280 × 720	720p	~46
Full HD (FHD)	1920 × 1080	1080p	~70
Quad HD (QHD)	2560 × 1440	1440p	~92
4K or ultra-HD (UHD)	3840 × 2160	2160p	~140
8K	7680 × 4320	4320p	~280

11.4 Basics of Video Transmission

With the availability of multiple video output formats in image processors, it is important to understand the basics of video signals and choose the best format for optimal video display quality.

Basic concepts to understand in video transmission include pixel, resolution and pixels per inch.

Pixel is the smallest unit of an image, which can be displayed on any digital device.

Resolution is defined as the number of pixels arranged horizontally and vertically on a given display screen. Resolution is represented as pixels in width x pixels in height as in 1920 × 1080. This resolution, commonly termed as 1080p, refers to a vertical resolution of 1080 pixels. The higher the resolution, the better the video clarity, but also dependent on display size.

Pixel per inch (ppi) refers to the number of pixels packed in one inch of monitor display. This parameter varies both with video resolution and display size. Minimum ppi requirement for medical grade monitor is 110 to ensure image clarity. Table 11.1

depicts the common video resolutions along with corresponding ppi values for a 32-inch monitor.

11.5 Video Transmission

Video transmission is broadly divided into two types: analog and digital.

The key difference between analog and digital video lies in how they transmit signals between devices. Analog cables transmit a continuous wave signal, while digital cables transmit discrete voltage signals representing binary data of value 0 or 1. Each possible combination of 0 and 1 translates into a different colour that can be displayed. In digital systems, images are encoded before transmission and decoded by the receiving device, such as a monitor. Commonly used 8-bit system of digital video contains a total of eight 0's and 1's (00000001 to 11111111) to represent the colour shade for each pixel. This 8-bit colour depth means that up to $2^8 = 256$ shade combinations per colour channel. Since there are three colour channels in RGB spectrum, this means that as many as $2^8 \times 3 = 16.77$ million different colour shades can be displayed for each pixel. This forms the basis of '16 million' colour advertised as 'True colour' in digital video devices. Since human eye cannot fully discern differences beyond 10 million colour shades, 10-bit and 12-bit encoding systems are used only in professional settings.

The main advantage of digital transmission is the accurate reproduction without degradation of image quality. This is because digital signals are encoded discretely and can be precisely decoded despite interference. In contrast, analog signals are continuous and susceptible to interference resulting in a loss of quality during transmission. Other advantages include higher resolution support, greater bandwidth and additional features like audio return channel, ethernet connectivity and support for multiple channels. Common video outputs available in laproscopic image processing units are shown in Figs. 11.3 and 11.4.

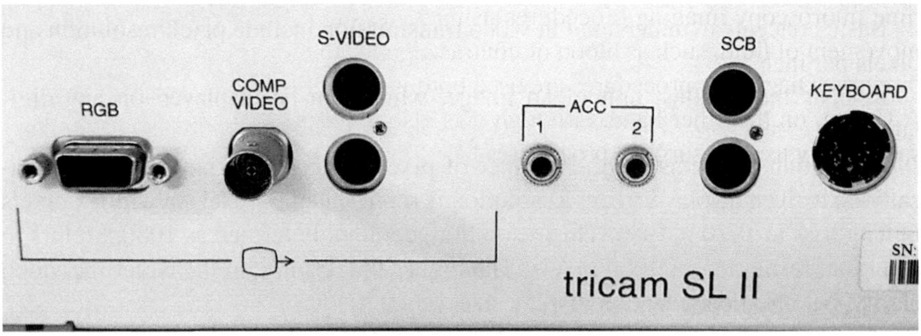

Fig. 11.3 Legacy image processor with analog video outputs

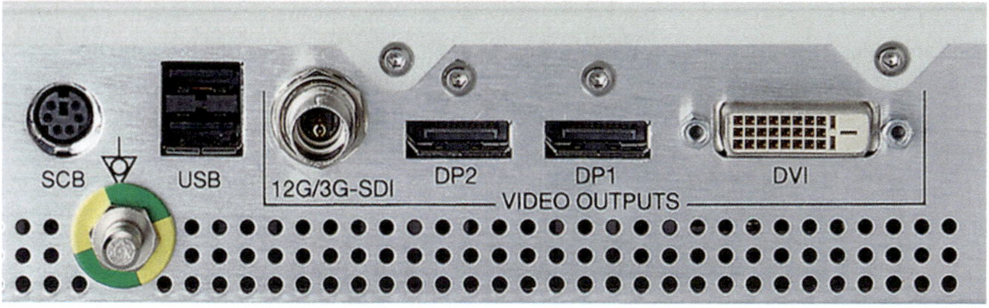

Fig. 11.4 Rear panel of a modern image processor with digital and analog video outputs

11.6 Analog Video Formats

11.6.1 Video Graphics Array (VGA)

VGA connector is currently the most popular analog format present in image processors. It has a three-row, 15-pin format also known as D15 or sub-D or HD15. Since it is an analog format, it does not support content protection restrictions and allows recording of protected videos (Fig. 11.5).

11.6.2 S-Video (Separate-Video/Super-Video)

S-video is an analog format that carries standard-definition video up to 576p resolution. There are 4-pin, 7-pin and 9-pin variants which can be identified based on pin layouts as shown in the figure. The 4-pin variant is the most common and supports standard-definition video. Seven-pin or 9-pin variants can be used to support other communication between devices, so matching connectors is important for compatibility (Fig. 11.6).

11.6.3 Composite Video

The name 'composite' video cable is derived from the fact that it combines multiple video signals into a single cable. In this case, all the video information, including the luminance (brightness) and chrominance (colour) are combined into a single yellow coloured cable. But this close proximity of signals can lead to interference that can degrade the image quality and lower the resolution. The red and white cables carry right and left stereo audio signals, respectively (Fig. 11.7).

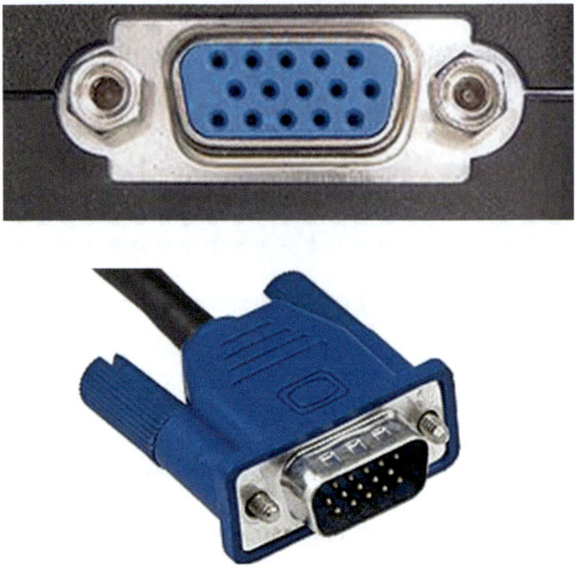

Fig. 11.5 VGA socket and cable adapter with screw lock

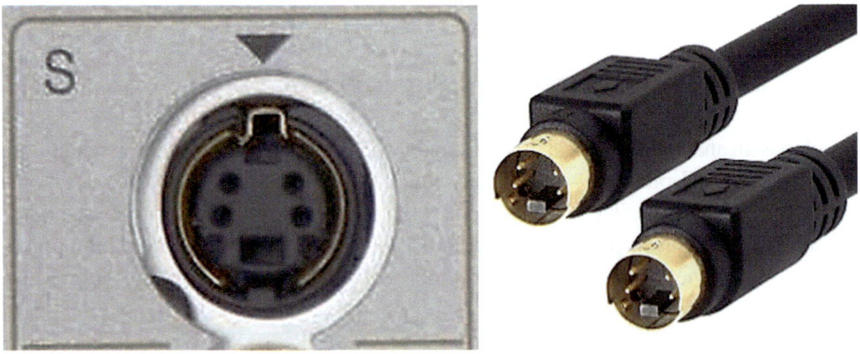

Fig. 11.6 S-video socket and cable ends

11.6.4 Component Video

Component cables separate the video signal into three components in three separate cables: Pr (red), Pb (blue) and Y (luminance). The Pr and Pb components carry the colour information, while the Y component green cable carries the brightness information. By splitting the signal into these components, component cables improve resolution with lesser interference. Figure 11.7 illustrates the ports and corresponding cables used for component video transmission.

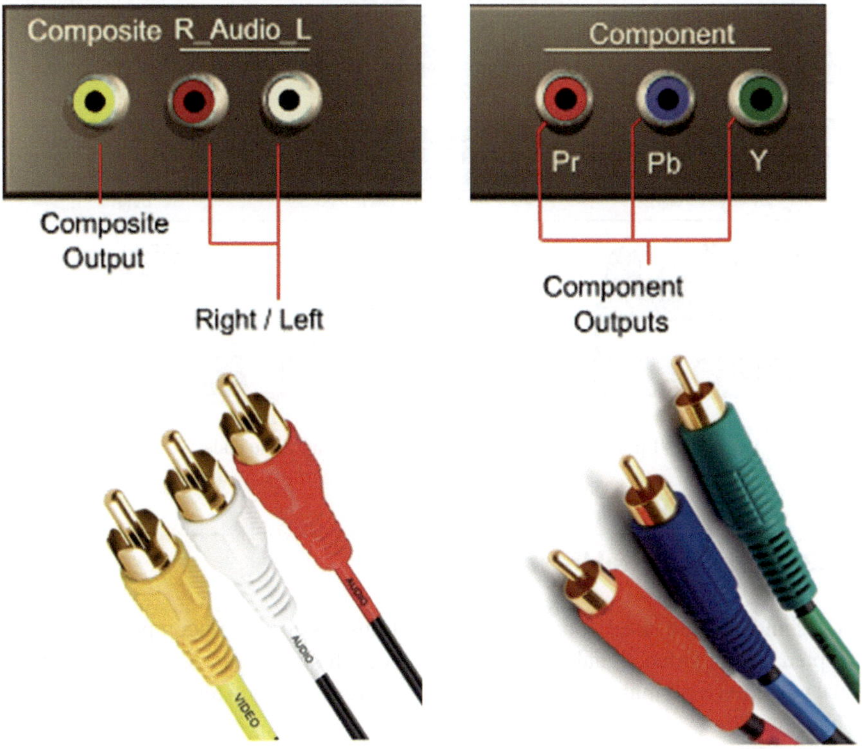

Fig. 11.7 Composite (left) and component (right) socket with corresponding cable ends

11.7 Digital Video Formats

11.7.1 Digital Visual Interface

Digital visual interface (DVI) was developed as an industry standard for the transfer of an uncompressed digital video signal. It does not carry an audio signal which is not important in laparoscopy. There are various types namely

- DVI-**D** is **D**igital (single link or dual link)
- DVI-**I** is **I**ntegrated (supports both digital and analog)
- DVI-**A** is **A**nalog interface

Single link cable supports resolutions up to 1920 × 1200 at 60 Hz while dual link adds six extra pins increasing the bandwidth to support resolutions up to 2560 × 1600. The layout can be identified based on the images in Fig. 11.8 and the appropriate cable is to be used. There is a screw lock mechanism to prevent the slippage of connectors.

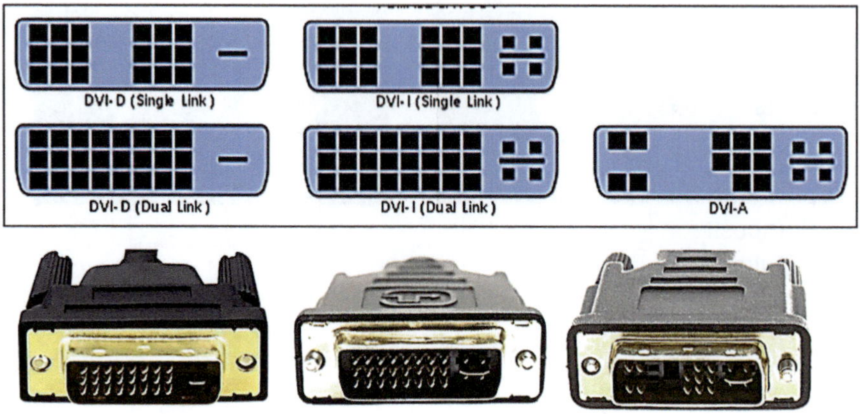

Fig. 11.8 Various DVI port configurations with corresponding cable ends

11.8 Serial Digital Interface (SDI)

SDI standards are used for unidirectional transmission of uncompressed, unencrypted digital video signals over long distances. It started as a standard SDI interface but underwent many revisions to cater to increasing video resolution bandwidth. These include

- SD-SDI: supports standard definition video
- HD-SDI: supports 1.5 Gigabits/sec with high definition 1080p video
- 3G-SDI: supports 3Gigabits/sec transmission in single cable
- 6G-SDI: supports 6Gigabits/sec including ultra-HD 4k displays
- 12G-SDI and 24G-SDI: supports 8k displays

SDI is used in professional settings where there is a lot of movement and risk of signal disconnection is undesirable as in an operation theatre. SDI is transmitted over coaxial cables with BNC (named after inventors Bayonet Neill-Concelman) connectors; hence often referred to as BNC cables. The lock-in mechanism of connectors makes it resistant to accidental disconnection (Fig. 11.9).

11.9 DisplayPort (DP)

DisplayPort interface was designed to replace VGA and DVI. It carries both video and audio signals and is backward compatible with HDMI and DVI through adapters. DisplayPort 2.1 is the latest standard incorporating the new DP40 and DP80 cables certified for 40 Gbit/s and 80 Gbit/s transmission, respectively.

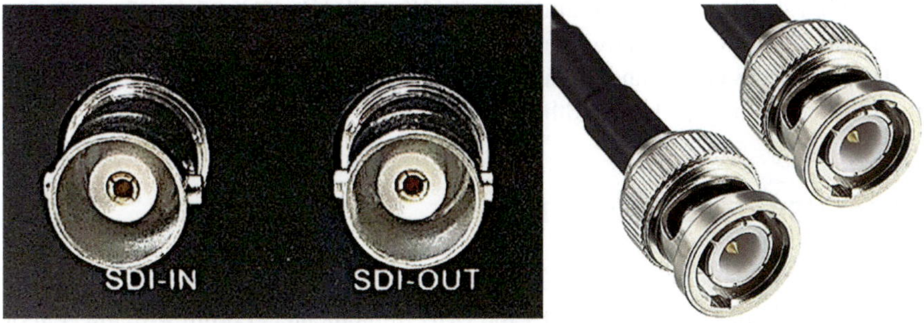

Fig. 11.9 Typical SDI port with corresponding BNC cable ends

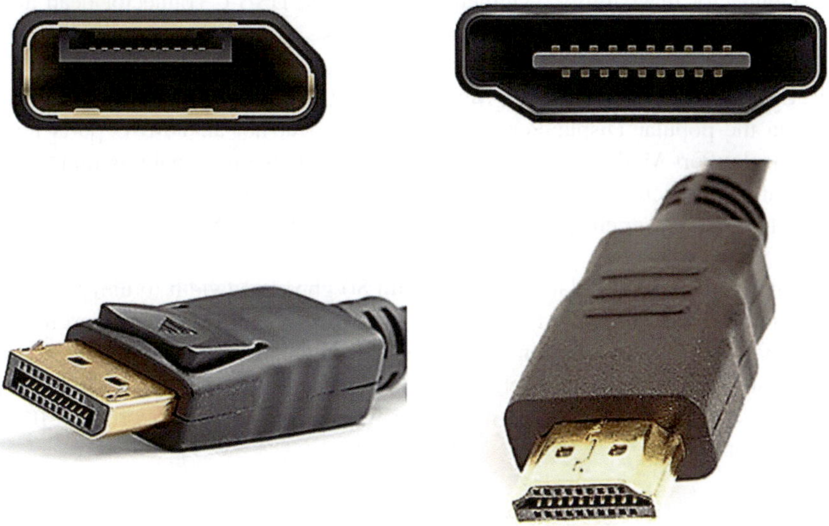

Fig. 11.10 Display port (left) and HDMI port (right) with cable ends

11.10 High-Definition Multimedia Interface (HDMI)

HDMI is a proprietary audio-video transmission format from an HDMI-compliant source to a compatible monitor with content protection enabled. High-bandwidth digital content protection (HDCP) is a form of digital encryption to prevent copying. It is widely used in commercial appliances and rarely in professional systems due to the requirement of licensing fees and royalty requirements. Moreover, it does not allow daisy chaining of monitors which is important in laparoscopy setup. Daisy-chaining refers to connecting multiple monitors serially one after another unlike plugging all cables into a single source (Fig. 11.10).

HDCP does not allow recording of protected content using video recording devices. This may be bypassed by using select HDMI splitters which strips the encryption and allows multiple outputs to monitors and recording devices.

- HDMI 1.4: 10 Gbps bandwidth supports 4K at 30 Hz
- HDMI 2.0: 18 Gbps bandwidth supports 4K at 60 Hz
- HDMI 2.1: 48 Gbps bandwidth supports 10K at 120 Hz
- HDMI 2.2: 96 Gbps bandwidth supports 16K at 60 Hz

11.11 USB-C with Display Mode

USB type-C is a physical connector for transmitting data, video and power, all in a single cable. USB-C is developed by the USB Implementers Forum with the goal of making USB-C as a universal port. Salient features include:

- Connector reversibility: symmetric oval-shaped USB-C connector head allows connection irrespective of orientation, unlike other asymmetric USB-A and B ports.
- USB-C DisplayPort (DP Alt Mode) allows USB-C ports to transfer video data via the popular DisplayPort video interface. But not all USB-C ports feature DisplayPort Mode functionality. The manufacturer must enable required hardware and specify compatibility in the product manual.
- Integrated power charging up to 240 W in Thunderbolt 5.

Thunderbolt 5 is the latest revision with 80 gbps bandwidth to unify all digital transmission into a standard USB-C interface (Table 11.2). It can support multiple external displays and is used mainly in the consumer space. Thunderbolt cables and ports are marked with the 'lightning bolt' logo as shown in Fig. 11.11. USB4 is another common USB-C implementation with 20–40 Gbps support seen in consumer computers.

11.12 Choosing the Right Cable

When selecting the appropriate video port for your laparoscopic setup, it is based on image quality and compatibility. Comparison of all the cable types is summarised in Table 11.3. Points to consider in decision-making include:

- Resolution of the camera system

Table 11.2 Comparing properties of various USB-C configurations

	Thunderbolt 5	Thunderbolt 4	USB4	USB 3.2
Connector	USB-C			
Minimum bandwidth	80 Gbps	40 Gbps	20–40 Gbps	5 Gbps
Monitor support	Dual 8k monitors	One 8K monitors	Two 4K monitors	One 4K monitor
Daisy-chaining	6 devices	6 devices	No	No

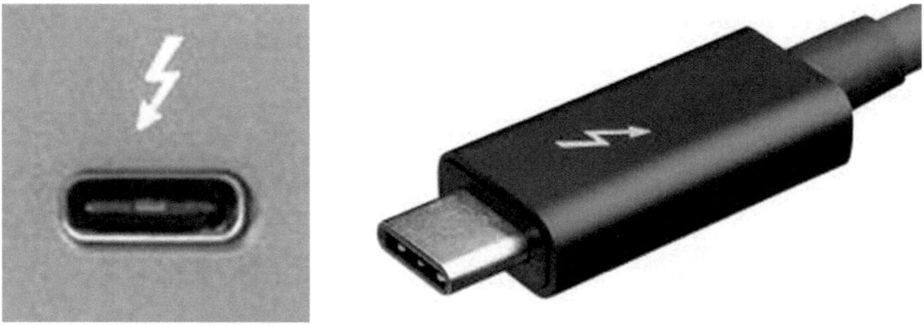

Fig. 11.11 Thunderbolt port with corresponding USB-C cable

- Resolution of the monitor
- Availability of corresponding output and input ports in the camera and monitor system, respectively
- Choosing the correct length and speed specifications for the selected cable
- Daisy chain connection to second monitor or video recording system

DisplayPort (DP): These digital ports offer high image quality and support resolutions up to 10K. They are widely compatible and provide audio transmission along with video.

HDMI: These are less commonly used in laparoscopic setup due to potential for signal interference (especially from use of electric cauterisation), lack of daisy chain support and absence of locking mechanism. Moreover, HDMI systems do not support video recording.

DVI: DVI ports provide high-quality digital video transmission, supporting resolutions up to 2560 × 1600 (Dual link). However, they do not carry audio signals.

SDI: SDI ports are commonly used in professional settings, offering various standards with increasing video resolution bandwidth. They are suitable for long-distance transmission and maintain signal integrity.

VGA, S-Video, Composite: These analog ports are older formats and have limited support for higher resolutions. VGA is the most widely used analog format.

11.13 Video Conversion Adapters

Video adapter refers to a device that converts one video protocol to another, such as DisplayPort to HDMI. This enables compatibility between different devices without needing to invest in new hardware.

Various aspects to consider are:

- Active (requires additional power source) or passive adapter: HDMI and DisplayPort are functionally similar video interfaces and allow passive conver-

Table 11.3 Comparison of common analog and digital cable features

Cable type	Cable end	Max resolution	Advantages	Disadvantages
Analog				
VGA	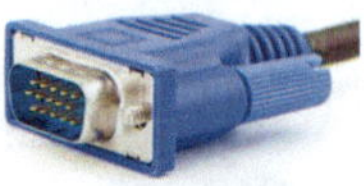	2048 × 1536 @ 85 Hz	Widely adopted, better image quality	No content protection
S-Video	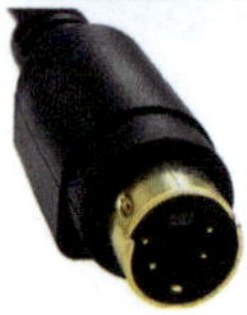	720 × 576 @ 50 Hz	Widely supported, low cost	Limited resolution
Composite	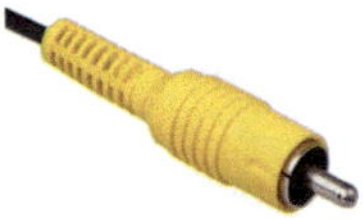	720 × 576 @ 50 Hz	Simple and widely compatible	Lowest image resolution, prone to interference
Component	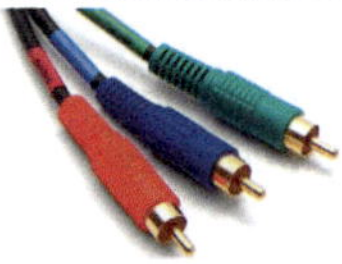	1920 × 1080 @ 60 Hz	Better image quality than composite	Bulky cables
Digital				
DVI	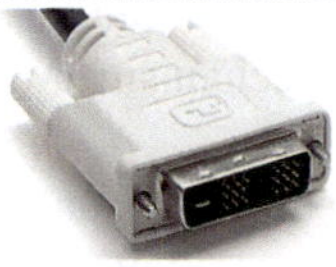	2560 × 1600 @ 60 Hz	High image quality, supports high resolutions	No audio support
SDI	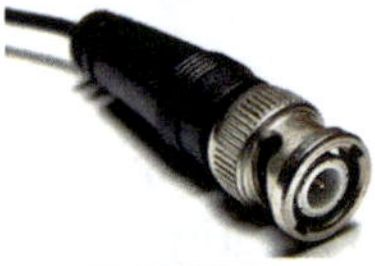	24g-SDI supports 8k at 30 hz	Long-distance support, used in recent 4K systems	Licensing prohibiting widespread use
DisplayPort	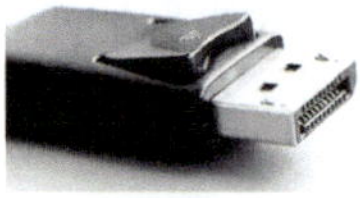	DisplayPort 2.1 supports 8k at 240 hz	High image and audio quality, backward compatibility	*Length of cable varies based on the speed certifications*
HDMI	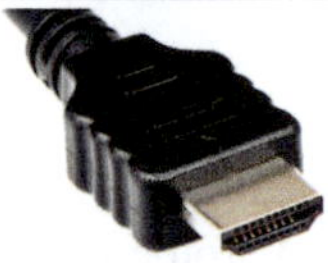	Hdmi 2.2 supports 16k at 60 hz	High image and audio quality, widely supported in consumer industry	No locking mechanism No daisy chain support. Licensing and royalty fees involved
USB-C	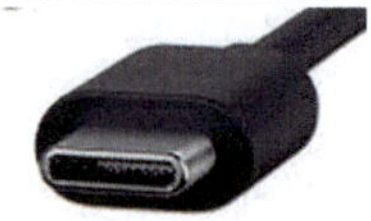	Thunderbolt 5 support DisplayPort 2.1	Versatile, combines video and data transmission	Limited adoption in laparoscopic systems

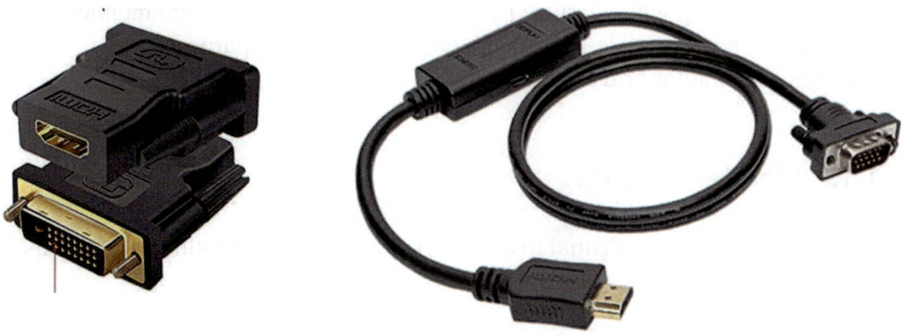

Fig. 11.12 A bidirectional DVI male-HDMI female adapter (left) and an HDMI male to VGA male adapter cable (right)

sion to other digital and even VGA analog formats. Converting from VGA to HDMI is not a straightforward process because HDMI is a digital signal, while VGA is an analog signal. This conversion requires an active adapter with a built-in analog-to-digital converter.

- Adapter is unidirectional or bidirectional: For instance, VGA to HDMI adapter will not support reverse HDMI to VGA conversion, whereas DVI to HDMI adapter allows signal conversion both ways.

Choose the correct 'male' or 'female' ends of the adapter. Male port refers to the plugging port and female port refers to the receiving port as shown in Fig. 11.12.

Also to note if the adapter is standalone or comes with inbuilt cable and whether the cable length is sufficient.

11.14 Troubleshooting Video Output Issues

Step-by-step approach in case of no image or corrupt display:

1. First check monitor and processor and light source 'powered on' status.
2. Check if camera cable and light source are slotted into their sockets properly. Clean and reinsert if necessary sequentially.
3. Check cable connection from 'video out' port of processor to 'video in' port of monitor. Ensure proper plug in.
4. Check if correct input port is selected in monitor setup panel. Most modern monitors support 'auto mode' to automatically detect input source. Otherwise manually select the input source.
5. In case of usage of adapters to connect different port formats, check for directional compatibility. For example, 'DP to HDMI' adapter cable may not support 'HDMI to DP' connection.
6. Check cables for damage, especially prone to damage at junction bends.

7. Try reconnecting with alternate ports of the image processor and monitor. Have a standby alternate cable like a VGA cable for checking purposes.
8. Restart the monitor or try connecting to a different monitor.

11.15 Maintenance Tips

Proper care of cables is essential to ensure their longevity and optimal performance. Here are some guidelines:

- Avoid sharp bends in the cables as it can break the internal wiring. Gently loop or coil the cables when storing them.
- Do not pull or yank the cables when unplugging them. Grasp the connectors firmly and pull straight out. Locked connections need to be unlocked before detachment.
- When plugging or unplugging cables, avoid applying excessive force can damage the connector pins.
- Keep cables away from heat sources, sharp objects, or areas with heavy foot traffic to prevent physical damage.
- Clean the connectors periodically using a soft, dry cloth to remove dust or debris that may affect the connection.
- Use cables with lock mechanisms to avoid accidental pulling of cables. All the newer cables like DVI and SDI have lock mechanism. Loose connections can lead to signal disruption issues.
- When routing or storing cables, use gentle curves and avoid tightly wrapping them. Correct way of storage is depicted in Fig. 11.13.
- Use cable organisers to avoid tangling of cables as shown in Fig. 11.14.
- Always keep standby equipment ready in case of sudden malfunctions of components.
- Regular inspection: Periodically inspect cables for any signs of wear, such as fraying or exposed wiring. Replace damaged cables promptly to prevent potential hazards or degraded performance.

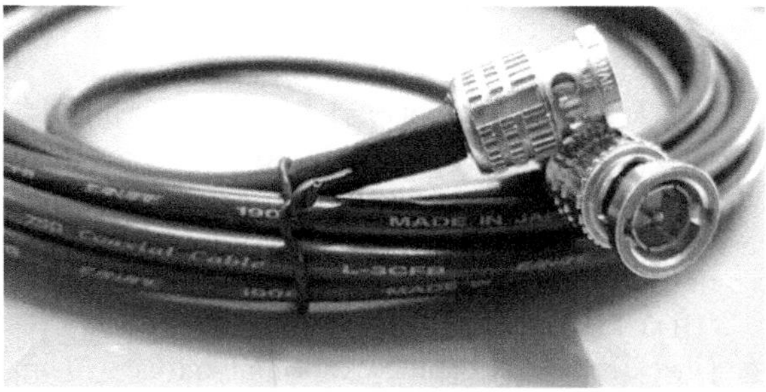

Fig. 11.13 Proper way of coiling a cable

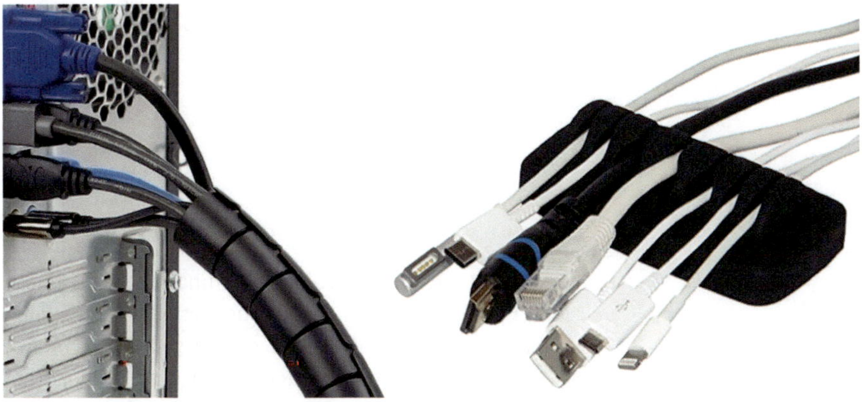

Fig. 11.14 Cable organisers and cord holders to avoid cable entanglement

Further Reading

John AS, Caturegli I, Kubicki NS, Kavic SM. The rise of minimally invasive surgery: 16 year analysis of the progressive replacement of open surgery with laparoscopy. JSLS J Soc Laparosc Robot Surg. 2020;24(4)

Alkatout I, Schollmeyer T, Hawaldar NA, Sharma N, Mettler L. Principles and safety measures of electrosurgery in laparoscopy. JSLS J Soc Laparoendosc Surg. 2012;16(1):130.

Poynton C. Digital video and HD: algorithms and interfaces. Elsevier; 2012.

Berci G, Schwaitzberg SD. The importance of understanding the basics of imaging in the era of high-tech endoscopy: Part II. Surg Endosc. 2002;16(11):1518.

Siddaiah-Subramanya M, Nyandowe M, Tiang KW. Technical problems during laparoscopy: a systematic method of troubleshooting for surgeons. Innov Surg Sci. 2017;2(4):233–7.

Camera and Monitor

12

Chakiev Aybek Moldosvich, Manoj Yadav,
and Gursehaj Singh Mehta

Minimal access surgery (MAS) has revolutionized the field of surgery by reducing trauma, enhancing precision, and expediting patient recovery. At the heart of this technique lies the laparoscopic camera system, a critical tool that provides surgeons with a magnified, high-definition view of the surgical field inside the body. It serves as the surgeon's eyes, transmitting real-time images to a monitor, allowing for precise dissection, suturing and manipulation of tissues. Over the years, advancements in optics, sensor technology and image processing have significantly improved visualization, making procedures safer and more efficient.

12.1 Laparoscopic Camera

It can be divided into:

1. Camera head: This part is the one that is connected to endoscope and is held in hand during surgery. It is connected to camera control unit (CCU) with a cable. Camera head consists of ocular coupler, focusing ring, zoom optics (25–50 mm), video sensor housing and program/function selector (Fig. 12.1).
2. Camera control unit (CCU): This part is usually kept on laparoscopic trolley or tower and it is connected to power source, monitor and camera head. Recorder can also be given video feed through this.

C. A. Moldosvich (✉) · M. Yadav · G. S. Mehta
Department of Surgery, International Higher School of Medicine, Bishkek, Kyrgyzstan

J. S. Ahluwalia (ed.), *User Manual for Minimally Invasive Surgical Equipment*,
https://doi.org/10.1007/978-981-95-9019-3_12

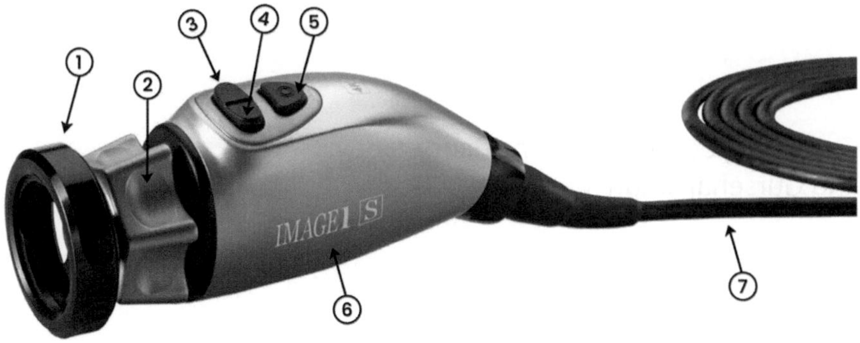

Fig. 12.1 Camera Head. (1—coupler, 2—focus adjustment ring, 3 to 5—user control buttons, 6—camera housing, 7—camera head cable)

12.1.1 Camera Head

1—Coupler: It connects the camera head to the laparoscope. It ensures that the image captured by the laparoscope is correctly transmitted to the camera sensor without distortion or loss of quality. The coupler maintains proper alignment, focuses the image, and magnifies (If this option is available). It can be a C-mount type or twist-and-lock mechanism type. Some couplers have an optical zoom build in them which can be changed using a rotatable ring.

2—Focus adjustment ring: User can rotate this ring to adjust the focus of the camera. Some camera systems have auto focus function.

3 to 5—User control buttons: These buttons can have different functions depending upon the make of the camera.

6—Camera housing: Houses the camera. If marked as autoclavable, it can be sterilized in an autoclave.

7—Camera cable: It attaches the camera head to the camera control unit.

12.1.2 Types of Sensors Used in Cameras

Two types of sensors are usually used in cameras.

1. *CCD (Charge-Coupled Device) Sensors*:

CCD sensors use an array of light-sensitive pixels to capture images. Photons striking the sensor generate an electrical charge, which is transferred across the chip and converted into a digital signal. The process is highly controlled, ensuring minimal noise and superior image quality.

Advantages:

- *Higher Image Quality*: Produces images with better dynamic range, colour accuracy and reduced noise.
- *Better Low-Light Performance*: More effective in dimly lit surgical fields.
- *Less Image Distortion*: No rolling shutter effect, ensuring smooth motion capture.

Disadvantages:

- *Higher Power Consumption*: Requires more energy, generating heat.
- *Expensive to Manufacture*: Costlier than CMOS sensors.
- *Slower Processing Speed*: Charge transfer is sequential, leading to higher latency.

2. *CMOS (Complementary Metal-Oxide-Semiconductor) Sensors*

CMOS sensors convert light into electrical signals directly at each pixel using an integrated circuit. Each pixel processes its own charge, allowing for faster image readout and real-time processing.

Advantages:

- *Lower Power Consumption*: Uses less energy, reducing heat generation.
- *Faster Processing Speed*: Direct signal conversion enables rapid image capture, ideal for real-time applications.
- *Cost-Effective*: More affordable to produce, making CMOS cameras more widely available.

Disadvantages:

- *Lower Image Quality*: May exhibit more noise, lower dynamic range and inferior colour fidelity compared to CCD.
- *Rolling Shutter Effect*: Can cause motion distortion in fast-moving scenes.
- *Reduced Low-Light Performance*: May struggle in low-light laparoscopic environments.

12.1.3 Which Is Better for Laparoscopy?

Advancements in *CMOS technology* have significantly improved its performance, narrowing the gap with CCD sensors. Many modern laparoscopic systems now use *high-end CMOS sensors* with sophisticated image processing to achieve near-CCD quality while benefiting from the advantages of CMOS technology.

Now, two new systems are the cutting edge of surgical video technology: 3D and 4K ultra-HD (UHD). These systems were developed with the goal of providing better imaging and better depth perception.

12.1.4 4K and 3D Systems

Modern advancements in laparoscopic imaging technology have led to the introduction of 4K ultra HD and 3D stereoscopic cameras, significantly enhancing visualization, depth perception and precision during minimally invasive surgeries (MIS). These technologies provide high-resolution images and improve the accuracy of surgical manoeuvres.

4K Camera 4K ultra-HD (UHD) cameras provide a resolution of 3840 × 2160 pixels, which is 4 times higher than full HD (1080p) systems. This offers greater detail, colour accuracy, and contrast. This also improves the overall perception of depth. Higher cost is the main limiting factor for these systems.

3D Camera The term '3D' originates from 'three-dimensional' as it adds depth to the length and breadth of a standard 2D image, such as those seen on surgical monitors. This overcomes the primary limitation of conventional imaging used in laparoscopy, the absence of depth, which contributes to the learning curve and remains a limiting factor to surgical performance even after this has been overcome. However, a different technology is required to add depth to a flat monitor which otherwise lacks it. The normal sense of three dimensions is perceived by the brain because our eyes view a slightly different aspect of each image as they are positioned at a distance from one another. The brain then combines these two aspects of the same image to create a sense of three-dimensionality. Similarly, for 3D imaging, different images are presented to each surgeon's eye to facilitate stereopsis (the sense of a three-dimensional image). This can be achieved using either of the following technologies:

Single-channel Laparoscope This system uses one lens to create a separate image for each eye digitally. This is likely to result in inferior 3D perception compared to a double-lens system.

Dual-lens Laparoscope This system features two lenses placed adjacent to each other capturing images from two perspectives as our eyes do. This creates a perception of 3D after processing and provides better stereovision.

Images from two separate perspectives must be presented to a surgeon or the staff involved in a manner that each eye sees only the intended image. Systems may achieve this by using:

Polarized Glasses These filter one image for each eye. They are lightweight, do not require power to operate and are also inexpensive.

Active Shutter Glasses These block the view of users' eyes alternately by synchronising with the monitor image and may create a better 3D effect. However, they require power to operate and are heavier and more expensive.

3D imaging may reduce the learning curve for novice surgeons. The main limiting factors are the higher cost, limited ability to rotate such laparoscopes, eye fatigue and the need to wear glasses.

12.1.5 Controller Unit

The image is captured by the image sensor placed inside the camera head or on the tip of the scope and is converted into electronic signals. These signals are carried by the camera head wire to this unit for further processing. After processing, the controller unit sends electronic signals to the monitor to display the final image. The camera cable usually attaches to this unit from a connector placed on its front panel, and connections for the video monitor are usually placed at its rear side (Figs. 12.2 and 12.3). Some newer controller units combine both image processor and light source functions in one unit.

12.1.6 CCU Front View

1. Power switch—to power on and off the console
2. White balance—to white balance the camera
3. Universal serial bus (USB) storage device output—for saving of images and videos in USB devices
4. Camera head connector—to connect camera head to CCU

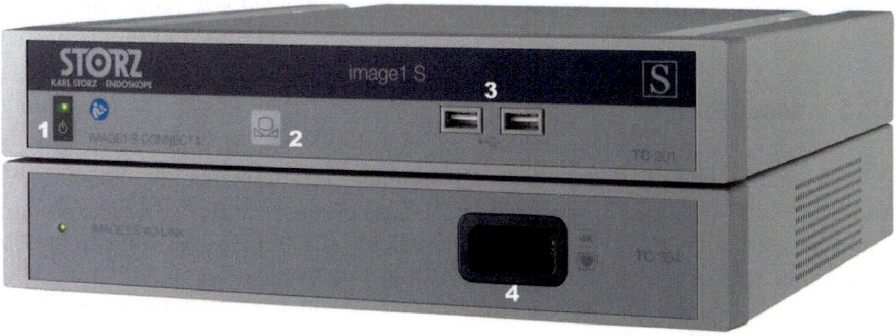

Fig. 12.2 Front view of CCU. (1—power button, 2—white balance, 3—USB for recording, 4—camera connector)

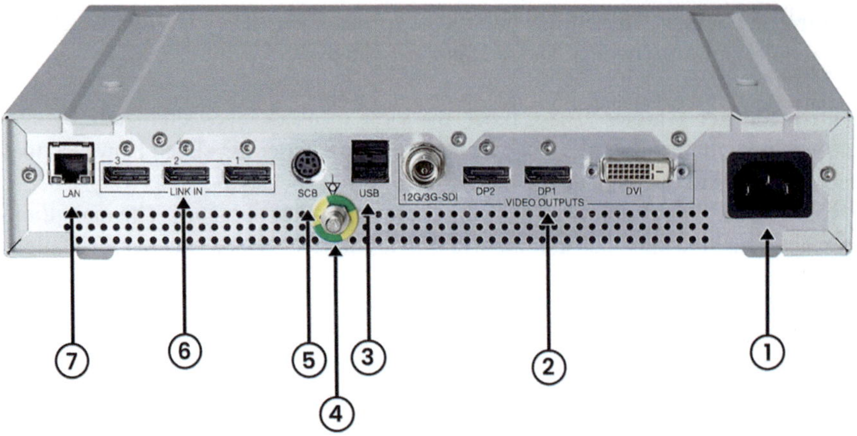

Fig. 12.3 Back view of CCU (labels are explained in the text)

12.1.7 Back View

1. Power cable connector—to connect power cable.
2. Video out ports—to attach compatible cables to carry video signal to monitor, recorder, etc.
3. USB connector—depending upon the model, USB ports can be used for keyboard, mouse, recording media, printer, foot pedal, software update, etc.
4. Potential equalization connector—this helps to reduce the risk of electrical shock to patients and medical personnel by minimizing potential differences between different equipment and conductive surfaces. The connector, usually a cable or a specific type of plug, can be plugged into the wall socket, ensuring that all equipment is connected to the same ground potential.
5. S video connector—used to connect S video cable to carry video signal.
6. Link In—to connect to various other devices that can be connected to this specific camera depending upon the model.
7. LAN—to connect LAN cable which can be used for different purposes depending upon the model.

12.2 Monitor

A laparoscopic monitor is an essential component in minimally invasive surgery, displaying high-resolution images from the laparoscopic camera. High-resolution liquid crystal display (LCD) or light-emitting diode (LED) monitors are suitable for the reproduction of endoscopic images. Their key differences are:

- *LCD (Liquid Crystal Display)*: Uses liquid crystals to produce images, but requires a backlight. Traditional LCDs use *CCFL (Cold Cathode Fluorescent Lamp)* backlighting.

- *LED (Light Emitting Diode)*: A type of LCD display that replaces CCFL back-lighting with LEDs, offering better brightness and contrast.

Feature	LED monitor	LCD monitor (CCFL)
Brightness	Higher, essential for bright operating rooms	Lower
Contrast ratio	Higher, providing clearer differentiation of tissues	Lower, less precise imaging
Colour accuracy	Better, crucial for distinguishing tissues and vessels	Moderate
Viewing angles	Wider, useful for multiple viewers in the OR	Narrower
Response time	Faster, reducing lag in real-time imaging	Slower
Energy efficiency	More efficient, generates less heat	Less efficient
Lifespan	Longer	Shorter
Size & thickness	Thinner and lighter	Bulkier

LED Monitors are Generally Preferred for Surgical Applications Because of:

- Better brightness
- Higher contrast
- More colour accuracy
- Lower heat emission
- Lesser energy consumption
- Faster response time, especially beneficial for endoscopic and robotic surgeries

12.2.1 Special Considerations for Surgical Displays

- *Anti-Reflective Coatings*: Reduces glare from surgical lights
- *Electromagnetic Interference (EMI) Shielding*: Prevents interference with other medical devices
- *Water & Dust Resistance*: For easy cleaning and disinfection
- *High Contrast, Brightness and Colour Accuracy*: For better representation and differentiation of tissues
- *Medical-grade Plastic or Metal*: Anti-bacterial and easy to clean
- *Sealed Buttons & Screen*: To prevent ingress of liquids and dust
- *Multiple Input/Output Ports*: HDMI, SDI, DVI, VGA, DisplayPort, USB, RS-232C, LAN, etc., for wide compatibility with different surgical devices

In general, the resolution capability of the monitor should match that of the video camera. Hence, HD monitor for HD camera and 4K monitor for 4K camera. Two separate monitors on each side of the table are commonly used for laparoscopic procedures.

Size and Pixels: A larger screen displaying the same number of pixels will have a lower spatial resolution compared to a smaller screen since the resolution is dependent on the pixel density. Most full HD monitors range from 26 to 32 inches in size (measured as diagonal of the screen). The advantage of UHD-4K technology in laparoscopy monitors is that it allows the image to be displayed on a larger screen of up to 55 inches without compromising the resolution. Larger 4K screens are available in different sizes ranging from 40 to 55 inches (Fig. 12.4).

Different monitors may have varying button layouts. This table presents a comprehensive overview of typical controls found in medical-grade monitors. It is important to note that not all buttons may be present in every monitor, and some monitors may have additional buttons.

Button	Function
Power button	Turns the monitor on/off
Input source selection	Switches between different input sources (e.g. HDMI, DVI, SDI)
Mode selection (e.g. endoscopy, fluoroscopy, etc.)	Optimizes display settings based on the procedure type
Brightness control	Adjusts screen brightness for optimal visibility
Contrast adjustment	Enhances differences between light and dark areas
Colour temperature	Modifies screen colour tone (e.g. warm, cool, neutral) to match surgeon preference
Sharpness control	Adjusts edge definition for a clearer image
OSD (on-screen display) menu	Opens monitor settings for advanced customization

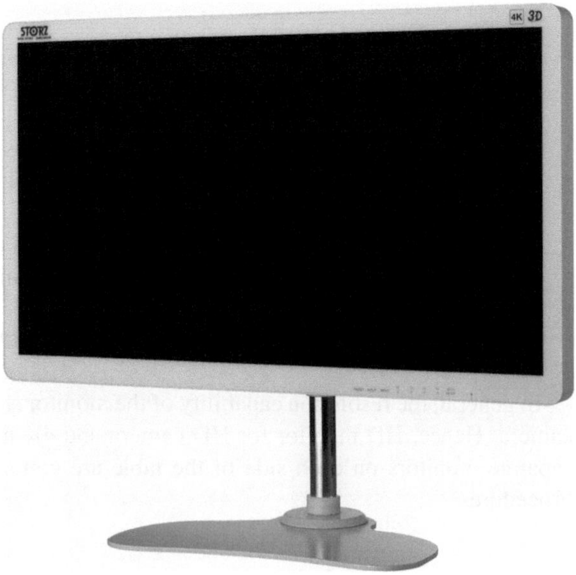

Fig. 12.4 Monitor

Button	Function
Mode selection (e.g. endoscopy, fluoroscopy, etc.)	Optimizes display settings based on the procedure type
Arrow buttons	Move menu items in respective direction and help in changing values of various settings
Picture-in-picture (PIP)/split screen	Displays multiple video feeds simultaneously.
Freeze frame	Holds the current image on-screen for closer examination

Monitors are equipped with a variety of rear connectors, as detailed in the subsequent table. It is crucial to acknowledge that not all monitors are compatible with all connectors, and some connectors may not be available on certain monitors. Technological advancements continually evolve, leading to changes in connector types.

Connector	Type	Function
HDMI (High-Definition Multimedia Interface)	Digital	Transmits high-definition video and audio
DVI (Digital Visual Interface)	Digital	Transfers high-quality video signals
SDI (Serial Digital Interface—3G, 6G, 12G SDI)	Digital	Provides long-distance, high-definition signal transmission
DisplayPort	Digital	High-resolution video with better bandwidth than HDMI
VGA (Video Graphics Array)	Analog	Transfers video signals, lower quality than digital interfaces
Composite Video (RCA—Yellow Plug)	Analog	Transmits standard-definition video signals
S-Video (Separate Video)	Analog	Better than composite video, separates colour and brightness signals
USB (Type-A, Type-B, Type-C)	Digital	Transfers data, video, and power in some models
RJ45 (Ethernet Port)	Digital	Network connection for remote monitoring and software updates
Audio In/Out (3.5mm Jack or RCA—Red & White Plugs)	Analog	Connects external audio devices or speakers
Fibre Optic Connector	Digital	High-speed data transfer with minimal signal loss

12.2.2 Placement

- Horizontal Placement: The monitor should be directly in front of the surgeon, aligned with the surgical field to minimize head and neck movement.
- Vertical Placement: The top of the monitor should be at or slightly below eye level (15–30° below horizontal eye level) to avoid excessive neck strain.
- Tilt: The monitor should be tilted slightly backward (10–15°) to reduce glare and improve visibility.

12.3 ICG Imaging in Laparoscopic Cameras

Indocyanine Green (ICG) imaging is a fluorescence-guided technology used in laparoscopic surgery. After intravenous injection, ICG binds to plasma proteins and emits fluorescence when exposed to near-infrared (NIR) light (~800 nm). Laparoscopic camera systems equipped with NIR capability can detect this fluorescence, allowing real-time visualization of structures such as bile ducts, blood vessels, ureters and lymph nodes.

These cameras allow surgeons to toggle between normal white light and fluorescence views, enhancing anatomical identification, improving safety and guiding decision-making in minimally invasive procedures.

12.3.1 ICG Administration Protocols for Laparoscopic Surgery

General guidelines for use of ICG are shown in the following table, but it must be borne in mind that different users have reported different protocols.

Procedure/use	ICG dose and route	Timing before imaging	Purpose
Laparoscopic cholecystectomy	2.5 mg IV	45 min to 2 h before surgery	Bile duct visualization to reduce injury risk
Liver resection	0.3–0.5 mg/kg IV	24 h before surgery (for tumour demarcation)	Segmental mapping and tumour margin detection
Colorectal surgery (perfusion check)	2.5–5 mg IV	Intraoperatively (just before or after anastomosis)	Assess bowel perfusion, reduce leak risk
Sentinel lymph node mapping	1–2 ml of 2.5 mg/ml ICG injected peritoneally	15–30 min before lymph node dissection	Guide lymphadenectomy in cancer surgery
Ureteral identification	25 mg ICG in 10 ml saline injected IV slowly	10–30 min before pelvic dissection	Enhances visualization of ureters to prevent injury
Endometriosis or peritoneal lesion detection	2.5–5 mg IV or diluted for peritoneal instillation	Intraoperative, shortly before exploration	Improves detection of endometriotic or ischemic tissues
Gastric/bariatric anastomosis	2.5–5 mg IV	Immediately before perfusion assessment	Evaluates blood flow to staple line or anastomosis
Nephrectomy/renal tumour surgery	0.25 mg/kg IV	10–20 min before vascular control	Assists in segmental perfusion mapping and tumour localization

12.4 Maintenance

As with all other medical equipment, regular maintenance plays a crucial role for monitors as well.

- Use approved disinfectants (alcohol-based or hospital-grade cleaners) to wipe the screen and control panel.
- Avoid abrasive materials, which may scratch the screen.
- Do not use excessive liquid to prevent moisture from entering the monitor.
- Use lint-free, soft microfibre cloths to clean the screen without leaving streaks.
- Avoid bending or twisting cables, as this can lead to signal loss or damage.
- Secure cables properly to prevent tripping hazards in the operating room.
- Maintain a dust-free, well-ventilated area around the monitor to prevent overheating.
- Avoid exposure to direct sunlight, which can degrade screen quality over time.
- Ensure proper electrical grounding to avoid static damage and power fluctuations.
- Turn off the monitor when not in use to extend its lifespan.
- Use protective covers when storing for long periods.
- Handle with care to avoid accidental screen cracks or internal damage.
- If applicable, update firmware/software to maintain compatibility with imaging systems.

12.5 Troubleshooting

Issue	Possible causes	Troubleshooting steps
No power/monitor not turn on	Loose or unplugged power cable Faulty power outlet or power adapter Internal hardware failure	Ensure the power cable is securely connected Try a different power outlet or adapter Check for any blown fuses or tripped circuit breakers
No image/blank screen	Incorrect input source selected Loose or damaged video cable Camera or imaging device not sending signal	Check and select the correct input source (HDMI, DVI, SDI, etc.) Inspect cables for damage and ensure firm connections Test with another monitor or device to rule out camera issues
Flickering or unstable image	Loose connection or faulty cable Electrical interference Refresh rate or resolution mismatch	Tighten or replace cables Move away from sources of electromagnetic interference (e.g. MRI, high-frequency devices) Adjust refresh rate and resolution in monitor settings

(continued)

Issue	Possible causes	Troubleshooting steps
Poor image quality (blurry, low contrast, washed out colours)	Incorrect brightness/contrast settings Dirty or damaged screen Camera focus issue	Adjust brightness, contrast, sharpness, and colour temperature Clean the screen with a soft, lint-free cloth Check and adjust the laparoscopic/endoscopic camera focus.
Frozen or lagging image	Overheating Software or firmware issue Hardware failure	Turn off the monitor and allow it to cool down Check for firmware updates Restart connected devices (camera, video processor)
Colour distortion (yellow/blue tint, unnatural colours)	Incorrect colour settings Damaged video cable Hardware fault in the monitor	Adjust colour settings (gamma, colour temperature) Replace the video cable Test with another input source to determine if the monitor or camera is at fault
Monitor turns off randomly	Overheating Power supply issue Automatic power-saving settings	Ensure adequate ventilation and no blockages in air vents Check for power fluctuations or loose connections Disable auto power-off settings if applicable

12.6 Future Directions

As the technology advances, we are likely to see many changes in the near future. Adoption of OLED and micro-LED for improved contrast, colour accuracy and reduced motion blur. Enhanced visualization in low-light conditions with better handling of dark areas in surgical fields. Flexible and curved displays for ergonomic positioning without compromising image quality. Touchscreen, voice-activated or gesture-controlled interfaces for easy access. Wireless video transmission to reduce cable clutter and improve OR mobility. Real-time AI-powered image processing to enhance clarity, detect structures and highlight anomalies.

12.7 Conclusion

Laparoscopic monitors play a critical role in modern minimally invasive surgery by providing high-resolution, real-time imaging essential for precision and efficiency. Proper selection, placement, maintenance and troubleshooting of these monitors significantly enhance surgical outcomes and reduce ergonomic strain on surgeons. Advances in display technology, image processing and connectivity continue to refine the surgical experience, ensuring improved visualization and patient safety.

Laparoscopes

13

Jun Liang Teh and Asim Shabbir

Since the first laparoscopic appendectomy in 1980, laparoscopic surgery has gained widespread acceptance, with minimally invasive surgery (MIS) now considered the gold standard for conditions such as appendicitis and cholecystitis. Advances in surgical hardware have greatly enhanced visualization and magnification of the operative field, enabling greater precision in dissection, improving safety, and making complex procedures more feasible.

This chapter explores the role of laparoscopes in MIS, the types of laparoscopes currently available, practical considerations during use, maintenance protocols and recent technological innovations.

13.1 Anatomy of the Laparoscope

The origins of endoscopic visualization can be traced to Philip Bozzini's early cystoscope, which used reflecting mirrors, candles, and a urethral cannula to examine the canine bladder. Key milestones in the development of modern laparoscopy include the incorporation of the electric bulb, cold light fibre optic illumination, gas insufflation for abdominal distension, and the introduction of the rod-lens system [6].

Two major types of laparoscopes are in use today:

J. L. Teh
Department of Surgery, JurongHealth Campus, National University Health System, Singapore, Singapore

A. Shabbir (✉)
Department of Surgery, National University Hospital, National University Health System, Singapore, Singapore
e-mail: Suras@nus.edu.sg

J. S. Ahluwalia (ed.), *User Manual for Minimally Invasive Surgical Equipment*,
https://doi.org/10.1007/978-981-95-9019-3_13

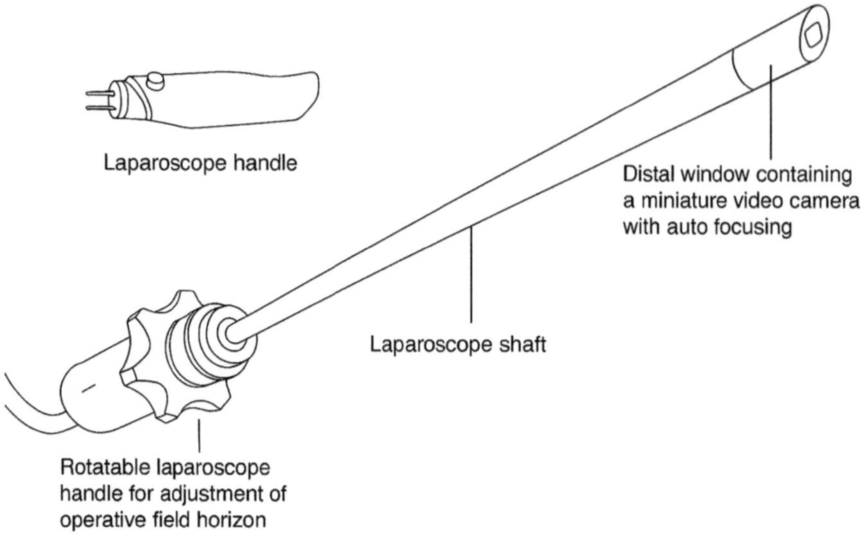

Image 13.1 Example of an all-in-one digital laparoscope system. (Depicted here is the Olympus Endo Eye System)

1. *Rod-Lens Laparoscopes*

   These have a rigid shaft containing a system of optical lenses, a light post, light cables, and an eyepiece. The image is captured by the objective lens at the distal tip and transmitted via a lens train to the camera head, where it is processed and displayed on an external monitor.
2. *Digital Laparoscopes*

   These devices integrate a camera sensor (CCD or CMOS) directly at the tip of the endoscope. Systems like the Olympus EndoEye eliminate the need for a separate camera head and offer features such as auto-focusing, creating a streamlined "all-in-one" design (Image 13.1). Despite this innovation, rod-lens systems remain widely used due to their image clarity and durability.

13.2 Choosing a Laparoscope

Laparoscope selection depends on the surgical procedure and surgeon preference, with factors such as scope diameter, angle of view, and specialized imaging capabilities influencing the choice. Generally, the principal considerations for laparoscope choice will be its size as well as the field of view required. Most laparoscopes utilize a fibre optic halogen or LED light source, but certain laparoscopes may have unique functions such as near infrared fluorescence (NIRF) for detection of indocyanine green (ICG), which may be indicated in certain clinical scenarios.

13.2.1 5 mm vs 10 mm Laparoscopes

Laparoscopes are manufactured in several diameters, and the most commonly used laparoscopes are the 10 mm and 5 mm laparoscopes. Traditionally, 10 mm laparoscopes were preferred as they offered higher resolution and sharper images, but in recent years, image quality for 5 mm laparoscopes has been comparable to their 10 mm counterparts with comparable working lengths. 5 mm laparoscopes fit into smaller laparoscopic ports, which offers benefits of a smaller incision which reduces post-operative pain and potentially reduces the risk of developing incisional port site hernias. Small randomized controlled trials have demonstrated that patients undergoing laparoscopic total hysterectomy [1] with 5 mm umbilical ports and laparoscopes had shorter operative times and lesser post-operative pain with similar complication rates and length of stay. Although uncommon, needlescopic surgery with the use of smaller (2–3 mm) [7, 8] laparoscopes has been described in the literature for various surgical procedures as well [14].

13.2.2 Angle of View

The most common angles of view offered by commercially available laparoscopes are the 0-degree, 30-degree (Image 13.2), and 45-degree laparoscopes. In recent years, with the advent of flexible tip digital laparoscopes, laparoscopes with angulation of up to 100 degrees have been available as well. Zero-degree laparoscopes provide a straight end-on view of the operative field. These laparoscopes provide a brighter and sharper image, but with a shallow depth of field and may not be ideal for overhead views. Zero-degree laparoscopes are useful in certain scenarios such as when optical entry is performed or in scenarios when the axis of the instruments and the laparoscope are similar such as in single incision laparoscopic surgery.

In most laparoscopic surgeries where triangulation of the laparoscopic ports is essential to facilitate traction and visualization of the operative field, 30-degree

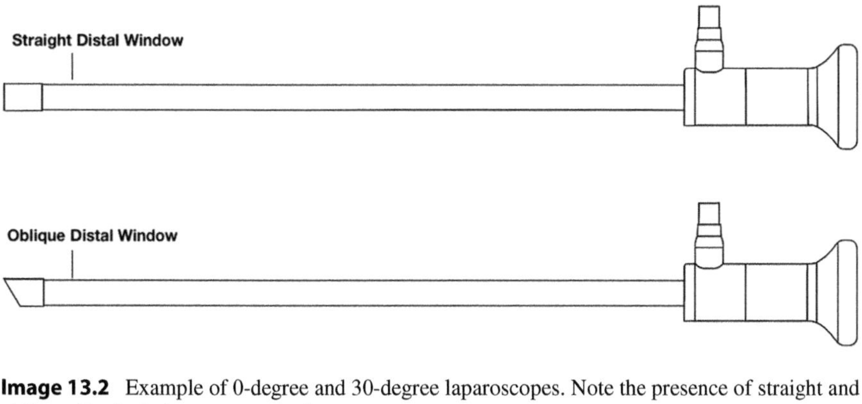

Image 13.2 Example of 0-degree and 30-degree laparoscopes. Note the presence of straight and oblique distal windows, respectively

cameras are preferred as these laparoscopes provide a greater range of view, facilitating instrument manipulation and laparoscopic suturing. Rotation of the fibre optics of the 30-degree laparoscope will offer better visualization in the lateral axis, and the fibre optics moves in the opposite direction to the rotation direction. That is, rotation of the fibre optic to the left will show more right-sided views of the operative field and vice versa. Rotation of the fibre optic 180 degrees will allow better visualization of the roof of the operative field and may be especially helpful in surgeries such as abdominal wall hernia repair.

Flexible tip laparoscopes offer an even greater range of view compared to traditional rigid laparoscopes and the articulating laparoscopes such as the ENDOEYE Flex provides a field of view up to 100 degrees in four directions (Image 13.3). Flexible tip laparoscopes usually have two controls, one for left-right movement and the other for up-down movements. Early in vitro studies found that flexible tip laparoscopes have no advantage over standard rigid 30-degree laparoscopes [11] in simulated surgical models. However, later studies demonstrated that flexible tip laparoscopes may reduce operating time in single incision laparoscopic cholecystectomy and reduce laparoscope contact with working instruments [10]. Flexible tip laparoscopes are also newer digital laparoscopes with the chip-in-tip technology with no need for manual focusing; however, the learning curve of learning how to handle a flexible tip laparoscope may present more challenges to a novice surgical assistant compared to the conventional rigid laparoscopes.

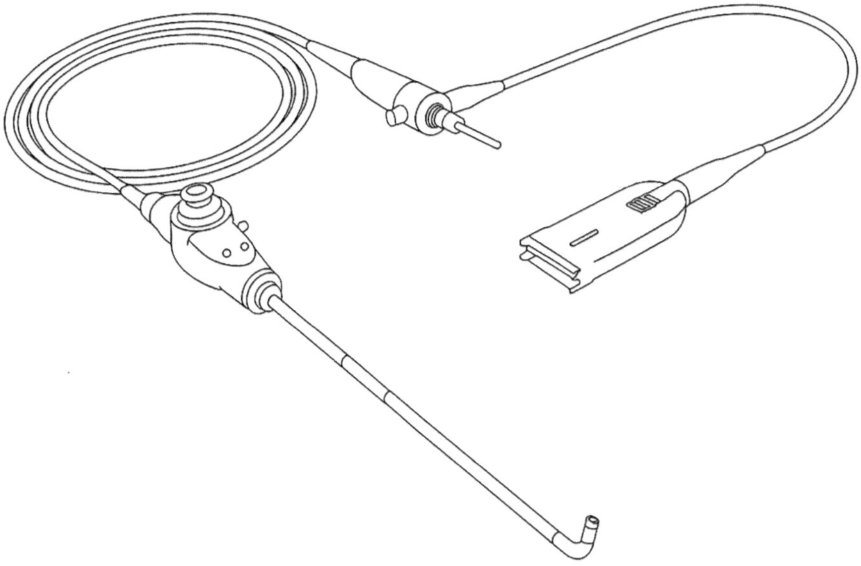

Image 13.3 Example of a flexible tip laparoscope

13.2.3 Three-Dimensional Imaging and 4 K Systems

Most laparoscopy systems utilize a two-dimensional display which provides the surgical team with mono-ocular view of the surgical field. The drawback of a two-dimensional system is that of loss of binocular vision which provides the operator with a stereoscopic depth perception; without depth perception, complex laparoscopic tasks can still be performed by adapting to other light cues such as object interposition, object size, and instrument parallax as a substitute for estimating depth [13], but may increase surgeon fatigue increasing the chance for mistakes.

Several 3D systems are now available on the market, such as the VISCERA ELITE II 3D® from Olympus or the IMAGE1 S™ 3D laparoscope from Karl-Storz. 3D laparoscopes are dual-channel laparoscopes (Image 13.4) which consist of either two separate rod lens or two separate chips to capture two slightly different images of the same object which are co-displayed on a stereoscopic display with oppositely polarized lights. Similar to how the human brain processes two retinal images to generate one image with depth perception, the surgeon now is able to perceive the operating field with depth perception after donning polarized 3D glasses which polarize alternate rows of pixels corresponding to left and right eye images. In a randomized controlled trial, the use of 3D imaging improved depth perception and reduced strain in both novice and experienced surgeons and reduced execution time for laparoscopic cholecystectomy amongst novice surgeons [5]. The EAES consensus development conference in 2018 concluded that with the use of

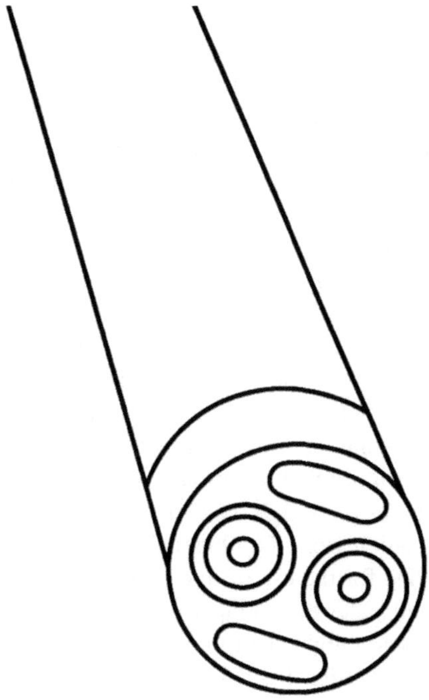

Image 13.4 Tip of 3D scope has two lenses to capture image in 3D format

3D, operative time was significantly shortened with significant reduction of operative complications, particularly in cases which required laparoscopic suturing [2].

Another recent innovation in laparoscopy is the adaptation of 4 K imaging technology into laparoscopes. 4 K systems provide high-resolution 2D images with quadrupled pixel count compared to a conventional 2D full high-definition system, allowing the projection of ultra-high-resolution images in the operating suite. The Olympus Visera Ultra HD 4 K system generates a wider colour gamut which adopts the 4 K colour format (BT2020), allowing greater contrast and appreciation of subtle differences in tissue colour as well as panoramic views and preserved resolution when the image is zoomed in. Several studies have studied the potential benefits of operating with a 4 K laparoscope. In a randomized cross-over trial comparing 3D versus 4 K display systems, 3D systems shortened operating time in operators regardless of their surgical expertise and reduced errors in novice operators [15]. A meta-analysis also concluded that utilization of 3D technology resulted in shorter operative time and better efficiency of movement as a result of better depth perception but may result in higher visual side effects compared to the 4 K group [12]. The adaptation of 4 K technology in 5 mm laparoscopes now allows the projection of high-quality images surpassing those offered by conventional 10 mm HD laparoscopes.

13.2.4 Near Infrared (NIFR) Laparoscopes

In recent years, the indications of fluorescence dye imaging have dramatically expanded in the field of surgery.

Fluorescence dye imaging can be used for localization of lesions during laparoscopic surgery to aid in surgical resection and tissue preservation, identification of the biliary system during hepatobiliary surgery, sentinel lymph node mapping in oncological surgery, and assessment of tissue perfusion and bowel viability amongst other uses. The most commonly used fluorescence dye is indocyanine green (ICG). ICG binds to plasma proteins and is excited by infrared radiation to emit a fluorescent light.

Traditional laparoscopic light sources utilize a xenon light source which provides a white light image. Modern infrared laparoscopes are able to combine white light images and fluorescence imaging under near infrared light in real time. These systems require the use of an infrared xenon light source. The laparoscope possesses an optical filter which can be turned on to suppress the infrared radiation when a white light image is required. In infrared mode, the optical filters allow the passage of infrared radiation and suppression of the red light wavelength. The emitted fluorescence light can then be visualized either with or without background illumination from the blue and green wavelengths of light. Recently, a consensus guideline for the use of fluorescence imaging in hepatobiliary has been published [16] and states that in laparoscopic cholecystectomy, the use of fluorescence imaging may highlight aberrant anatomy and accessory biliary ducts, thereby aiding the surgeon in safer dissection of the Calot's Triangle. ICG also increases the lymph node yield in gastric cancer patients undergoing D2 lymphadenectomy [4] and improved visualization of the common hepatic duct during hepatobiliary surgery [9].

13.3 Laparoscope Maintenance

Maintenance of the laparoscope will include the following: careful use of the laparoscope and examination of the endoscope before and after each use and adequate reprocessing of the laparoscope to ensure that the equipment is sterile before it is used for the next patient. As the laparoscope is a delicately built system of lens and or electrical components, the shaft of the endoscope should not be bent, and the scope should be handled with care. The team should pay attention not to leave the laparoscope at the edge of the sterile trolley or the operating table where it may be prone being dropped. While handling the laparoscope, one should also take care not to violently shake the scope as this may displace the lens train in the laparoscope resulting in image quality degradation.

Before and after each case, the endoscope should also be examined thoroughly to inspect for any obvious scratches and shaft damage which might compromise image quality. The surgeon should inspect the lens by looking through the eye piece at the proximal end of the endoscope and rotate the instrument clockwise to check for any image distortion, haziness of the image, or presence of condensation in the rod lens system.

The steps to clean the laparoscope will include dismantling, decontamination, pre-cleaning, cleaning and rinsing, drying, sterilization followed by storage. After each use, the laparoscope should be removed from the camera head, and any adapters that were used to connect the light cables should also be removed to be cleaned separately. The cleaning process starts in the operating room when any visible blood and body fluids on the laparoscope are wiped off by the nursing staff. The instruments are then soaked in a pH-neutral disinfectant solution up to an hour. Pre cleaning is then performed in the Central Sterile Supplies Department (CSSD) with the use of enzymatic solutions to dissolve any body fluids that were not removed by the initial decontamination and cleaning process. If stains persist on the optical surface after the use of enzymatic solution, we can attempt to clean the surfaces with the use of cotton swab moistened with 70% alcohol. It is imperative to rinse the optical surface and equipment thoroughly with distilled water to remove any excess enzymatic or cleaning solutions. The use of distilled water is important for two reasons; the use of tap water may result in a hard layer of lime deposits forming on the instruments overtime which is not easily removable; furthermore, the water used needs to be free of micro-organisms to minimize the risk of infection. The use of ultrasonic cleaners on laparoscopes is to be avoided as the lens position may be displaced during the ultrasonic cleaning process, again resulting in degradation of image quality.

The final step of reprocessing for laparoscopes is sterilization, following thorough cleaning of the laparoscope. Most scopes can undergo gas sterilization with ethylene oxide, with conditioning, sterilization, and aeration parameters specified by the individual manufacturer. Certain laparoscopes marked "AUTOCLAV" can undergo autoclaving, otherwise known as steam sterilization using the pre-vacuum or gravity displacement method.

13.4 Troubleshooting

13.4.1 Fogging of the Laparoscope

Fogging of the laparoscope lens occurs frequently, especially at the beginning of the operation. It occurs because the shaft and the lens of the laparoscope are at a lower temperature compared to that of the abdominal cavity, thereby promoting condensation on the shaft and the objective lens. This usually improves when the laparoscope is gradually warmed up to the temperature of the abdominal cavity. Condensation can also occur when the laparoscope is near energy devices resulting in surgical plume condensation on the laparoscope lens. Furthermore, the proximity of the lens to the surgical field predisposes contact with blood and tissue fluid onto the lens, obscuring the view of the surgical field. When this happens, the assistant usually must remove the laparoscope for cleaning of the scope lens. To reduce fogging due to temperature differences between the scope and abdominal cavity, it is also common practice to warm the laparoscope temperature in a flask of saline or water maintained at around 50 degrees [3] before reapplication of anti-fog solution to the lens. It is also common for fluid to pool around the valve of the trocar port and in the port itself, hence the entry site of the trocar and the inside of the port should also be cleaned to minimize recontamination of the camera lens.

When tissue fluid obscures the view on the laparoscope lens, one common practice by the surgical assistant is to clean the lens on the surface of the liver or the bowel to remove the fluid. Although sometimes this may be successful in restoring the view of the surgical field, tissue fluid containing proteins can dry on laparoscopic lens, necessitating more force to clean the lens to remove these proteinaceous stains. This may lead to the removal of the optical coating on the objective lens, thereby hastening the degradation of the image quality provided by the laparoscope. Apart from anti-fogging solutions and warm saline, commercial all-in-one products such as Clearify® are also available to aid cleaning and visualization. The Clearify® system has a multi-functioning hub which warms up the laparoscope, cleans the objective lens, helps with white balancing, and has a micro pad for cleaning debris off the laparoscope.

13.4.2 Poor Visualization with Blood in the Surgical Field

The presence of blood in the surgical field causes the dimming of surgical field as light emitted from the laparoscope is absorbed by the blood in the field. Ways to circumvent this problem will include increasing the light intensity of the laparoscope, suctioning of blood clots, and lavage of the surgical field. Increasing the light intensity of the laparoscope will sometimes result in excessive lens glare which

Table 13.1 Troubleshooting common problems

Problem	Possible causes	Solutions
Fogging of the lens	Cold laparoscope entering a warm cavity Insufflation cooling the scope Lens contamination with fluids or fat	Pre-warm the laparoscope using warm saline or light source and use anti-fog solution or defogging wipes Use warmed and humidified CO_2 insufflation Clean the lens with warm saline as needed
Blurry image	Improper focus Lens contamination Poor camera settings	Adjust focus on the camera coupler Remove and clean the scope Ensure proper white balance and camera settings
Dark or dull image	Light source issue Fibre optic cable or scope damage Wrong light cable connection	Increase light intensity on the light source Check fibre optic cable and scope for damage and replace if needed Ensure proper connection of the light cable to the laparoscope

again may compromise the view. Furthermore, one should also be aware of the high temperature of the laparoscope which may result in inadvertent tissue burns when the light intensity is increased, especially if the laparoscope is in contact with tissue. A temporizing measure is to place a piece of white gauze in the surgical field over the area with the blood clots so that less light is absorbed by the blood in the field. This will allow the surgeon to continue the operation or to suction the clots with continued illumination of the surgical field.

Table 13.1 provides some common problems with their possible causes and solutions.

13.5 Conclusion

The laparoscope is an integral part of laparoscopic surgery, and without it, minimally invasive surgery will not be possible. The last two decades have seen a tremendous improvement in imaging technology in laparoscopes, and the advent of 3D and 4 K technology has shortened operative time, reduced surgical error, and facilitated the conduct of more complex surgeries through a laparoscopic approach. Laparoscopes, however, are delicate and expensive equipment, and there is a need for the surgical team to understand how to maintain and troubleshoot these laparoscopes so that the longevity of this delicate equipment can be lengthened.

Acknowledgements The authors would like to thank Ms. Sophia Eng, Assistant Manager, Olympus Singapore Pvt. Ltd. for providing and approving the use of the images in this chapter.

References

1. Acton JN, Salfinger SG, Tan J, Cohen PA. Outcomes of total laparoscopic hysterectomy using a 5-mm versus 10-mm laparoscope: a randomized control trial. J Minim Invasive Gynecol. 2016;23(1):101–6.
2. Arezzo A, Vettoretto N, Francis NK, Bonino MA, Curtis NJ, Amparore D, Arolfo S, Barberio M, Boni L, Brodie R, Bouvy N, Cassinotti E, Carus T, Checcucci E, Custers P, Diana M, Jansen M, Jaspers J, Marom G, Momose K, Muller-Stich BP, Nakajima K, Nickel F, Perretta S, Porpiglia F, Sanchez-Margallo F, Sanchez-Margallo JA, Schijven M, Silecchia G, Passera R, Mintz Y. The use of 3D laparoscopic imaging systems in surgery: EAES consensus development conference 2018. Surg Endosc. 2019;33(10):3251–74.
3. Brown JA, Inocencio MD, Sundaram CP. Use of a warming bath to prevent lens fogging during laparoscopy. J Endourol. 2008;22(11):2413–4.
4. Chen QY, Xie JW, Zhong Q, Wang JB, Lin JX, Lu J, Cao LL, Lin M, Tu RH, Huang ZN, Lin JL, Zheng HL, Li P, Zheng CH, Huang CM. Safety and efficacy of Indocyanine green tracer-guided lymph node dissection during laparoscopic radical gastrectomy in patients with gastric cancer: a randomized clinical trial. JAMA Surg. 2020;155(4):300–11.
5. Curro G, La Malfa G, Lazzara S, Caizzone A, Fortugno A, Navarra G. Three-dimensional versus two-dimensional laparoscopic cholecystectomy: is surgeon experience relevant? J Laparoendosc Adv Surg Tech A. 2015;25(7):566–70.
6. Gordon AG, Magos AL. The development of laparoscopic surgery. Baillieres Clin Obstet Gynaecol. 1989;3(3):429–49.
7. Kanehira E, Tanida T, Kamei A, Nakagi M, Yoshida T, Touma S. Needlescopic intragastric surgery facilitated by newly developed 2mm instruments. Minim Invasive Ther Allied Technol. 2016;25(4):210–4.
8. Lai EC, Fok M, Chan AS. Needlescopic cholecystectomy: prospective study of 150 patients. Hong Kong Med J. 2003;9(4):238–42.
9. Lim SH, Tan HTA, Shelat VG. Comparison of indocyanine green dye fluorescent cholangiography with intra-operative cholangiography in laparoscopic cholecystectomy: a meta-analysis. Surg Endosc. 2021;35(4):1511–20.
10. Matsui Y, Ryota H, Sakaguchi T, Nakatani K, Matsushima H, Yamaki S, Hirooka S, Yamamoto T, Kwon AH. Comparison of a flexible-tip laparoscope with a rigid straight laparoscope for single-incision laparoscopic cholecystectomy. Am Surg. 2014;80(12):1245–9.
11. Perrone JM, Ames CD, Yan Y, Landman J. Evaluation of surgical performance with standard rigid and flexible-tip laparoscopes. Surg Endosc. 2005;19(10):1325–8.
12. Singla V, Bhattacharjee HK, Gupta E, Singh D, Mishra AK, Kumar D. Performance of three-dimensional and ultra-high-definition (4K) technology in laparoscopic surgery: a systematic review and meta-analysis. J Minim Access Surg. 2022;18(2):167–75.
13. Sinha RY, Raje SR, Rao GA. Three-dimensional laparoscopy: principles and practice. J Minim Access Surg. 2017;13(3):165–9.
14. Tagaya N, Kubota K. Reevaluation of needlescopic surgery. Surg Endosc. 2012;26(1):137–43.
15. Wahba R, Datta R, Busshoff J, Bruns T, Hedergott A, Gietzelt C, Dieplinger G, Fuchs H, Morgenstern B, Moller D, Hellmich M, Bruns CJ, Stippel DL. 3D versus 4K display system – influence of "state-of-the-art"-display technique on surgical performance (IDOSP-study) in minimally invasive surgery: a randomized cross-over trial. Ann Surg. 2020;272(5):709–14.
16. Wang X, Teh CSC, Ishizawa T, Aoki T, Cavallucci D, Lee SY, Panganiban KM, Perini MV, Shah SR, Wang H, Xu Y, Suh KS, Kokudo N. Consensus guidelines for the use of fluorescence imaging in hepatobiliary surgery. Ann Surg. 2021;274(1):97–106.

Light Source and Light Cable

14

Laurent A. Layani and Alpa Morawala

14.1 Light Source

Laparoscopic surgery, also known as minimally invasive surgery, has revolutionized the field of surgical procedures since its introduction in the late 1980s. One crucial aspect of laparoscopic surgery is the use of light sources to illuminate the surgical field and provide clear visibility to the surgeon. In this chapter, we will delve into the historical evolution of light sources in laparoscopic surgery, examining their development over time and gaining a comprehensive understanding of their relationship with equipment to optimize their utilization. Additionally, we will address the significance of maintaining and troubleshooting these light sources to ensure optimal performance.

14.2 Introduction

A good laparoscopic light source should emit light as near as possible to natural sun light. A typical light source consists of:

- A lamp (bulb).
- A heat filter.
- Manual or automatic intensity control circuit (shutter).

L. A. Layani
Department of Surgery, Minimal Access Surgery and Bariatric Surgery, Alsharq Hospital, Fujairah, UAE

A. Morawala (✉)
General Surgery, Barts Health NHS Trust, London, UK
e-mail: A.morawala@nhs.net

J. S. Ahluwalia (ed.), *User Manual for Minimally Invasive Surgical Equipment*,
https://doi.org/10.1007/978-981-95-9019-3_14

Light originates from an object when it is heated sufficiently, and the colour (wavelength) of the light emitted varies with the temperature of the source, and this phenomenon is described by Planck's law of black-body radiation [1]. This colour property of temperature is measured in degrees Kelvin (K°).

Light sources with higher K° contain more high-frequency (blue) wavelengths, resulting in a brighter and more accurate image. Quality of the image obtained during the laparoscopic procedure depends on the quantity of light available at each step of the optical and electronic system. It is imperative for the laparoscopic team, particularly the surgeon, to be well-versed in the intricacies of the light source.

(a) Lower temperatures (lower kelvin values, e.g. 2000 K to 3000 K): These light sources appear more reddish or "warmer" in colour. They emit a higher proportion of longer-wavelength light, including red and orange hues. Incandescent light bulbs are an example of light sources with lower colour temperatures [2].
(b) Higher temperatures (higher kelvin values, e.g. 5000 K to 6500 K and above): These light sources appear bluish or "cooler" in colour. They emit a higher proportion of shorter-wavelength light, including blue and white hues. Daylight and many LED light sources fall into this category [2].

The concept of laparoscopy began in the early twentieth century, with early pioneers like Georg Kelling (1901) and Hans Christian Jacobaeus (1910) using incandescent bulbs mounted on cystoscopes for illumination. These early light sources were inefficient, producing heat and poor lighting. The introduction of fibre optic technology in the 1950s revolutionized laparoscopic lighting. Harold Hopkins and Karl Storz developed cold light sources, utilizing fibre optics to transmit light from an external source, reducing heat exposure and improving brightness.

In the 1980s, halogen and later xenon light sources became the standard. These sources were integrated with light cables and endoscopes, making laparoscopy more effective. Halogen bulbs, while widely used initially, produce a yellowish light with lower intensity and generate more heat, which can pose risks of overheating and tissue damage. They also have a shorter lifespan, requiring frequent replacements. In contrast, xenon light sources offer a much brighter, whiter light that closely mimics natural daylight, enhancing colour accuracy and tissue differentiation, which is crucial in laparoscopy. Additionally, xenon bulbs are more energy-efficient and have a longer lifespan than halogen, making them a superior choice for modern surgical procedures despite their higher cost.

The early 2000s witnessed a significant breakthrough with the introduction of light-emitting diode (LED) technology in laparoscopic surgery [3]. LED light sources offered several advantages over their predecessors. They were compact, energy-efficient, and had a longer lifespan. LED lights also produced a wide spectrum of light, enabling better colour representation and enhancing tissue differentiation during surgery. Furthermore, LED lights generated less heat, improving patient safety and reducing the risk of thermal injury.

14.2.1 Lamp

The lamp or bulb is the most important part of the light source. When the bulb fails, the entire system fails.

Three common types of lamps used as laparoscopic light sources include:

1. Halogen.
2. Xenon.
3. LED.

14.2.1.1 Halogen [4]

Halogen light sources operate by passing an electric current through a tungsten filament enclosed in a halogen gas-filled bulb. The filament heats up to produce visible light, while the halogen gas helps recycle tungsten deposits back onto the filament, extending its lifespan compared to traditional incandescent bulbs. However, halogen bulbs generate a significant amount of heat and emit a yellowish light with lower intensity, which can affect colour accuracy in laparoscopic surgery. They require additional cooling mechanisms, such as fans or heat sinks, to prevent overheating of fibre optic cables and endoscopic instruments.

14.2.1.2 Xenon Lights [5]

Xenon light sources use a high-voltage electrical arc between two electrodes inside a xenon gas-filled bulb to produce a bright, white light that closely resembles natural daylight. The high-intensity arc excites xenon gas molecules, generating a continuous, broad-spectrum light with excellent colour rendering, which is crucial for distinguishing tissues accurately during surgery. Xenon bulbs provide higher brightness and better illumination depth compared to halogen lamps, making them the preferred choice for laparoscopic procedures. Additionally, xenon bulbs have a longer lifespan and operate at a cooler temperature than halogen, reducing the risk of overheating and improving safety. However, they require specialized power supplies and cooling systems to maintain stable performance.

14.2.1.3 LED [6, 7]

Light-emitting diode (LED) sources work by passing an electric current through a semiconductor material, which excites electrons and releases energy in the form of photons. Unlike halogen and xenon lamps, LEDs do not rely on filaments or gas discharges, making them highly energy-efficient and durable. LED light sources emit a bright, white light with excellent colour accuracy and minimal heat production, eliminating the need for complex cooling systems. Their long lifespan, low energy consumption, and ability to provide consistent illumination without degradation make them the most advanced option in modern laparoscopy. Additionally, some LED systems incorporate tunable wavelengths and fluorescence imaging capabilities, further enhancing surgical visualization and precision.

14.3 Comparison of Light Sources

Feature	Halogen	Xenon	LED
Light intensity	Moderate	Very high	High
Colour temperature (K)	~3000 to 3500 K (yellowish)	~5600 to 6000 K (daylight white)	~5000 to 6500 K (cool white)
Brightness consistency	Decreases over time	Stable but degrades gradually	Very stable over long time
Lifespan	500 to 1000 hours	500 to 1000 hours	20,000 to 50,000+ hours
Heat generation	High	High	Low
Energy efficiency	Low	Moderate	High
Warm-up time	Short	Short	Instant
Size & portability	Bulky	Bulky	Compact
Cost	Low (initial), higher replacement	High (initial and maintenance)	High (initial), low maintenance cost
Safety (thermal risk)	Potential burns	Higher risk due to heat	Very low risk
Usage in modern surgery	Declining	Still common in many systems	Increasingly popular

14.4 Concept of LED RGB

LED RGB (red, green, blue) light technology in laparoscopic surgery is an advanced illumination system that enhances visualization by allowing adjustable light wavelengths for better tissue differentiation and improved contrast. Unlike traditional white light sources such as halogen or xenon, RGB LED systems generate light by combining red, green, and blue LEDs in varying intensities to produce a broad spectrum of colours, including pure white light. This allows surgeons to customize the lighting conditions based on the specific surgical need.

One of the key advantages of RGB LED technology in laparoscopy is enhanced tissue contrast and differentiation. Different tissues absorb and reflect specific wavelengths differently; for example, haemoglobin in blood absorbs more blue and green light, making vascular structures more distinct when these colours are adjusted. By tuning the RGB light components, surgeons can highlight specific anatomical features, improving their ability to identify structures like nerves, tumours, and blood vessels with greater precision.

Additionally, RGB LED light sources are often integrated with *fluorescence-guided surgery* techniques, such as *near-infrared (NIR) imaging* with indocyanine green (ICG). By optimizing green and near-infrared light wavelengths, surgeons can visualize perfusion, lymphatic drainage, and tumour margins more effectively.

Another benefit of RGB LED systems is reduced eye strain and improved colour rendering, as they provide a more natural and customizable illumination environment. This reduces surgeon fatigue during long procedures and enhances overall surgical efficiency.

14.4.1 Heat Filter

Heat filters in laparoscopic light sources are essential components designed to reduce thermal energy transmission while maintaining optimal illumination. Since traditional high-intensity light sources like halogen and xenon generate significant heat, direct exposure to this thermal energy can damage fibre optic cables, overheat laparoscopic instruments, and potentially cause tissue injury inside the body. Heat filters help mitigate these risks by selectively blocking infrared (IR) radiation, which is responsible for heat generation, while allowing visible light to pass through.

One common type of heat filter used in laparoscopic light sources is the *infrared (IR) cutoff filter*, which consists of specialized glass or coatings that absorb or reflect IR wavelengths while transmitting visible light. Another advanced technology is the *cold light filter*, which redirects heat away from the fibre optic cable, ensuring that only cool, bright light reaches the endoscope.

With the advent of LED light sources, the need for heat filters has significantly reduced since LEDs produce minimal infrared radiation compared to halogen and xenon lamps.

14.4.2 The Intensity Control Circuit (Manual or Automatic)

The intensity control circuit of a laparoscopic light source can be either manual or automatic, depending on the design of the light source and the specific needs of the surgical procedure. Both types of control circuits serve the purpose of adjusting the brightness of the light output to optimize visibility during laparoscopic surgery.

14.5 Manual Intensity Control

User-Operated: Manual intensity control involves the surgeon or an assistant adjusting the light source's brightness settings manually. This can be done through knobs, dials, or buttons on the control panel of the light source.

User Flexibility: Manual control provides the surgical team with the flexibility to tailor the light intensity to their preferences and the specific requirements of the procedure. Surgeons can adjust the brightness in real-time to enhance visualization.

Real-time Adjustments: Surgeons can increase or decrease the light intensity as needed during different phases of the surgery, such as when moving from a deep tissue dissection to a more superficial view.

14.6 Automatic Intensity Control

Closed-Loop Systems: Some laparoscopic light sources are equipped with automatic intensity control mechanisms. These systems often use feedback from sensors to adjust the light output automatically.

Brightness Stabilization: Automatic control ensures that the light intensity remains stable, even if there are changes in the working distance or the condition of the surgical field. Sensors can monitor the brightness and make real-time adjustments to maintain a consistent level.

Reduce Surgeon Distraction: By offloading the intensity control to an automatic system, surgeons can focus more on the surgical procedure without the need to constantly adjust the light source.

The choice between manual and automatic intensity control may depend on several factors, including the surgeon's preferences, the complexity of the procedure, the specific laparoscopic equipment being used, and the available technology. Some advanced laparoscopic light sources may offer both manual and automatic control options, allowing the surgical team to choose the method that best suits their needs.

14.7 Description of Light Source (Fig. 14.1)

14.7.1 How to Connect

1. Plug in the AC power cord to the AC Inlet on the rear console panel.
2. Plug in the other end of the AC cord to a hospital-grade outlet.
3. The output from the light source is conducted to the telescope by light cables.

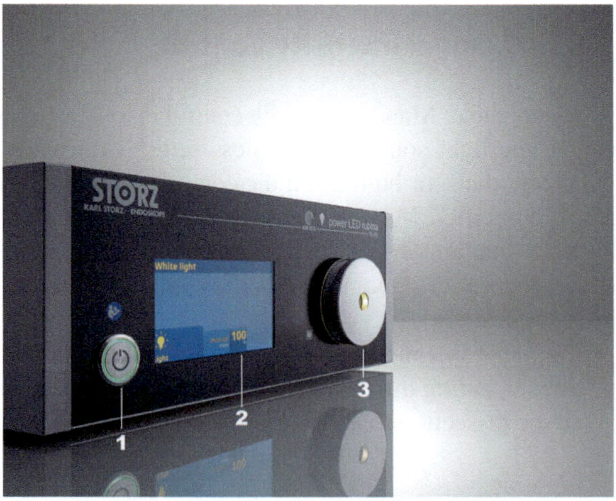

Fig. 14.1 Light source (1—power on/off, 2—adjustment screen, 3—light cable connector). (Courtesy: Karl Storz)

14.7.2 Buttons and Controls in a Laparoscopic Light Source

Due to the diverse nature of light sources manufactured by various companies, a comprehensive overview of potential features present on a given machine is provided. Please bear in mind that all features may not be available in all such machines.

1. *Power Button*:
   - Turns the device on/off. Some units have a standby mode for quick reactivation.
2. *Standby Mode Button*:
   - Temporarily reduces light output without turning off the unit, allowing quick reactivation.
3. *Light Intensity Control (Brightness Adjustment)*:
   - Dial or digital buttons adjust the brightness level based on surgical needs.
   - Higher intensity is used for deep cavities, while lower intensity reduces glare on shiny tissues.
4. *Colour Temperature Adjustment*:
   - May be available in some LED systems to modify the light spectrum for optimal visualization.
   - Adjusting between warm (yellowish) and cool (bluish) tones enhances tissue differentiation.
5. *Auto/Manual Mode Selection*:
   - Auto Mode: Adjusts light intensity dynamically based on feedback from the camera.
   - Manual Mode: Allows surgeons to set a fixed brightness level.
6. *White Balance Button*:
   - Calibrates the light source to ensure accurate colour representation in the surgical field. This is available in camera control unit, camera head, and or in light source, depending upon the manufacturer.
7. *Filter Selection (IR or UV Filters)*:
   - Some systems allow toggling of infrared (IR) filters to minimize heat exposure.
   - Certain models also have fluorescence imaging filters (e.g. near-infrared for ICG fluorescence).
8. *Fibre Optic Cable Locking Mechanism*:
   - A rotary or push-lock system secures the fibre optic cable in place.
9. *Display Screen (On Digital Models)*:
   - Shows real-time settings such as intensity level, lamp status, and filter mode.
   - Some units include touchscreen controls for precise adjustments.

10. *Lamp Life Indicator*:
    - Displays remaining lifespan of the light source bulb (especially in xenon and halogen models).
11. *Remote Control Connectivity*:
    - Some models allow integration with laparoscopic camera systems for synchronized adjustments.

14.8 Light Cable

Light cables are essential components in laparoscopic surgery, responsible for transmitting high-intensity light from the light source to the laparoscope. They ensure *optimal illumination* of the surgical field while minimizing heat transfer. The quality, material, and design of light cables significantly impact the clarity and brightness of the image during surgery (Fig. 14.2).

1. Fibre-optic cable.
2. Liquid crystal gel cable.

14.8.1 Fibre Optic Light Cable

14.8.1.1 Structure and Working Principle

Fibre optic cables consist of thousands of thin glass or polymer fibres bundled together to transmit light efficiently. Each fibre acts as a waveguide, using total internal reflection to guide light from the source to the laparoscope without significant loss.

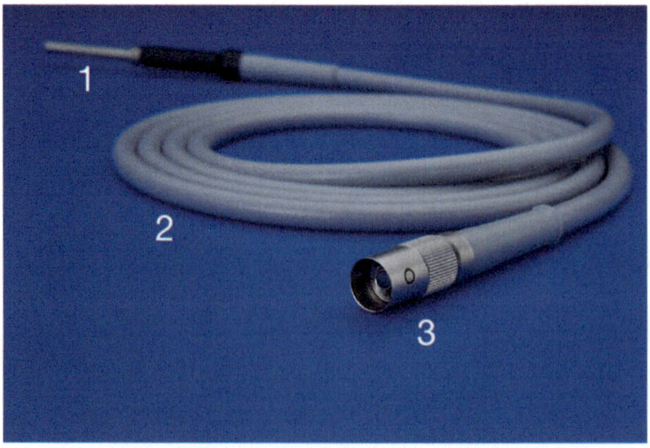

Fig. 14.2 Fibre optic light cable (1—light source end, 2—cable containing fibre optic fibres with protective covering, 3—laparoscope connector)

Advantages

- *High Light Transmission*: Ensures bright and clear illumination with minimal loss.
- *Durability*: Resistant to bending, but excessive kinking can break individual fibres.
- *Minimal Heat Transfer*: Does not retain or transfer excessive heat to the laparoscope.
- *Compatibility*: Available with various connectors for Storz, Olympus, Wolf, ACMI, and universal adapters.

Disadvantages

- *Fragility*: The glass fibres can break over time, reducing efficiency.
- *Cost*: High-quality fibre optic cables can be expensive.

14.8.2 Liquid Crystal Gel Cable

14.8.2.1 Structure and Working Principle

Liquid crystal gel cables use a hollow core filled with a transparent liquid or gel to guide light. Instead of reflecting light through individual fibres, they allow light to pass directly through the liquid medium with minimal scattering or loss.

Advantages

- *Superior Light Transmission*: Offers higher brightness and efficiency than standard fibre optics.
- *Minimal Light Scattering*: Provides more uniform and stable illumination.
- *Heat Resistance*: The liquid medium absorbs heat, reducing the risk of overheating laparoscopic instruments.
- *Flexibility*: Unlike fibre optic cables, they are less prone to fibre breakage.

Disadvantages

- *Fragility*: The liquid medium can degrade or leak over time if the cable is damaged.
- *Higher Cost*: More expensive than standard fibre optic cables.
- *Limited Availability*: Less commonly used than fibre optics.

14.8.3 Maintenance

Proper maintenance of laparoscopic light cables is essential to ensure optimal light transmission, prevent damage, and extend the lifespan of the cable. Since light cables are responsible for delivering high-intensity illumination from the light source to the laparoscope, any deterioration can lead to reduced visibility, poor image quality, and increased risks during surgery.

1. *Handling and Storage*
   - *Avoid excessive bending or twisting*: Light cables, especially fibre optic cables, contain delicate glass fibres that can break if over-flexed. Always maintain a smooth curve when handling the cable.
   - *Do not coil tightly*: Loose coiling prevents internal fibre breakage. A diameter of at least 15 cm (6 inches) is recommended for coiling.
   - *Store in a dry and dust-free environment*: Humidity and dust can degrade the cable's outer sheath and internal fibres. Keep cables in protective cases when not in use.
   - *Avoid heavy loads*: Do not place objects on the cable, as pressure can crush or misalign the fibres, reducing light transmission.
2. *Cleaning, Disinfection and Sterilization*
   - *Clean after each use*: Wipe the outer surface with a soft, lint-free cloth and a mild detergent solution.
   - *Use approved disinfectants*: Follow manufacturer guidelines to prevent damage from harsh chemicals. Common disinfectants include glutaraldehyde, peracetic acid, and enzymatic cleaners.
   - *Avoid immersion in liquids*: Fibre optic cables should not be submerged, as moisture can seep into the connectors and degrade internal components.
   - *Sterilization*: Use EtO or plasma sterilization if the cable is heat sensitive.
3. *Regular Checks*:
   - *Check for external damage*: Look for cuts, cracks, or abrasions on the cable sheath, which can expose internal fibres to contamination or breakage.
   - *Inspect light transmission*: Connect the cable to a light source and check for uniform brightness at the distal end. If dark spots or reduced brightness appear, internal fibre damage may be present.
   - *Perform periodic light intensity checks*: Compare the brightness output of older cables with new ones. If there is a significant drop, replacement may be necessary.

14.8.4 Troubleshooting

The following table provides quick troubleshooting guidance for common issues related to laparoscopic light sources and cables, ensuring optimal illumination during surgery.

Problem	Possible cause	Solution
No light output from the source	Power cable disconnected or faulty power supply Blown fuse or lamp failure Light source in standby mode	Check power cable and connections Replace fuse or lamp Disable standby mode
Dim or weak light output	Light intensity set too low Cable damaged or broken fibres Lamp nearing end of life	Increase light intensity Inspect and replace the cable Replace lamp if old
Flickering light	Loose fibre optic cable connection Faulty bulb or power fluctuations Overheating of the light source	Secure the cable properly Replace the lamp Ensure proper ventilation and cooling
Uneven brightness or dark spots	Internal fibre breakage in the cable Dirt or debris on lens or connectors Light source optical components misaligned	Replace damaged fibre optic cable Clean lens and connectors with lint-free cloth Get light source serviced
Light source overheating	Fan or cooling system blocked Prolonged use without standby mode High-intensity setting for long periods	Ensure proper airflow and clean cooling vents Use standby mode during pauses Lower intensity when possible
Cable getting excessively hot	Heat-resistant filter missing or faulty Use of non-compatible cable Light source left on at full intensity for too long	Check if IR/heat filter is intact Use heat-resistant fibre optic cable Reduce intensity when not in use
Connector does not fit properly	Incorrect connector type Debris inside the connector port Damaged connector end	Use the correct connector adapter Clean connector port carefully Replace cable if connector is damaged
Light turns off suddenly	Overheating safety shutdown Faulty power connection or internal issue Lamp failure	Allow time for cooling before restarting Check power cables and connections Replace the lamp if needed

References

1. The Theory of Heat Radiation | SpringerLink [Internet]. https://link.springer.com/book/9780883185971
2. Quint R. Physics of light and image transmission. Laparosc Baltim Williams Wilkins. 1977;18–23.

3. Nakamura S, Pearton S, Fasol G. The blue laser diode: the complete story. Springer Science & Business Media; 2000. p. 390.
4. Wallace H. A different kind of chemistry: a history of tungsten halogen lamps. IEEE Ind Appl Mag. 2001 Nov;7(6):10–7.
5. Wayback Machine [Internet]. 2013. [https://web.archive.org/web/20130718003525/http://assets.sylvania.com/assets/documents/ENGR_BLTN11.161355cc-1d94-4996-b6cd-a3001fea6f1a.pdf
6. HJ Round Started It All By Discovering Electroluminescence. https://web.archive.org/web/20201028074225/http://www.myledpassion.com/History/hj-round.htm
7. Zheludev N. The life and times of the LED — a 100-year history. Nat Photonics. 2007;1(4):189–92.

Insufflator

15

Jasmeet Singh Ahluwalia

A carbon dioxide insufflator is a crucial piece of equipment in maintaining an optimal field of view during minimally invasive surgery by maintaining the cavity of interest in a distended state. Usually, a typical laparoscopic surgery would start with the creation of pneumoperitoneum and a good insufflator goes a long way in establishing safe entry into the abdomen, as its accurate readings can predict if one is in the right space. As the procedure proceeds, the maintenance of CO_2 pressure at the desired level is also the responsibility of this machine. There are many hidden meanings between various readings on insufflator and many points of potential fault from the source of CO_2 to patients cavity of interest. If properly understood, this will enhance the safety of the patient as well as enable the surgical team to troubleshoot changes in abdominal pressure quickly.

15.1 Identify Controls

Identify the following controls (either present as physical buttons or on a touch screen depending upon make) on the front side of your insufflator (Fig. 15.1):

- *Power*: This switch is to power on and off the unit. It is advisable to power on the unit after establishing CO_2 connections with the insufflator. Also, before powering off the unit, one should stop insufflation.
- *Start/Stop*: This is used to start the supply of CO_2 from the insufflator into the connected tube towards the patient. After power is turned on by switching on the power button, this switch is in "off" state by default. One must press it once to start insufflation. If there is a power loss while the unit is running, this switch

J. S. Ahluwalia (✉)
Department of Bariatric & Minimal Access Surgery, STAR Superspeciality Hospital, Jalandhar, Punjab, India

J. S. Ahluwalia (ed.), *User Manual for Minimally Invasive Surgical Equipment*,
https://doi.org/10.1007/978-981-95-9019-3_15

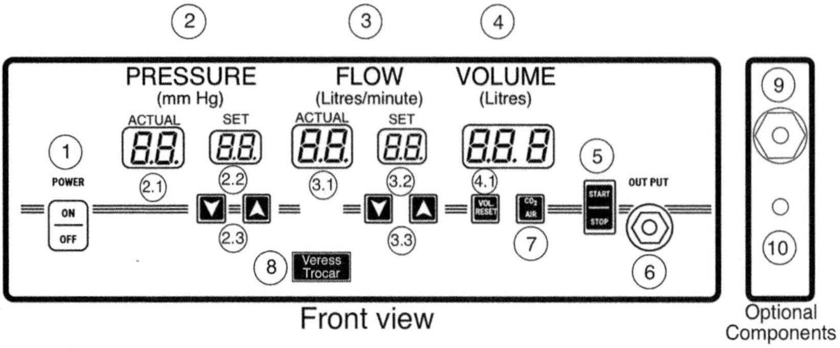

1. Power button
2. Pressure display and settings
   2.1 Actual Pressure
   2.2 Set Pressure
   2.3 Buttons to increase or decrease pressure
3. Flow display and settings
   3.1 Actual flow rate
   3.2 Set flow rate
   3.3 Buttons to increase or decrease flow rate
4. Volume
   4.1 To reset volume to zero
5. Start / Stop button
6. Output connector to CO2 gas pipe
7. Button to switch to air insufflation in case of emergency
8. Veress / Trocar insufflation mode switch button
9. Connector for smoke evacuator
10. Connector for heating element

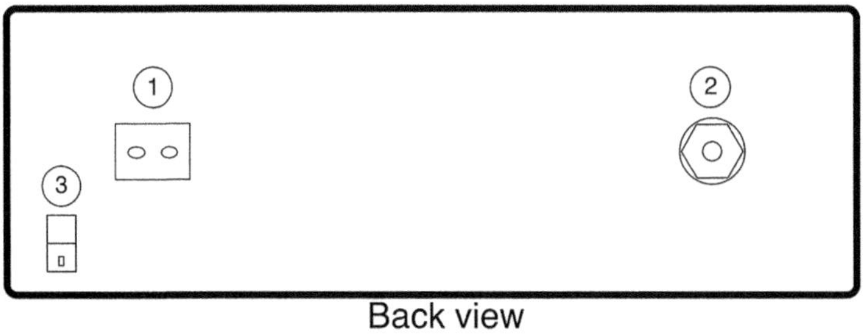

1. Power cable connector
2. CO2 pipe connector
3. Power on / off switch

Fig. 15.1 Front and back of Insufflator with physical buttons

may turn to off position (as it is its default setting) once the power supply resumes. So be aware to turn it on again in case of a power shut down during the procedure.

- *Pressure*: Insufflator has two readings for pressure (measured in mm of Hg) inside the abdomen (or any given working space).

  - *Actual*: The reading shows actual pressure inside the cavity during the procedure at a given time.
  - *Set*: This is the maximum pressure at which you wish to perform the procedure, and the insufflator will maintain this pressure throughout the procedure. It will keep on insufflating till this pressure is reached and re-insufflate whenever there is a fall in pressure due to gas leakage. The nearby up and down controls are used to increase and decrease the set pressure.
  - Most insufflators have a range of set pressure from 0 to 30 mmHg. Some special purpose and newer ones can go up to 50 mmHg. Usually, a pressure of 12 to 15 mmHg is used in adults. It may be decreased in paediatric laparoscopy and increased in surgeries on morbidly obese.
- *Flow*: Insufflator has two readings for flow rate in litres per minute (L/min).
  - *Actual*: This shows the rate of flow of CO_2 from the insufflator at a given time.
  - *Set*: This is the maximum flow rate that the insufflator will use to attain the set pressure. Most insufflators provide at least flow rates up to 20 L/min, but for some special procedures like bariatric surgery, high flow insufflators with flow rates up to 50 L/min are also available. The nearby up and down controls are to increase and decrease the set flow rate.
- *Volume*: This indicates the total volume of CO_2 that has been inserted in litres. This may reset to zero on its own after switching off the machine or may have a separate control button to do so (Fig. 15.2).
- *Volume Reset*: To reset volume reading to zero at the start of another procedure.
- *Cylinder pressure*: This shows information about the pressure of CO_2 inside the CO_2 cylinder connected to the back of the insufflator. This may show just full and empty status in some models and real-time pressure in others. One should note that the supply of gas from the cylinder to the insufflator must be switched on by rotation of the control valve before this indicator can show a reading. If the inlet valve is closed, this will show empty status falsely.
- *Output connector for CO_2 tube*: The tube used for CO_2 insufflation is connected here. A disposable filter must be used before the tube to avoid contamination. Use a silicon tube as it is more durable, flexible, sterilisation-friendly and inert.
- *Heating element connector*: Some insufflators may have a separate connection for connecting the heating element. Such elements are coiled around the gas-carrying tube to keep CO_2 warm as it is transferred inside the patient's abdomen (Fig. 15.3).
- *Smoke evacuation connector*: Some insufflators have a built-in mechanism for the evacuation of smoke produced by energy devices. Such a tube can be connected here and the other end to one of the ports.

15.2 On the Back Side of the Equipment, One Can Find the Following Connectors

- *Power cord connector*: To connect the power supply cable. Always ensure power supply comes via a power backup system which ensures continuous power supply to the insufflator even during a power failure.

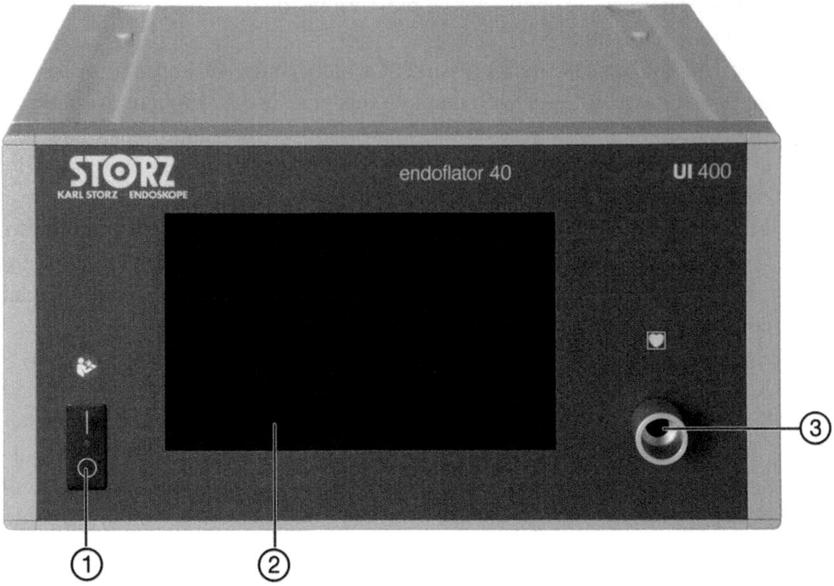

ENDOFLATOR 40 (UI400) – Front view

1 Power switch
2 Touch screen
3 Insufflation connection to the patient

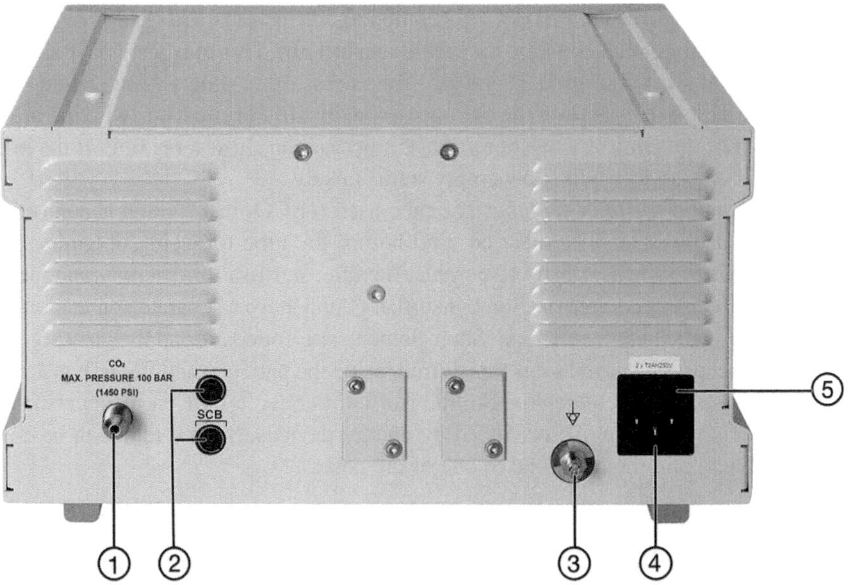

ENDOFLATOR 40 (UI400) – Rear view

1 Gas connection (standard American type)
2 SCB sockets
3 Potential equalization connector
4 Power socket
5 Line fuse holder

Fig. 15.2 Front and back of Storz Insufflator (Endoflator 40 (UI400))

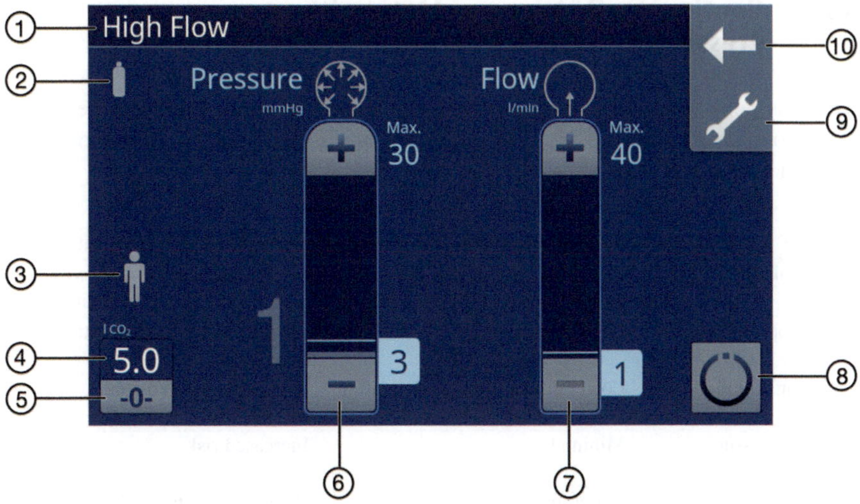

1	Mode	6	Set pressure values
2	Gas bottle pressure display	7	Set flow values
3	Mode symbol (High Flow, Pediatrics)	8	Start insufflation, stop insufflation
4	Gas consumption display	9	Settings
5	Reset gas consumption display	10	Browse back

Fig. 15.3 Storz Insufflator (Endoflator 40 (UI400)) display screen showing various readings and settings

- *CO_2 inlet connector*: To connect the metallic tube which will connect with CO_2 cylinder or its supplying tube at the other end. There should be a pressure regulator in-between CO_2 and the insufflator to prevent high CO_2 pressure at inlet connector which can damage the equipment. Some insufflators have an inbuilt pressure regulator. Check with the manufacturer to ensure what the optimal pressure is that can be used at this inlet, as higher pressure can damage the equipment and lower pressure may not allow it to function well. A filter can be used before CO_2 gas is let inside the insufflator. This is separate from the front filter.
- *Veress/trocar*: Some insufflators have additional settings to choose between Veress needle vs trocar insufflation. Veress needle insufflation will limit the flow rate to a low level as most Veress needles will not allow a flow rate over 3 L/min. This can be used as a safety at the start of insufflation.
- *CO_2/air*: Some insufflators have a provision to provide air as an insufflation medium in case of emergency if CO_2 supply is finished during a procedure. Air is not safe as it can lead to air embolism and does not suppress combustion, so this mode should be reserved for a very rare emergency only.

15.3 Continuous Pressure and Intermittent Pressure Insufflators

Previous generation insufflators will deliver intermittent gas so as to take a short pause to measure pressure. Newer generation ones do real-time pressure monitoring without taking any pause.

Feature	Continuous pressure insufflators	Intermittent pressure insufflators
Mechanism	Real-time, continuous pressure monitoring and adjustment	Intermittent gas delivery with periodic pressure reassessment
Pneumoperitoneum stability	Highly stable	Fluctuates due to intermittent gas delivery
CO_2 consumption	Lower due to efficient regulation	Higher due to frequent reinjections
Risk of pressure spikes	Minimal	Increased risk
Patient comfort	Better, due to steady pressure maintenance	Reduced, due to sudden pressure changes
Response time	Fast and automatic adjustments	Slower response to pressure variations
Cost	Higher	Lower
Best use cases	Complex and prolonged laparoscopic surgeries	Basic and short-duration laparoscopic procedures

15.4 Assembling

Insufflator should be placed along with other laparoscopic instruments on a trolley or pendant in a horizontal position at a height where its readings are clearly visible to surgical team members during the entire procedure. Since one may need to stop and start or change set pressure and flow rate during surgery, the controls must be accessible at all times during the procedure.

Supply of CO_2 to the inlet valve must be very well secured to avoid any leakage of gas. Open the valve to start the supply of CO_2 from the cylinder towards the insufflator.

Switch on the power supply. The insufflator will do a self-diagnostic test. All numbers and LED panels will be lit up to show there are no faulty elements involved which may misrepresent readings. Make sure none of the LCD or LED parts miss to illuminate. After this insufflator goes into standby mode, we need to press the start button to start the flow of gas once everything else is ready.

15.5 Initialise

Check the pressure of CO_2 cylinder to make sure it is enough for the planned surgery. Always keep an extra cylinder of CO_2 ready as it is not easy to ascertain the amount of CO_2 remaining inside the cylinder.

After connecting the insufflation tubing (along with a disposable filter) to the insufflator, turn the insufflator to high flow (>6 L/min). Keep the other end of the tube open to air and let some CO_2 escape to wipe out any air inside tubing. At this time pressure should read 0 as CO_2 is escaping into the air. Now block the outlet of the tube with your thumb and the pressure reading should hit its highest (30 mmHg to 50 mmHg depending on the make of insufflator). These checks will ascertain that the insufflator pressure sensors are working properly.

Insufflator is now ready to be connected to the sterile silicon gas pipe via the filter. The tube must be ready and the insufflator switched on with proper gas pressure before entry into the abdomen is attempted. Once entry is established, the tube (from which air has been expelled already as described before) is connected to the Veress needle if it is being used (in Veress mode if the insufflator has one) or directly to the trocar in case of open entry. Use a flow rate of 1 L/min to inflate the abdomen slowly till at least 1 L of CO_2 has been insufflated. This will decrease the negative effects of pneumo-peritoneum on the patient's body. After this flow rate can be increased to the desired level depending upon the type of patient and procedure.

- *Disassembling*: At the end of the procedure, disconnect the silicon tube from the trocar first and then from the insufflator. Turn the inlet valve to the closed position and let the remnant CO_2 to flush out of the insufflator. Then switch off the "on/off" switch followed by pushing the power button to the off state. Cut the power supply to the equipment from the mains.
- *Maintenance*: After use, the power supply must be disconnected by switching off the plug where the power cable is connected. Rear CO_2 inlet connection may remain connected, but the supply of CO_2 must be stopped by turning off the gas valve. Ensure the insufflator stays away from any water spillage. Outer surface must be cleaned as per the disinfection protocols of the hospital. Keep equipment in a horizontal position at all times.
- *Troubleshooting*: The following table lists various reasons for insufficient pressure inside the working area.

Cause	Solution	Comments/hints	Pressure reading	Flow rate reading
Low pressure inside the abdomen				
Problem at insufflator level				
Leak at level of metallic tube connected to CO_2 cylinder or at CO_2 inlet of insufflator	Need to tighten the joint	Audible gas leak sound at back of insufflator	↓	↑
Low or no CO_2 in cylinder	Replace CO_2 cylinder	CO_2 cylinder pressure indicating red light, very low CO_2 level or empty level and CO_2 cylinder was not changed recently—Likely to be empty	↓	↓
Closed valve at inlet Clogged inlet filter	Need to open it Need to change filter	CO_2 cylinder pressure indicating red light, very low CO_2 level or empty level and cylinder was changed recently—Unlikely to be empty	↓ ↓	↓ ↓
On/off switch at off position as it resets to off position on every restart	Push it once more to bring it to on position	Always check this if there was break in power supply to insufflator during procedure	No Reading	No Reading
Set pressure or flow too low	Increase set pressure and flow	Always check set pressure and flow at start of each procedure	↓	↓
Breakdown of insufflator	Replace the machine	Always keep spare insufflator ready in close vicinity	–	–
Problem at tube level				
Outflow gas tube not connected to insufflator or to port gas channel	Pipe needs to be connected	This can happen any time during procedure. Ensure both ends of pipe fits snuggly	↓	↑
Break in tube	Plug the break with a sterile tape or change the tube soon	Always keep a spare sterile tube ready inside OR	↓	↑
Kink in tube	Kink needs to be located and removed	Use a sturdy tube if possible to avoid kink	↑	↓
Problem at port level				
Valve of port closed	Open the valve	Port should be rotated to keep valve upwards so it doesn't close by itself due to movement of port during surgery	↑	↓

(continued)

Cause	Solution	Comments|hints	Pressure reading	Flow rate reading
Leak from instrument channel while instrument is inside port	Make sure washer is properly placed Reducer is used where needed If washer has cracks—need a replacement	Washers are made of delicate material which makes them vulnerable to breakdown over time. Extra sterile washers must be available inside OR at all times	↓	↑
Leak from instrument channel only when there is no instrument inside port	Some tissue stuck inside valve—open the head and clean if from inside Breakdown of spring or silicon seal of valve—change port to continue procedure and send for repair later	This is due to leakage from valve that checks CO_2 escaping back once instrument is out	↓	↑
Leak from head of port	Tighten the port	This usually happens because technician has not tightened to port enough after cleaning it	↓	↑
Leak around the port	Apply towel clip or a suture to secure gas leak	This usually happens after enlargement of port for specimen delivery	↓	↑
Port CO_2 outlet blocked	CO_2 outlet hole not inside peritoneal cavity—Push port little more inside CO_2 outlet hole blocked by some tissue like momentum—change position	CO_2 outlet valve must lie freely inside abdomen for gas to pass through it. If blocked, insufflator will reflect high pressure even though there is little gas inside the abdomen	↑	↓
Inserted instrument too wide for the port	Change gas connection to another port	Sometimes instruments like ligature or harmonic are too wide for a given port and block flow of CO_2	↑	↓
Gas valve of another port is open	Needs to be closed	Always remember to close another valve after it is opened to clear fumes	↓	↑
Excessive use of suction	Suction must be used intermittently during procedure	One may use lesser pressure of suction if it is leading to loss of pressure very quickly	↓	↑

(continued)

Cause	Solution	Comments|hints	Pressure reading	Flow rate reading
Excess pressure from smoke evacuator	Decrease its pressure setting	Proper pressure selection is important to avoid unnecessary loss of pressure	↓	↑
High pressure inside the abdomen				
Insufflation pressure set at high level	Lower the set pressure	Always ensure to check set pressure and flow at the start of every procedure	↑	↓
Patient is not relaxed	Ask anaesthetist to relax the patient	Improper relaxation will decrease available space for procedure	↑	↓
Faulty equipment	Send for service or replace	A faulty equipment that is not able to stop flow once set pressure is reached can lead to serious injury to patient. Open of the ports to evacuate gas immediately if pressure is high	May show normal set pressure reading if machine is at fault	May vary if machine is at fault

Pressure	Flow	Inference
A glance at insufflator readings can give idea about location of a problem		
Normal	Zero or low	No problem
Normal	High	Leak being compensated by high flow
Low	High	Leak not being compensated by high flow
High despite collapsed cavity	Low	Block in gas flow

15.6 Recent Trends

Newer insufflators are coming up with advancements in all elements of a basic CO_2 insufflator like:

- High flow rates of about 50 L/min to insufflate larger abdomens, especially in morbidly obese patients. This is helpful during the surgery whenever there is loss of pressure due to suction or otherwise, adequate exposure can be gained back quickly.
- Large touch screens in modern insufflators make it easier to change settings as well as to observe readings.
- Different settings for different types of procedures and patients like visceral surgery, bariatric surgery, paediatric surgery, endoscopic vein removal proce-

dures, endoscopic cardiac surgery, etc., make it easier to change settings quickly.

- Integrated smoke evacuation systems are becoming better with time and are helping in maintaining a clear field of view. Now users can select different rates of smoke evacuation to meet their requirements.
- Smoke evacuation is being combined with better filtration of gas to avoid the release of harmful products inside OR.
- Gas heating is being improved to deliver more optimised temperature to the abdominal cavity to prevent hypothermia and fogging of lens. But their significant impact on patient outcomes remains debated.
- Humidification has been combined with heated CO_2 in an effort to decrease tissue damage, decrease inflammatory response, and decrease adhesion formation. All this is to improve patient outcomes, but again, their impact on clinical outcomes remains debated.
- Newer systems are incorporating auto deflation in case excess pressure is detected inside the abdomen due to certain conditions like the patient losing muscle relaxation, excess abdominal pressure from outside, etc.

15.7 Conclusion

The insufflator plays a crucial role in laparoscopic surgery by creating and maintaining a stable pneumoperitoneum, which is essential for optimal visualisation and safe surgical manipulation. By delivering a controlled flow of carbon dioxide (usually CO_2) into the abdominal cavity, the insufflator ensures adequate working space while minimising the risks associated with excessive intra-abdominal pressure. Understanding its function, settings, and potential risks allows surgeons to optimise surgical outcomes while ensuring patient well-being.

Electrosurgery

16

Sónia Ribas, Ionica Stoica, and Raquel Rodrigues

Electrosurgery is the most widely used form of surgical energy in both open and laparoscopic surgery, owing to its broad availability, cost-effectiveness and versatility. Over recent years, the rapid expansion of minimally invasive surgical techniques has been accompanied by an increasing number of reported adverse events and procedure-specific complications related to the use of electrosurgical energy. These reports have understandably raised concerns regarding the safe application of electrosurgery in laparoscopic surgery [1–3].

When used appropriately, electrosurgery is both safe and highly effective, enabling surgeons to operate with efficiency and precision. By allowing controlled tissue division and effective haemostasis, it facilitates the performance of complex procedures while minimizing operative times. However, the prevention of complications critically depends on a thorough understanding of the technology and the correct use of instruments and generators. It is therefore essential that laparoscopic surgeons develop a comprehensive familiarity with the principles, applications, and safety considerations of the energy sources employed during minimally invasive surgery [1–5].

Given the wide variety of available devices, this chapter focuses on the fundamental principles of electrosurgery. A reference electrosurgical unit is described in the concluding section to illustrate key components and operational features.

S. Ribas (✉)
ULS Póvoa de Varzim – Vila do Conde, Porto, Portugal

Hospital Lusíadas Braga, Braga, Portugal

I. Stoica
Evelina Children's Hospital, London, UK

R. Rodrigues
ULS Póvoa de Varzim – Vila do Conde, Porto, Portugal

J. S. Ahluwalia (ed.), *User Manual for Minimally Invasive Surgical Equipment*,
https://doi.org/10.1007/978-981-95-9019-3_16

16.1 History

The origins of electrosurgery can be traced back approximately 5000 years. Historical evidence suggests that Egyptians used cautery to treat tumours as early as 3000 BC [4, 5]. The development of electrosurgery has been closely linked to advances in the use of electricity. In the early nineteenth century, Becquerel introduced electrocautery, using direct electric current to heat a wire for haemostasis without any electricity passing through the patient. In 1881 Morton demonstrated that alternating current with a frequency of 100 kHz did not produce neuromuscular stimulation or electric shock when applied to the human body. Subsequently, d'Arsonval showed that high-frequency alternating current generated tissue heating [1, 2].

Modern electrosurgery emerged in the late 1920s following collaboration between the physicist William T. Bovie and the neurosurgeon Harvey Cushing. In 1926, they performed the first neurosurgical procedure using an electrosurgical generator. This early model remained in use until 1968, when Valleylab introduced a smaller and more practical unit, forming the basis of contemporary electrosurgical platforms [2, 4].

16.2 Biophysics of Electrosurgery

Electrosurgery is often incorrectly referred to as electrocautery; however, the two are fundamentally distinct. Electrosurgery involves the application of high-frequency electricity to tissue to produce thermal effects, whereas electrocautery uses a heated instrument without electrical current passing through the tissue. The electric current can be direct, when it flows in one direction, or alternating, when it changes its direction regularly. Electrosurgery utilizes alternating current, while electrocautery employs direct current [2–4].

The principles of electrosurgery are grounded in basic electrical physics. There is a direct relationship between current, voltage and resistance. Current represents the flow of electrical charge and it is measured in amperes (A) and its source is the electrosurgical generator. Voltage, measured in volts (V), is the electromotive force that drives the current through a circuit. Resistance, expressed in ohms (Ω), often referred to as impedance, opposes current flow. These variables are related by Ohm's law: Current (I) = Voltage (V)/Resistance (R). Energy (power), expressed in watts is defined as the product of voltage and current; $W = V \times I$.

The electrosurgical circuit is formed by a generator, two electrodes and the patient [1]. During surgery, the patient's tissues act as the conductor, with different tissue types (e.g. fat, muscle, liver, bone) exhibiting variable impedance [4].

High-frequency alternating current causes oscillation of intracellular ions, generating frictional heat and converting electrical energy initially into mechanical and then into thermal energy at the tissue level [1].

Modern electrosurgical generators convert standard electrical power into high-frequency currents (typically 500 kHz to 3 MHz) and regulate wattage, voltage and duty cycle to achieve the desired tissue effects [1, 3].

16.3 Understanding the Waveform

Tissue response to electrosurgery is primarily determined by the waveform type delivered by the generator. Three principal waveforms are used in electrosurgery: cutting, coagulation and blended modes. The electrosurgical generator has "cut," "coag" and "blend" settings (Fig. 16.1).

16.4 Cutting Waveform

The cutting waveform is sinusoidal, unmodulated and utilizes high-frequency continuous current delivered at relatively low voltage (power setting of 50–80 W). It produces a rapid temperature rise (>100 °C), resulting in vaporizing of intracellular water, rupture of cell membranes and precise tissue division. Lateral thermal spread and depth of tissue necrosis are minimal, and smoke production is relatively low. However, because it is a non-contact waveform, there is considerable energy into air.

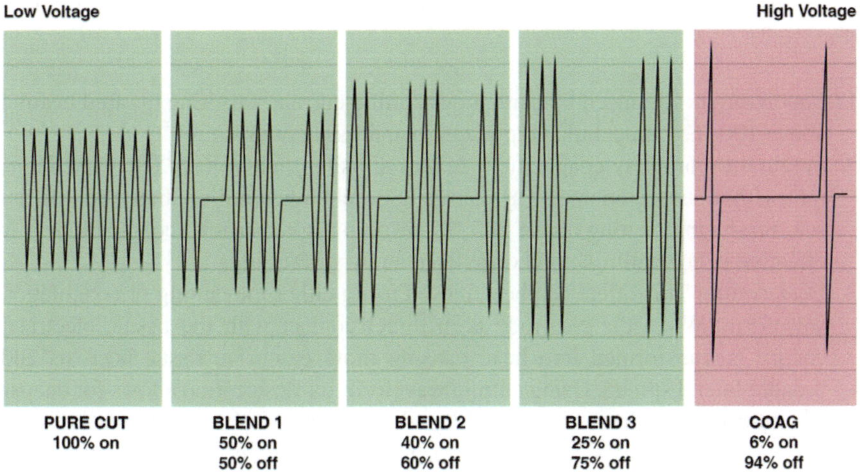

Fig. 16.1 Basic current waveforms

16.5 Coagulation Waveform

Coagulation waveform is low-frequency, high-voltage, modulated current with periods of activation and de-activating. Intermittent energy delivery allows heat to dissipate into surrounding tissues, resulting in protein denaturation, dehydration and coagulum formation at temperatures between 60 and 95 °C. Coagulation produces wider thermal injury, greater tissue charring, and increased smoke compared with cutting waveform. Power settings of 30–50 W are commonly effective.

The duty cycle describes the proportion of time during which a current is delivered. Cutting currents typically have a 100% duty cycle, whereas coagulation currents may be active for only 6% of the time.

16.6 Blended Waveform

A blended waveform is a modification of the cutting waveform by introducing periods of interruption to enhance haemostasis. It consists of a combination of both cutting and coagulation waves. Higher blend settings correspond to lower duty cycle and increased coagulation effects. As duty cycle decreases, voltage must increase to maintain constant power output [1–5].

16.7 Tissue Effect of Energy Sources

Electrosurgical tissue effects depend on the type of current waveform used (Fig. 16.2):

1. Vaporization: Produced by continuous cutting current, resulting in rapid heating above 100 °C, intracellular vaporization and tissue division.
2. Fulguration or spray coagulation: Achieved using high-voltage interrupted current without tissue contact. The electrode is held a few millimetres from the tissue, producing heating above 200 °C, resulting in superficial coagulation. It is effective in controlling blood ooze from a raw surface area.
3. Desiccation: This effect can be achieved using either the cutting or coagulation waveform. When the electrode is in direct contact with the tissue, electrical energy is transformed into heat, causing more extensive tissue necrosis and broader lateral spread. Using cutting waveform for desiccation allows for deeper penetration with less charring. A gradual increase in temperature between 60–95 °C leads to desiccation and coagulation instantaneously. The process of desiccation results from the loss of water from cells through their membrane, while coagulation is caused by the denaturation of proteins due to heat [1–5].
4. Coaptation (sealing of small to medium vessels <2 mm): can be accomplished with either cutting or coagulation current, when the electrode is in contact with the vessel and compression is applied. It is associated with considerable lateral spread of thermal effect (Fig. 16.3) [5].

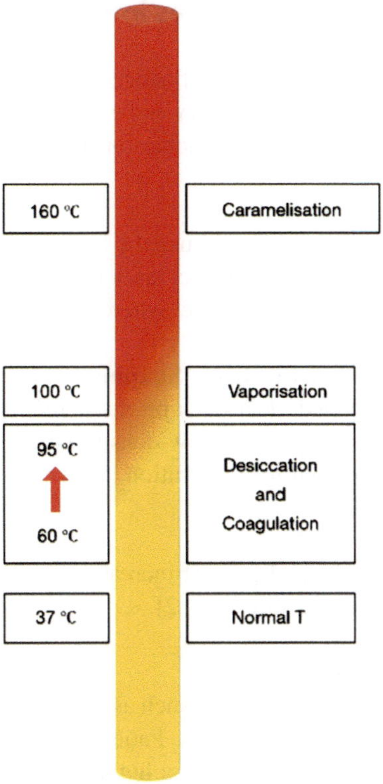

Fig. 16.2 Thermal tissue effects

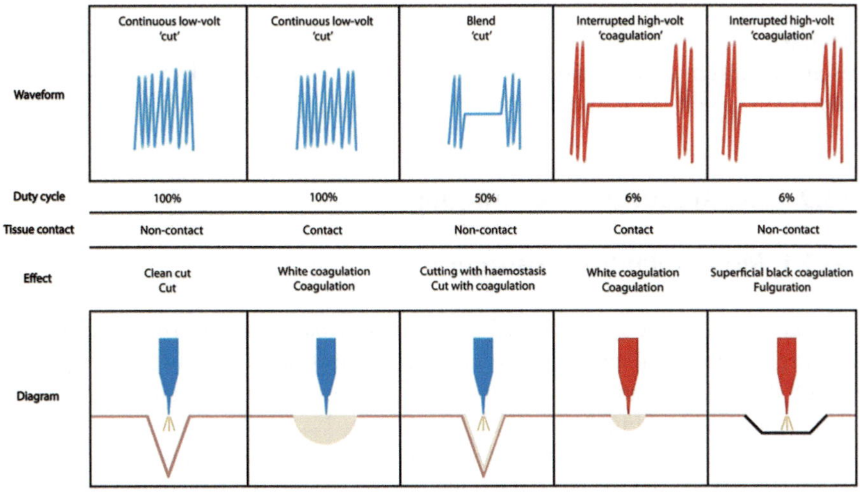

Fig. 16.3 Waveforms and tissue effects

16.8 Variables Influencing Tissue Effects

Several factors influence electrosurgical tissue response, including power settings, electrode geometry and current density, dwell time, electrode-tissue interface, tissue impedance and eschar formation.

Power Setting
Surgeons should use the lowest effective power output to minimize complications. Higher current increases tissues effects. A power of 50–80 W for the cut mode is generally effective, whereas 30–50 W is effective for the coagulation mode [1, 3].

Active Electrode Shaping (Current Density)
Pointed electrodes produce high-density current effective for cutting; broad electrodes produce low-density current effective for coagulation; spherical electrodes are used for fulguration [1–4].

Dwell Time
Prolonged contact increases tissue injury; optimal cutting speed minimizes lateral thermal spread [1, 2].

Tissue Factors
High impedance, such as fat, bone and scar tissue, requires higher power to achieve the desired effects. Patient's characteristics are also important, as in high BMI or emaciated patients a higher power output should be employed to achieve the same tissue effects as in lean and muscular patients [1, 2].

Eschar
Eschar build-up on the active electrode increases impedance; electrodes should be kept clean or non-stick variants used (Teflon or silicone coated) [1].

16.9 Electrosurgical Techniques

16.9.1 Monopolar Electrosurgery

It is the most commonly employed technique in laparoscopy. Current is generated by the electrosurgical unit, flows from an active electrode at the surgical site (handpiece), through the patient to a return electrode (dispersion pad), and returns to the electrosurgical unit (Fig. 16.4) [2–5].

Understanding the circuit is important in order to prevent complications. Tissue effects occur only at the active electrode, where the current density is highest. The density of electrons diminishes as the distance from the electrode increases. If resistance is encountered at the level of the tissue, the current will take the path of least resistance, which is provided by the return electrode. Proper placement and secure contact of the dispersive electrode are essential to prevent patient burn. Modern

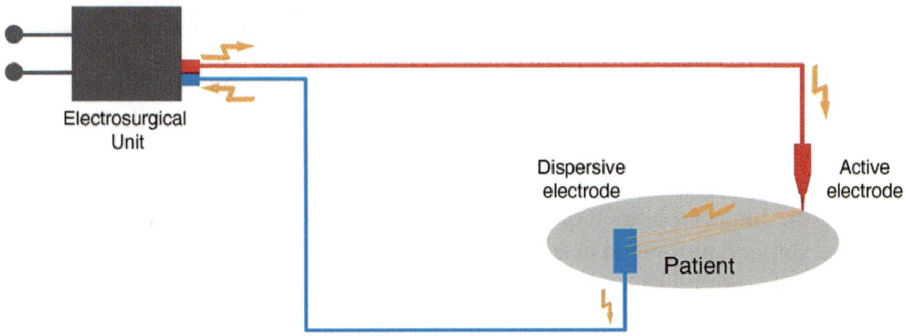

Fig. 16.4 Monopolar electrosurgery

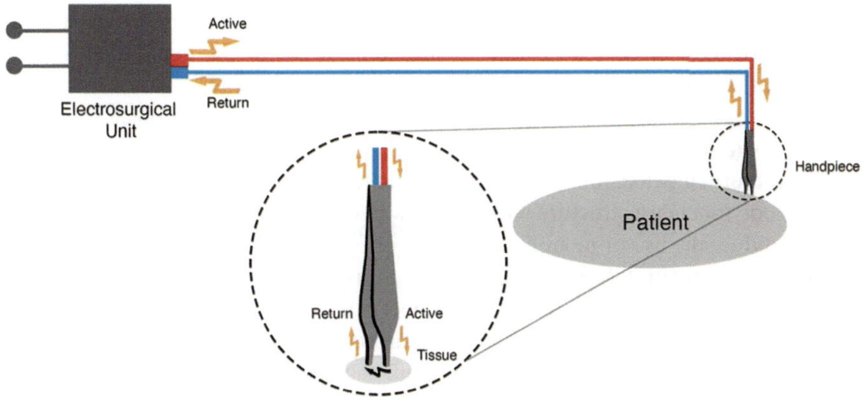

Fig. 16.5 Bipolar electrosurgery

generators incorporate contact-quality monitoring systems that interrupt the current flow if unsafe conditions are detected [1–5].

16.9.2 Bipolar Electrosurgery

In bipolar systems, both active and return electrodes are integrated into a single instrument. Current passes only through the tissue grasped between electrodes (instrument tips), eliminating the need for a dispersive pad (Fig. 16.5). Bipolar electrosurgery produces less thermal spread, less smoke and reduces the risk of interference with implanted devices. Although generally safer, bipolar instruments may be less reliable for haemostasis in some situations and require longer activation [1–5].

16.10 Complications and Hazards in Laparoscopic Surgery

Electrosurgical complications account for approximately 25% of laparoscopic complications. Despite technological advances, serious thermal injuries still occur leading to increased morbidity and potential mortality, especially if the injury is not recognized intraoperatively. In addition to the impact on the patient, these events increase the financial burden on the healthcare system as they are associated with repeated surgery, prolonged hospitalization and malpractice claims [1, 2, 4, 5].

Mechanisms of injury include:

- Lateral thermal spread—represents one of the most important hazards with laparoscopy energy sources and risk of injury varies with the device used, power output, dwell time and tissue impedance.
- Residual heat—energy devices can retain heat after activation for a variable period of time. A period of time should be allowed for the instrument to cool down after activation, before touching important structures [1, 2].
- Inadvertent activation—instruments should be kept in a secure place such as a dry plastic holster when not in use [1–3, 5].
- Direct thermal extension (pedicle effect, funnelling)—can occur when the active electrode touches a structure with a narrow pedicle. Prevention can be employed by avoiding the use of monopolar devices or by using the lowest effective power with short activation time (2–3 s) in areas at risk [1].
- Direct Coupling—occurs when active electrode is in close proximity or in contact with another metal instrument (laparoscope, grasper or clip/stapler line) allowing current to be conducted through the second instrument/device. This may cause unintended tissue injury, often outside the visual field. To prevent this, the electrode should only be activated under direct vision and in contact with the target tissue (Fig. 16.6) [1–5].

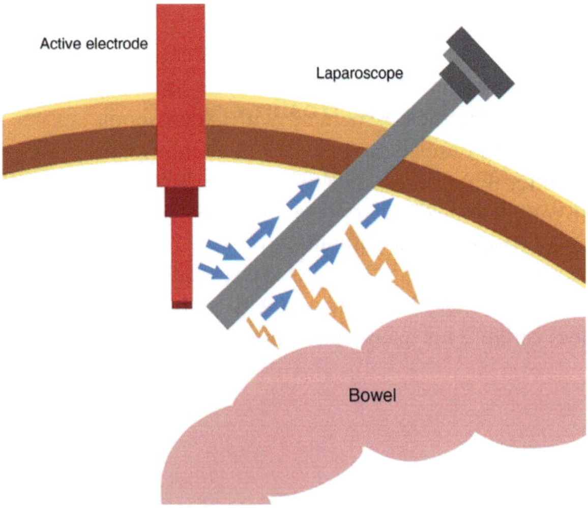

Fig. 16.6 Direct coupling effect

- Capacitive Coupling—occurs when electrical current is transferred from an active electrode to a nearby metal instrument running parallel, despite the absence of direct contact. This arises when two conductors are separated by an insulation layer and a potential difference exists, when an active electrode is placed within a trocar. Current may then pass through the adjacent conductor and into surrounding tissues, causing injury (Fig. 16.7) [1–5].

This risk can be reduced by using all-metal trocars, which allow dissipation of stored energy over the large surface of the patient's skin. The risk is increased by the use of hybrid cannulas (part plastic, part metal), proximity of the two conductors, high voltage, prolonged activation, longer instruments, thin insulation, and narrow trocars.

Active electrode monitoring technology (AEM) was introduced in the 1990s. mitigate this risk by incorporating a conductive shield that detects and diverts stray current and also by interrupting energy delivery when unsafe levels are detected (Fig. 16.8) [1–4].

- Insulation Failure—is the leading cause of electrothermal injury. Small defects in instrument insulation creates alternative current pathway, allowing arching to adjacent tissues, often outside the surgeon's field of view, leading to undetected damage (Fig. 16.9).

Defects most commonly occur in the distal third of laparoscopic instruments and are more frequent in reusable instruments due to repeated trocar passage and sterilization; reported rates are approximately 20% in reusable and 3% in single-use laparoscopic instruments. Robotic instruments demonstrate higher rates of

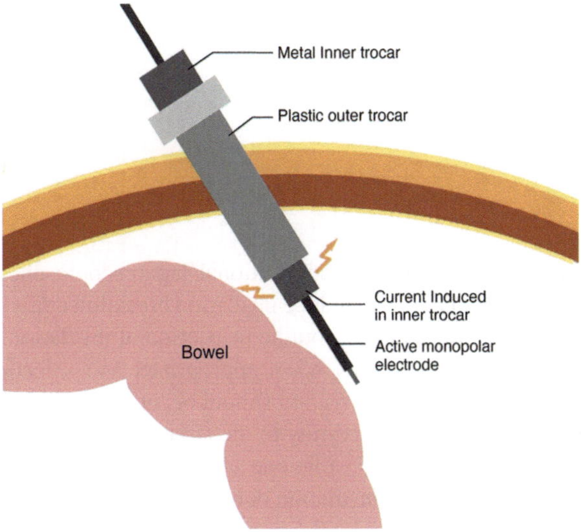

Fig. 16.7 Capacitive coupling effect

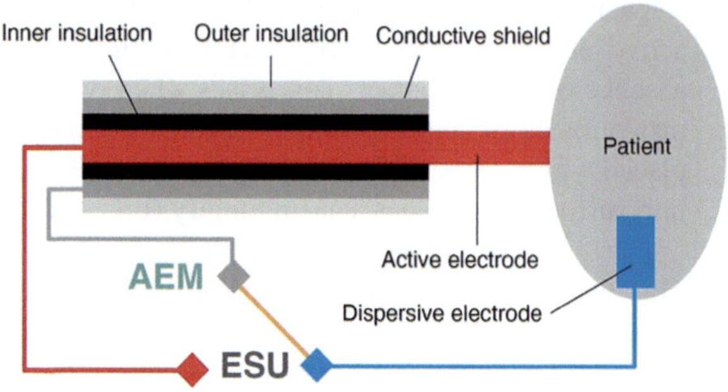

Fig. 16.8 Active electrode monitoring circuit

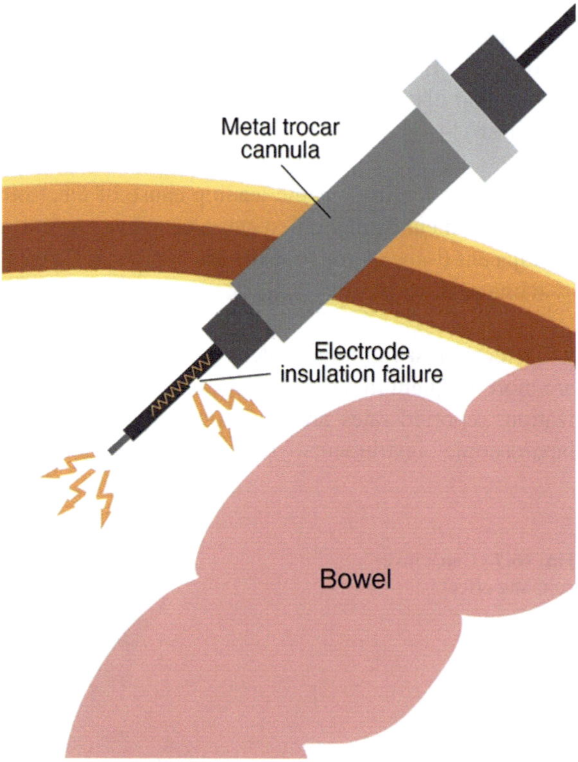

Fig. 16.9 Insulation failure

insulation failure than conventional laparoscopic ones. High-voltage coagulation waveform may rarely induce insulation breakdown in a previously intact instrument.

Prevention relies on routine inspection of insulation integrity, preferential use of disposable instruments when appropriate, and selection of lower-voltage cutting waveform. Energy activation should occur only when the active electrode is in contact or immediate proximity to the target tissue, as this will reduce the incidence of "blowing holes" in insulation, and also reduce the chance of the current to take alternative paths if insulation defects already exist.

As referred before AEM technology is designed to reduce the risk of injury from insulation failure and capacitive coupling [1–5].

- Dispersive electrode burns—occur when the dispersion pad is improperly applied, with inadequate skin contact, resulting in the current to return via alternative routes, such as electrocardiogram (ECG) leads, towel clips, stirrups or head frames, resulting in skin burns. Prevention relies on correct dispersion pad placement on well-perfused, dry, hairless skin, avoiding bony prominences and joints, and ensuring a sufficiently large contact area to maintain low current density. Modern contact-quality monitoring systems use split pads to detect poor contact or high impedance and automatically interrupt energy delivery if risk factors are detected [1–3, 5].
- Antenna coupling—occurs when electromagnetic energy from an active electrode cord (emitting antenna) is captured by a nearby inactive cord (receiving antenna), such as ECG wires, neuromonitors or camera cord (Fig. 16.10).

This mechanism is similar to capacitive coupling and may result in patient burns. Risk is reduced by separating the electrosurgical generator from laparoscopy tower, avoiding parallel cord alignment, and by using the lowest effective voltage [1].

- Electrical shock and glove burns—electrical injury to the surgeon may occur via three mechanisms, when current can pass through the gloves: direct current conduction (hydration with low resistance conduction), capacitive coupling (induced charge from the haemostat to the sweating conductive skin of the surgeon) and high-voltage dielectric breakdown (holes in glove). Risk reduction includes use of the lowest effective power, avoidance of prolonged and open activation and routine double gloving or glove replacement during lengthy procedures [1–3].
- Surgical smoke—is a common by-product of energy device use and consists predominantly of water vapour (95%) carrying fine particulate matter (5%). It impairs visibility which can lead to complications. Bipolar and ultrasonic devices are associated with less smoke production than the monopolar. Surgical smoke can cause irritation to the eyes and upper respiratory tract of the surgical team. Particles smaller than 5 μm can reach the distal airways and may contain toxic substances, bacteria, viruses or viable malignant cells. Risk mitigation includes minimizing tissue charring, routine smoke evacuation and use of appropriate per-

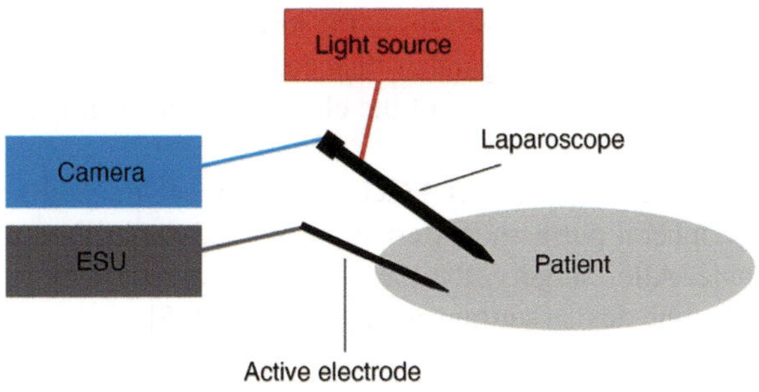

Fig. 16.10 Antenna coupling due to the close proximity and parallel arrangement of the cords

sonal protective equipment, particularly highlighted during the COVID-19 pandemic [1, 2, 5].
- Explosions—surgical explosions are rare, but potentially fatal and require the presence of three factors: oxygen, fuel and an ignition source. Early cases were linked to flammable bowel gases during endoscopy or inappropriate insufflation gases during laparoscopy. The exclusive use of carbon dioxide to achieve pneumoperitoneum and adequate bowel preparation minimized this risk [1].
- Surgical fires—operating-room fires, although considered never events, continue to occur and can have devastating outcomes. Similar to explosions, fires occur when all three elements of the fire triangle are present: oxidizer, ignition source and fuel. Supplemental oxygen concentrations above 30% markedly increase the risk, particularly involving surgical drapes. Immediate management includes cessation of oxygen delivery, extinguishing flames with saline (in case of airway fires removal of the endotracheal tube and saline instillation in the airway) and wet towels, removal of burning material, re-establishment of airway control in a safe environment [1].

16.11 Electromagnetic Interference (EMI) with Other Devices

16.11.1 Implantable Electronic Devices

Electrosurgery generates electromagnetic fields that may interfere with implantable electronic devices, including pacemakers, cardioverter-defibrillators, and neurostimulators, potentially causing adverse effects such as arrythmias, hypotension, myocardial injury or device malfunction. Clinical impact effect depends on the patient's dependency on the device. Therefore, management should be patient-specific and multidisciplinary.

The use of monopolar devices below the umbilicus is unlikely to interfere with cardiac devices. When surgery is performed near an implanted device, bipolar or ultrasonic instruments are preferred. If the use of monopolar devices is required, precautions include:

- Appropriate dispersive electrode placement to divert the current path away from the implanted device
- Positioning the generator at a distance from the implanted device
- Using short activations at the lowest effective power
- Selecting cutting rather than coagulation mode (less voltage)
- Avoiding activation of the electrode over the implanted device

As EMI can affect ECG, an additional method should be used to check the peripheral pulse and external pacing and defibrillation equipment should be available. After surgery, the patient should remain under continuous monitoring until baseline device settings are restored [1, 4, 5].

16.11.2 Electrocardiography (ECG)

In addition to the possible burns at the level of the ECG electrodes, electrosurgery can also distort ECG signal primary due to electrical arcing. Interference can be reduced by:

- Maximizing the distance between electrosurgical and ECG cables
- Using the lowest effective power
- Employing short activation in the cutting mode
- Avoiding open activation [1]

16.11.3 Video Imaging System

High-frequency electrosurgical currents generate electromagnetic waves that can interfere with laparoscopic video system, particularly at high power, higher voltage, or when equipment is in close proximity. Modern generators and imaging systems incorporate power regulation and electromagnetic shielding to reduce the interference. Simple separation of the electrosurgical unit and the video system further minimizes interference [1].

16.12 Best Practice Recommendations

General safety measures for preventing electrosurgical complications include [2, 3]:

- Careful inspection of instrument insulation
- Use the lowest effective power setting
- Preference for low-voltage waveform (cut)
- Short, intermittent activation
- Avoidance of open-circuit activation
- Avoidance of activation in close proximity or in direct contact with another instrument
- Preference of bipolar electrosurgery when appropriate
- Selection of all metal cannula system
- Utilization of electrosurgical accessory safety equipment (active electrode monitoring, tissue response technology)
- Utilization of smoke evacuation system

16.13 Description of a Reference Electrosurgery Machine

Electrosurgical machines vary between manufacturers. A machine is described below as a reference to explain its features and how to use it (Fig. 16.11).

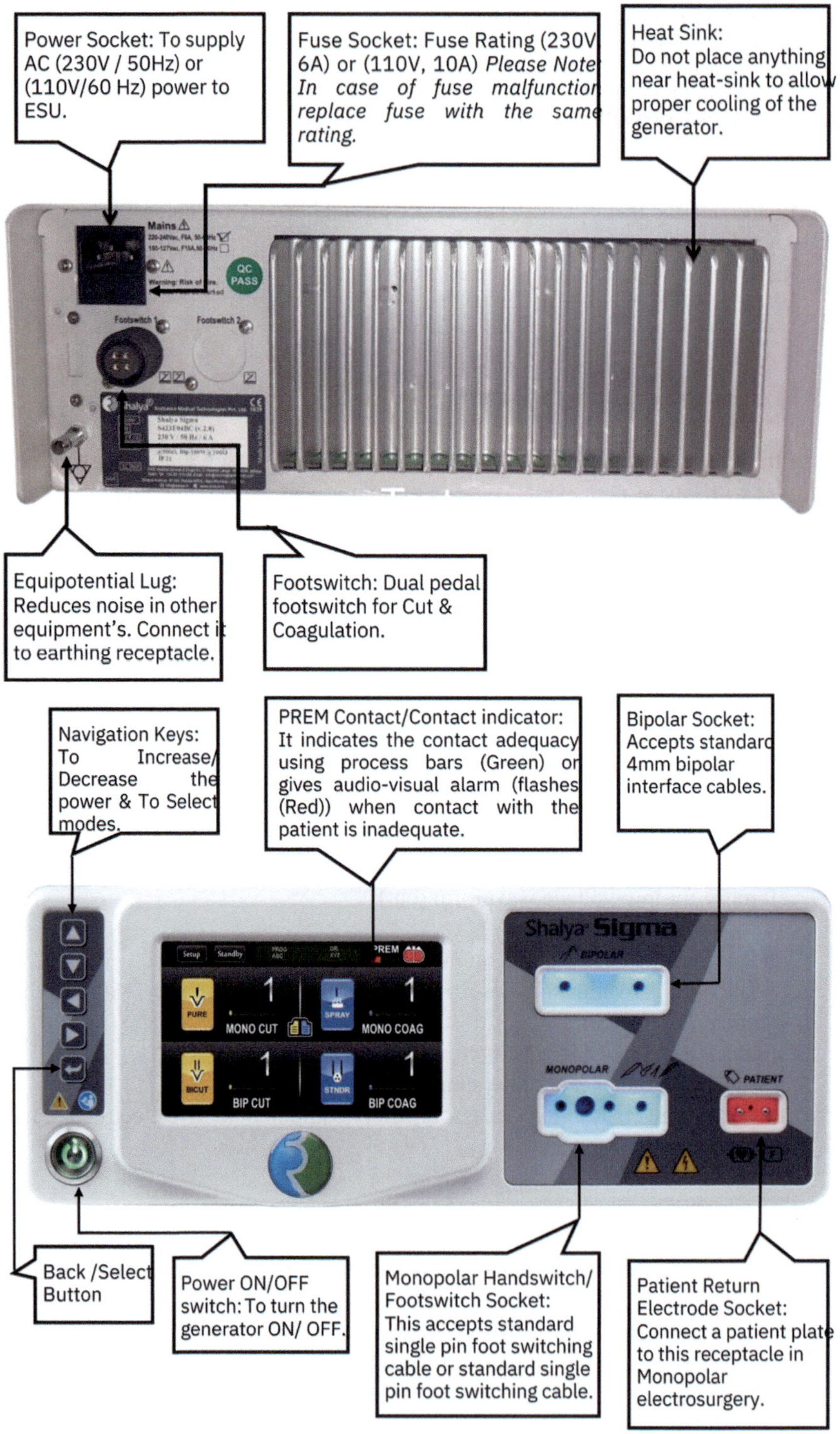

Fig. 16.11 Front and rear side of an electrosurgical machine

1. *Power button*: Turns the machine on and off. It is usually accompanied by an LED light that illuminates when the unit is powered on.
2. *Mode selection button/knob*: Allows the selection of different electrosurgical modes like cut, coagulation, blend, fulguration, etc. Some machines need to switch between monopolar and bipolar modes.
3. *Power adjustment controls*: Help to change power output of the given mode.
4. *PREM contact indicator*: Indicates whether patient return electrode is properly connected to the patient through patient plate.
5. *Monopolar socket*: To attach monopolar instrument cable.
6. *Bipolar socket*: To attach bipolar instrument cable.
7. *Foot-switch socket*: To attach foot-switch cable.
8. *Patient return electrode socket*: To attach patient plate cable.
9. *Touch screen*: To change settings.
10. *Fuse*: To prevent machine from damage due to voltage fluctuation or short-circuit.
11. *Equipotential nug*: Reduces noise in other equipment like monitor.
12. *Power socket*: To connect three pin high power cable.
13. *Seat sink*: For dissipation of heat. Should always be kept free of any blockage.

16.14 Conclusion

Electrosurgery remains an indispensable tool in modern surgery. Advances in technology have improved safety. Comprehensive training in electrosurgical principles and safe practice is crucial to prevent adverse events. The Society of American Gastrointestinal and Endoscopic Surgeons (SAGES) has developed a validated training program in electrosurgery—"SAGES Manual on the Fundamental Use of Surgical Energy (FUSE)." Mastery of electrosurgery basic principles is essential for optimizing outcomes and minimize risks [2, 4].

References

1. El-Sayed MM, Saridogan E. Principles and safe use of electrosurgery in minimally invasive surgery. Gyn Pelvic Med. 2021;4:6. https://doi.org/10.21037/gpm-2020-pdf-10.
2. Alkatout I, Schollmeyer T, Hawaldar NA, Sharma N, Mettler L. Principles and safety measures of electrosurgery in laparoscopy. JSLS. 2012;16:130–9.
3. Wu M-P, Ou C-S, Chen S-L, Yen YET, Rowbothom R. Complications and recommended practices for electrosurgery in laparoscopy. Am J Surg. 2000;179:67–73.
4. Harrell AG, Kercher KW, Heniford T. Energy sources in laparoscopy. Semin Laparosc Surg. 2004;11(3):201–9.
5. Ahmad A, Nigam A, Kaur A. Principles of electrosurgery in laparoscopy. Pan Asian J Obs Gyn. 2019;2(1):22–9.

Advanced Bipolar Devices

17

Jasmeet Singh Ahluwalia

While standard bipolar electrosurgery has already been discussed in the previous chapter, surgical technology has since evolved to produce a new generation of advanced bipolar devices. These systems go beyond simple bipolar coagulation by incorporating precise energy delivery, tissue sensing, and vessel sealing capabilities that enable safe and reliable sealing of vessels up to several millimetres in diameter. Their ability to combine cutting and sealing in a single step makes them particularly valuable in laparoscopic surgery, where efficiency, precision, and minimal thermal spread are critical.

For both the surgeon and the operating theatre staff, an in-depth understanding of these devices—their working principles, limitations, and correct handling—is essential. Proper knowledge ensures maximised surgical performance, minimises the risk of device-related complications, and promotes the best patient outcomes in minimally invasive procedures.

These devices are "advanced" compared to conventional bipolar because they not only pass electric current between two electrodes (as in bipolar forceps) but also continuously monitor tissue properties and modulate energy delivery to achieve a permanent, safe seal with minimal collateral damage.

Working principle As with standard bipolar devices, the energy passes only through the tissue grasped between the jaws—not through the rest of the body. The goal is to denature and fuse collagen and elastin fibres in the vessel wall. This creates a coaptive seal strong enough to withstand blood pressure without clips or sutures. As tissue desiccates and collagen melts, impedance rises. The generator constantly measures tissue impedance (resistance to electrical current). When optimal sealing temperature and tissue state are reached, the system automatically stops energy flow.

J. S. Ahluwalia (✉)
Department of Bariatric & Minimal Access Surgery, STAR Superspeciality Hospital, Jalandhar, Punjab, India

J. S. Ahluwalia (ed.), *User Manual for Minimally Invasive Surgical Equipment*,
https://doi.org/10.1007/978-981-95-9019-3_17

Role of Tissue Compression The jaws apply precisely calibrated pressure to thin and align collagen fibres, while heat bonds them permanently. Hence, vessel sealing requires both energy and optimal compression.

Advantages over Conventional Bipolar

- Seals larger vessels (up to 5 or 7 mm, sometimes more) reliably
- Minimal lateral thermal spread (<2 mm)
- Automated shutoff to prevent overcooking and charring
- Integrated cut function—can seal and divide in one step
- Less instrument exchange in laparoscopic surgery enabling lesser surgical time

There are various such devices available:

1. LigaSure™—Medtronic (formerly Covidien)
2. ENSEAL®—Ethicon, Johnson & Johnson
3. Caiman® AESCULAP®—B. Braun Melsungen AG
4. POWERSEAL™—Olympus Corporation
5. Voyant—Applied Medical
6. Vessel Sealer Extend—Intuitive Surgical (da Vinci)
7. marSeal—KLS Martin
8. CoolSeal®—Bolder Surgical (HOLOGIC)
9. BiCision—Erbe Elektromedizin GmbH
10. ERGO—TissueSeal®—BOWA MEDICAL
11. BiSeal®—HEBUmedical
12. Axer—XcelLance Medical Technologies Pvt. Ltd. (Shalya)

The detailed description of every such instrument is beyond the scope of this book. Therefore, we have chosen to provide a comprehensive overview of two specific instruments: LigaSure and Enseal. We trust this will provide readers with a comprehensive understanding of various devices, irrespective of their specific applications.

17.1 Medtronic Devices

Medtronic has produced different energy platforms over time and the ones in common use are described in this chapter.

17.1.1 Valleylab™ LS10 Generator

Unlike other systems detailed later in the chapter, this generator is designed to provide vessel sealing application alone [1]. It detects the LigaSure instrument attached to it automatically and configures the device accordingly. It has been shown to be effective for sealing vessels up to 7 mm, tissue bundles and lymphatics.

Front Panel Various elements on front side of the device are detailed below (Fig. 17.1):

1. Power button: To power on, just push and release, and to power off, push and hold for 3 s.
2. System error indicator: This indicator illuminates upon detection of a system error within the generator.
3. System status indicator: Changes motion and colour to show various statuses.
   White:
      In motion—System is performing a self-test.
      Constant—System is now ready for use, insert desired LigaSure instrument.
      Flashing—Indicates service mode, power cycle system for clinical use.
   Purple:
      In motion—Sealing is in process.
      Constant—Ready for sealing/seal cycle complete.
   Amber:
      Seal cycle incomplete alert. Inspect, re-grasp, and reactivate sealing to complete the sealing cycle.
4. Usage limit indicator: Illuminates when inserted device has already been used
5. Instruments status or switch stuck indicator

Red—The inserted instrument may be invalid, damaged, or incompatible and also illuminates when hand or foot-switch is stuck. Check that the compatible LigaSure instrument is in proper working condition and that no activation switches are depressed.

6. Instrument Port: Connect LigaSure instruments when the system status indicator is white.

17.1.1.1 LS10

Back Panel Various elements on the back side of the equipment are detailed below (Fig. 17.2):

1. Volume knob: Used to adjust feedback volume of the device.
2. Foot-switch port: It is to connect foot-switch for activation of device.

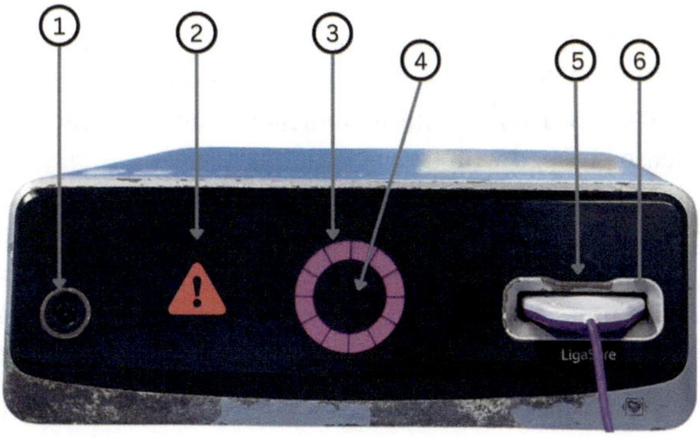

Fig. 17.1 Front panel of Valleylab LS10

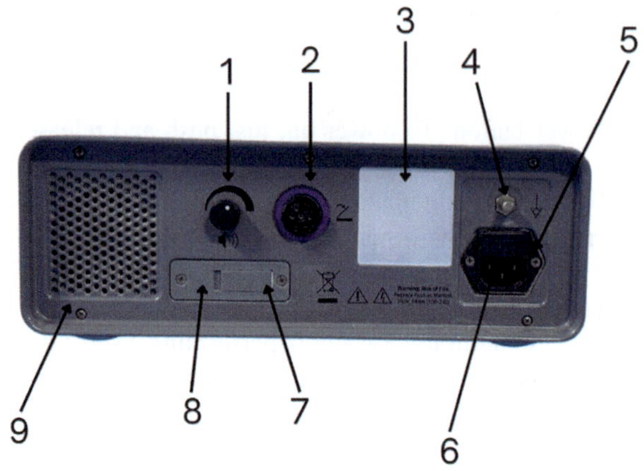

Fig. 17.2 Back panel of Valleylab

3. Serial label showing various details of the machine.
4. Potential equalisation conductor terminal that can be connected to the earth wire in case of earthing failure.
5. Fuse: It can be replaced if it gets burnt due to electrical disturbances.
6. AC mains receptacle: This is for connecting the power cord to give electricity supply to the machine.
7. ECG blanking connector which is provided to signal to external devices that the generator is delivering RF energy. Open the door to the USB/ECG blanking port cover to access the ECG blanking port. The receptacle is a 2.5 mm mono jack. It is electrically isolated from the internal ground referenced electronics with the shell electrically connected to the chassis for ESD protection.
8. USB port: Provides communications interface for communicating with an externally connected device.
9. Vent to maintain machine's temperature.

17.1.1.2 System Setup

Place the generator on a flat, stable surface such as a table, platform, or cart. Plug the system power cord into the rear-panel AC mains receptacle. Plug the system power cord into a grounded power outlet.

Turn on the system by pressing the power on/off button. The system status indicator illuminates in white colour and shows rotating motion indicating boot up and self-test. A beep is heard upon completion of the self-test and system indicator illuminates constant white to indicate system is ready. If it does not pass self-test, please proceed with troubleshooting.

Insert the LigaSure connector into the receptacle. The system status indicator illuminates purple, indicating that the system is ready for surgical use. Activate the LigaSure instrument by pressing and holding the activation button on the instrument or by pressing and holding the foot-switch pedal. During the duration of energy delivery, the system status indicator illuminates purple, rotating segment by segment, and an activation tone sounds. When the two-pulse seal cycle completes, the activation tone is emitted, and the system status indicator illuminates solid purple, indicating that the seal cycle has been completed. Release the activation button or foot-switch. One may cut the tissue using in built knife if desired.

17.1.1.3 Troubleshooting

Table 17.1 shows some common problems that one may encounter and their solutions.

17.1.2 ForceTriad Energy Platform

The name is derived from the fact that it has three types of energies built into single machine—monopolar, bipolar, and LigaSure (Fig. 17.3).

The touch screens on the device adapt their displays in response to the attached instruments. The device identifies the distinctive electrical signature of each instrument and reacts accordingly [2].

Description:

1. Monopolar 1 Accessory Touchscreen: A dedicated touch interface enables the selection, monitoring, and adjustment of settings for the Monopolar 1 output and any connected accessory tools. This interface facilitates the modification of power levels, modes (cut/coagulation), and waveform types without requiring navigation away from other settings.

Table 17.1 Troubleshooting LS10 device

Indicator	Description	Solution
Amber colour on system status along with four pulse tones	Incomplete seal cycle	Reactivate to complete seal cycle
Red instrument status indication and three pulse tone	Invalid instrument or stuck hand switch or stuck foot switch	Change instrument or release stuck switch
No energy delivered and single pulse tone heard	Foot switch activation disabled	Use hand switch or replace instrument with foot switch compatible instrument
Amber or red usage limit indicator	Inserted hand instrument is already used	Replace the instrument
No tone on pressing foot switch	Faulty foot switch	Confirm instrument is fully inserted and foot switch plug is also properly
Red system error indicator illuminated and three pulse tone heard	System error	Power cycle the generator. If persists, contact technical service team
White colour system status indicator illuminated and flashing	System in service mode	Cycle the power to exit this mode

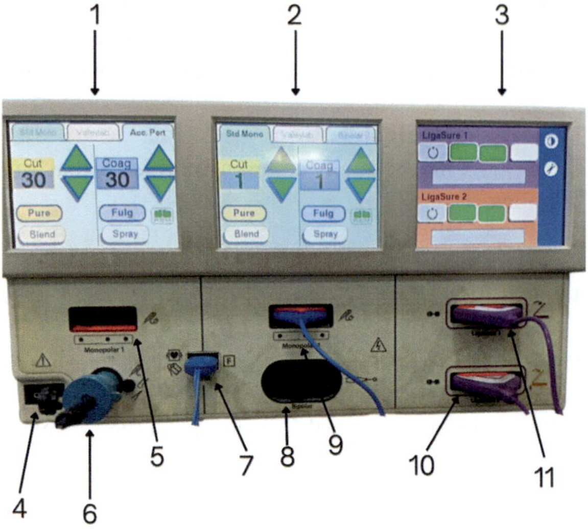

Fig. 17.3 ForceTriad energy platform (front view)

2. Monopolar 2 and Bipolar Touchscreen: Controls both Monopolar 2 and Bipolar modes from a single touchscreen. Useful when both energy types are in use during the same surgery, allowing quick switching and fine adjustments from a dedicated touchscreen for each device type.
3. LigaSure and System-Tray Touchscreen: A dedicated touchscreen interface for LigaSure vessel sealing functionalities, facilitating the activation of seal cycles, adjustment of seal settings, and monitoring device performance. It serves as the primary system tray interface for setup, calibration, and other platform-wide functionalities.
4. Power Switch: The main on/off control for the ForceTriad unit, conveniently located at the front for quick access during emergencies or start-up/shutdown procedures.
5. Monopolar Instrument Receptacle: This receptacle is designed to connect the wire from a monocular hand instrument and facilitates the delivery of monopolar energy from the generator to the tip of the instruments.
6. Foot-switch Receptacle: Provides attachment for foot switch supplied with the machine to provide foot-controlled activation for energy delivery without using hand controls. This can enhance ergonomics and control for the operator.
7. Patient Return Electrode (REM) Receptacle: Provides connection for the return electrode (grounding pad). This completes the electrical circuit in monopolar modes and is essential to use device in this mode. REM monitoring technology continuously checks contact quality to prevent accidental patient burns.
8. Bipolar-Instrument Receptacle: For connecting bipolar surgical instruments. This port supplies energy without the need for a return electrode as energy has to pass between two tips on the same instrument in this case.

9. Monopolar 2 Instrument Receptacle: Another monopolar device can be attached here for procedures requiring multiple monopolar tools without replugging devices.
10. LigaSure 2 Receptacle: Another LigaSure device can be connected here to be used simultaneously or as a standby during the procedure.
11. LigaSure 1 Receptacle: Primary connector for LigaSure vessel sealing instruments for providing controlled, feedback-regulated bipolar energy optimised for vessel sealing and division.

These three touchscreens can display a variety of symbols which are described in Fig. 17.4.

Back side of the machine has the following connectors (Fig. 17.5):

1. USB Port: It is a network connection interface for software updates and system integration. Only authorised personnel should be allowed to use this port.
2. Ethernet Port: This port is used for diagnosing errors, service, and communication with external systems (e.g. integration with OR systems or data collections).
3. RS232 Port: It is used for communication with external devices, specifically for software updates and data transfer related to system maintenance and diagnostics. Only authorised personnel should be allowed to use this port.
4. LigaSure 1 Foot-switch Receptacle: For connecting foot-switch of primary LigaSure device.
5. LigaSure 2 Foot-switch Receptacle: For connecting foot-switch of secondary LigaSure device.
6. Bipolar Foot-switch Receptacle: For connecting foot-switch of bipolar device.
7. Interlink Cable Port: Used to connect compatible devices like smoke evacuator to work in conjunction with this device.
8. Expansion Port: The expansion port serves as a connecting mechanism, facilitating the integration of the generator with various systems and accessories like remote controls or connection to integrated OR.
9. Monopolar Foot-switch Receptacle: For connecting monopolar instrument foot-switch. Please note that it requires adapter to connect standard four-pin monopolar foot-switch.
10. Power Entry Module (with fuse): Enables the connection of a power cord. It incorporates an integrated fuse holder for overcurrent protection.

17.1.2.1 System Setup

Start with system in off position. Place the device on a flat and stable surface or on a ForceTriad cart that can be bought from the manufacturer. Plug the system power cord into the rear panel receptacle. Plug the system power cord into a grounded power receptacle.

Turn on the system by pressing the power switch on and observe the following during the power-up self-test:

- The Covidien (company logo) logo appears on all three screens.

Symbol	Name	Description
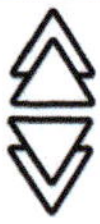	Page Up Page Down	Scroll through blocks of options that cannot be displayed on a single screen.
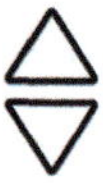	Up/Down	Pressing once increases/decreases the associated value or moves highlighted selection up/down one line. Pressing and holding scrolls up/down.
	Next/Back	Progresses/regresses to the next screen.
	Back Space	Regresses one character.
	Bipolar Mute On/Off	Turn on/off the audio tones produced by the system that indicate the increase or decrease of current during a bipolar procedure.
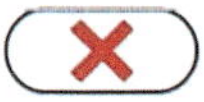	Cancel	Cancels current screen and returns to the previous screen.
	Enter	Accepts and initiates current selections.
	System Tray	The system tray contains controls that allow you to access and adjust system settings including screen brightness and main menu options.
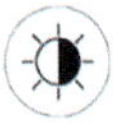	Brightness	Each selection of this button adjusts the screen brightness to the next of the two available brightness settings. When maximum brightness is reached, next selection resets to the least bright setting.
	Wrench	Select access to the main menu, which provides user-selected options for language, appearance, and operation.
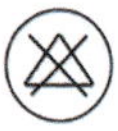	Errors Disabled	This indicates that error warnings have been disabled using the ervice menu. The generator will not alarm or give error condition hen this symbol is activatec.

Fig. 17.4 ForceTriad energy platform common symbols

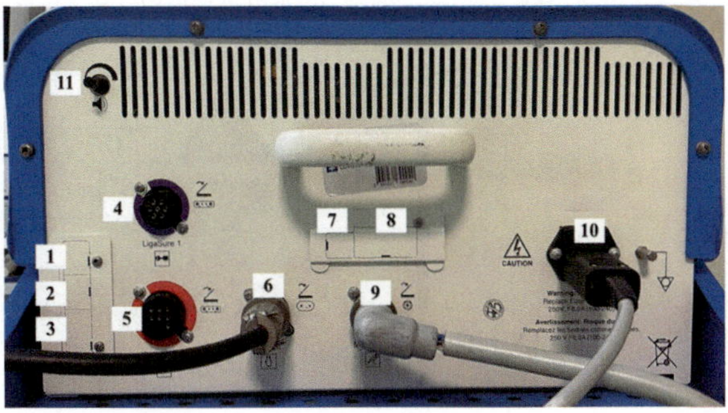

Fig. 17.5 ForceTriad energy platform rear panel

- A blue status bar indicates progress of the startup.
- An hourglass icon indicates activity after the status bar disappears.
- The system revision code appears on the centre screen.
- A tone sounds upon completion of self-test.

In case the system is unable to pass the power-up self-test and an error code is displayed, refer to the troubleshooting section.

17.1.2.2 Standard Monopolar Mode

Functions available in this mode are (Fig. 17.6):

1. Power Output Mode Display: Displays set power in Watts.
2. Green Power Control Arrows: Up and down arrows to increase or decrease power, respectively.
3. Power Output Mode Waveform: To select various modes available according to the application. The waveforms available in the cut mode are Pure and Blend. In the coagulation mode, the waveforms available are Fulgurate and Spray.
4. REM indicator: Green indicates a complete and functional circuit. Red signifies an open circuit and prevents power output.

17.1.2.3 Valleylab Mode

Valleylab mode offers following settings (Fig. 17.7):

1. Power Output Modes: Shows power setting in watts.
2. Power Bar Indicators: The five gold bars situated in the centre of the Valleylab tab signify the five available power bars for the specific instrument connected to the energy platform receptacle. The system automatically selects the default power bar setting for each instrument. Power bar modifications can only be made via the touchscreen interface on the energy platform.

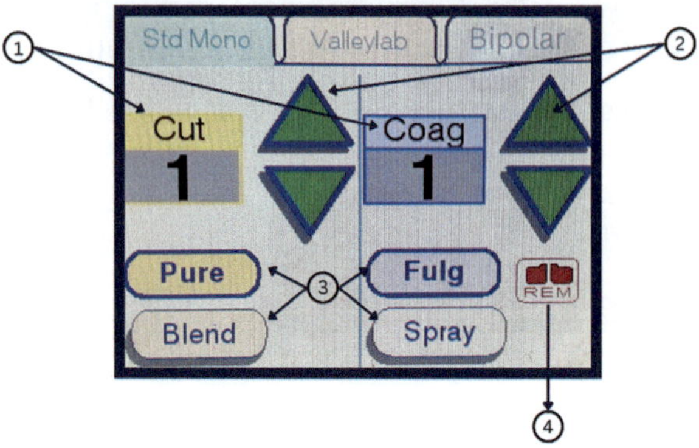

Fig. 17.6 Screen showing standard monopolar mode

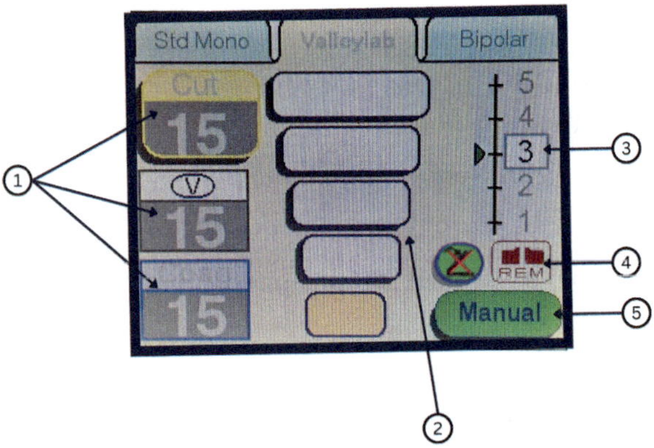

Fig. 17.7 Screen showing Valleylab mode

3. Slider Position Indicator: The energy platform continuously monitors the current position of the instrument's slider switch. The slider position indicator, situated on the right side of the Valleylab tab, promptly displays this information. It is crucial to emphasise that only the instrument user is authorised to modify the slider position within the sterile field.
4. REM Indicator: Green indicates a complete and functional circuit. Red signifies an open circuit and prevents power output.
5. Manual Selector Button: Manual mode enables the user to operate the energy platform independently of the predefined power ranges accessible on the Valleylab tab. In manual mode, any slider on the electrosurgical instrument is disabled, and power can only be adjusted by the touchscreen interface. It is important to note that manual mode is the sole available mode for instruments lacking a slider.

17.1.2.4 Accessory Port Mode

The Accessory Port tab displays the available accessory port options. Instruments with 8 mm pins connect directly to the accessory port on the ForceTriad Energy Platform. Instruments with pin diameters less than 8 mm may necessitate the use of an adapter. Remove the adapter when not in use.

When a single pin electrosurgical instrument is attached to the universal foot switching accessory port, the ForceTriad Energy Platform identifies the instrument and displays the Accessory Port tab on the touchscreen. The Accessory Port tab enables the user to control the power mode and power output level at the system interface for any foot-switching instrument connected.

17.1.2.5 Bipolar Mode

Bipolar mode offers following features (Fig. 17.8):

1. Power Output Modes: Shows the set power in watts.
2. Power Output Mode Waveforms: The waveforms available in the bipolar mode are Low, Standard, and Macro.
3. Green Power Control Arrows: Desired power can be set by pressing up and down arrows.
4. Virtual Ammeter: The virtual ammeter on the bipolar tab indicates the current being delivered during bipolar-instrument activation. The ammeter registers current values between 1 and 1050 milliamps. An audio tone is emitted to signify fluctuations in current delivery. A mute button enables the user to silence the ammeter tone, while the activation tone remains audible.

17.1.2.6 Autobipolar Function

This feature enables the user to configure the system for automatic activation and deactivation of bipolar energy. Before the autobipolar function can be utilised, the Autobipolar mode must be enabled in the feature menu. When the autobipolar mode

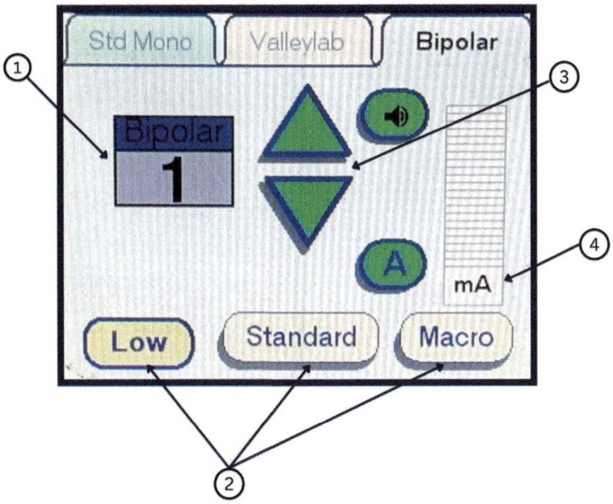

Fig. 17.8 Screen showing bipolar mode

is enabled, a green button "A" button appears on the Bipolar tab. User can select power output modes waveform, set desired output power and change auto bipolar activations parameters in this mode.

17.1.2.7 LigaSure Mode

The LigaSure touchscreen comprises two distinct functional components: the LigaSure 1 control panel, which governs instruments connected to the LigaSure 1 receptacle; and the LigaSure 2 control panel, which controls instruments connected to the LigaSure 2 receptacle (Fig. 17.9). Two LigaSure instruments can be simultaneously set up via this touchscreen interface, but only one instrument can be activated at a time. Upon instrument activation, the corresponding LigaSure control panel status bar illuminates blue, accompanied by a sound indicating the duration of energy delivery.

The green bars on the display indicate varying degrees of desiccation. Two green bars are the default configuration for all LigaSure tissue-fusion instruments. By selecting one bar, surgeons anticipate a gentler and typically extended fusion cycle, potentially more effective for thinner tissue bundles and smaller, isolated vessels. Conversely, selecting three bars indicates a longer fusion cycle, potentially more effective for thicker tissue bundles. The instrument settings can be modified by pressing one of the three setting buttons on the corresponding LigaSure 1 or LigaSure 2 control panel. The button pressed in conjunction with the buttons to its left undergoes a visual transformation, turning green, while the standby button transitions to a grey colour.

Note that a standby button is preceded by three green bars, which can be pressed to set the instrument to standby mode until the user is ready to use it to prevent accidental damage.

17.1.2.8 Activating the Instrument

Activate the LigaSure instrument by pressing and holding the activation button on the instrument or by pressing and holding the foot-switch pedal. During instrument activation, the status bar in the corresponding LigaSure control panel illuminates

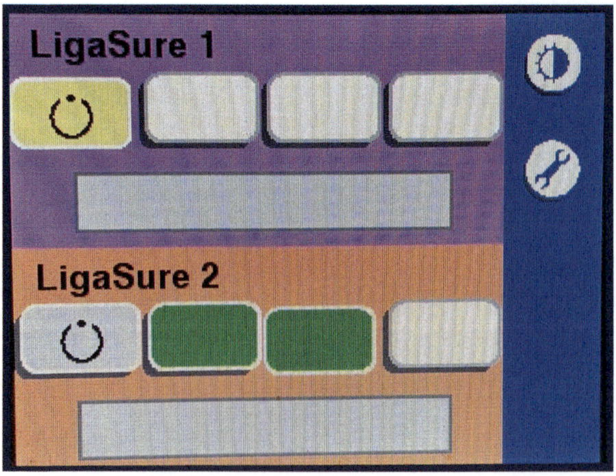

Fig. 17.9 Screen showing LigaSure mode

blue, and an activation tone sounds for the duration of energy delivery. Upon hearing the end tone, release the activation button or foot-switch pedal. In the event of an alert condition, refer to the following section.

17.1.2.9 Alerts

A pulsed tone will sound when an alert condition occurs, and the LigaSure touchscreen will display an alert message that instructs the user on the corrective actions to be taken.

Reactivate A four-pulsed tone will sound when the reactivate screen is displayed. Either the endpoint was not reached or the seal cycle was interrupted before completion. The user should release the foot-switch pedal or hand switching button and reactivate the seal cycle without repositioning the instrument.

Check Instrument A six-pulsed tone will sound when the Check Instrument screen is displayed. The user should release the foot-switch pedal or activation button. Open the instrument jaws and inspect for a successful seal. Follow the suggested corrective action on the screen.

17.1.2.10 Troubleshooting

Table 17.2 provides quick troubleshooting steps for common issues encountered with the Valleylab ForceTriad energy platform.

17.1.3 Valleylab FT10 Energy Platform

This is the latest iteration of Medtronic vessel sealer (Fig. 17.10) [3]:

1. On/Off Button: This button enables the system to be turned on and off. Upon activation, the device executes a brief self-test before commencing its operational cycle.
2. Restore Settings Button: Resets the platform to its default factory settings. This button is useful when incorrect adjustments have been made and you wish to begin anew with safe defaults.
3. Audio Volume Control Button: This button enables surgeons and staff to adjust the alarm and activation sound levels. By increasing or decreasing audio alerts, they can enhance their audibility in the operating room.
4. Service/Settings Button: Accesses the system settings menu, enabling customisation, diagnostics, and service functionalities.
5. Return Electrode Monitoring (REM) Indicator: The indicator illuminates to indicate the status of patient return electrode monitoring. This ensures the safe dispersal of electrical energy, thereby preventing burns resulting from inadequate patient pad contact.

Table 17.2 Troubleshooting Valleylab ForceTriad energy platform

Situation	Possible cause	Solution
Energy platform does not respond when turned on	Disconnected/faulty power cord or wall outlet; blown fuses; internal malfunction	Check/replace power cord, fuses, outlet; contact service if needed
System is on but did not complete self-test	Software malfunction; internal component failure	Restart system; if persists, contact biomedical/service team
System on, instrument activated, but no output	Malfunctioning footswitch/ instrument; low power setting; alarm condition; internal malfunction	Check instrument connections, replace instrument, increase power, resolve alarm, contact service
System does not detect instrument	Loose or incorrect connector insertion	Reinsert connector properly
Check instrument alert, tone, RF disabled	Dirty electrode tips; loose electrodes; metal object in jaws; too thin tissue; fluid around tip	Clean electrodes; reseat electrodes; avoid grasping metal; use sufficient tissue; remove fluids
Reactivate screen and tone	Seal cycle interrupted (handswitch/footswitch released early)	Reactivate seal cycle without repositioning instrument
Continuous monitor interference	Faulty monitor or ground connections; equipment grounded differently	Replace monitor; correct ground wiring; plug equipment into same line; contact service
Interference with other devices	Metal sparking; high fulguration settings; faulty grounding	Check connections; lower settings; correct ground wiring; contact service if persists
Pacemaker interference	Electrosurgical current near pacemaker; poor electrode placement	Reprogram pacemaker if needed; use bipolar if possible; place return electrode close to site; monitor patient

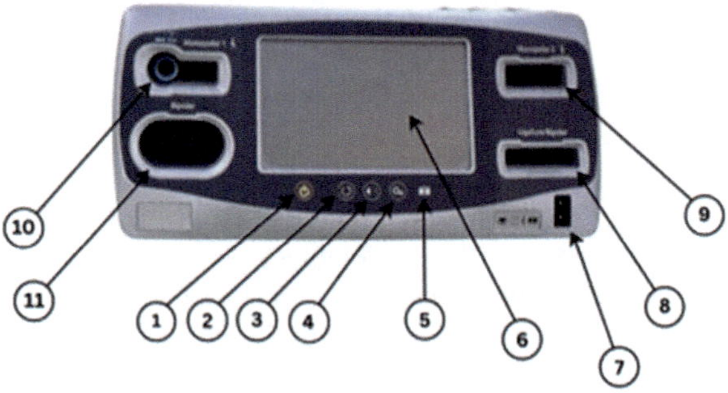

Fig. 17.10 Valleylab FT10 energy platform front view

6. Interface Touchscreen: The primary control display on the FT10 enables surgeons to select energy modes, modify power settings, and monitor system performance.
7. REM Patient Return Electrode Receptacle: Connector port for the patient return electrode (grounding pad). It monitors the contact quality of the pad and alerts if there is an unsafe situation.

8. LigaSure™/Bipolar Receptacle: This receptacle is designed to accommodate LigaSure instruments (vessel sealing devices) or bipolar instruments, providing advanced energy for vessel sealing or precise bipolar coagulation.
9. Monopolar 2 Instrument Receptacle: This receptacle serves as a connector for a second monopolar surgical instrument, enabling the support of both cutting and coagulation modes, irrespective of the Monopolar 1 instrument.
10. Monopolar 1 Universal Foot Pedal Port (UFP) Receptacle: This receptacle facilitates the connection of foot-switches to Monopolar 1 instruments, facilitating hands-free activation of monopolar energy functions.
11. Bipolar Instrument Receptacle: This receptacle is specifically designed to connect standard bipolar instruments, such as bipolar forceps, facilitating delicate coagulation between forceps tips with minimal current spread.

The Monopolar 1 UFP-receptacle, distinguished by a blue ring, accommodates UFP connectors with diameters ranging from 4 to 8 mm and lengths from 15.2 to 41.7 mm. UFP connectors with a diameter less than 4 mm necessitate the use of an adapter to connect to the Monopolar 1 UFP receptacle.

Back side of the machine (Fig. 17.11) has:

1. Monopolar 2 foot-pedal receptacle (requires included adapter to connect standard four-pin monopolar foot pedal)
2. Monopolar 1 foot-pedal receptacle
3. LigaSure/Bipolar foot-pedal receptacle (requires included adapter to connect bipolar resection foot pedal)
4. Bipolar foot-pedal receptacle
5. Fuse drawer
6. Power cord receptacle
7. Equipotential ground connection
8. WiFi antenna (Covered. For service only.)
9. Ethernet receptacle (Covered. For service only.)
10. Interlink cable receptacles for EKG blanking and smoke-evacuation control (independently linked to Monopolar 1 and Monopolar 2 activation)

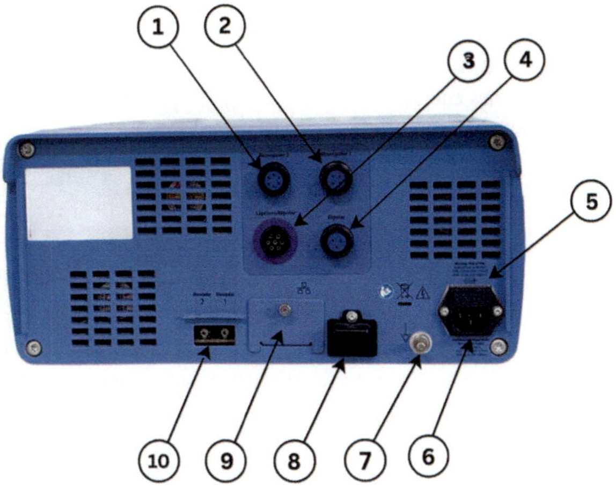

Fig. 17.11 Valleylab FT10-FT series energy platform series back view

17.1.3.1 The Touchscreen

This device features a touchscreen interface to control system functions. The touchscreen is divided into quadrants (Fig. 17.12); each of the four sections is associated with an adjacent instrument receptacle. Quadrant 1 and 2 are for settings of monopolar instruments attached to monopolar receptacle 1 and 2 respectively. Quadrant 3 is for bipolar instrument and quadrant 4 is for LigaSure and bipolar resection devices.

17.1.3.2 Troubleshooting

Table 17.3 shows steps to troubleshoot some common Valleylab ForceTriad energy platform problems.

17.1.4 LigaSure Instrument

LigaSure instruments come in different shapes and sizes, and the Maryland jaw laparoscopic sealer/divider is described here for reference (Fig. 17.13):

1. Jaws: This is the working end of the instrument. It is designed to grasp tissue and vessels. It delivers bipolar energy between the two jaws to seal blood vessels and tissue bundles. It also has a cutting mechanism to divide sealed tissue, which can be triggered by pressing the cutting trigger.
2. Shaft: Long, insulated tube connecting the jaws to the handle. Provides reach inside the abdominal cavity during laparoscopic surgery. Insulated to prevent stray current and ensure safe energy delivery.
3. Rotation Wheel: Allows 360° rotation of the shaft and jaws and helps the user to position the jaws precisely without changing hand grip, thereby improving ergonomics during laparoscopic procedures.
4. Handle: Provides for ergonomic grip to the user and houses control mechanisms for activation and cutting.
5. Activation Button: Triggers bipolar energy delivery when pressed. In this model of instrument, this button will be pressed automatically on grasping the tissue hard enough. Used to seal vessels and tissue between the jaws.

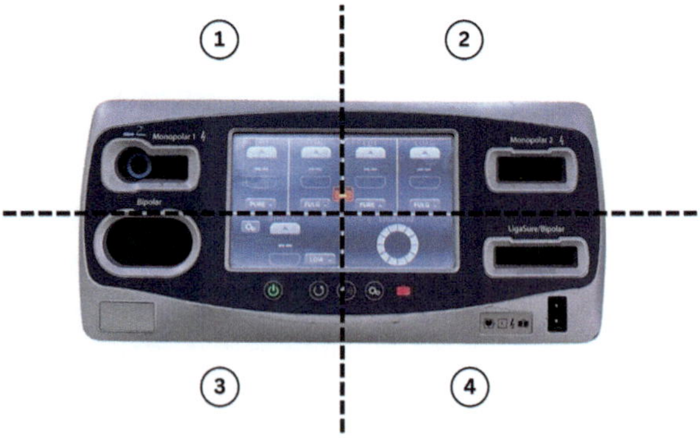

Fig. 17.12 Valleylab FT10-FT series energy platform touchscreen quadrants

Table 17.3 Troubleshooting Valleylab FT 10 energy platform

Situation	Possible cause	Solution
Abnormal neuromuscular stimulation (stop surgery immediately)	Metal-to-metal sparking	Check all connections to platform, patient return electrode, and active electrodes
	High power settings	Use lower power setting
Energy platform does not respond when turned on	Disconnected/faulty wall outlet	Check power cord and outlet
	Faulty power cord	Replace power cord
	Blown fuses/open fuse drawer	Replace fuse(s), close drawer
	Internal component malfunction	Use backup platform and call service
System on, but no self-test completion	Software malfunction	Restart the platform
	Internal component malfunction	Note error code, use backup platform, call service
Platform on and instrument activated, but no output	Malfunctioning foot pedal or hand switch	Turn off, check connections, replace instrument if needed
	Power set too low/off	Increase setting
	Alarm condition	Note error code, refer to alarms section, check REM
	Internal malfunction	Contact service
System does not detect tissue-fusion (LigaSure) instrument	Loose/incorrect connector	Reinsert LigaSmart connector, check detection on screen
System does not detect monopolar instrument	Loose/incorrect connector	Reinsert monopolar connector, check quadrant indicator
System does not detect bipolar instrument	Loose/incorrect connector	Reinsert bipolar connector, check detection on screen
Check LigaSure instrument pop-up and tone	Tissue/eschar on jaws	Clean jaws with wet gauze
	Electrodes loose/bent	Reinsert or replace electrodes
	Metal/foreign body grasped	Avoid staples/clips/sutures
	Tissue too thin	Insert sufficient tissue, retry
	Pooled fluids	Remove excess fluids
Reactivate LigaSure pop up and tone	Seal cycle interrupted (released early, jaws opened early, extra time needed)	Reactivate cycle without repositioning instrument
Continuous monitor interference	Malfunctioning monitor	Replace monitor
	Faulty grounding	Check ground connections for monitor and generator
	Different ground sources in OR	Plug equipment into same power source
Interference with devices only when activated	Metal-to-metal sparking	Check all electrode and platform connections
	High power settings	Use lower settings
	Inconsistent OR grounding	Verify all grounds connect to same point
Pacemaker interference	Sparking or intermittent connections	Check all cords, may need pacemaker reprogramming
	Current path near pacemaker	Use bipolar if possible, reposition return electrode

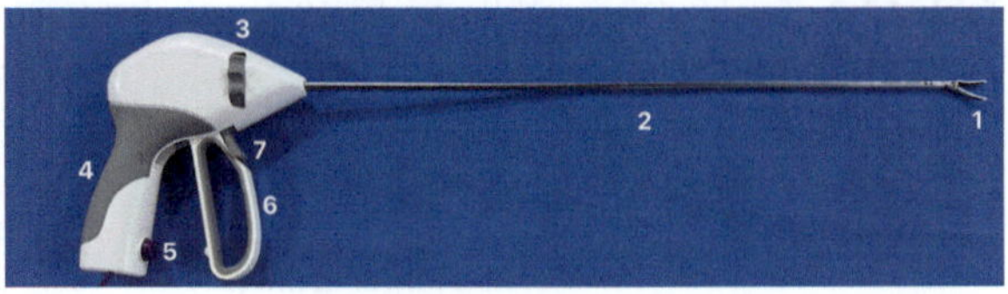

Fig. 17.13 LigaSure Maryland jaw laparoscopic sealer/divider

6. Lever: Mechanical lever used to open and close the jaws to provide controlled grasping of tissue.
7. Cutting Trigger: Engages the cutting mechanism (integrated knife) within the jaws. Activated after sealing, allowing surgeons to divide tissue safely. Provides a one-step seal-and-cut function, reducing instrument exchanges.

LigaSure hand instruments are available in a variety of configurations designed for different surgical needs and specialties. The primary configurations include variations in:

1. Jaw Design and Shape
   Straight jaws—standard type for general tissue sealing
   Curved/Maryland jaws—improve visibility and access in confined spaces
2. Length
   Short (23 cm)—For open or superficial surgeries
   Standard (37 cm)—Common in laparoscopic procedures
   Long (44 cm)—For deep or bariatric surgeries
3. Diameter
   5 mm instruments—Standard for most laparoscopic procedures
   10 mm instruments—For more robust vessel sealing and tissue handling
4. Special Uses
   LigaSure Atlas—10 mm, blunt-tip laparoscopic sealer with integrated cutting, ideal for sealing large vessels and tissue bundles
   LigaSure Maryland Tip—5 mm curved, fine-tip sealer designed for precise dissection, sealing, and cutting in tight or delicate areas
   LigaSure Retractable L-Hook—A versatile instrument combining vessel sealing with a retractable L-shaped electrosurgical hook for dissection
   LigaSure Exact—Open-surgery sealer designed for precise and ergonomic handling, combining sealing and cutting
   LigaSure Maryland Thoracic Sealer/Divider—A specialised sealer with a long shaft and curved Maryland jaw, optimised for thoracic surgeries

17.2 User Manual for Ethicon Devices

Ethicon manufactures different models of energy platforms, but we will elaborate on the Gen 11 model as a reference for this chapter (Fig. 17.14). It combines ultrasonic shears (Harmonic) with an advanced bipolar device (Enseal) [4].

Front of the generator has a large touchscreen for various functions:

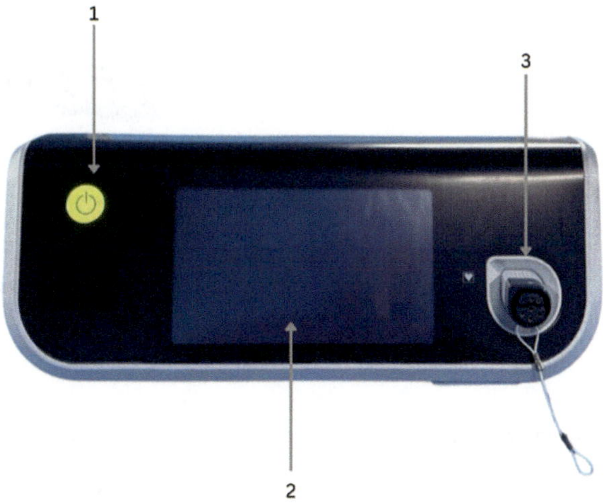

Fig. 17.14 Ethicon Gen 11 generator front view

1. Power On/Off Switch: Turns the generator on or off. When powered on, it glows green, indicating the system is active and ready for use.
2. Touch Screen: Serves as the main user interface and displays system information such as generator status, instrument recognition, settings, and error/warning messages. It also allows the user to adjust controls, select modes, and configure energy delivery settings.
3. Connector/Instrument Receptacle: A receptacle used to connect surgical instruments (e.g. Harmonic scalpel, Enseal devices, or other Ethicon advanced energy instruments).

Back side of generator has following components (Fig. 17.15):

1. Power cord Receptacle: Socket for attaching the generator's power cord. It supplies mains electrical power to the unit.
2. Foot-switch Receptacle: Connection port for the surgical foot-switch to allow hands-free activation of instruments.
3. Potential Equalisation Terminal: This is a grounding point to connect a potential equalisation conductor. This ensures the generator and other equipment share the same ground potential and minimises the risk of electrical interference or shock.

17.2.1 Footswitch

Foot-switch has two pedals for activation of device depending on the instrument connected (Fig. 17.16):

1. MIN (Left Pedal): Activates power for Enseal instruments. When used with HARMONIC instruments, it delivers minimum power output. Provides more coagulation and slower cutting speed.

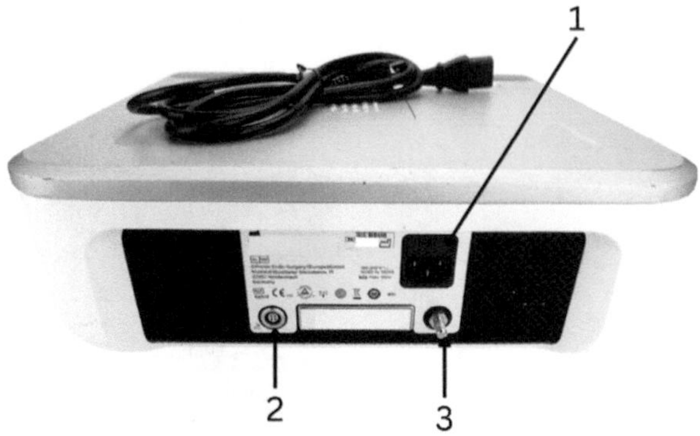

Fig. 17.15 Ethicon Gen 11 generator back view

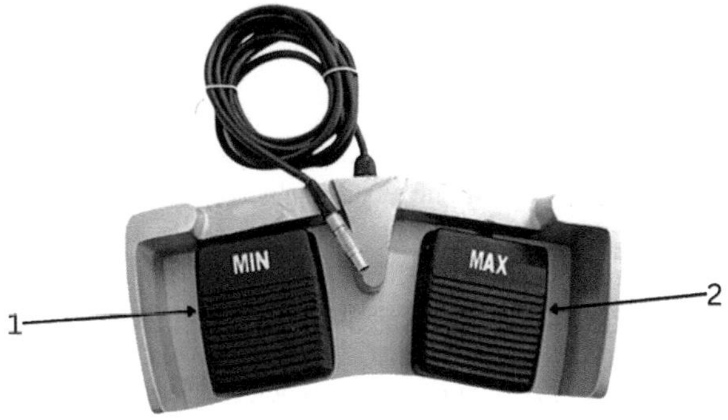

Fig. 17.16 Ethicon GEN11 foot pedal

2. MAX (Right Pedal): Activates maximum power for Harmonic instruments. Used when higher energy is required for faster cutting.

17.2.2 Enseal Tissue Sealer

Enseal has various hand instruments for different needs. G2 tissue sealer is explained here (Fig. 17.17):

1. Jaws: The working end of the instrument that is used to grasp, compress, and seal tissue or vessels. It is integrated with a cutting mechanism to divide tissue after sealing.
2. Shaft: Long insulated portion of the device that connects jaws to the handle and is designed for laparoscopic access (5 mm diameter).
3. Rotation Knob: Allows 360° rotation of the shaft and jaws to enable optimal positioning of the instrument without changing hand grip. This improves ergonomics and access to difficult angles during surgery.
4. Energy Activation Button: This triggers the delivery of bipolar energy.
5. Closing Handle: Mechanical handle that opens and closes the jaws and allows the surgeon to grasp and secure tissue before energy activation.

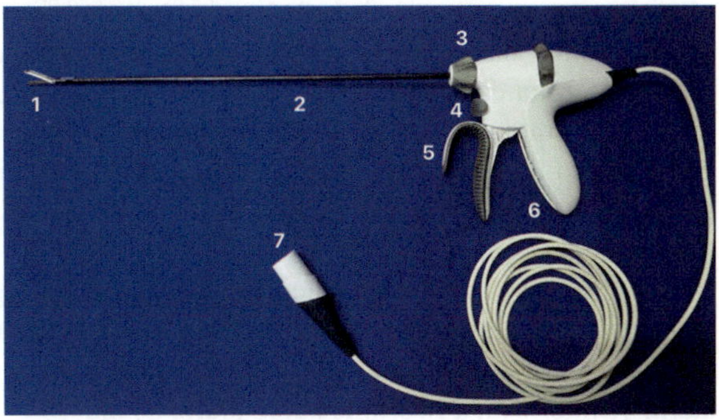

Fig. 17.17 Enseal G2 tissue sealer

6. Grip Housing: The main body/handle of the device that is ergonomically designed for comfort and stability during long procedures. It houses the mechanical and electrical controls.
7. Connector: Connects the instrument to the Ethicon Gen11 Energy Generator and transmits bipolar energy from the generator to the jaws.

17.2.2.1 Setup

1. Check the generator and instrument for damage. Don't use damaged devices.
2. Secure the generator on its cart or suitable fixture in the right place.
3. Connect the power cord to the back panel of the generator in power cord receptacle and a grounded electrical outlet.
4. Connect the foot-switch connector to the generator's back panel foot-switch receptacle if needed.
5. Connect the instrument to the generator. You may need an adapter to do so depending on the make of your instrument.
6. Turn on the generator using the On/Off switch.
7. The green standby indicator lights up, and the system initiates. A tone plays during the sequence. After the sequence ends, the Enseal ready screen appears, and the generator is ready to use.

17.2.2.2 Types of Hand Instruments Available

X1 series: Newer generation with more efficient sealing with bigger jaw length.

G1 series: Older generation and is also available in articulating design.

X1 large jaw is available in 20 cm length only as it is intended for open surgery, whereas other models are available in lengths from 14 to 45 cm (not all lengths are available in all models) to use in different types of patients.

Jaw Shape: Jaw tip can be straight or curved depending upon the model.

17.2.2.3 Troubleshooting

The user interface for this generator has a number of informative screens to guide the efficient use of the generator. Informative screens are of dark background to differentiate them from the alarm screen which look significantly different. Generator monitors its operation and flashes either informative screens or alarms with no delay. Audible alarm sounds are also produced. Alarm settings are not adjustable by the operator nor can priority be reassigned. The Power on Self Test (POST) verifies that the generator is operational. During the POST an audio tone is emitted from the generator so the user can verify that the audio output is operational. Alarm audio cannot be paused but audio automatically ends when the user discontinues activation of the instrument.

Low Priority Alarms: Indicate an issue that will not generally progress to a hazardous condition even if not addressed promptly but must be addressed to continue the procedure. The screen shows a solid yellow background with a low priority alarm symbol with a two-tone audio alarm sound.

Medium Priority Alarms: Ignoring this alarm can result in a serious injury or death. Screen shows a solid yellow background with a flashing medium priority alarm symbol along with a three-tone audio alarm sound. This requires prompt attention.

Note that there are no alarms classified as high priority in this generator.

The alarms are usually self-descriptive with help of text and diagrams on the screen and the solution is also usually mentioned on the screen. Also not that when an alarm sounds, the generator output stops. If the jaws are closed on tissue and an alarm sound, do not advance the knife. If the knife is advanced, do not release the instrument. Add additional clamping as necessary to prevent blood loss before releasing the instrument.

17.2.2.4 Best Practices to Ensure Best Outcomes

To achieve optimum results with advanced bipolar instruments surgeons should carefully select appropriate vessels within the recommended size range (up to 5 or 7 mm depending on the instrument) and ensure the tissue is fully and evenly placed within the jaws without overloading. Complete jaw closure and steady compression are essential before activating energy and the sealing process should be carried out in a single continuous cycle until the generator confirms seal completion. This avoids repeated short activations that weaken seal strength and increase thermal spread. During activation the jaws should remain steady without twisting or movement and a brief pause should be allowed for the seal to cool and solidify before cutting. The cutting blade should only be advanced once the seal is confirmed complete and if an alarm interrupts sealing cutting should not be attempted until the issue is resolved. For consistent performance the jaws should be kept clean of tissue debris and activation should never occur over metal objects such as clips or retractors. Using compatible generators with preset energy algorithms ensures optimal output. Finally, seals should be visually inspected for integrity. In the case of large pedicles two adjacent seals with staggered cuts may be applied to enhance security and ensure reliable vessel sealing, minimal thermal injury and patient safety.

17.3 Conclusion

Advanced bipolar instruments have revolutionised laparoscopic surgery by providing reliable vessel sealing with precision, safety, and efficiency. Their effectiveness, however, depends significantly on correct usage. This includes proper vessel selection and tissue handling adherence to recommended activation techniques and generator settings. By following best practices such as ensuring complete jaw closure, maintaining instrument cleanliness, and avoiding activation on inappropriate tissues or metal objects, surgeons can achieve consistent seal integrity with minimal thermal spread. As technology continues to evolve, these devices will become more refined, but their success in the operating room will always depend on a combination of advanced design and meticulous surgical technique.

References

1. Covidien. Valleylab LS10, LS series single channel vessel sealing generator: user's guide. https://everymed.eu/api/viewFile?file=/_userfiles/everymed/image/product_images/00/00/00/00/03/24/document_370.
2. Covidien. ForceTriad Energy Platform software v3-8 service manual. https://www.scribd.com/document/789828764/Forcetriad-Energy-Platform-Software-v3-8-Service-Manual-1. Accessed 27 Nov 2025.
3. Valleylab. Valleylab FT10 FT Series Energy Platform user's guide. Part No. PT00093618, Scribd. n.d. https://www.scribd.com/document/624855630/FT10-ug-sw-v-4.
4. Ethicon Endo-Surgery. Generator G11 operator's manual. Document No. A001490 Rev B. 2018.

Conclusion

Ultrasonic Shears 18

Jaideep Rao and Danson Yeo Xue Wei

Ultrasonic devices were developed in the 1980s and have gained widespread adoption with the rise of laparoscopic surgery. Compared to conventional electrosurgery, ultrasonic energy offers several advantages, including include faster cutting and coagulation [1, 2], reduced thermal damage, improved haemostasis with reduced blood loss [3, 4] and decreased surgical plume production [5]. Over the past decade, ultrasonic devices have gone substantial refinement and evolution, resulting in improved efficiency, safety and ergonomics.

An ultrasonic shear (US) typically comprises a generator, a transducer and an active blade. The generator provides electrical energy, and in modern systems, dynamically adjusts voltage to maintain consistent frequency and blade displacement in response to changes in tissue impedance. The transducer converts electrical energy from the generator to mechanical motion in the blade via piezoelectic crystals. Within the transducer, the electrical energy excites the piezoelectric ceramics causing them to expand and contract, thus transforming the electrical energy into ultra-high frequency ultrasonic waves resulting in linear oscillation of the active blade (Fig. 18.1). The wave of ultrasonic motion is sometimes referred to as a harmonic wave. The displacement is maximum in the distal tip of the blade.

Tissue dissection and coagulation occur through a combination of computation and cavitation [6]. Coaptation involves compression of tissue between the jaws, with frictional heat leading to protein denaturation and vessel sealing [7]. Cavitation results from vaporisation of intracellular fluid, generating microbubbles that expand and disrupt tissue planes. The balance between cutting and coagulation effects is influenced by the power setting of the electrical energy, tissue tension, blade

J. Rao (✉)
Mount Elizabeth Novena Hospital, Singapore, Singapore

D. Y. X. Wei
Mount Elizabeth Novena Hospital, Singapore, Singapore

Department of General Surgery, Tan Tock Seng Hospital, Singapore, Singapore

J. S. Ahluwalia (ed.), *User Manual for Minimally Invasive Surgical Equipment*,
https://doi.org/10.1007/978-981-95-9019-3_18

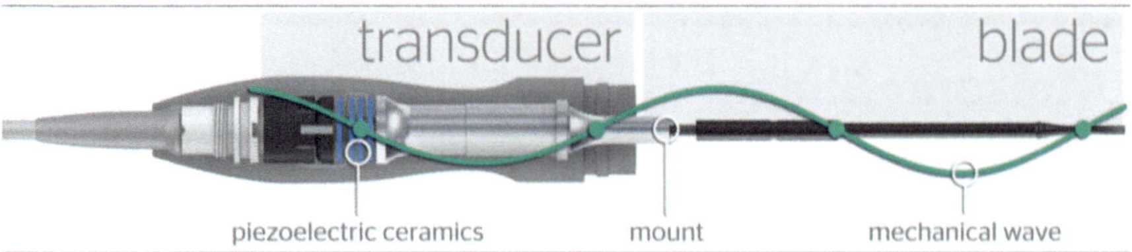

Fig. 18.1 Conversion of electrical energy to mechanical motion in the hand piece

Table 18.1 Factors affecting cutting and coagulating effect

Power	Increasing the power increases the displacement of the blade and increases the cutting effect while decreasing the power improves coagulation effect
Tissue tension	Maximizing tissue tension increases cutting effect and minimizes coagulation. When sealing large vessels, tension on the tissue should be released
Blade pressure	Increasing blade pressure increases the cutting effect
Blade position	The distal part of the blade has a larger displacement as the blade vibrates and has better cutting effect while the proximal part of the blade has less displacement and has better coagulation effect

pressure, blade sharpness and blade position [8]. Increasing power, tissue tension, or blade pressure enhances cutting efficiency but reduces coagulative effect, and vice versa (Table 18.1).

Compared to traditional advanced bipolar devices, which generally have larger and blunter jaws, ultrasonic shears are narrower and better suited for dissection. Heat generation occurs via mechanical energy ather than electrical energy, resulting in reduced lateral thermal spread compared to advanced bipolar devices [9]. However, with the advent of hybrid devices combining advanced bipolar energy and ultrasonic technology, the distinction between advanced bipolar devices and ultrasonic shears is increasingly blurred.

While much focus is on the evolution of the ultrasonic handpiece, the accompanying generators play an important role and have gone through many updates over the years. The current generators are smaller and use sophisticated software that continuously detects changes in tissue and optimizes the energy delivered [8]. This enables less energy to be used, reducing the temperature of the active blade and minimizing thermal damage.

Common ultrasonic shears are the Harmonic (Ethicon Endo-Surgery Inc., Cincinnati, OH, USA), Sonicision (Covidien, Mansfield, MA, USA) and the Thunderbeat (Olympus Corporation, Tokyo, Japan). In this chapter, we provide an overview of the ultrasonic shears currently available. Most of the available comparative clinical studies on ultrasonic shears were carried out using older generations of devices or with non-ultrasonic shears. Given the rapid evolution and release of subsequent generations of ultrasonic shears, many studies are obsolete soon after they are published. Some of the areas that are commonly compared in clinical studies include lateral thermal spread, maximum blade temperature and cooling time, surgical plume production and vessel burst pressure.

18.1 Overview of Devices

18.1.1 Harmonic (Ethicon Endo-Surgery Inc., Cincinnati, OH, USA)

The Harmonic platform has undergone multiple iterations since its introduction as UltraCision in 1988. Subsequent developements include the Harmonic ACE in 2005, followed by Harmonic ACE+ in 2012, Harmonic HD 1000i in 2016 and Harmonic 1100 in 2021 (Fig. 18.2). The Harmonic HD 1000i has a blade length of 19 mm. The longer, tapered blade mimics a mechanical dissector and enables sealing of vessels up to 7 mm in diameter. While the Harmonic 1100 is mechanically identical to the previous generation Harmonic 1000i shears, the difference lies in the generator. The generator of the Harmonic 1100 incorporates Adaptive Tissue Technology with enhanced thermal control. Adaptive Tissue Technology continuously modulates energy delivery based on real-time feedback, resulting in significantly lower peak blade temperatures while maintaining, cutting efficiency and sealing performance [10]. Lower blade temperatures help to lower the risk of thermal tissue injury while retaining the benefits of the current Harmonic 1000i shears. The device enables sealing of vessels up to 7 mm in diameter, with adjustable power settings allowing the surgeon to balance cutting speed against haemostatic effect. Higher power settings favour rapid dissection, whereas lower settings improve coagulation. Assembly and setup have been simplified in newer generations, with plug-and-play functionality and automated system checks. Earlier models required manual assembly and testing, whereas current systems perform self-calibration upon connection.

18.1.1.1 Harmonic Ace 7+ Ultrasonic Shears Assembly and Testing

The Harmonic Ace 7+ ultrasonic shears is a single-use device. The instrument and the hand-piece must be assembled and tested before use. Hold the hand-piece and

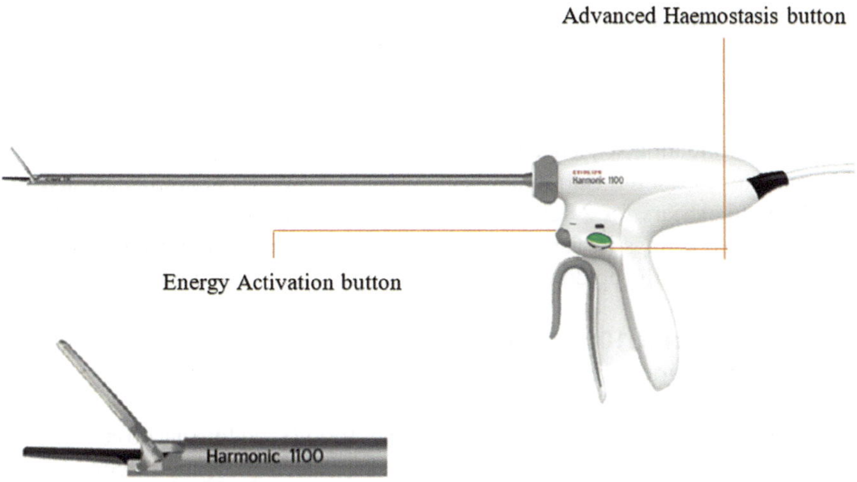

Fig. 18.2 HARMONIC 1100 shears with next-generation adaptive tissue technology

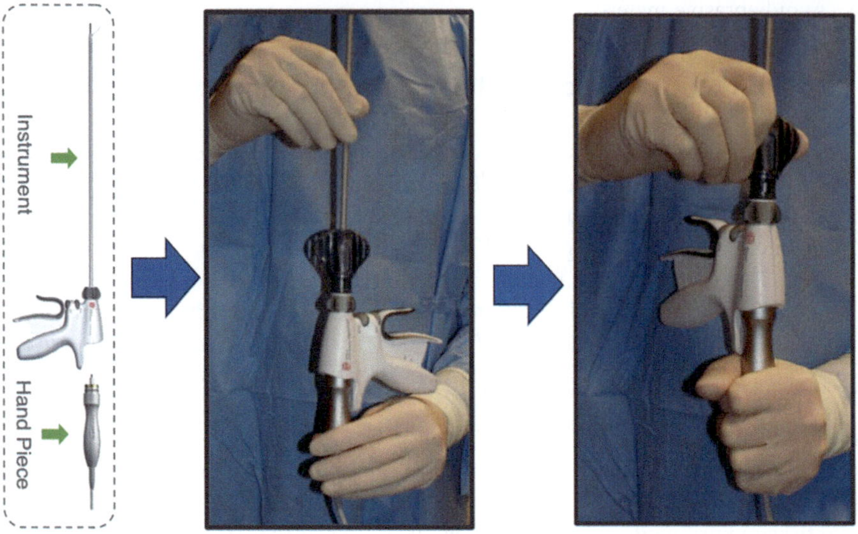

Fig. 18.3 Harmonic Ace 7+ assembly

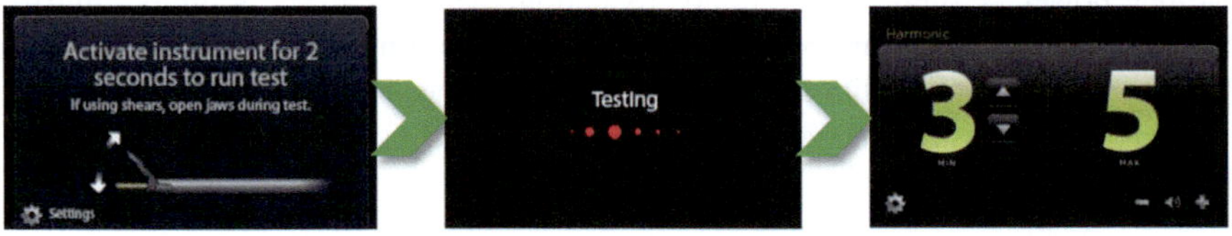

Fig. 18.4 Harmonic Ace 7+ testing

instrument vertically, attach the components together by rotating the instrument onto the hand-piece in a clockwise rotation (Fig. 18.3). The grey torque wrench comes already mounted onto the shaft. Tighten the torque wrench clockwise until it clicks twice, and remove it thereafter. Hold only the grey torque wrench and not the shaft of the instrument when tightening. Connect the wire of the hand-piece to the generator and turn the power on. Follow the on-screen instructions for testing.

Once the initiation sequence is complete, a prompt will appear on the screen of the generator to test the Harmonic shears (Fig. 18.4). With the jaws open, activate the Harmonic shears for 2 seconds to run the test until the ready screen with the default energy settings is displayed. The minimum power setting can be increased or decreased using the up/down buttons on the touch screen of the generator.

18.1.1.2 Harmonic 1000i/1100 Ultrasonic Shears and Generator Set-Up

The Harmonic 1000i/1100 shears is a single-use device. Unlike earlier generations of Harmonic ultrasonic shears, the Harmonic 1000i/1100 shears do not require assembly or manual testing of the ultrasonic shears after plugging in. Simply turn on the generator, remove the Harmonic shears from the box and plug the attached

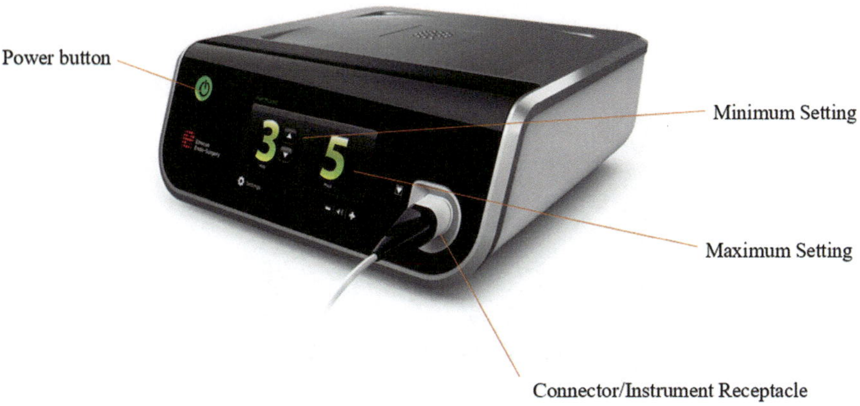

Fig. 18.5 Ethicon Generator G11

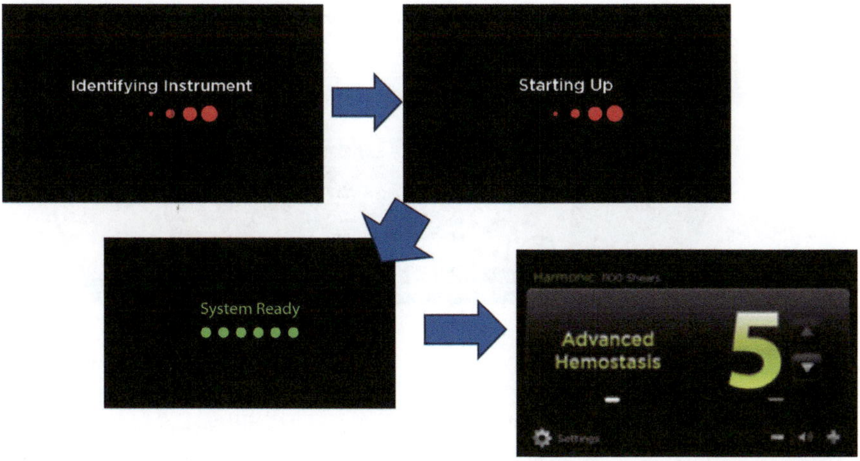

Fig. 18.6 Ethicon generator with software version 2018-1 or later, Screen images during set-up

cable from the Harmonic shears into the front of the generator as shown in Fig. 18.5. Once plugged in, the screen on the generator will show "Identifying Instrument", followed by "Starting Up", followed by a transient green "System Ready" before displaying "Advanced Haemostasis" and a default power setting of 5 (Fig. 18.6). During this time, the generator will automatically test the device and prepare it for use, no input is necessary from the surgical team.

The Harmonic 1000i/1100 ultrasonic shears have two buttons, an energy activation button, and an advanced haemostasis button at the side. The energy activation button is indicated to seal up to 5 mm vessels while the advanced haemostasis button is indicated to seal vessels up to 7 mm. The Harmonic shears can also be activated using a foot switch (Fig. 18.7) connected to the back of the Harmonic generator (Fig. 18.8). The Min button of the footswitch activates the advanced haemostasis functionality.

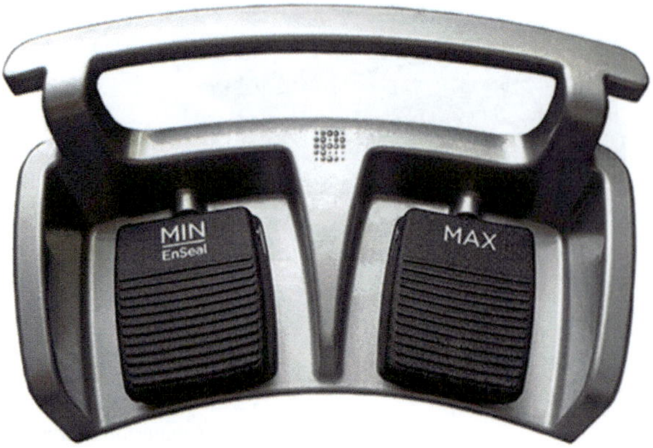

Fig. 18.7 Foot pedal for Harmonic Ultrasonic shears

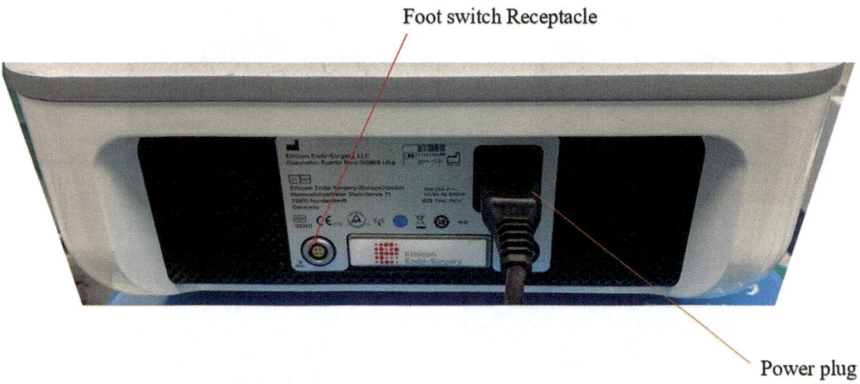

Fig. 18.8 Back of the Ethicon Harmonic Generator

The advanced haemostasis mode is not adjustable. The power level for the energy activation button can be adjusted using the up/down buttons on the touch screen of the generator. The power level can be adjusted from 1 to 5, power level 5 is the default setting and the highest power level. Lowering the power level changes the displacement of the blade and increases the haemostatic seal of the harmonic shears. Use a higher generator power level for greater tissue cutting speed, and a lower generator power level for greater coagulation. For thicker tissue types such as liver parenchyma, the recommended power setting is three when activating the Harmonic shears while gradually closing the jaws.

18.1.1.3 Ethicon Generator G11 Features

The Generator G11 supplies energy to the Harmonic ultrasonic shears. The generator uses a touchscreen display interface. Do not use sharp metal objects on the touch screen as it is very sensitive. Before cleaning, turn the generator main power off and unplug the power cord. The generator can be cleaned with a soft, clean cloth moistened with a neutral pH detergent, or chemical disinfectants such as Isopropyl

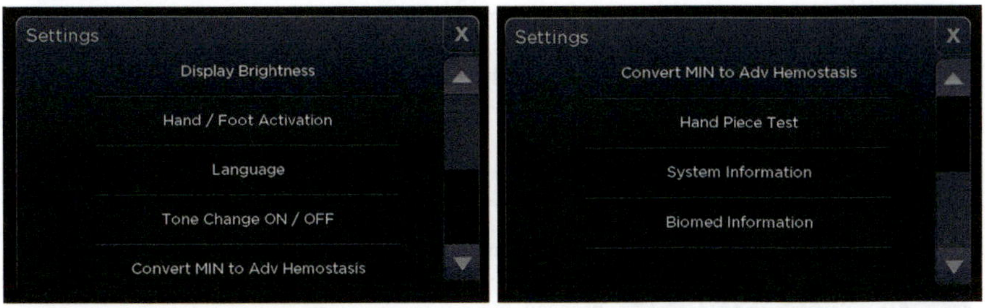

Fig. 18.9 System settings options

Alcohol 70%. Do not sterilize the Generator G11 as it will damage the unit. Ensure that the opening at the bottom and the back of the generator are not covered as they are necessary for airflow cooling of the generator and to avoid generator overheating.

When the Harmonic ultrasonic shears are connected and read for use, the screen of the generator will show the default power settings (Figs. 18.4 and 18.6). The top left corner of the screen indicates the instrument in use. The number displayed indicates the power level; the default power level is five and can be adjusted between one and five. The up/down buttons on the right of the number can be used to increase or decrease the level of the power. The bottom right buttons on either side of the volume icon can be used to adjust the volume of the activation tones. The default volume setting is five. A tone is heard to indicate the volume selected.

The bottom left button is for system settings. Touch the "Settings" button to make adjustments in the system settings and access system information. After the settings screen opens (Fig. 18.9), scroll down for further options. System settings can be used to change the brightness of the screen, hand/foot activation, the preferred language, tone change, convert minimum to advanced haemostasis, test the hand piece, display system or biomed information. System information reveals high-level information about the generator and the instrument currently connected to the generator. Biomed information allows technicians to access information about each error that has occurred on the generator.

Troubleshooting the "Remove Instrument from Patient" alert screen sequence
One may see various prompts on the screen of the generator during use of the Harmonic 1000i/1100

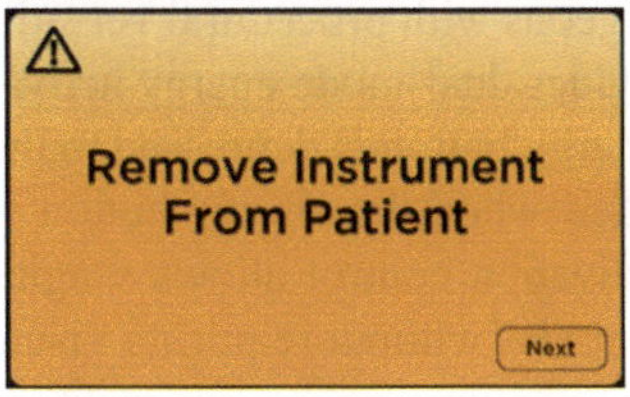	When this instruction appears on the screen, it is a prelude to further diagnostics Remove the instrument and press the "Next" button on the bottom left corner of the screen

(continued)

<table>
<tr><td>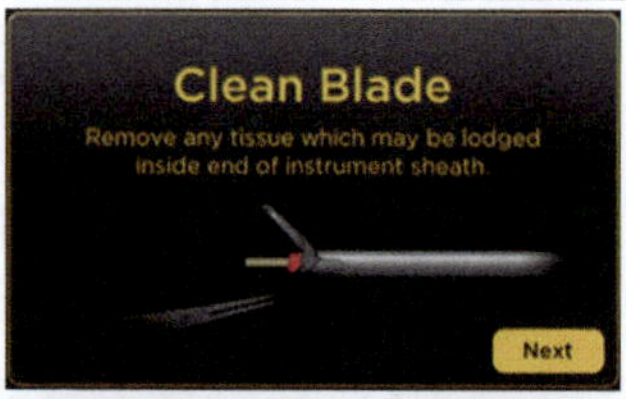
</td><td>After thoroughly cleaning the blades and removing any residual tissue, press the "Next" button on the bottom left corner of the screen</td></tr>
<tr><td>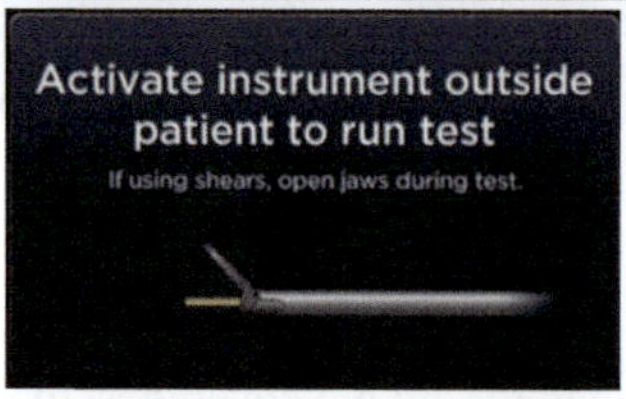
</td><td>Activate the instrument with the jaws open to run test
If the test is completed successfully, the procedure may proceed</td></tr>
<tr><td>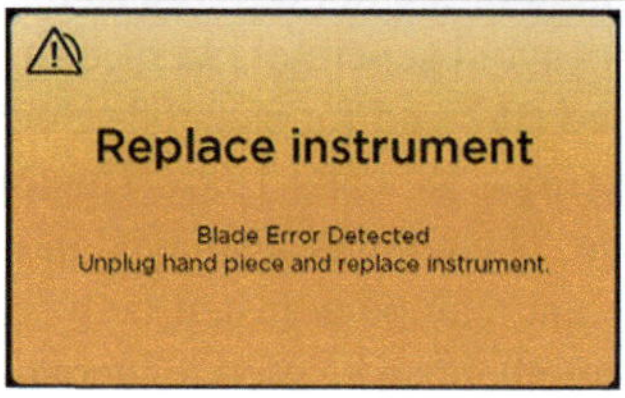
</td><td>If the test is unsuccessful, the harmonic instrument may be damaged and cannot be activated
Discontinue use, unplug the handpiece and replace the instrument</td></tr>
</table>

18.1.2 Sonicision™ (Covidien, Mansfield, MA, USA)

Sonicision is a cordless ultrasonic dissection device. It is a hand-held, battery-powered surgical device that is indicated for a wide variety of surgical procedures. Its unique cordless design and simplified set-up of the Sonicision system allow for more freedom of movement and facilitates instrument exchange, reducing cable clutter and results in better efficiency in the operating room (Fig 18.10).

The active blade of second-generation Sonicision has a length of 14.5 mm and is indicated for coagulating vasculature up to 5 mm in diameter. The curvature of the jaw allows better visualization in the operating space and easier access in confined spaces. Compared to the first-generation Sonicision, the Sonicision (2G) has a tapered curved jaw. The Sonicision 7 is the third-generation device and is capable of dissection and coagulating vessels up to and including 7 mm in diameter. The length and curvature of the Sonicision 7 are identical to the second-generation device.

The Sonicision (2G) and Sonicision 7 provide surgeons with procedural versatility and efficiency by having a single button that provides dual-mode energy activation. Minimum power mode is activated when the energy button is depressed to the first position, and maximum power mode is activated when the energy button is fully depressed. The intuitive dual-mode energy activation control allows seagles transition between minimum and maximum energy modes without requiring visual attention away from the operative field.

The blade and pistol grip of the Sonicision are single-use, while the battery and generator are reusable. The generator of the Sonicision 7 uses a three-phased algorithm (preheat, coagulate, cut) allowing for improved coagulation and haemostatic

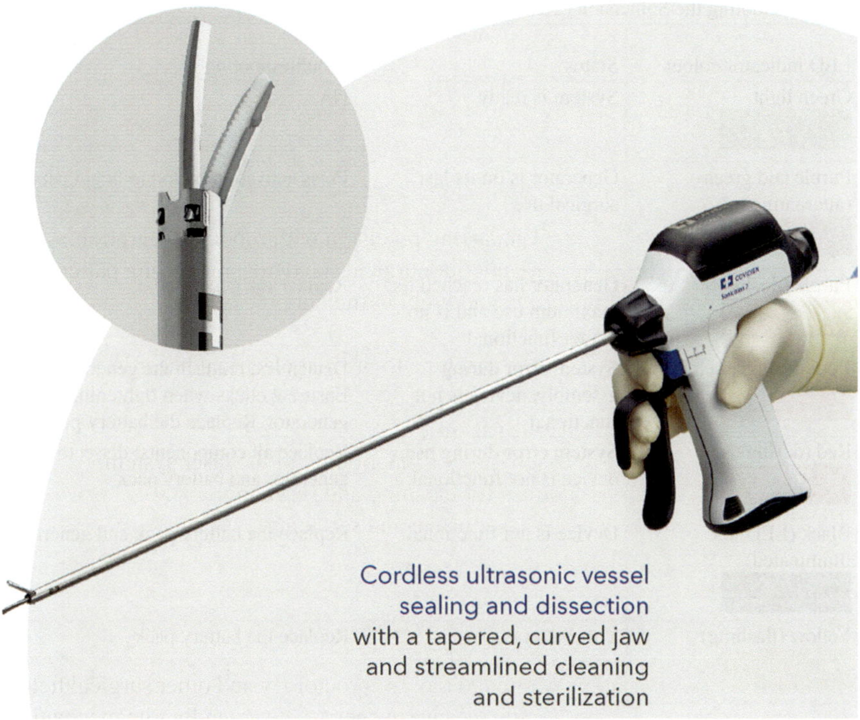

Fig. 18.10 Sonicision 7 curved jaw device (third generation)

dissection of vasculature up to 7 mm in diameter. The reusable generator is autoclavable and can be used for 150 procedures before needing to be replaced. The battery and charger of the Sonicision (2G) and Sonicision 7 have an 88% increase in battery capacity and double the procedural reusability from 100 to 200 procedures.

18.1.2.1 Assembly of Sonicision (2G) and Sonicision 7

After assembly, the device should be tested. With the jaw open, first activate the minimum power mode, followed by the maximum power mode. Assembly is completed and the device is ready for use when the device emits different tones for minimum/maximum power mode and the LED is green.

After each procedure, the battery pack should be removed, cleaned and disinfected with a disinfectant wipe containing isopropyl alcohol (70%) < ethyl alcohol or hydrogen peroxide. Ensure that the battery is completely dry before inserting into the generator or the charger. The generator should be removed, and together with the battery insertion guides, undergo cleaning with warm (32–40 °C/90–104 °F) water. After drying, place the generator and battery insertion guides in a sterilization tray. Load it into an autoclave for steam sterilization.

Troubleshooting the Sonicision (2G)/Sonicision 7

LED indicator colour	Status	Troubleshooting
Green light	System is ready	NA
Purple and green (alternating)	Generator is on its last surgical use	Press activation button to begin use
Purple (flashing)	Generator has reached its maximum use and is no longer functional	Replace the generator
Red (during assembly)	System error during assembly, device is not functional	Detach and reattach the generator. Ensure 2 clicks when tightening the generator. Replace the battery pack
Red (during use)	System error during use, device is not functional	Replace all components; dissector, generator and battery pack
Black (LED not illuminated)	Device is not functional	Replace the battery pack and generator
Yellow (flashing)	Low battery	Replace the battery pack

18.1.2.2 Decontamination, Cleaning, and Sterilization of Sonicision Battery and Generator

Decontamination

Under warm (32–40 °C, 90–104 °F) running tap water for a minimum of 1 min. Scrub all components with a small, soft, nylon-bristle, general instrument cleaning brush to remove surgical debris. For hard-to-reach crevices, use a 4.0 mm soft nylon-bristle brush for the battery insertion guide, and use a 12.0 mm soft nylon-bristle brush for the generator and sterilization tray.

Prepare a cleaning solution according to the manufacturer's instructions. Use a cleaning solution of pH-neutral, pH-neutral enzymatic, or alkaline detergent to clean the generator, battery insertion guides, and sterilization tray.

Manual Cleaning

Immerse the battery insertion guides, generator, and sterilization tray in a warm (32–40 °C; 90–104 °F) detergent bath for 10 min. Scrub each component in the detergent bath for a minimum of 1 min. Rinse each component under warm (32–40 °C; 90–104 °F) running tap water for a minimum of 1 min. Perform a final rinse under warm purified water for a minimum of 1 min for each component. Use a clean, soft, lint-free cloth to dry the components.

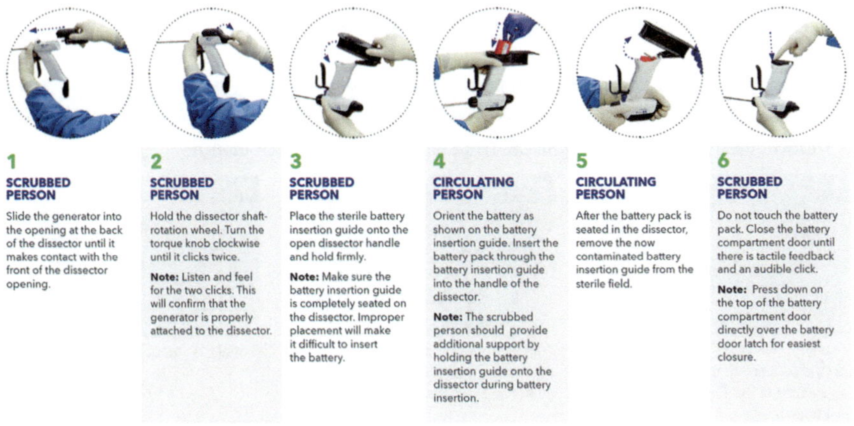

Fig. 18.11 Getting Sonicision ready for use

Sterilization with a Sonicision Reusable Sterilization Tray
After cleaning, place one generator and as many as two battery insertion guides in the base of the sterilization tray. Secure the lid of the sterilization tray. Use the manufacturer's instructions for the sterile barrier selected: single polypropylene wrap or double polypropylene wrap or rigid steam sterilization container.

Place the loaded sterilization tray into the autoclave. Select one of the sterilization cycles in the following Steam Sterilization Cycles table. To ensure adequate cool down time to 48 °C (118 °F) for handling of the sterilization tray and its contents, the sterilization tray should be allowed to cool down on a rack after sterilization for a minimum of 30 min.

Kindly refer to Medtronic's website https://www.medtronic.com/en-us/index.html for the latest information and improvements.

18.1.3 Thunderbeat® (Olympus Corporation, Tokyo, Japan)

The Thunderbeat Type S (Fig. 18.11) is the latest generation device of the Thunderbeat family, and a hybrid device that combines ultrasonic energy and advanced bipolar energy within a single instrument. The Thunderbeat has two modes. The combined seal-and-cut mode (purple button) delivers simultaneous ultrasonic and bipolar energy, and a seal-only mode (blue button) using advanced bipolar energy without the cutting effects of ultrasonic energy for precise haemostasis. The combined energy mode allows for sealing of vessels up to 7 mm in diameter with faster cutting speeds, and the advanced bipolar mode allows for haemostasis by spot coagulation without cutting. The instrument tip of the Thunderbeat has atraumatic serrations along the edges of the upper jaw that allow it to grasp tissue effectively, while the high tip-opening force enables blunt tissue dissection.

Thunderbeat device has an Intelligent Tissue Monitoring (ITM) safety system that regulates energy delivery for improved temperature profile of the instrument. ITM also incorporates an auto-stop mechanism once transection is complete, enhancing safety and thermal control.

It is a single-use device that requires assembly and activation test.

18.1.3.1 Assembly of Thunderbeat (Fig. 18.12)

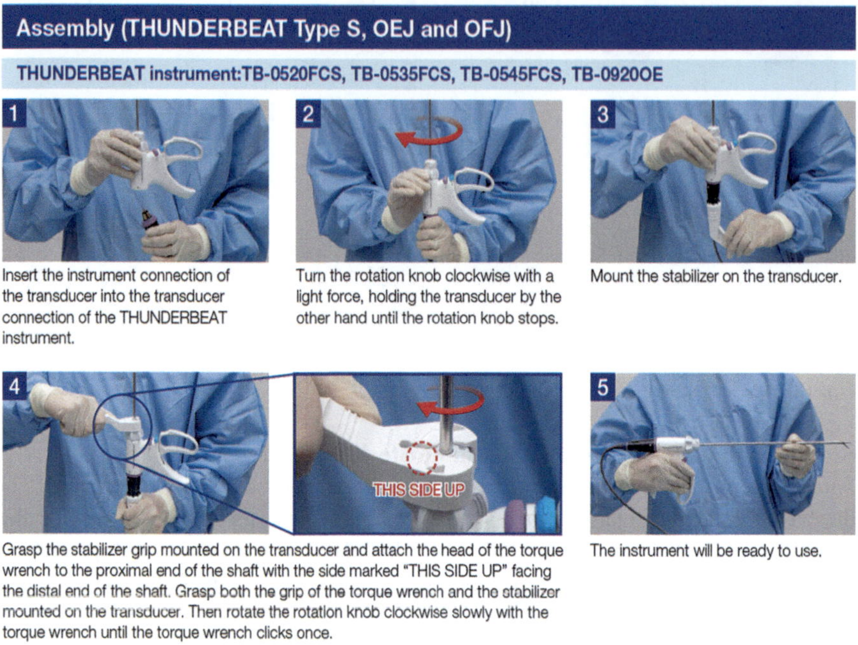

Fig. 18.12 Assembly of Thunderbeat Type S

18.1.3.2 Activation Test for Ultrasonic Output

1. Connect Thunderbeat and tap the "Test" button.
   Caution: Do not apply the instrument on patients during activation test.
2. Activate instrument with jaws opened following the instructions on the screen.
3. When the activation test result is displayed, release the hand switch and confirm with OK.
4. After a successful test, the instrument can be used safely.

18.1.3.3 The Thunderbeat Generator (USG-410)

Ultrasonic Bipolar Generator (USG-410) (Fig. 18.13) is the latest Thunderbeat generator. The USG-410 activates both ultrasonic and bipolar energy simultaneously in a single unit, while maintaining 7 mm reliable sealing and fast tissue-cutting capability generators.

When used together with Olympus insufflators (UHI-3 or UHI-4), the generator communicates intelligently with the insufflators to evacuate any smoke and mist whenever required during laparoscopic surgery, helping improve visualization.

The USG-410 offers three levels under the seal & cut mode and one level under the seal mode.

Fig. 18.13 Olympus Ultrasonic Bipolar Generator (USG-410)

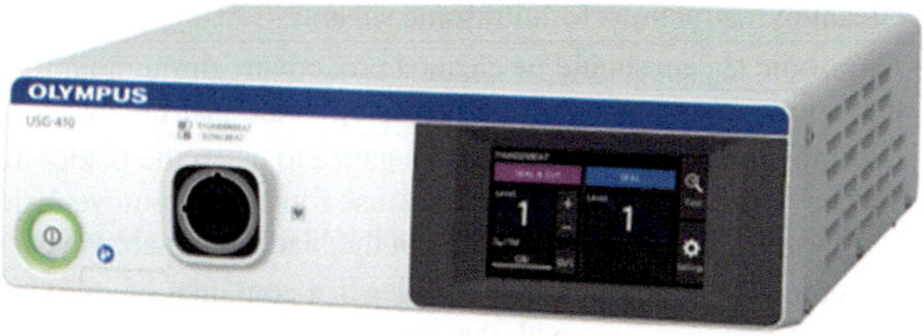

Instrument	Mode	Energy	Level	Standard settings	Characteristics	Vessel sealing	ITM
THUNDERBEAT	Seal & cut	Ultrasonic RF bipolar	1–3	1	Fastest cutting speed at level 1; constant sealing performance over all levels	Up to 7 mm	Available
	Seal	RF bipolar	1	1	Shorter sealing time by improved SEAL algorithm compared to ESG-400 & USG-400	Up to 7 mm	Not available

18.1.3.4 Tips and Tricks

Tips and tricks for using ultrasonic shears:	
1.	Use the distal tip of the ultrasonic shear while dissecting as energy is maximum at the tip, and this will minimize plumes
2.	Maintain visual awareness of the active blade orientation to minimise inadvertent injury. Keep the active blade facing you at all times.
3.	Apply appropriate tissue tension to optimise cutting efficiency. The direction of motion should be forward or against the active blade.
4.	Avoid contact with any and all metal or plastic instruments. Activating the active blade while in contact with other instruments can lead to cracked or broken blades and premature blade failure
5.	Do not activate the device without tissue between the blades to avoid instrument damage
6.	Regularly clean the jaw and blade throughout the procedure to maintain optimal device performance
7.	Fully close the jaws of the ultrasonic device before activating energy delivery
8.	Minimize tissue tension and ensure tissue is fully within the jaws for optimal haemostasis. Failure to do so may result in bleeding. 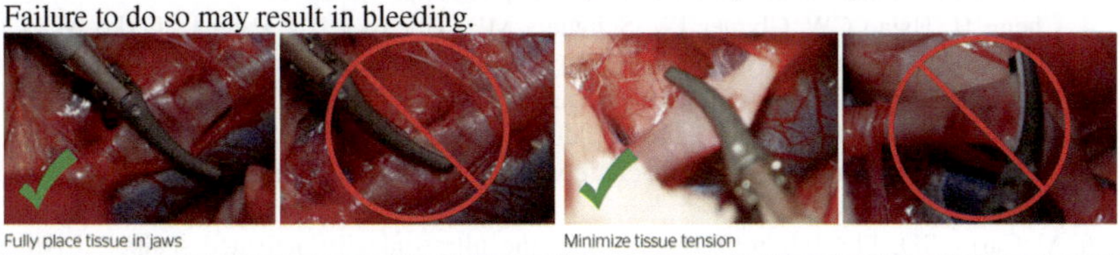

(continued)

Cleaning instructions for ultrasonic shears:	
Ultrasonic shears should be cleaned proactively throughout the procedure for optimal device performance and to avoid tissue sticking to the instrument	
Cleaning with moist gauze	Use a moist gauze to clean the blades and remove tissue If necessary, use forceps to remove residual tissue Do not clean the blades with abrasives
Cleaning with saline	Dip the blades in a container of sterile saline and activate the instrument with the jaws open Avoid contact between the active blade and the container

18.2 Conclusion

The current available ultrasonic shears are different in terms of clinical performance, and it is essential for a surgeon to fully appreciate the limitations of the device at hand. Such is the rate of technological evolution that much of the clinical evidence compares previous generations of ultrasonic shears, and as such no longer relevant. The surgeon must decide which is the most suitable ultrasonic shear based on the cost-benefit ratio and the device he is most comfortable with. Advances in generator technology, real-time energy modulation, and hybrid energy platforms continue to expand the role of ultrasonic devices in minimally invasive surgery. As device performance improves, distinctions between ultrasonic and bipolar systems are diminishing, with modern instruments offering increasingly versatile and efficient solutions for both dissection and haemostasis. Ongoing innovation is likely to focus on further reducing thermal spread, enhancing precision, and integrating intelligent feedback systems to optimise surgical outcomes.

References

1. Jiang HP, Liu YD, Li YS, Shen ZL, Ye YJ. Ultrasonic versus electrosurgical device for laparoscopic cholecystectomy: a systematic review with meta-analysis and trial sequential analysis. Int J Surg. 2017;40:24–32.
2. Lei H, Xu D, Shi X, Han K. Ultrasonic dissection versus conventional dissection for pancreatic surgery: a meta-analysis. Gastroenterol Res Pract. 2016;2016:6195426.
3. Revelli L, Damiani G, Bianchi CB, Vanella S, Ricciardi W, Raffaelli M, Lombardi CP. Complications in thyroid surgery. Harmonic scalpel, harmonic focus versus conventional Hemostasis: a meta-analysis. Int J Surg. 2016;28(Suppl 1):S22–32.
4. Cheng H, Hsiao CW, Clymer JW, Schwiers ML, Tibensky BN, Patel L, Ferko NC, Chekan E. Gastrectomy and D2 lymphadenectomy for gastric cancer: a meta-analysis comparing the harmonic scalpel to conventional techniques. Int J Surg Oncol. 2015;2015:397260.
5. Devassy R, Gopalakrishnan S, De Wilde RL. Surgical efficacy among laparoscopic ultrasonic dissectors: are we advancing safely? A review of literature. J Obstet Gynaecol India. 2015;65(5):293–300.
6. McCarus SD. Physiologic mechanism of the ultrasonically activated scalpel. J Am Assoc Gynecol Laparosc. 1996;3(4):601–8.

7. Amaral JF. The experimental development of an ultrasonically activated scalpel for laparoscopic use. Surg Laparosc Endosc. 1994;4(2):92–9.
8. McCarus SD, Parnell LKS. The origin and evolution of the HARMONIC(R) scalpel. Surg Technol Int. 2019;35:201–13.
9. Hayami M, Watanabe M, Mine S, Imamura Y, Okamura A, Yuda M, Yamashita K, Toihata T, Shoji Y, Ishizuka N. Lateral thermal spread induced by energy devices: a porcine model to evaluate the influence on the recurrent laryngeal nerve. Surg Endosc. 2019;33(12):4153–63.
10. Singleton D. Intelligent ultrasonic energy: new adaptive tissue technology in harmonic shears. J Surg. 2020;8:178.

Morcellator

19

Rajesh Modi

A morcellator is a medical device used in minimally invasive surgical procedures, particularly in gynecological surgeries. Its primary function is to divide or fragment large masses of tissue into smaller pieces, facilitating their removal through small incisions. There are two types of gynecological applications.

1. Laparoscopic morcellators
2. Hysteroscopic morcellators/shavers

19.1 Mechanism of Action

The morcellators usually consist of a motorized, cylindrical blade or cutter that rotates or oscillates. When the tissue (e.g., fibroids, uterus, kidney, or spleen) is engaged with the device, the blade cuts it into smaller fragments. Some morcellators are equipped with an integrated suction system to simultaneously remove the fragmented tissue pieces, reducing the risk of scattering within the surgical site.

19.2 Laparoscopic Morcellators

Laparoscopic morcellators are used for procedures such as laparoscopic hysterectomy and myomectomy (Fig. 19.1).

Benefits of Morcellation:

- No large abdominal incision to retrieve specimen
- Lower risk of surgical infection

R. Modi (✉)
Gynaecology and Robotic Surgery, Akola Endoscopy Center, Akola, Maharashtra, India

J. S. Ahluwalia (ed.), *User Manual for Minimally Invasive Surgical Equipment*,
https://doi.org/10.1007/978-981-95-9019-3_19

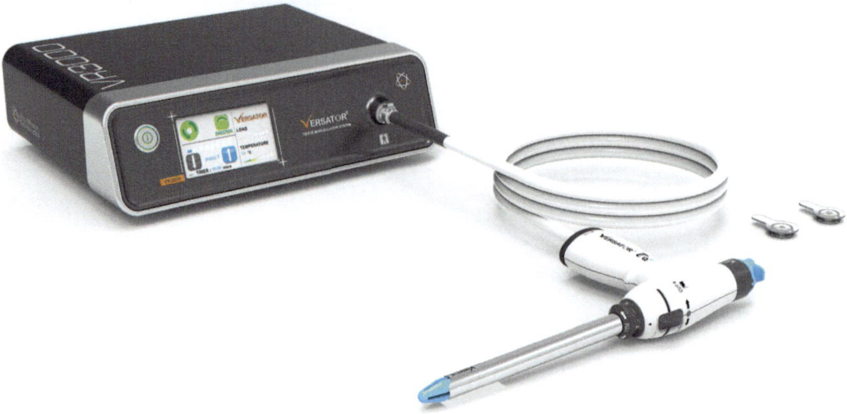

Fig. 19.1 Laparoscopic morcellator

- Lesser postoperative pain
- Better cosmetic result
- Faster healing and recovery

The choice of morcellator type depends on the surgical procedure, the surgeon's preference, and the specific characteristics of the treated tissue. While features may vary between different models and types of morcellators, common attributes typically present in all morcellators are:

19.3 Components

1. *Drive unit*: This device is placed on a laparoscopic tower or on another trolley. It powers and controls the rotation of the cutting blade. It houses the electrical supply and circuit, switches to power on the system, controls the speed of rotation, and also the direction of rotation of the blade. Some models may have a touchscreen for controls. Some models have a motor built into the drive unit, while others have a motor inside the handpiece. The advantage of having a motor built into the drive unit is that it makes the handpiece much lighter, making it more ergonomic and also decreasing the fatigue on the operator's hand and body.
2. *Cable*: This could be an electric cable transferring power if the motor is located in the handpiece. Alternatively, it could be an internally rotating cable if the motor is situated in the drive unit, thereby transmitting the rotation of the motor to the handpiece.
3. *Handpiece*: Provides grip to the surgeon and acts as an interface between drive unit and tissue. It must be ergonomically designed to allow comfortable handling during long procedures and often includes buttons or switches to control the

blade's operation—its activation and speed. It has a removable blade. Some handpieces offer different blade positions like:

Partially exposed blade: Provides a peeling effect around the surface of the tissue as the blade is partially exposed.

Fully exposed blade: Provides a coring effect as the blade is fully exposed.

Off mode: Blade is fully retracted for patient safety.

4. *Safety Guard*: Some morcellators are equipped with protective guards designed to shield the blade when not in use or during insertion and withdrawal from the abdominal cavity. This minimizes the risk of damaging the port and prevents inadvertent injury to organs in case the blade is accidentally activated.
5. *Tissue holding forceps*: A sturdy toothed forceps is used to hold tissues to be morcellated. This instrument is passed through the hollow blade so as to hold and pull the tissue towards the morcellator blade.
6. *Foot switch*: Some models have a dedicated foot switch to activate the morcellator.

19.4 How to Use

1. Place the drive unit on a flat and secure surface.
2. Make sure cable and hand piece (including all its accessories) are appropriately sterilized before usage.
3. Connect the free end of the power cord to the AC inlet, and connect the other end of the power cord to the power socket. Then, connect the cable to the drive unit.
4. Connect the handpiece to the cable at the other end and power on the drive unit by pressing the power button.
5. The speed of the motor can be adjusted by tapping touch screen or using the buttons/switches on drive unit.
6. Select the appropriate mode.
7. Hold the tissue to be morcellated with toothed forceps (usually supplied with the system) and pull towards the blade under vision.
8. Press the foot switch or button on handpiece to activate the cutter blade.
9. The rotation of the cutter can be halted by releasing the Foot Switch or handpiece button.
10. Make sure not to activate the blade unless one has a clear vision of the tip of the blade and the tissue being cut.
11. Keep a steady traction on tissue as it is being morcellated. Stop the blade as soon as the blade comes out of the specimen at the other end and pull out the blade from port to extract the morcellated tissue.
12. The steps need to be repeated several times depending upon the size of the specimen.
13. After completing tissue morcellation, switch the cutter blade to an unexposed position and disconnect the power cord, footswitch, and rotor. Next, turn off the machine and the mains supply.

19.5 In-Bag Morcellation

In-bag morcellation or contained morcellation is a technique used during laparoscopic surgery, especially in gynecological procedures like hysterectomy or myomectomy. This approach involves inserting the tissue, often a fibroid or the uterus itself, into a containment bag before morcellating it. The bag functions as a protective barrier, preventing any tissue fragments or cells from spreading within the abdominal cavity. This method is designed to enhance safety by containing and minimizing the potential dissemination of tissue during the morcellation process (Fig. 19.2).

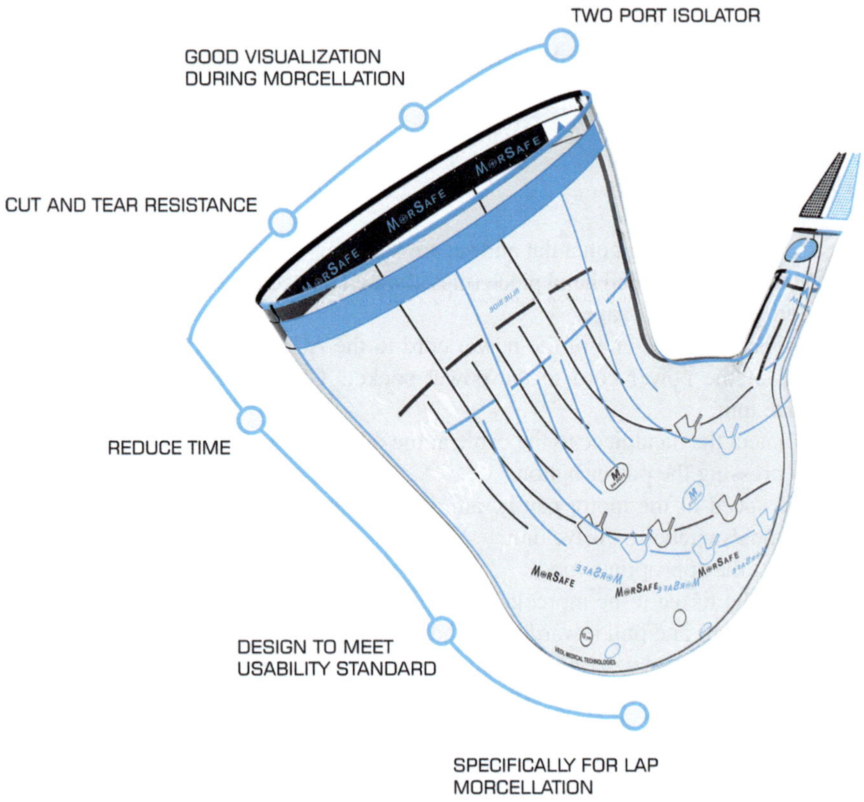

Fig. 19.2 Bag specially designed for in-bag morcellation

19.6 Hysteroscopic Morcellators

A hysteroscopic morcellator is used during hysteroscopic procedures to remove intrauterine tissues, such as fibroids, polyps, etc. Unlike laparoscopic morcellators, these devices combine visual system (hysteroscope), shaving system (morcellator), and irrigation system into a single device that can be inserted into uterus per vagina.

For ease of understanding, TruClear™ system is being used here as a reference (Figs. 19.3, 19.4, and 19.5).

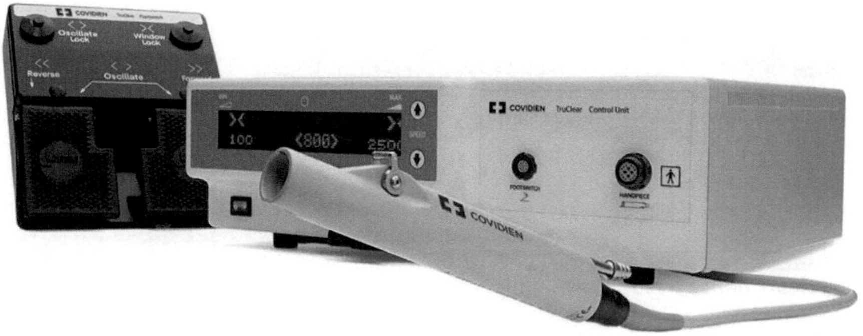

Fig. 19.3 TruClear™ system—control unit, handpiece, and footswitch

Fig. 19.4 Elite mini and plus scope

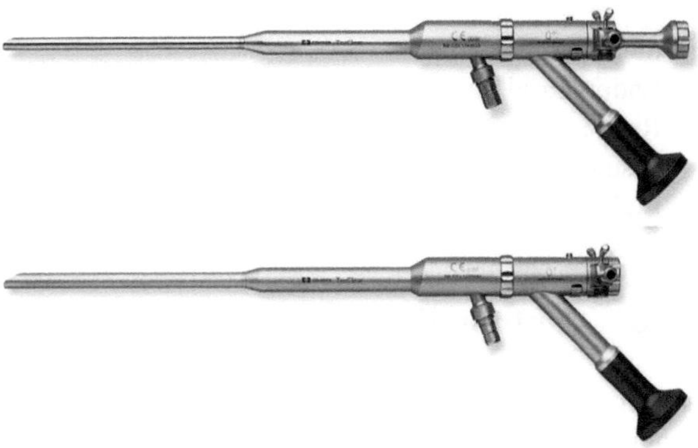

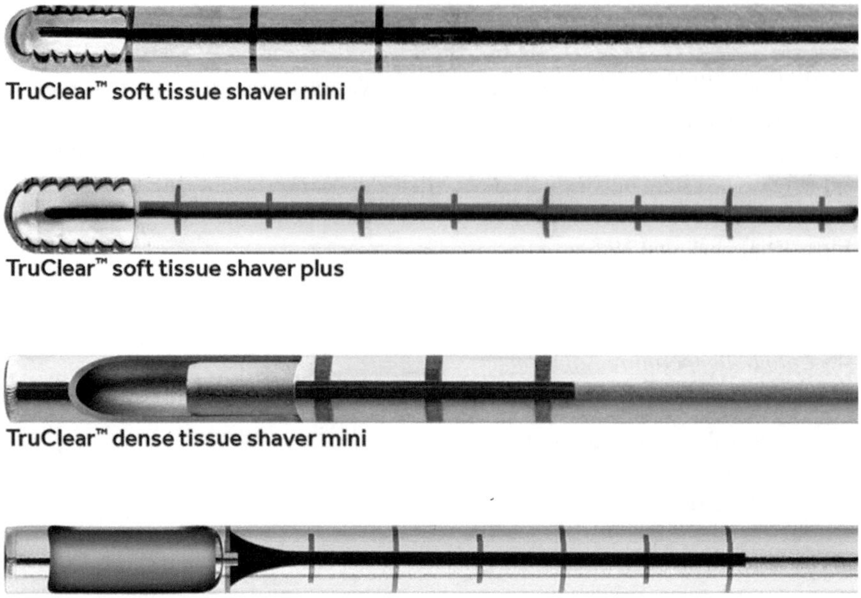

Fig. 19.5 Pathology optimized shavers for soft and dense tissue

19.7 Indications for Use

- Submucous myomas
- Endometrial polyps
- Retained products of conception Intrauterine adhesions
- Visual D&C
- Endometrial biopsy

19.8 Contraindications

The TruClear™ hysteroscopic tissue removal system should not be used with pregnant patients or patients exhibiting pelvic infection, cervical malignancies, or previously diagnosed endometrial cancer.

19.9 Components

Control Unit:

- Controls the motor in the handpiece, which drives the shavers
- Handpiece and footswitch both plug into the front
- Displays minimum, maximum, and set speeds, handpiece motor direction, diagnostic information, and length of resection time

Footswitch:

- Controls the tissue shaver rotation and the initial setup of the shaver
- Has two foot pedals, has capability to perform window lock, and change mode

Handpiece (Autoclavable):

- Is a hand-held motor drive unit that is electrically connected to the control unit via a 3-m cable
- Is activated by a footswitch
- Has a stainless-steel barbed connector for the suction tubing
- Has a suction lever to provide manual control of the suction rate

Scopes

TruClear™ Elite hysteroscopes are reusable instruments for use in visualizing the uterine cavity and performing diagnostic and operative hysteroscopy. The hysteroscopes are designed with optical lenses, optical fibers for illumination, and a working channel to permit introduction of instrumentation. There are two TruClear™ Elite hysteroscopes and a disposable seal:

6 mm TruClear™ Elite hysteroscope mini with 3 mm working channel
7.25 mm TruClear™ Elite hysteroscope plus with 4 mm working channel

A single-use hysteroscope seal is supplied separately from the hysteroscope. The hysteroscope seal is located on the proximal end of the hysteroscope and secured by a removable retaining cap. The seal prevents fluid leakage from the proximal end of the hysteroscope during the procedure and provides a fluid barrier around the tissue removal device.

TruClear™ Elite hysteroscope mini:

- 6 mm outside diameter (OD)
- 3 mm working channel
- 201.1 mm working length

TruClear™ Elite hysteroscope plus:

- 7.25 mm outside diameter (OD)
- 4 mm working channel
- 201.1 mm working length

Shavers

These come in many variations for different types of tissues: TruClear™ disposable shavers, TruClear™ soft tissue shaver plus, TruClear™ soft tissue shaver mini, TruClear™ dense tissue shaver plus, and TruClear™ dense tissue shaver mini. These are single-use instruments used specifically with the TruClear™ hysteroscopic tissue removal system for resection of intrauterine tissue (Fig. 19.6).

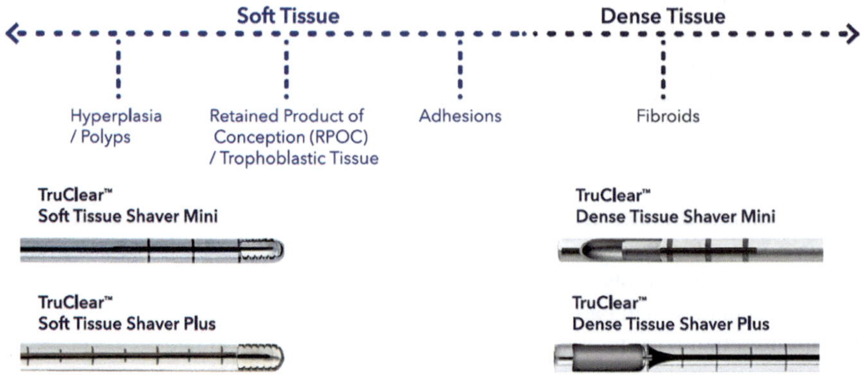

Fig. 19.6 Choosing the shaver as per tissue type

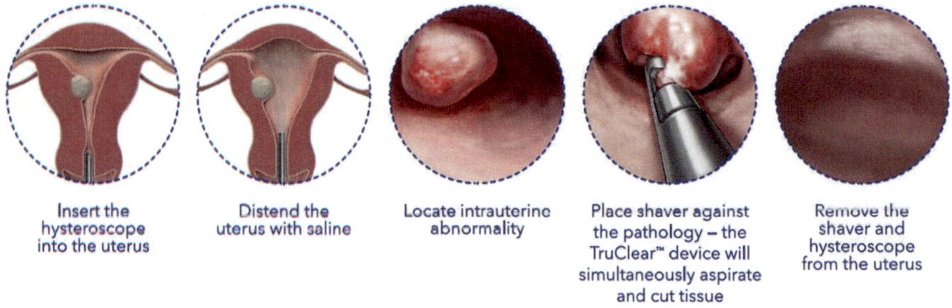

Fig. 19.7 Working of hysteroscopic shaver

19.10 Working

The TruClear™ system uses a tissue shaver device that is inserted through a hysteroscope to simultaneous cut and aspirate the tissue (Fig. 19.7).

19.11 Maintenance

1. Cleaning and Sterilization
    - Disassemble all parts after each use.
    - Rinse thoroughly to remove blood and tissue debris.
    - Use enzymatic detergent to clean and prevent biofilm formation.
    - Autoclave as per the manufacturer's guidelines.
2. Lubrication and Inspection
    - Lubricate moving parts to reduce friction and wear.
    - Inspect cutting blades for dullness and replace if necessary.
    - Check the motor for any unusual noise or vibration.

3. Electrical Safety

   - Ensure the power cord and connectors are intact.
   - Verify that the foot pedal functions correctly.
   - Test the motor unit for any electrical leakage.

4. Calibration and Testing

   - Perform calibration to maintain consistent rotation speed.
   - Test blade rotation and speed to ensure smooth functioning.
   - Confirm that safety features (such as blade guards) are working properly.

5. Preventive Maintenance

   - Schedule regular preventive maintenance as per manufacturer's guidelines.
   - Keep a log of usage and service history.
   - Replace consumable parts periodically.

19.12 Troubleshooting

Problem	Possible causes	Solutions	Blade rotation	Motor sound
Blade not rotating	Motor malfunction or jammed	Check motor and clean debris	No rotation	Unusual/no sound
Dull cutting or tissue jamming	Blade wear or debris accumulation	Replace or clean blade	Slow or uneven	Normal
Motor not starting	Power supply or foot pedal fault	Check power and foot pedal	No rotation	No sound
Excessive vibration	Misaligned blade or loose parts	Tighten or replace blade	Uneven rotation	Loud noise
Erratic speed	Faulty control or calibration	Recalibrate or replace control	Irregular	Variable sound
Overheating	Continuous use or motor strain	Allow cooling, check lubrication	Slow or erratic	Buzzing noise
Tissue not morcellated properly	Incorrect blade installation	Check and reinstall the blade	Slow or jammed	Normal

19.13 Conclusion

Laparoscopic and hysteroscopic morcellators have revolutionized the field of minimally invasive surgery, offering surgeons tools that enhance precision, efficiency, and safety. These devices have significantly reduced procedure times, minimized patient recovery periods, and improved overall surgical outcomes. By allowing targeted removal of tissues through small incisions or natural orifices, they preserve surrounding structures and reduce the physical and emotional toll on patients. A proper understanding of such instruments will go a long way in making an efficient and safe surgeon.

Bibliography

1. Emanuel MH, Womstaker K. A new hysteroscopic operating technique to remove intrauterine polyps and myomas. J Minim Invasive Gynecol. 2005;12(1):62–6.
2. Smith PP, Middleton LJ, Connor M, Clark TJ. Hysteroscopic morcellation compared with electrical resection of endometrial polyps. Obstet Gynecol. 2014;123(4):745–51. https://doi.org/10.1097/AOG.0000000000000187.
3. HysteroLux™ fluid management system instructions for use. New Haven: Medtronic; 2017.
4. TruClear™ operative hysteroscopes IFU.
5. Hooker A, Aydin H, Brohlmann H, Huirne J. Long-term complications and reproductive outcome after the management of retained products of conception: a systematic review. Fertil Steril. 2016;105(1):156–64.

Irrigation System 20

Mandeep Kaur

Laparoscopic surgery has revolutionized the field of surgery by allowing surgeons to perform complicated procedures through small incisions, resulting in reduced patient trauma, quicker recovery times, and lesser complications compared to traditional open surgeries.

One crucial aspect of laparoscopic surgery is irrigation, which involves the controlled delivery of fluids to the surgical site to maintain visibility, rinse tissues which helps in dissection and control bleeding.

Some systems may feature manual buttons (Fig. 20.1), while others may employ a touchscreen interface (Fig. 20.2) to control various functions.

Given the diverse range of irrigation system manufacturers, this chapter will provide an in-depth analysis of various settings by giving examples of some machines only. By extrapolating this knowledge from the provided examples, readers can gain insights into their existing irrigation systems, enabling them to explore the functions and settings of irrigation devices utilized in laparoscopic and hysteroscopic surgeries. This understanding will also shed light on the mechanisms and roles of these devices in enhancing surgical outcomes. Also note that sine irrigation devices come with suction functions as well, and some do not.

20.1 Intended Use

Irrigation systems provide delivery of fluid to and from (if the system has a suction facility) the patient at a set pressure and/or flow rate to allow the performance of the following procedures:

M. Kaur (✉)
Department of Fertility Services, STAR Hospital, Jalandhar, Punjab, India

J. S. Ahluwalia (ed.), *User Manual for Minimally Invasive Surgical Equipment*,
https://doi.org/10.1007/978-981-95-9019-3_20

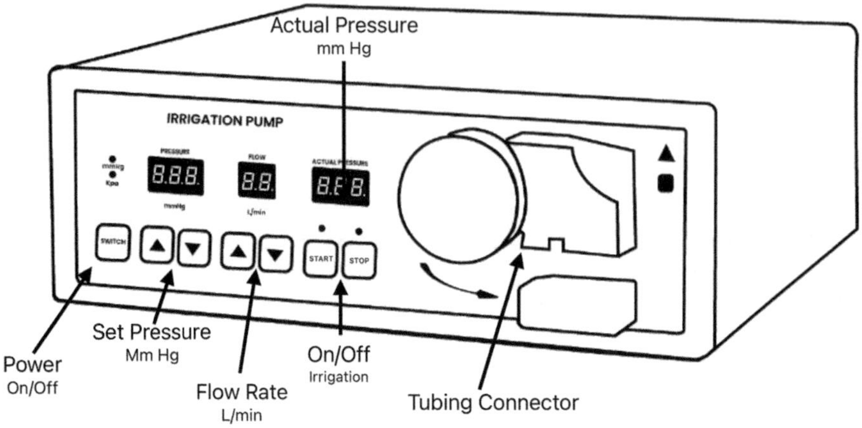

Fig. 20.1 Irrigation system with basic features

Fig. 20.2 Storz Endomat select irrigation system

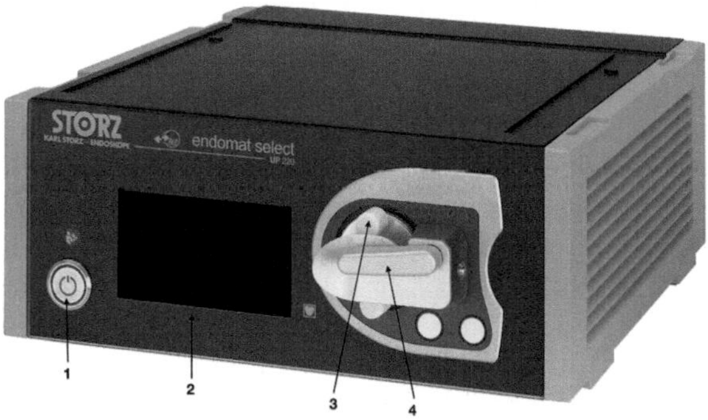

- Laparoscopy/thoracoscopy: used to flush blood and debris from the operating field. This improves visibility and also helps in washing away unwanted debris (blood, pus, bile, bowel contents, etc.).
- Hysteroscopy: distends the uterine cavity to permit the visualization and the performance of endoscopic procedures in the uterine cavity.
- Urology: distends the urinary tract to permit the visualization and the performance of endoscopic procedures inside the urinary tract.
- In addition, such systems can be used for arthroscopy, ENT, and certain neurological procedures as well, but their discussion is beyond the scope of this book.

1. Power on/off.
2. Touch screen interface for various settings.
3. Pump roller—for controlling motion of liquid.
4. Pump lever—for attaching/removing irrigation tubing.

Placement It is important to note that irrigation and suction systems should be placed at the level of the patient (table height) to avoid pressure gradient between them [1].

20.2 Working Principle

As the rotor turns, the part of the tube under compression is pinched, thus forcing the fluid to be pumped and moved through the tube. Typically, four rollers occlude the tube and trap a body of fluid between them. The body of fluid is then transported, at ambient pressure, towards the pump outlet. Peristaltic pumps run continuously, or at partial revolutions to deliver the desired amount of fluid into the surgical site. The flow rate is calculated through motor revolutions.

For suction, some machines have vacuum pump which is used to create vacuum. This vacuum pressure is maintained inside a canister which aspirates the fluid from surgical site into the canister. Other machines reverse the direction of rotor pump to use it as suction apparatus instead of irrigation. In this type of arrangement, connecting tube has to be changed every time so as to connect it to canister when suction mode is used.

The suction irrigation unit consists of the following parts:

- Suction irrigation pump unit [2].
- The tubing set connected to irrigation machine on one side and to irrigation/suction instrument on the other (Figs. 20.3 and 20.4).

20.3 How to Attach the Irrigation System to the Pump

This is equipment specific, but a general guideline is:

Insert one connector of tube guide connector set in the cavity of the top or bottom side of the tube guide (Fig. 20.5 No. 1). Then gently stretch the silicone tube over rotor and lock the other connector of tube guide connector set in the opposite cavity on the upper side of tube guide (Fig. 20.5 No. 2). The two connectors may be of different size and shape to prevent wrong connections. Attach pressure sensor end of pipe to the pressure sensor port (Fig. 20.5 No. 3 & 4). Suction pipe can be connected to suction connector in case machine has suction function. Some models use reverse direction of rotor for suction and do not have separate suction connector. Irrigation and suction function can be reversed using button or touch screen in them. Spikes of tubing set are to be connected to irrigation fluid and Leur lock side to the laparoscopic instrument.

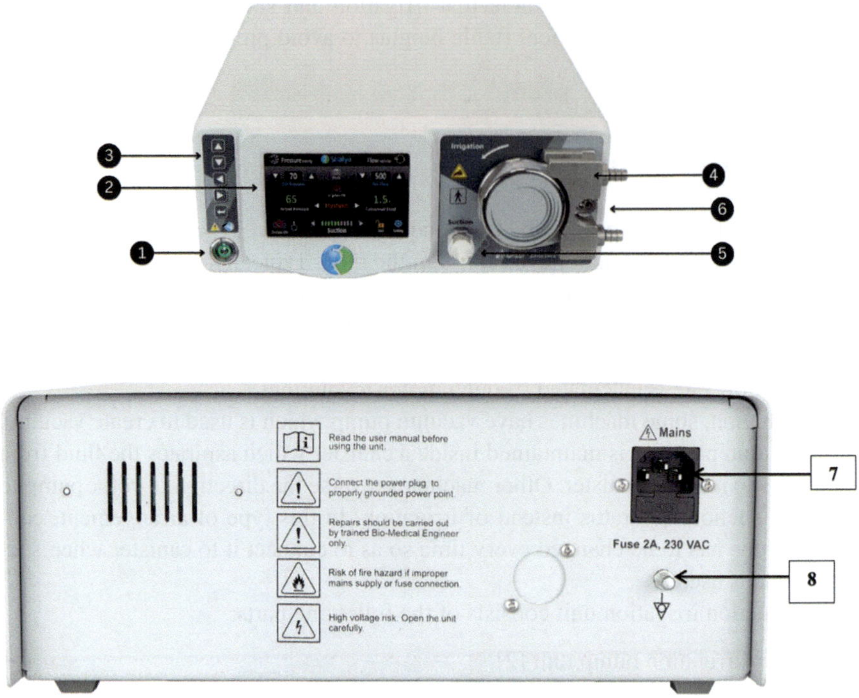

Fig. 20.3 Shalya Aquaflow: front and back

20.4 Basic Settings

Most modern machines equipped with a graphical user interface offer predefined modes that allow direct manipulation of flow and pressure parameters for specific procedures. Users typically have the option to select between laparoscopy, hysteroscopy, urology, arthroscopy, and ENT. However, it is crucial to exercise caution when utilizing these settings. Lower values may result in insufficient visualization of the operative field, while higher settings can lead to severe tissue damage. The pressures may vary depending on the scope used, diameter, and the length of the scope. Some examples of default settings are given below:

Hysteroscopy:

Pressure: 80 mmHg; flow: 500 mLPM

Max pressure: 400 mmHg; max flow: 1000 mLPM

Laparoscopy:

Pressure: 200 mmHg; flow: 1000 mLPM

Max pressure: 400 mmHg; max flow: 2000 mLPM

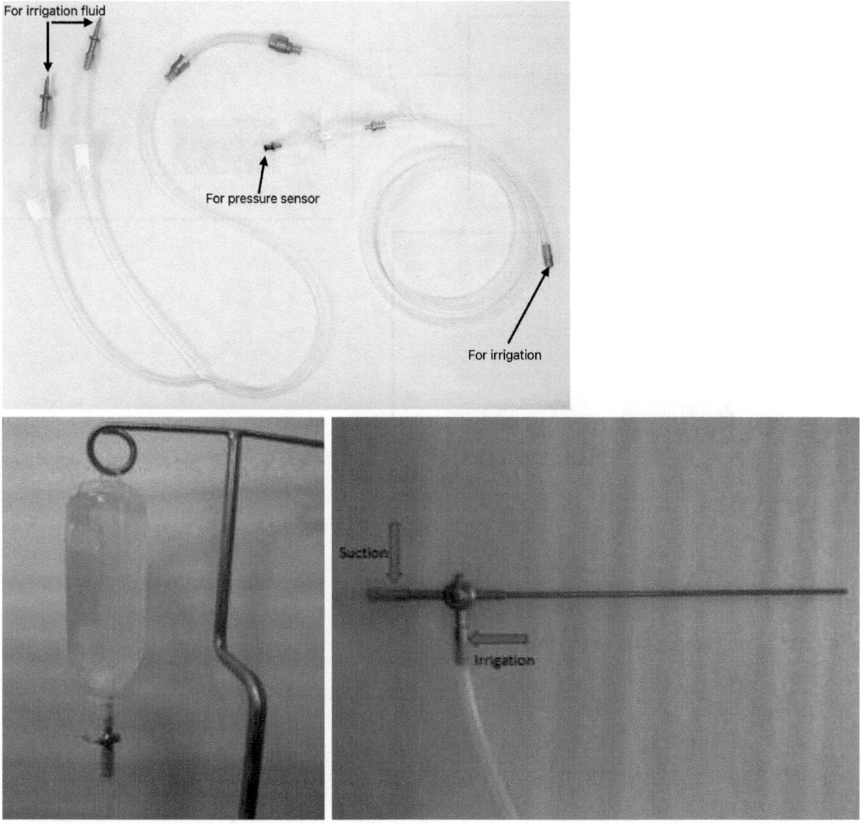

Fig. 20.4 Irrigation tubing set and its connection

1	Power button	The power switch is used to turn on and to turn off the system
2	Touch screen	Provides user controls and system feedback
3	Keypad	User controllable touch keys
4	Tubeguide for attaching irrigation tubing set	Peristaltic mechanism is used for irrigation. Tubeguide is used to hold the peristaltic tube on roller
5	Suction port	Vacuum or negative pressure is created in this port for suction
6	Pressure sensor inlet port	Senses the irrigation pressure
7	Mains connector with fuse compartment	For main electricity connector cord
8	Equipotential	Can be used to connect it to the earth receptacle if needed

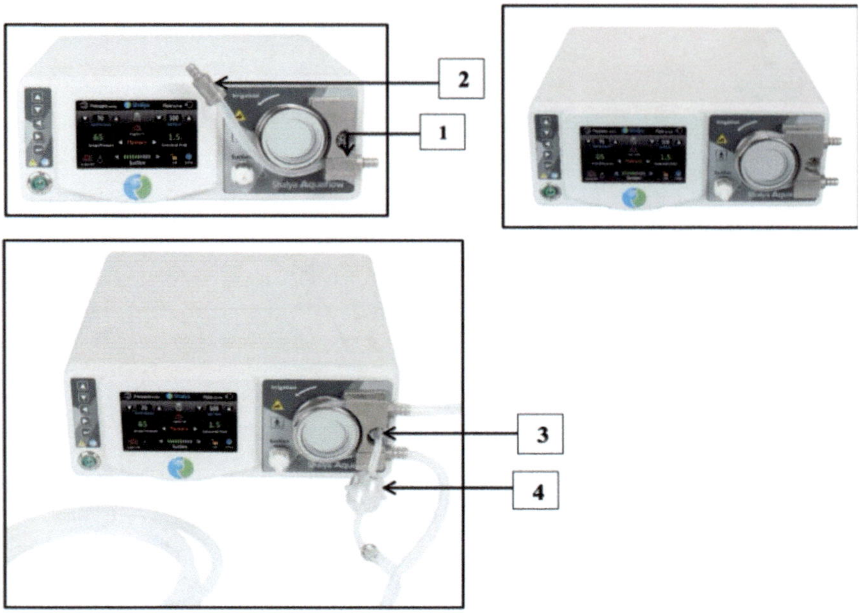

Fig. 20.5 Attaching tubing set to machine

Urology:
Pressure: 120 mmHg; Flow: 800 mLPM.
Max Pressure: 400 mmHg; Max Flow: 1000 mLPM.
Arthroscopy:
Pressure: 100 mmHg; Flow: 1200 mLPM.
Max Pressure: 400 mmHg; Max Flow: 2000 mLPM.

Set Flow This refers to the flow rate at which the machine delivers fluid to attain the desired pressure. It is advisable to commence with lower settings for a specific procedure and progressively increase them to accommodate the requirements of the procedure.

Set Pressure This represents the maximum pressure the machine will attain before ceasing the flow. Commence with the lower settings for a specific procedure and progressively increase them.

Actual Pressure This represents the current pressure reading of the fluid.

20.5 Advanced Settings (Fig. 20.6)

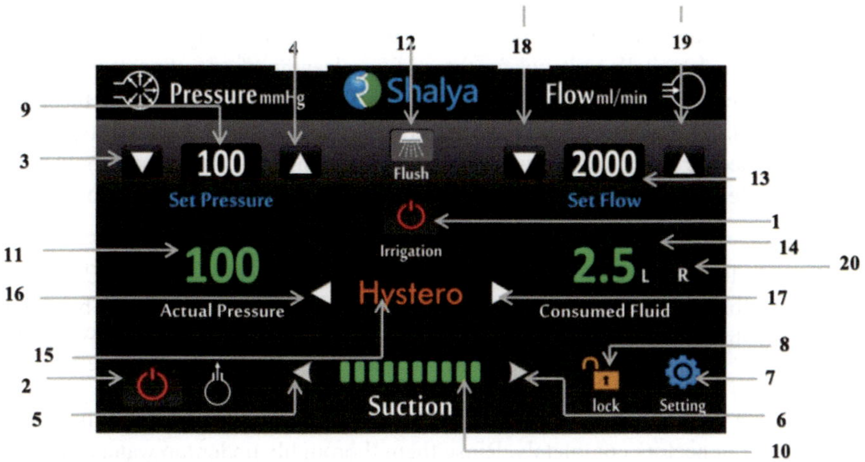

Fig. 20.6 Details of settings and functions

Sr. No.	Name	Description
1	Irrigation power button	Enable or disable the irrigation system
2	Suction power button	Enable or disable the suction function
3	Decrease irrigation pressure	Allows user to decrease irrigation pressure
4	Increase irrigation pressure	Allows user to increase irrigation pressure
5	Decrease suction level	Allows user to decrease suction level
6	Increase suction level	Allows user to increase suction level
7	Settings	Opens advanced settings
8	Lock & unlock	Locks the equipment to the user-set mode and values until unlocked
9	Irrigation pressure display	Displays irrigation pressure
10	Suction level display	Displays suction level
11	Actual pressure	Displays actual pressure in mmHg
12	Flush	It is used for removing the air from tubing set
13	Set flow	Allows user to set flow rate in ml/min
14	Consumed fluid	Displays consumed fluid in L
15	Mode display	Allows user to see the current working mode of surgery
16	Mode level forward	Allows user to change the mode in forward direction through single step
17	Mode level backward	Allows user to change the mode in backward direction through single step
18	Irrigation flow decrease	Allows user to increase irrigation flow with step of 100 ml
19	Irrigation flow increase	Allows user to decrease irrigation flow with step of 100 ml
20	Consumed fluid reset	Allows the user to reset the consumed fluid

20.6 Maintenance

1. *Cleaning*

   The outer body of the irrigation machine should be periodically cleaned in accordance with the hospital's protocol for the surface cleaning of operating room equipment. Before touching the machine with a wet cloth, the power cord must be disconnected. The machine should be allowed to dry completely before use to prevent the risk of electric shock and damage to the machine. Single-use tubing sets should not be reused. Reusable tubing sets must be cleaned before being sent for sterilization.

2. *Rinsing*

   Rinse the tubing set along with tube-guide connectors with tap water (<40 °C/104 °F) until all visible accumulations of the dirt is removed. Remove the stuck dirt by using a small brush or cloth. Enzymatic detergent may be used to further clean the tubes.

3. *Bathing*

   Prepare a thorough cleaning solution. Submerge the tubing set with its included tube-guide connectors completely. Rinse them thoroughly under tap water to eliminate any remaining cleaning agents. Allow the tubing set to dry completely. If any dirt persists, repeat the cleaning process.

4. *Disinfection*

   Glutaraldehyde may be used to disinfect the tubes and connectors. Prepare a disinfectant bath and immerse the tubing set along with tube-guide connector completely in it for the prescribed time. Rinse the tubing set with tube-guide connector in deionized/distilled water to remove the disinfectant without any residue. Allow the tubing set to dry completely.

5. *Sterilization*

   Autoclaving, EtO or plasma sterilization can usually be used with silicon tubing and its metallic connectors for sterilization.

   Power cable should not be sterilized by EtO gas or autoclaving. These methods can cause deformation & damage that can render the cable useless. After each procedure, wipe with a soft, clean, lint-free cloth. If dirt persists, moisten the cloth with 70% ethyl or isopropyl alcohol and wipe again. Dry thoroughly after wiping. A cable that is not completely dry may cause an electric shock.

20.7 Storage

Do not store these devices in humid and unventilated environments, as this may encourage the growth of microorganisms and pose an infection control risk. Do not store the unit in a location exposed to direct sunlight, x-ray, radioactivity, liquids, or strong electromagnetic radiation.

Do not apply excessive bending, straining, or squeezing force to any cords during storage as it may cause malfunction. Always disconnect the power cord while storing the device. Store the equipment at room temperature in the horizontal position in a clean, dry, and stable location.

20.8 Check for Tubing Set Before Each Use

- Check tubing set for leaks. Change set if there is a leak anywhere.
- Make sure that the tubes of the tubing set are not kinked.
- Fasten the tubes before starting irrigation as fluid under pressure can cause the tube to move on its own.
- Ensure distal end is connected to hand instrument before starting irrigation as otherwise fluid will escape under pressure from tube which may lead to water damage of sensitive operating room equipment.

20.9 Risks Involved with Irrigation Fluid

The following risks have been identified in clinical literature to be related to the use of irrigation fluid for distention of body cavities:
Hypothermia.
Fluid overload/extravasation.
Gas embolism.
Hypotensive bradycardic events in arthroscopy.
Pain during hysteroscopy.
Peri-renal hematoma.
The side effects described above relate to the use of irrigation fluid for distention of body cavities.

20.10 Troubleshooting

Follow a systematic approach to identify and resolve common issues. Below are general checks and tips to help you troubleshoot quickly:

1. Pump Not Turning On
    - Switch operation: Confirm that the power switch has been turned on and functioning properly.
    - Faulty cables or connectors: Inspect the cables for any signs of damage or loose connections.
    - Overheating protection: If the pump has overheated, it may automatically shut off if it has such a feature built into it. Allow it to cool down and try turning it on again.
2. Low or No Flow
    - Blockages: Check the tubing for kinks or blockages. Ensure the inlet and outlet are free from debris.
    - Tubing installation: Verify that the tubing is connected correctly and securely to the pump and cannula.
    - Clogged filters: Some pumps have filters that may become clogged. Clean or replace the filters if necessary.
    - Pump pressure settings: Ensure the pump's flow rate and pressure settings are adjusted correctly for the procedure.
3. Fluid Leaks
    - Damaged tubing: Replace punctured or worn tubing.

- Inspect connections: Check for any loose tubing connections. Tighten or replace any faulty parts.

4. Inconsistent Flow or Pressure
   - Air in the system: Air bubbles can cause irregular flow. Prime the system to remove any air trapped in the tubing.
   - Obstructions in the cannula: Ensure the cannula is not clogged with tissue or debris, which can impede the flow.
   - Pump wear or malfunction: Check for any signs of wear in the pump mechanism. Irregular pressure may indicate a failing pump motor or internal components.
5. Noisy Operation
   - Pump lubrication: If the pump produces unusual noise, it may require lubrication or maintenance.
   - Worn-out parts: Noises may indicate wear on mechanical components that could need replacement.
6. Alarm or Error Codes
   - Consult the manual: If the pump has an alarm system, refer to the user manual for details on the specific error code and the recommended troubleshooting steps.
   - Reset the system: Power cycle the device by turning it off and on to reset the system and clear minor software issues.
7. Software Issues
   - Firmware or software updates: If applicable, check for any updates to the pump's software that may resolve glitches or operational problems.
   - Otherwise, one may ask the manufacturer to reinstall software if it is giving repeated unexplained errors.

If these steps do not resolve the issue, consulting the manufacturer or a biomedical technician may be necessary for more complex repairs or recalibration.

20.11 Conclusion

Irrigation machines play a critical role in maintaining clear visibility during laparoscopic procedures by providing a continuous flow of sterile fluid to flush debris and maintain intra-cavitary pressure. Proper maintenance, regular calibration, and timely troubleshooting of these machines ensure optimal performance and prevent surgical complications. Regular training of operating staff on handling and identifying potential errors further enhances patient safety. As technology advances, modern irrigation systems are incorporating intelligent monitoring and auto-regulation to improve efficiency and reduce human error, ensuring safer and more effective surgical outcomes.

References

1. Karl Storz Se & Co. Kg. endomat select up220 — instructions for use (upp220_en_v1.1_01_2022_ifu_cemdd). 2022. https://stopler.nl/uploads/media/637eecd13774c/http-www-stoplerftp-comwebsitemanualsstz-up220-manual1-upp220.pdf.
2. Shalya Medical. Shalya Aquaflow1: Instructions for use. Document No. XMT/IFU/AQF/01, Version 1.7, November 2023.

Endoscopes

21

Hari Sellappan

21.1 Introduction

Endoscopes have become an essential adjunct during laparoscopic surgery with the advent of endo-laparoscopic surgical techniques. Modern endoscopes have undergone a transformative revolution over the past two decades, driven by advancements in optics, digital image sensors and processors, endoscope bodies that exhibit versatility and resilience, multiple working channels, and light sources capable of varying wavelengths, enabling chromoendoscopy [1, 2]. These technological advancements promote evolution in endo-laparoscopic techniques while expanding their application into clinical practice.

The endoscopes commonly used in the operating theatre include gastroscopes, colonoscopes, duodenoscopes and choledochoscopes. This chapter provides a comprehensive technical description and specifications of the endoscopes. It also covers cleaning and maintenance procedures, as well as troubleshooting common issues that may arise during their use. It is important to note that the description of surgical techniques falls outside the scope of this book.

Although many different endoscope manufacturers are currently available in the market, we will use Olympus (Tokyo, Japan) endoscopes for reference. The content in this chapter will be generic and can be applied to most endoscopes.

H. Sellappan (✉)
Hepatopancreatobiliary Unit, Department of General Surgery, Queen Elizabeth Hospital, Kota Kinabalu, Sabah, Malaysia
e-mail: hari.vs@moh.gov.my

J. S. Ahluwalia (ed.), *User Manual for Minimally Invasive Surgical Equipment*,
https://doi.org/10.1007/978-981-95-9019-3_21

21.2 Endoscopy Workstation: Technical Details and Specifications

The endoscopy workstation incorporates a modular design that can be customized according to required specifications. In a dedicated endo-laparoscopic operating theatre, the endoscopic workstation can be set up on an equipment boom which creates a more versatile and efficient working space. Alternatively, a mobile workstation on a trolley cart can allow the equipment to be transported to different operating rooms with ease [3–6]. (Fig. 21.1).

The standard workstation consists of a video system centre, light source, electrosurgery unit, water container, suction pump, water-jet, CO2 insufflator, high-definition monitor, keyboard and image printer.

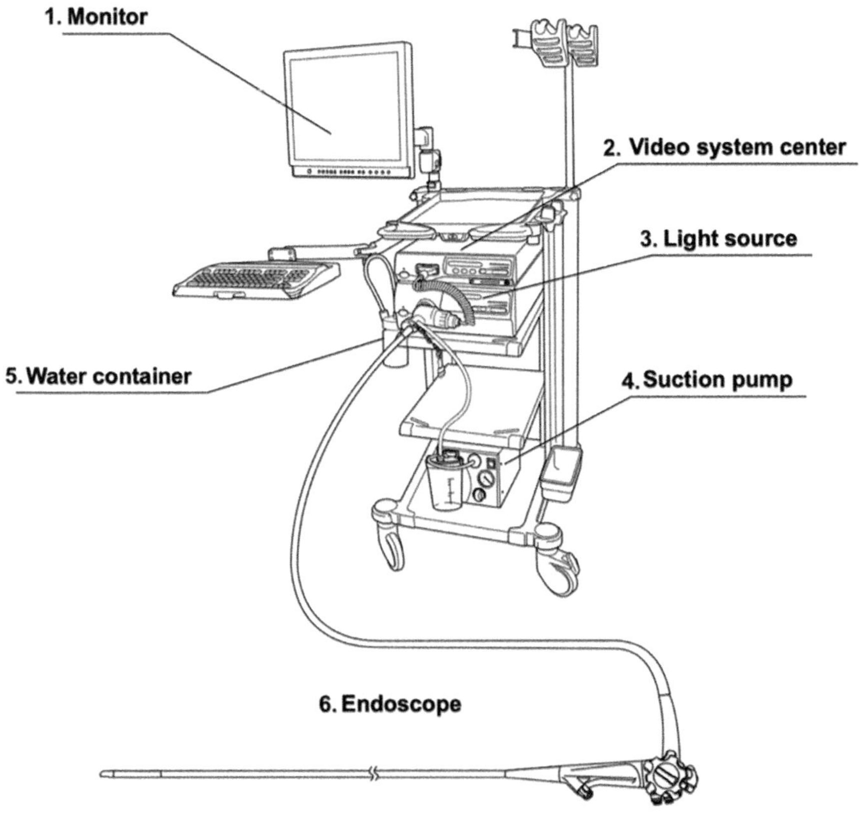

Fig. 21.1 Layout of endoscopic equipment on a mobile workstation

Description of Components of an Endoscopic Workstation (Fig. 21.1)

1. *Monitor*: HD monitor mounted on an adjustable bracket.
2. *Video system centre*: Video processing system that captures, processes and transmits image from the endoscope to the monitor.
3. *Light source*: High-intensity light source from either Xenon or LED bulb, and enables advanced image-enhanced endoscopy. Also contains an air insufflator.
4. *Suction pump*: Suction pump that is connected to the endoscope and can be controlled using the suction valve.
5. *Water container*: Stores water used to flush and cleanse the lens at the endoscopic tip.
6. *Endoscope*: Variety of endoscopes including gastroscopes, colonoscopes, duodenoscopes and enteroscopes can be connected to the video processing system and light source.

21.2.1 Video Processing System

The endoscopy image processing unit usually comes in 2 parts; the video processing system (Fig. 21.2) and light source (Fig. 21.3). Some manufacturers combine both functions into a single unit, e.g. Evis X1 (Olympus, Tokyo, Japan).

Features of the video processing system:

- White balance.
- Image enhancement.
- Variable iris mode.
- Storage of video and still images.

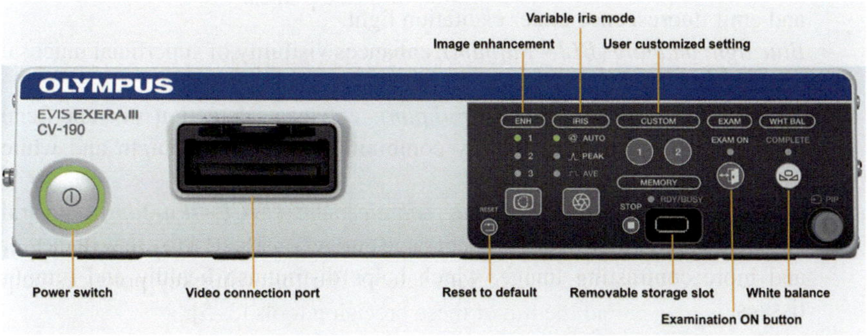

Fig. 21.2 Video processing system

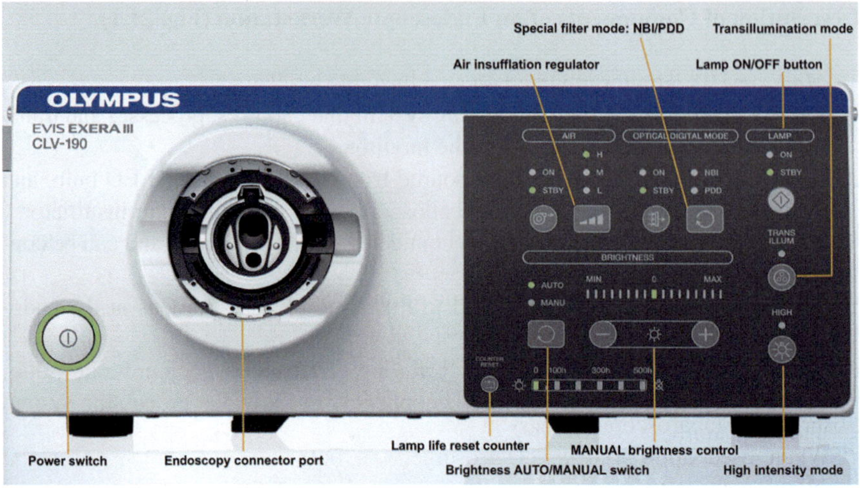

Fig. 21.3 Light source

21.2.2 Light Source

Features of the light source unit (Fig. 21.3):

- Lamp: Xenon or LED.
- Lamp life reset counter: after replacing the Xenon lamp, the lamp life counter can be reset back to 0 hours.
- Advanced image-enhanced endoscopy: improves detection of benign, pre-malignant and malignant lesions.
  - *Narrow-band imaging (NBI—Olympus)*: enhances visibility of mucosal & submucosal vessels and mucosal surface patterns with the use of narrow wavelength light.
  - *Photodynamic diagnostic (PDD—Olympus)*: enhances detection of gastric and colorectal tumours by using 5-aminolevulinic acid (5-ALA), a precursor to protoporphyrin IX (PpIX), which selectively accumulates in tumour cells and emit fluorescence under excitation light.
  - *Blue light imaging (BLI—Fujifilm)*: enhances visibility of superficial mucosal patterns and vessels with the use of narrow wavelength light.
  - *Linked colour imaging (LCI—Fujifilm)*: enhances detection of superficial mucosal patterns and vessels by combining narrow wavelength and white light imaging.
  - *Flexible spectral imaging colour enhancement (FICE—Fujifilm)*: spectral component of colour images is separated and reconstructed to create a clearer and more contrasting image, which helps distinguish healthy and tumour tissues.

  – *i-Scan and optical enhancement (Pentax)*: enhance visibility of mucosal surface and vascular patterns with the use of optical filters.
- Dual focus: switch from normal focus to near focus mode during enhanced endoscopic assessment.
- Automatic light intensity adjustment.
- Transillumination mode: emits intense light for 7 seconds that transmits through the patient's abdominal wall for the endoscopist to confirm position of the distal end of an endoscope.
- High intensity mode: emits brighter illumination light than usual.
- Air insufflator: regulates the flow of air for insufflation.

21.2.3 CO_2 Insufflator

Although most endoscopy systems come with a built-in air insufflation mechanism, a CO_2 insufflator (Fig. 21.4) is highly recommended during endo-laparoscopic surgery or intra-operative endoscopy. Benefits of CO_2 vs air insufflation during intra-operative endoscopy: [7].

- Rapid absorption of CO_2.
- Improves intra-operative exposure.
- Less post-operative bowel distension.
- Earlier commencement of post-operative enteral feeding.

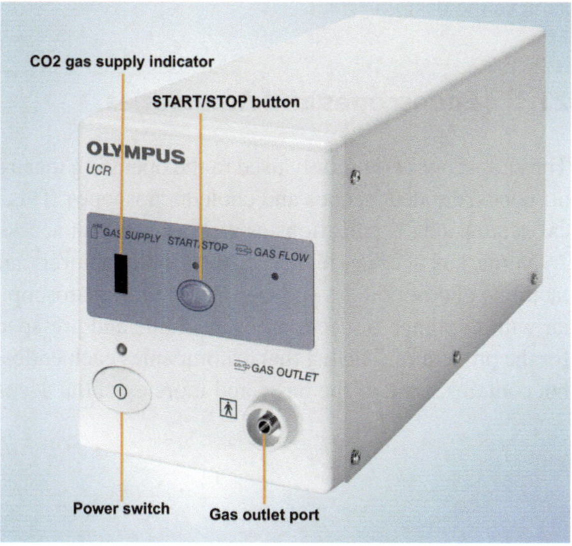

Fig. 21.4 CO_2 insufflator

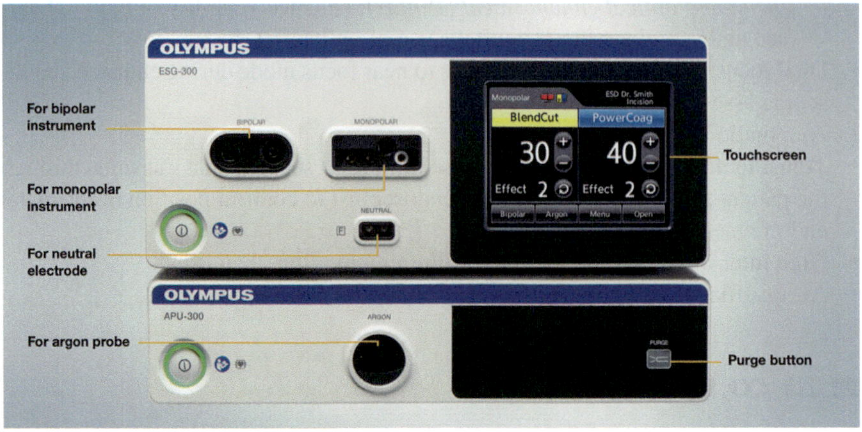

Fig. 21.5 Electrosurgery and argon plasma generator

21.2.4 Electrosurgery and Argon Plasma Generator

The electrosurgical generator (Fig. 21.5) provides both monopolar and bipolar function, whereas the argon plasma generator provides monopolar argon plasma coagulation. The monopolar spectrum ranges between pure cutting, deep coagulation and various combinations in between including endocut, pulsed cut, forced coag and soft coag. These electrosurgical devices are commonly used during endoscopic procedures such as polypectomy, endoscopic mucosal resection (EMR), endoscopic submucosal dissection (ESD), sphincterotomy, peroral endoscopic myotomy (POEM), tissue ablation and haemostasis [8]. Settings for specific procedures should follow the manufacturer's guidelines and the endoscopist's preference to achieve the desired effect.

21.3 Endoscopes and Accessories

The endoscopes commonly used in the operating theatre include gastroscopes, colonoscopes, duodenoscopes and choledochoscopes. This section describes the technical details and specifications as well as common accessories used.

Numerous accessories by various manufacturers are available in the market to facilitate endoscopic procedures. The endo-laparoscopic surgeon needs to be familiar with the range of accessories available and pre-specify the accessories required for the procedure. The list that accompanies each endoscope type is non-exhaustive, but contains some of the basic and more essential accessories commonly used.

21.3.1 Gastroscope and Colonoscope

Description of Components of an Olympus Endoscope Connector (Fig. 21.6) [3–5]

1. *Suction connector*: Connects the endoscope to the suction tube of the suction pump.
2. *S-cord connector mount*: Connects the endoscope with the Olympus electrosurgical unit via the S-cord. The S-cord conducts leakage current from the endoscope to the electrosurgical unit.
3. *Water supply connector and air supply connector*: Connects the endoscope to the water container via the water container tube to supply water to the distal end of the endoscope.
4. *Endoscope connector*: Connects the endoscope to the output socket of the light source and transmits light from the light source to the endoscope.
5. *Electrical connector*: Connects the endoscope to the video system centre via the videoscope cable. The endoscope contains a memory chip that stores information about the endoscope and communicates this information to the video system centre.

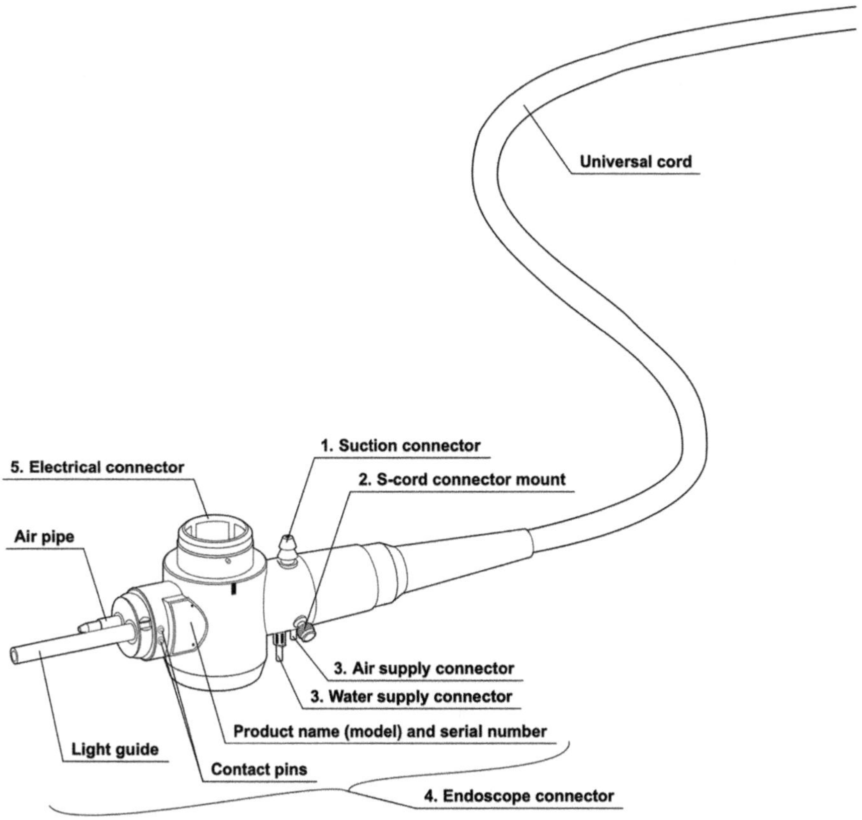

Fig. 21.6 Endoscope connector

Description of Components of an Olympus Video Gastroscope and Colonoscope (Fig. 21.7 and 21.8) [3, 4]

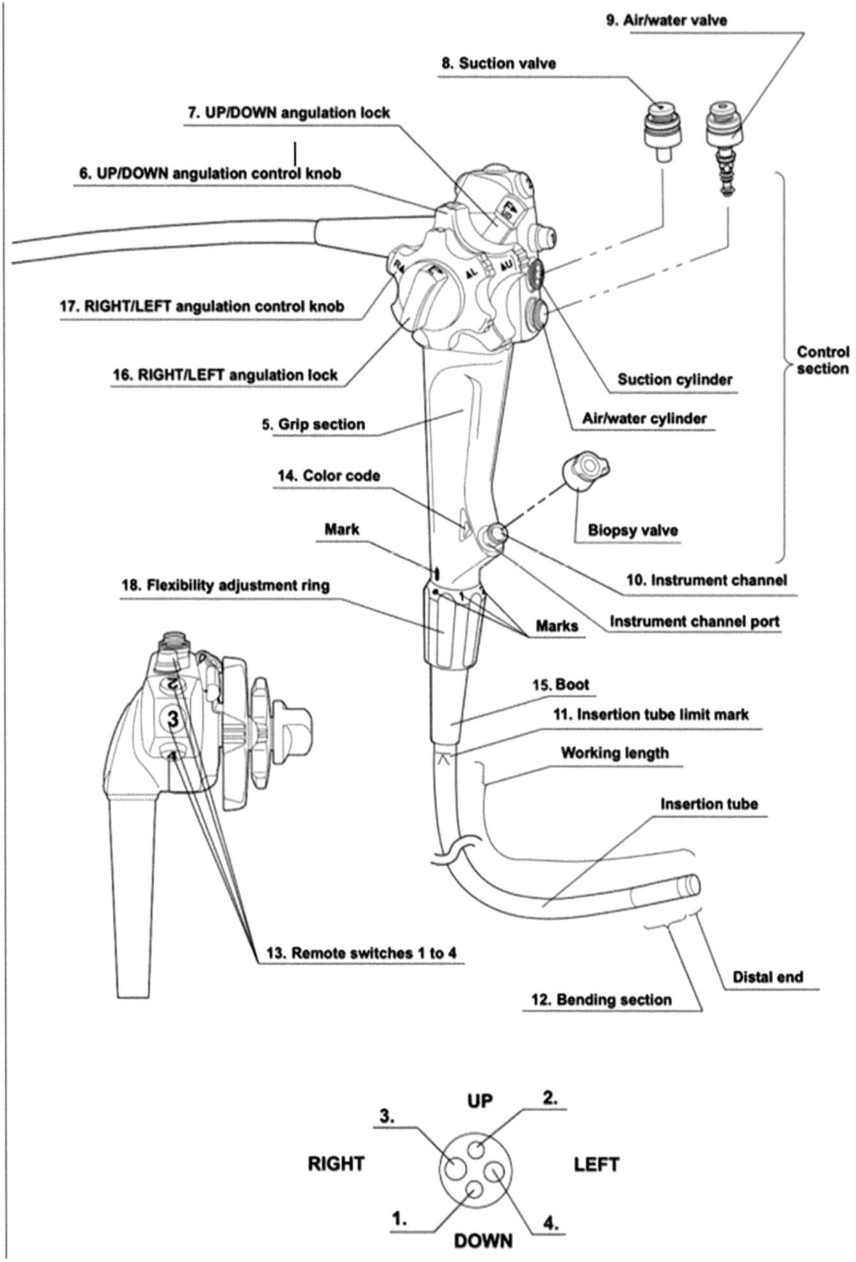

Fig. 21.7 Endoscope control section and insertion tube—gastroscope and colonoscope

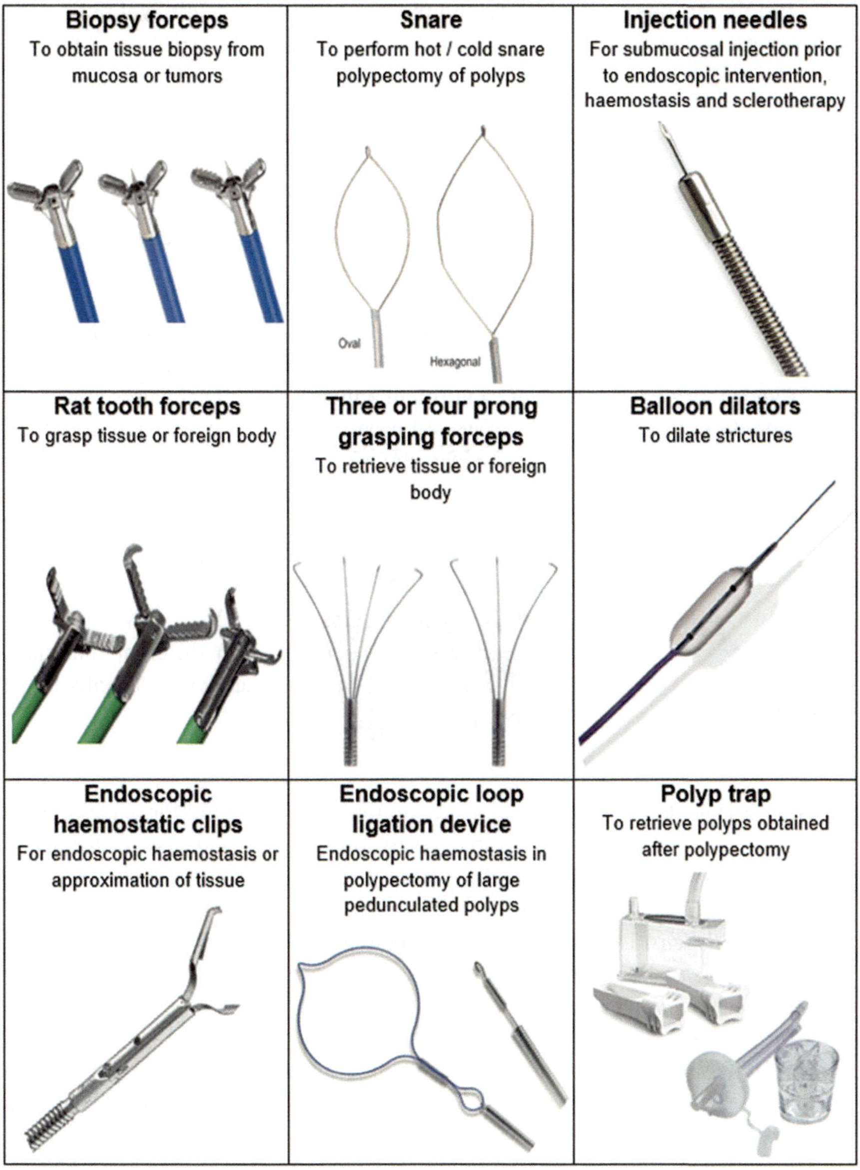

Fig. 21.8 Accessories for gastroscopy and colonoscopy

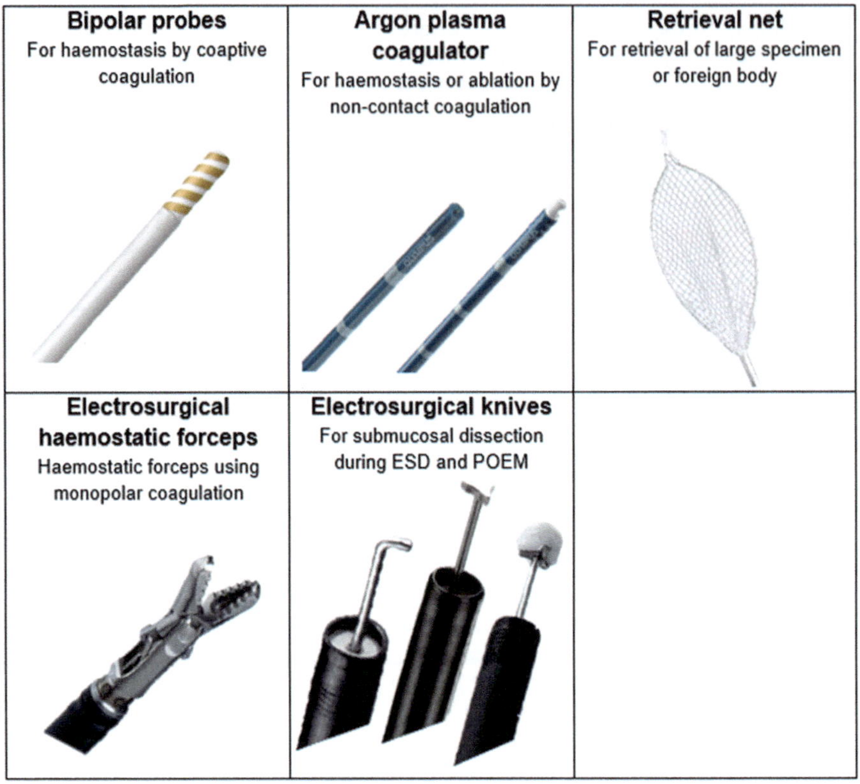

Fig. 21.8 (continued)

1. *Air/water nozzle*: Nozzle that allows passage of air for insufflation and water to cleanse the lens.
2. *Light guide lens*: Light source for illumination.
3. *Objective lens*: Lens through which the image is transmitted.
4. *Instrument channel outlet.*
5. *Grip section.*
6. *UP/DOWN angulation control knob*: When this knob is turned in the "U" direction, the bending section moves UP; when the knob is turned in the "D" direction, the bending section moves DOWN.
7. *UP/DOWN angulation lock*: Moving this lock in the "F" direction frees angulation. Moving the lock in the opposite direction locks the bending section at any desired position.
8. *Suction valve*: This valve is depressed to activate suction. The valve is used to remove any fluids, debris, flatus, or air from the patient.
9. *Air/water valve*: The hole in this valve is covered to insufflate air and the valve is depressed to feed water for lens washing. It also can be used to feed air for removing any fluids or debris adhering to the objective lens.

10. *Instrument channel*: The instrument channel functions as channel for the insertion of accessories, suction and fluid feed (from a syringe via the biopsy valve).
11. *Insertion section limit mark*: This mark shows the maximum point to which the endoscope may be inserted into the patient's body.
12. *Bending section*: This section moves the distal end of the endoscope when the UP/DOWN and RIGHT/LEFT angulation control knobs are operated.
13. *Remote switches*: The functions of remote switches 1 to 4 can be selected on the video system centre.
14. *Colour code*: The endoscope can be used with accessories that have the same colour code.
15. *Boot.*
16. *RIGHT/LEFT angulation lock*: Turning this lock in the "F" direction frees angulation. Turning the lock in the opposite direction locks the bending section at any desired position.
17. *RIGHT/LEFT angulation control knob*: When this knob is turned in the "R" direction, the bending section moves RIGHT; when the knob is turned in the "L" direction, the bending section moves LEFT.
18. *Flexibility adjustment ring (if available)*: Turn this ring to adjust the flexibility of the insertion tube.

21.3.2 Duodenoscope for ERCP

Description of Components of an Olympus Video Duodenoscope for ERCP (Fig. 21.9 and 21.10) [5]

1. *Air/water nozzle*: Nozzle that allows passage of air for insufflation and water to cleanse the lens.
2. *Objective lens*: Lens through which the image is transmitted.
3. *Light guide lens*: Light source for illumination.
4. *Instrument channel outlet.*
5. *Forceps elevator*: Elevator at the tip of scope allows angulation of instruments and forceps.
6. *Guidewire-locking groove*: Groove along forceps elevator allows guide-wire to be locked in position in an elevated position.
7. *Grip section.*
8. *Suction valve*: This valve is depressed to activate suction. The valve is used to remove any fluids, debris, flatus, or air from the patient.
9. *Air/water valve*: The hole in this valve is covered to insufflate air and the valve is depressed to feed water for lens washing. It also can be used to feed air for removing any fluids or debris adhering to the objective lens.
10. *Instrument channel*: The instrument channel functions as channel for the insertion of accessories, suction and fluid feed (from a syringe via the biopsy valve).
11. *Insertion section limit mark*: This mark shows the maximum point to which the endoscope may be inserted into the patient's body.

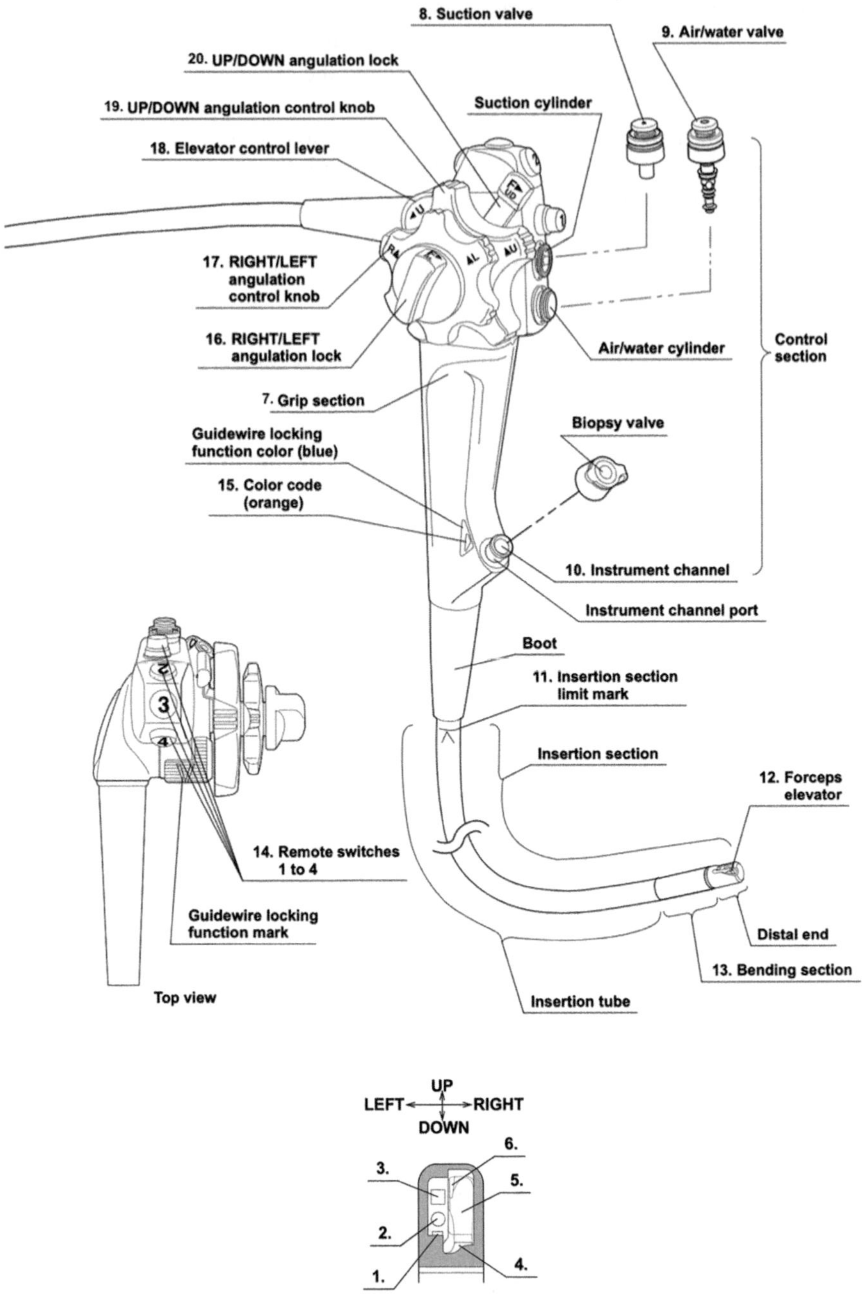

Fig. 21.9 Endoscope control section and insertion tube—duodenoscope

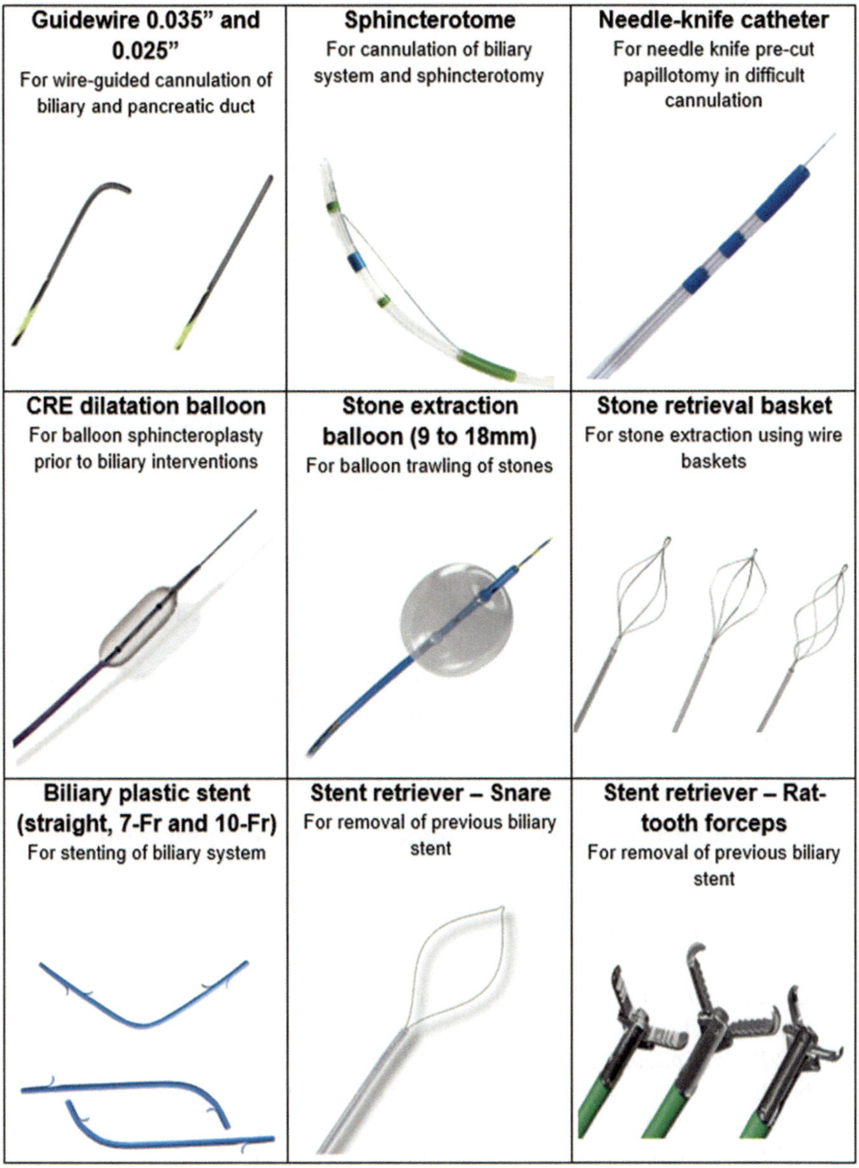

Fig. 21.10 Accessories for endoscopic retrograde cholangio-pancreatography (ERCP)

12. *Forceps elevator*: The elevator moves accessories when the elevator control lever is operated. In addition, the elevator is used to assist the locking function of the guidewire while inserting/withdrawing the wire-guided type accessories.
13. *Bending section*: This section moves the distal end of the endoscope when the UP/DOWN and RIGHT/LEFT angulation control knobs are operated.
14. *Remote switches*: The functions of remote switches 1 to 4 can be selected on the video system centre.
15. *Colour code*: The endoscope can be used with accessories that have the same colour code.
16. *RIGHT/LEFT angulation lock*: Turning this lock in the "F" direction frees angulation. Turning the lock in the opposite direction locks the bending section at any desired position.
17. *RIGHT/LEFT angulation control knob*: When this knob is turned in the "R" direction, the bending section moves RIGHT; when the knob is turned in the "L" direction, the bending section moves LEFT.
18. *Elevator control lever*: When this lever is moved in the "U" direction, the forceps elevator is raised. When the lever is turned in the opposite direction, the forceps elevator is lowered.
19. *UP/DOWN angulation control knob*: When this knob is turned in the "U" direction, the bending section moves UP; when the knob is turned in the "D" direction, the bending section moves DOWN.
20. *UP/DOWN angulation lock*: Moving this lock in the "F" direction frees angulation. Moving the lock in the opposite direction locks the bending section at any desired position.

21.3.3 Choledochoscope for Common Bile Duct Exploration

Description of Components of an Olympus Video Choledochoscope (Figs. 21.11, 21.12 and 21.13) [6]

1. *Bending section*: The bending section moves the distal end of the endoscope when the UP/DOWN angulation control lever is operated.
2. *UP/DOWN angulation control lever*: When turned in the "U" direction, the bending section moves UP; when turned in the "D" direction, the bending section moves DOWN.
3. *UP/DOWN angulation lock*: Pushing this lever in the "F" direction frees the angulation. Pushing the lever in the opposite direction locks the bending section at any desired position.
4. *Single-use suction valve*: The suction valve is depressed to activate suction. The valve is also used to remove any fluid or debris adhering to the objective lens.
5. *Forceps/irrigation plug (Isolated type)*: Accessories are inserted through the forceps port. Fluid can be fed through the irrigation port.
6. *Instrument channel port*: This channel is used for the insertion of accessories and for feeding fluid.

7. *Colour code*: The colour code is used to quickly determine the compatibility of accessories. The endoscope can be used with accessories that have the same colour code.
8. *Remote switches "1" to "4"*: The functions of remote switches 1 to 4 can be selected on the video system centre. When selecting the functions, refer to the instruction manual for the video system centre.

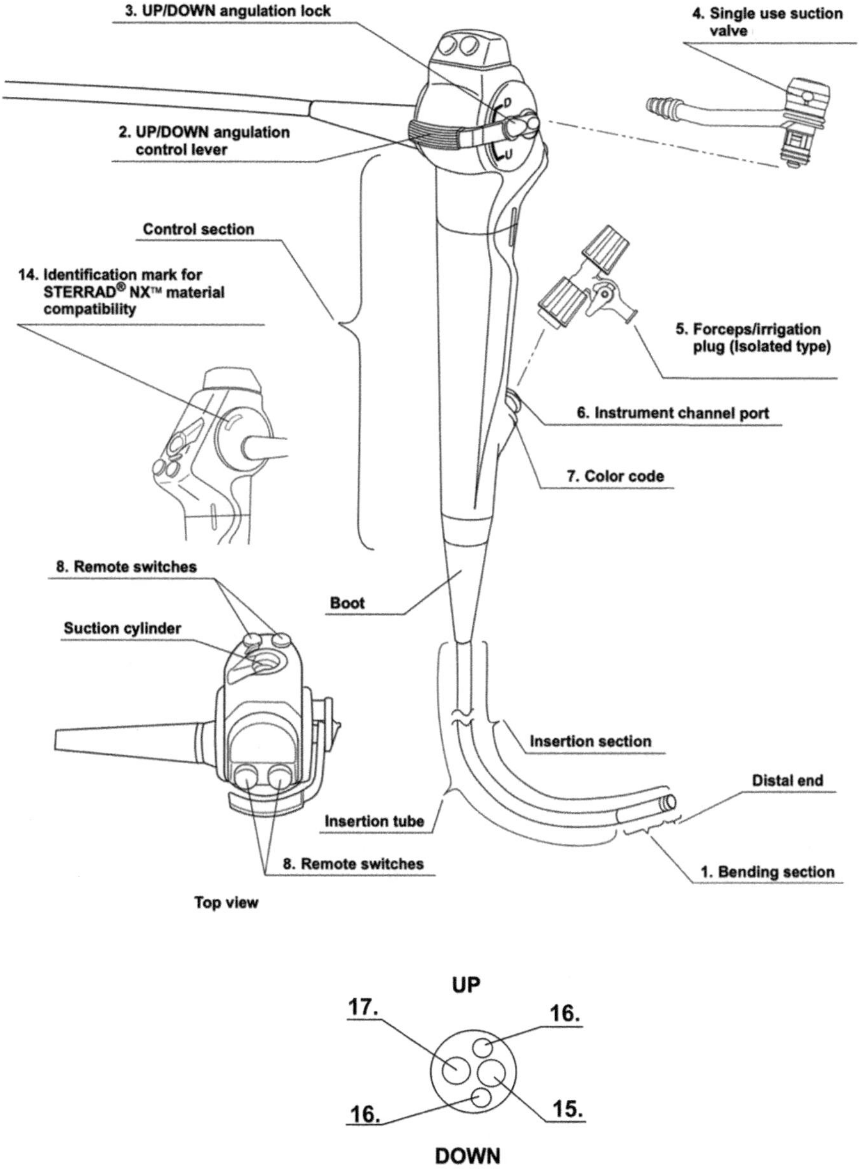

Fig. 21.11 Endoscope control section and insertion tube—choledochoscope

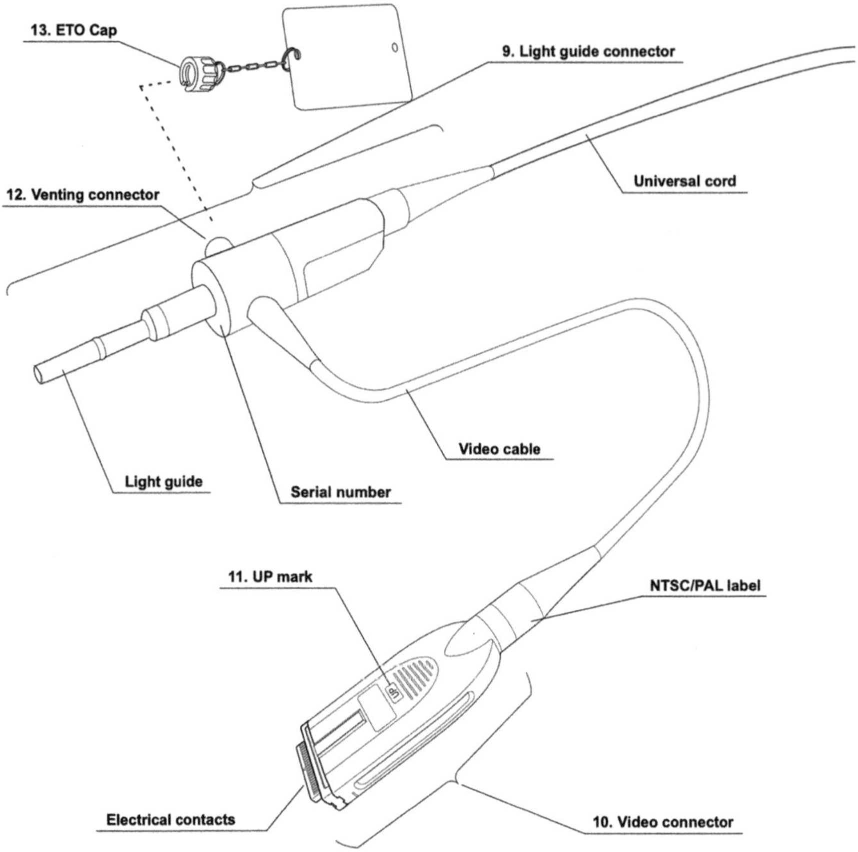

Fig. 21.12 Endoscope connector—choledochoscope

9. *Light guide connector*: The light guide connector connects the endoscope to the output socket of the light source and transmits light from the light source to the endoscope.
10. *Video connector*: The video connector connects the endoscope to the output socket of the video system centre so that the endoscopic image becomes visible.
11. *UP mark*: When the video connector is connected to the video system centre, this mark is facing upward.
12. *Venting connector*: Attach the ETO cap or leakage tester here.
13. *ETO Cap*: The ETO cap must be installed prior to ethylene oxide sterilization and removed prior to immersion or clinical examination. The cap must also be attached when the endoscope is transported outside the healthcare facility (shipment, return for repairs, etc.).
14. *Identification mark for STERRAD NX material compatibility.*
15. *Objective lens*: Lens through which the image is transmitted.
16. *Light guide lens*: Light source for illumination.
17. *Instrument channel outlet.*

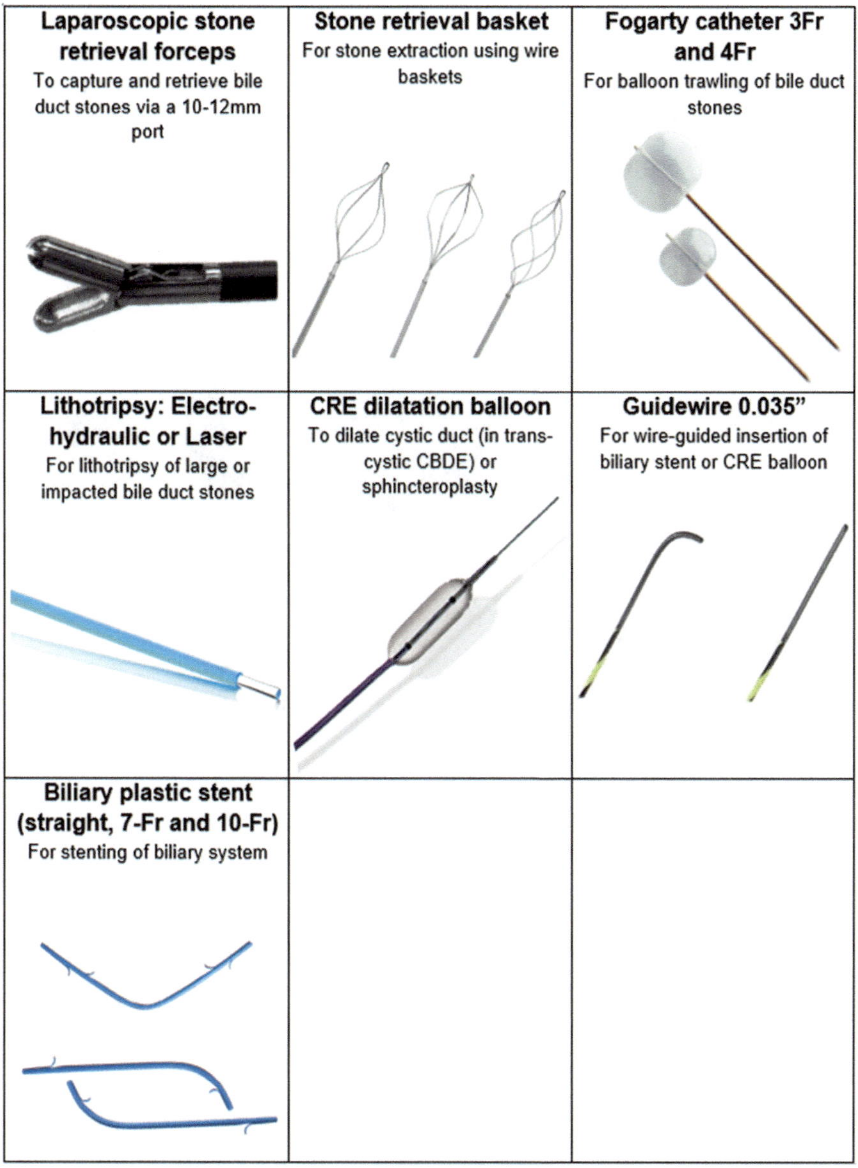

Fig. 21.13 Accessories for common bile duct exploration [9]

21.4 Cleaning and Maintenance

Endoscopes and their accessories are exposed to bodily fluids, tissue and blood during use, and carry the potential for cross-contamination between patients. Hence strict cleaning, disinfection or sterilization process needs to be observed to protect the patients undergoing the procedure as well as the healthcare providers handling the equipment. Adhere to cleaning, disinfection or sterilization standards and policy at your local institution. The cleaning and maintenance steps below [10] are only a guide and can be modified to suit your local practice (Figs. 21.14 and 21.15).

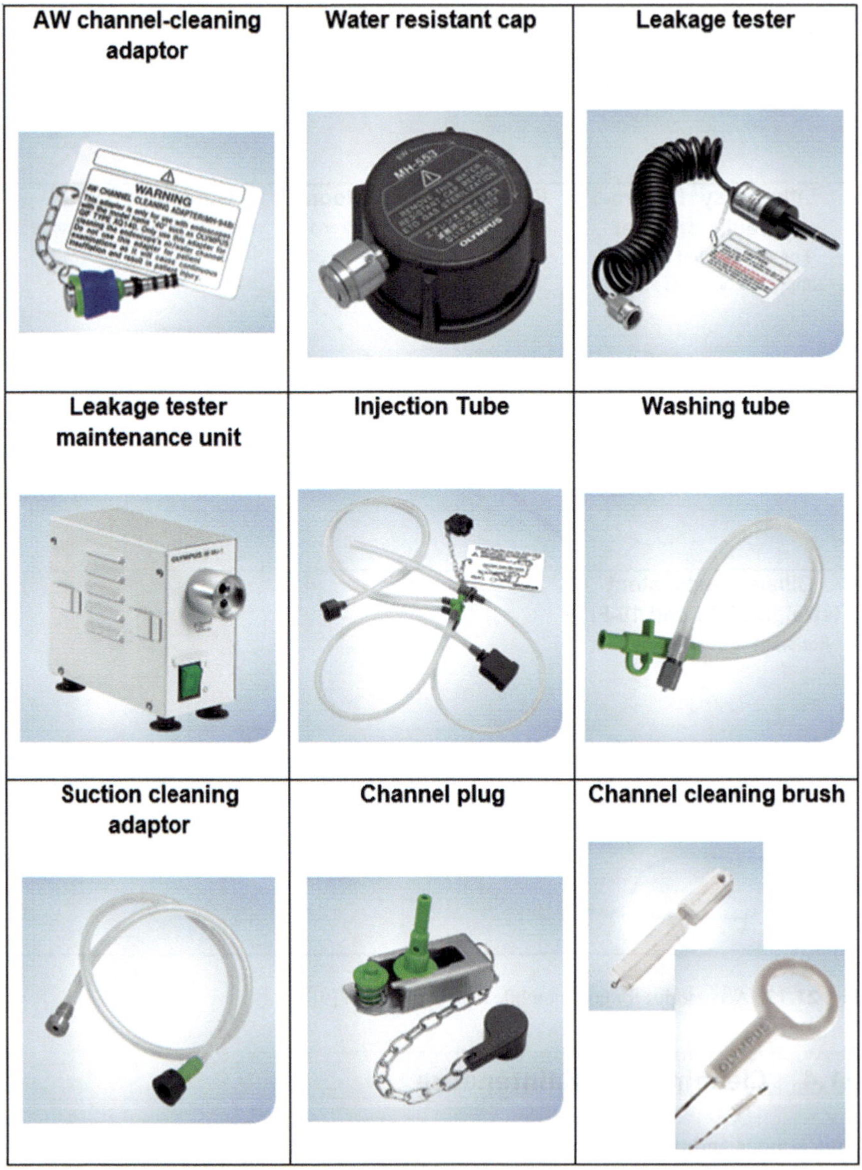

Fig. 21.14 Accessories for cleaning and disinfection

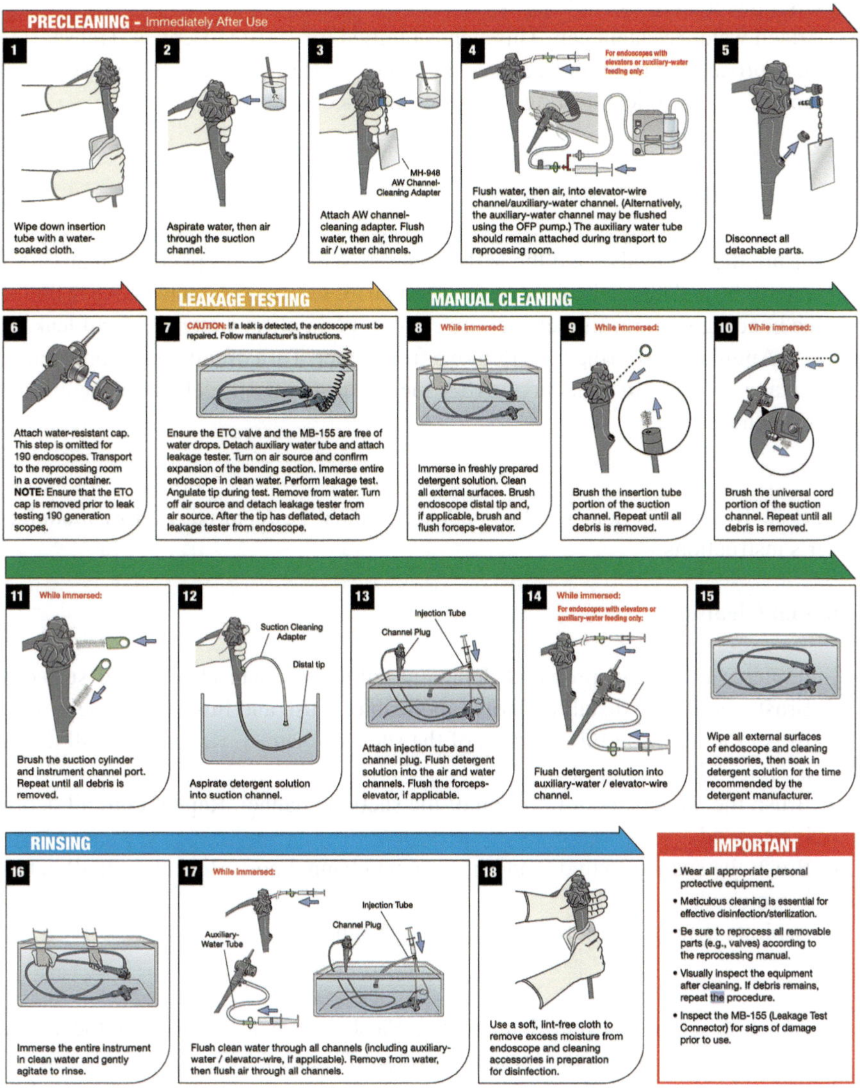

Fig. 21.15 Cleaning the endoscope—a pictorial guide

Pre-cleaning: Immediately After Use

1. Wipe down insertion tube with a water-soaked cloth.
2. Aspirate water, then air through the suction channel.
3. Attach AW channel-cleaning adapter. Flush water, then air, through air / water channels.
4. Flush water, then air, into elevator-wire channel/auxiliary-water channel. The auxiliary water tube should remain attached during transport to reprocessing room.

5. Disconnect all detachable parts.
6. Attach water-resistant cap. This step is omitted for 190 endoscopes. Transport to the reprocessing room in a covered container. NOTE: Ensure that the ETO cap is removed prior to leak testing 190 generation scopes.

Leakage Testing

7. Ensure the ETO valve and the MB-155 are free of water drops. Detach auxiliary water tube and attach leakage tester. Turn on air source and confirm expansion of the bending section. Immerse entire endoscope in clean water. Perform leakage test. Angulate tip during test. Remove from water. Turn off air source and detach leakage tester from air source. After the tip has deflated, detach leakage tester from endoscope.

Caution If a leak is detected, the endoscope must be repaired. Follow manufacturer's instructions.

Manual Cleaning

8. Immerse in freshly prepared detergent solution. Clean all external surfaces. Brush endoscope distal tip and, if applicable, brush and flush forceps-elevator.
9. Brush the insertion tube portion of the suction channel. Repeat until all debris is removed.
10. Brush the universal cord portion of the suction channel. Repeat until all debris is removed.
11. Brush the suction cylinder and instrument channel port. Repeat until all debris is removed.
12. Aspirate detergent solution into suction channel.

13. Attach injection tube and channel plug. Flush detergent solution into the air and water channels. Flush the forceps-elevator, if applicable.
14. Wipe all external surfaces of endoscope and cleaning accessories, then soak in detergent solution for the time recommended by the detergent manufacturer.

Rinsing

15. Immerse the entire instrument in clean water and gently agitate to rinse.
16. Flush clean water through all channels (including auxiliary water/elevator wire, if applicable). Remove from water, then flush air through all channels.
17. Use a soft, lint-free cloth to remove excess moisture from endoscope and cleaning accessories in preparation for disinfection.

Drying

18. After disinfection, the endoscope should be thoroughly dried to prevent the growth of microorganisms.
19. The endoscope should be hung vertically in a drying cabinet or on a drying rack.

Storage Room

20. Endoscopes should be stored in a designated storage room that is clean, dry, and well-ventilated.
21. The storage room should be kept at room temperature and away from direct sunlight.
22. Keep the cabinet door closed to prevent environmental contamination or accidental contact.

21.5 General Troubleshooting

The endoscope is a complex equipment that has many fixed as well as detachable components that are subject to wear and tear. As a result, many of these parts may fail or malfunction over time. An endoscopist needs to be familiar with all the common problems that may potentially arise during a procedure, quickly assess the situation, narrow down possible causes and find solutions.

The non-exhaustive list below contains common problems encountered, possible causes and potential solutions [3–6]. In the event that the problem persists and the issue cannot be resolved, the endoscopist may decide to abandon the procedure and withdraw the endoscope in safe manner without causing any harm or injury to the patient.

21.5.1 General Troubleshooting

Issues	Possible causes	Solution
Angulation		
Resistance during rotation of angulation control knobs	Angulation lock is engaged	Rotate angulation lock to the "F" direction
Air/water feeding		
No air feeding	Air pump on the light source is not operating	Set air pump to "LOW", "MED" or "HIGH" setting on the light source
	Air/water valve is damaged	Replace air/water valve
No water feeding	Air pump on the light source is not operating	Set air pump to "LOW", "MED" or "HIGH" setting on the light source

(continued)

Issues	Possible causes	Solution
	There is no sterile water in the water container	Fill water container with sterile water till the specified level
	Air/water valve is damaged	Replace air/water valve
Air/water valve is sticky	Air/water valve is dirty	Clean the valve
	Air/water valve is damaged	Replace air/water valve
Air/water valve cannot be attached	An incompatible air/water valve is used	Use a compatible air/water valve
	Air/water valve is damaged	Replace air/water valve
Air is continuously fed	Air/water valve is damaged	Replace air/water valve
Water is continuously fed	Air/water valve is damaged	Replace air/water valve
Suction		
Suction is absent or weak	Biopsy valve is not attached properly	Reattach biopsy valve correctly
	Biopsy valve is damaged	Replace biopsy valve
	Suction pump is set incorrectly	Adjust suction pump setting
	Suction valve is damaged	Replace suction valve
	Suction valve is blocked	Clean suction valve
	Working channel is blocked	Flush working channel through biopsy valve and/or suction cylinder
Suction valve is sticky	Suction valve is dirty	Clean suction valve
	Suction valve is damaged	Replace suction valve
Suction valve cannot be attached	An incompatible suction valve is used	Use a compatible suction valve
	Suction valve is damaged	Replace suction valve
Liquid leaks out of biopsy valve	Biopsy valve is not attached properly	Reattach biopsy valve correctly
	Biopsy valve is damaged	Replace biopsy valve
Suction cannot be stopped	Suction valve is damaged	Replace suction valve
Image quality/brightness		
No video image	Power switch not turned ON	Check main power switch, and power switch for monitor, video system Centre and light source
	Endoscope connector is not connected securely	Insert the endoscope connector securely until it stops and clicks

(continued)

Issues	Possible causes	Solution
	Electrical contacts on the endoscope connector are dirty	Wipe the electrical connectors on the endoscope connector with 70% isopropyl alcohol and allow to dry completely
	Light source not turned ON	Turn ON light source from standby mode
Image is not clear	Objective lens at the distal end of the endoscope is dirty	Activate water valve to clean lens
Image is excessively dark or bright	Light source is not set properly	Adjust light source setting
	Light guide lens at the distal end of the endoscope is dirty	Wipe the light guide lens with 70% isopropyl alcohol
	Glass at the endoscope connector end is dirty	Wipe the glass with 70% isopropyl alcohol
Image is out of focus	Focus setting is on near focus mode	Switch from near focus to normal focus mode
Endotherapy accessories		
Accessories do not pass through working channel smoothly	Incompatible accessory is being used	Use accessory that is compatible with the endoscope to avoid damage to working channel

21.5.2 Troubleshooting: Duodenoscopes for ERCP

Issues	Possible causes	Solution
Endotherapy accessories		
Guidewire cannot be locked	Guidewire is not locked at the stiff part	Lock guidewire at its stiff part
	Guidewire with a diameter less than 0.64 mm is used	Select guidewire with a diameter of 0.64 mm or more
	Guidewire locking groove is dirty	Clean guidewire locking groove

21.5.3 Troubleshooting: Choledochoscopes for CBD Exploration

Issues	Possible causes	Solution
Irrigation fluid feeding		
No irrigation fluid	Instrument channel is blocked	Clean the channel with a channel cleaning brush
	The forceps/irrigation plug is incorrectly assembled.	Reassemble it correctly as described in its instruction manual.
	The biopsy valve of the forceps/irrigation plug is worn out.	Replace it with a new one.

(continued)

Issues	Possible causes	Solution
Irrigation fluid leaks.	The instrument channel is obstructed.	Clean the channel with a channel cleaning brush.
	The forceps/irrigation plug is incorrectly assembled.	Reassemble it correctly as described in its instruction manual.
	The biopsy valve of the forceps/irrigation plug is worn out.	Replace it with a new one.
	The forceps/irrigation plug is incorrectly assembled.	Turn the tightening ring so that the ends of the biopsy valve and tightening ring are aligned.
Suction		
Suction is absent or insufficient.	The forceps/irrigation plug is not assembled properly.	Reassemble it correctly
	The biopsy valve of the forceps/irrigation plug is worn out.	Replace it with a new biopsy valve.
	The stopcock of the forceps/irrigation plug is opened.	Close the stopcock.
The suction valve does not return to its original position.	The aspiration pressure is too high.	Lower the aspiration pressure.
Endotherapy accessories		
The endotherapy accessory does not pass through the instrument channel smoothly.	The forceps/irrigation plug is incorrectly assembled.	Turn the tightening ring so that the ends of the biopsy valve and tightening ring are aligned.

21.5.4 Withdrawing an Endoscope with an Irregularity

If you encounter an irregularity while the endoscope is in use, and cannot be resolved with the troubleshooting guide above, you may need to withdraw the endoscope. However, please ensure the following precautions have been taken to avoid any injury to the patient during withdrawal:

- Remove or retract any accessory back into the working channel.
- Disconnect accessories from any electrosurgical units.
- Release the UP/DOWN and RIGHT/LEFT angulation locks by turning towards "F" position.
- If applicable, lower the elevator by turning in the opposite direction of "U".
- Gently suction any air, blood or mucus.
- Carefully withdraw the endoscope while observing the image on the monitor OR under fluoroscopy guidance if necessary.
- Do not withdraw the endoscope forcibly if you encounter any resistance.

21.6 Conclusion

The role of endoscopy during laparoscopic surgery continues to expand and will remain an essential tool in the armamentarium of an endo-laparoscopic surgeon. It is vital for surgeons and surgical trainees to be accustomed with the available tools, specifications and function, cleaning and maintenance as well as troubleshooting tips in order to gain maximal benefit during any endoscopic intervention.

References

1. Boese A, Wex C, Croner R, et al. Endoscopic imaging technology today. Diagnostics. 2022;12(5):1262. https://doi.org/10.3390/diagnostics12051262.
2. Rey JW, Kiesslich R, Hoffman A. New aspects of modern endoscopy. World J Gastrointest Endosc. 2014;6(8):334–44. https://doi.org/10.4253/wjge.v6.i8.334.
3. Operation Manual: Evis Extra III Colonovideoscope Olympus CF-HQ190L/I. Olympus Medical Systems Corporation; Japan, 2012.
4. Operation Manual: Evis Extra III Gastrointestinal Videoscope Olympus GIF-HQ190. Olympus Medical Systems Corporation; Japan, 2012.
5. Operation Manual: Evis Extra II Duodenovideoscope Olympus TJF Type Q180V. Olympus Medical Systems Corporation; Japan, 2015.
6. Operation Manual: Choledocho Videoscope Olympus CHF-Type V. Olympus Medical Systems Corporation; Japan, 2008.
7. Souma Y, Nakajima K, Takahashi T, et al. The role of intraoperative carbon dioxide insufflating upper gastrointestinal endoscopy during laparoscopic surgery. Surg Endosc. 2009;23(10):2279–85. https://doi.org/10.1007/s00464-008-0309-y.
8. Tokar JL, Barth BA, Banerjee S, et al. Electrosurgical generators. Gastrointest Endosc. 2013;78(2):197–208. https://doi.org/10.1016/j.gie.2013.04.164.
9. Bac NH, Hai PM, Tuan LQA. Laparoscopic choledochotomy for bile duct stones. In: Mastering endo-laparoscopic and thoracoscopic surgery. Singapore: Springer Nature; 2023. p. 315–8. https://doi.org/10.1007/978-981-19-3755-2_45.
10. Day LW, Muthusamy VR, Collins J, et al. Multisociety guideline on reprocessing flexible GI endoscopes and accessories. Gastrointest Endosc. 2021;93(1):11–33.e6. https://doi.org/10.1016/j.gie.2020.09.048.

22 Surgical Videos: Recording and Editing

Ramakrishnan Parthasarathi, Ramasamy Venkatachalam, and Shankar Balasubramanian

Video documentation of surgical videos serves a multifaceted role in the healthcare industry, benefiting medical education, patient care, research, and quality improvement. They help disseminate knowledge, improve surgical techniques, and ultimately contribute to better patient outcomes and safety. It is a good learning tool for the surgeon in their laparoscopic surgical career. The surgeon can periodically review the surgeries performed by him, again and again, till he attains perfection. Surgical videos can be used to create case studies and contribute to medical publications and conference presentations. Besides, surgical videos can serve as legal and ethical documentation. They provide a clear record of surgical procedures, ensuring transparency and accountability in the event of disputes or complications. The importance of video documentation is further highlighted by the Indian Medical Association's recommendation of taking video consent, especially for cancer surgeries and other major procedures.

22.1 Anatomy of a Surgical Video

An ideal surgical video should be very clear and of high resolution. The length of the video should be kept to a minimum while incorporating all the key surgical steps. Audio narration is essential to make it easier for the viewer to understand. The file size, quality and format should be appropriate for online uploading and viewing.

A properly edited surgical video should have the following components as shown in Table 22.1. The video should begin with the title and a brief introduction about the procedure which includes the indication for the surgery along with the details of

R. Parthasarathi (✉) · R. Venkatachalam · S. Balasubramanian
Department of Esophagogastric Surgery, GEM Hospital & Research Center, Coimbatore, Tamil Nadu, India
e-mail: drparthu@geminstitute.in

J. S. Ahluwalia (ed.), *User Manual for Minimally Invasive Surgical Equipment*,
https://doi.org/10.1007/978-981-95-9019-3_22

Table 22.1 Anatomy of a surgical video

Surgical video: Anatomy
Title and indication of the procedure
Relevant investigation (e.g. CECT chest and abdomen video/ endoscopy video)
Team setup and ports
Steps of the procedure
Voice narration
Specimen/HPE images
Post-operative period details
Conclusion

the relevant investigations like CT, MRI, or endoscopy. The video should have a voice narration with clear audio. Next, an explanation about the operating team setup and ports position should be given. The surgery part should be divided into multiple steps highlighting the importance of each step. For instance, while recording a cholecystectomy procedure, after achieving critical view of safety, it is a good practice to clean the dissected area and give a panoramic as well as close-up view of the hepatocystic triangle area emphasizing the importance of proper dissection to avoid bile duct injuries. At the end of the surgical procedure, a photograph of the surgical specimen captured in the correct anatomical orientation with a ruler by the side depicting the dimensions should be shown. The histopathology images are shown next before giving details of the post-operative period. Finally, the video should end with a conclusion.

Nowadays, it is very essential that the laparoscopic surgeon has a good knowledge about video documentation and editing. A properly edited high-quality video that contains the entire procedure along with the external view is almost equivalent to witnessing live laparoscopic surgeries in the operating room.

22.2 Laparoscopic Equipments

Laparoscopic surgery necessitates the use of specialized equipment, and the quality of the surgical video is significantly influenced by the performance of the telescope, camera systems, and light source. Therefore, laparoscopic surgeons must possess a fundamental understanding of the functionalities of these equipment components.

22.2.1 Camera Head

The clarity of the recorded videos is directly proportional to the resolution of the cameras. Single-chip cameras usually have a resolution of around 400 lines, the clarity of the video output being measured in terms of the number of horizontal lines. Three chip cameras have a higher resolution of 720–850, while the new generation high-definition cameras have a higher resolution of 1920x1080 pixels, 50 or 60 frames. The output from the laparoscopic camera can either be in digital format or analog format. The days of analog are gone and all the presently available camera systems have digital outputs. Some of the newer generation laparoscopic digital cameras even have the option of ethernet output for direct connection to computer networks.

22.2.2 Full HD

Full HD cameras have a resolution of 1920 × 1080 pixels or dots, 1920 horizontal and 1080 vertical resolution. These cameras' display is 60/30 frames or 50/25 frames depending on the video standards of the country.

1080i Interlaced scan: Displays frame twice, in a way—the first pass is 1920 × 540 for the even scan line field and the second pass is 1920 × 540 for the odd scan line field. The process by which this occurs is called interlacing. It contributes to a sense of motion and reduces perceived flicker.

1080p Progressive scan: In this format, 1920 × 1080-pixel high-definition movies are progressively drawn line after line, so they're not interlaced. All the lines of the image are visible at the same time. Images appear sharper and more defined than 1080i, particularly during scenes with a lot of fast motion.

Karl Storz, Image one HD, Stryker, Spice, Olympus S190, and S200 cameras are some of the full HD systems commercially available presently.

22.2.3 4 K and UHD

4 K camera head has 4096 x 2160 pixels resolution. 4 KUHD (ultra-HD) has 3840 x 2160 pixels resolution. Recently, 8 K UHD imaging technology with 7680 x 4320 pixels resolution has been introduced which offers 16-fold higher resolution compared to HD cameras.

22.2.4 3D Camera

Nowadays, full HD 3D camera systems with 3D monitors are used for depth perception. It has three formats—side by side, line by line, and top/bottom. The glasses being used are passive polarized glasses. Three-dimensional vision during laparoscopic surgery is found to be ergonomically superior compared to the conventional 2D cameras. Surgeons accustomed to 3D cameras find it easier when switching over to robotic surgery which has 3D vision as a standard.

22.2.5 Laparoscope

The laparoscope or the lens can be rightly called as the eye of the laparoscopic surgeon as it is through which the surgeon sees the internal organs. The rod Hopkins lens system offers better clarity when compared to the older generation laparoscopes. 0° laparoscopes give higher clarity than the 30° laparoscopes. 10 mm laparoscopes have better views and are ideal for recording purposes. Even though 5 mm and 3 mm scopes offer decent clarity during surgery, these are not usually as good as 10 mm scopes.

22.2.6 Light Sources and Cable

Though various light sources are available, Xenon 300 light sources are ideally suited for recording purposes as these provide a uniform distribution of light that is very similar to the sunlight. LED light sources are almost equally good. Light cables are optical cables that form an important part of video documentation. Even if the surgeon is using the best laparoscopic camera system, the quality of the video will not be good if low-quality light cables are used. The fluid-filled cables are capable of transmitting the maximum amount of light without any loss. But these cables are rigid and difficult to manipulate during the surgery. This difficulty is more appreciated when 30° scopes are used. Though flexible cables transmit little lesser amount of light than the fluid-filled cables, these are ideal for routine use. These cables are more affordable and easier to handle. Adequacy of light can be checked by focusing the laparoscope towards the right hypochondrium. If the light is adequate, the surface of the liver and the diaphragm are seen with uniform illumination; otherwise, the diaphragm will not be seen properly.

22.3 Video Signal Interfaces

There are various types of video input/output interfaces that are used to transfer the video from video source to other destinations, for example, from laparoscopic camera to displays, the recorder, or computer. Each of these interfaces has its own advantages and disadvantages. These can be broadly classified as those carrying analog video signals or digital video signals.

22.3.1 Digital Video Interfaces

Some of the earlier digital cameras had digital video inputs like DV, digital video, output through the interfaces called as Firewire, 1394, iEEE that connect directly to computers for recording. Nowadays, newer interfaces like Digital Video Interface (DVI), Serial Digital Interface (SDI), and High-Definition Multimedia Interface

(HDMI) are commonly seen to handle Full HD and 4 K. Among all these interfaces, SDI offers better handling.

22.3.1.1 Digital Video Interface (DVI)

This handles an uncompressed high-bandwidth digital video signal. This signal can be used for real-time display during live surgery due to its uncompressed nature. DVI-compatible flat monitors are now available in the market. These signals offer the same clarity as that of the RGB (Red-Green-Blue) in digitized format. It is also possible to record the DVI videos on computers using capture converters.

22.3.1.2 Serial Digital Interface (SDI)

This interface handles an uncompressed high-quality digital format like DVI. This can also be used for real-time display monitors. SDI can handle broadcast quality videos and can carry signal, unlike others, to long distances of about 100 meters.

22.3.1.3 HDMI Interface

High-Definition Multimedia Interface (HDMI) is the most common interface to handle Full HD and 4 K videos for use in displays and has a maximum signal carrying distance of up to 20 meters.

22.4 Video Recording and Editing

Video recording involves capturing video signals from the laparoscopic camera system output to the computer hard drive. This requires a device, called a capture card, in between the video source and the computer. These capture cards can be internal to the PC or external to the PC or laptop. The external capture cards are usually connected to PC/Laptop through USB. Stand-alone video recorders are also available.

Video editing of digital video requires video editing software like: iMovie, Adobe Rush, etc., for basic editing and Adobe Premiere, FinalCut Pro, etc., for professional editing. Digital video editing can appear complex and time-consuming to a surgeon, especially in the beginning. It needs a higher degree of patience and dedication to properly edit a surgery. It approximately takes more than 3 times the duration of the surgery for producing a high-quality short video of an advanced procedure. For example, producing a 10-minute video of a 2-hour-long surgery like a gastrectomy requires approximately 6 hours of dedicated editing in front of the computer. Even this is possible only if the operating surgeon himself edits the procedure. If the surgeon seeks professional help, then this duration will extend more as the audio-video professionals are not well versed with the surgical procedures and surgeons are not well versed in the editing lingo. Most of the time is spent in explaining the procedures to these professionals. If the surgeon learns the technique of editing, the quality of the edited video would be to the satisfaction of the audience, besides a reduction in editing time. This editing time will decrease as the surgeon becomes more comfortable with the software.

22.4.1 Advantages

When compared to basic analog recording and editing, there is practically no loss of clarity in digital video recording and editing. The quality of the video remains the same irrespective of the number of edits a particular video passes through.

Addition of titles, graphics, photos, illustrations, and ‘Picture in Picture’ has become easier with digital editing as compared to older times of VCR recordings. The final digitally edited version of the video can be copied in any of the available devices like SSD, HDD, CD, DVD, USB drives, etc., and/or uploaded directly to the website of the publisher or conference.

22.5 Recording Devices

The videos can be recorded either in the digital format or in analog format. The common recording devices for analog signals are the video cassette recorders but they are obsolete now. Numerous devices are available for recording digital video signals.

22.5.1 In-Built Recording in Camera System

Many laparoscopic camera manufacturers now provide a USB port for direct recording into USB drive or external hard disk drive. Usually, camera head or a keyboard provides access to functions for managing such recordings. User manual of such camera system can be referred to understand such recording process.

22.5.2 External Video Capturing Devices

Various self-contained devices are available from many brands like Blackmagic Design, AJA, MATROX, ATOMOS, etc., that record videos directly onto a flash card or hard disk drive without the need of a computer. The surgeries are recorded by connecting the camera through HDMI or SDI connectors to external capturing device for capture at a resolution of 1080i or 1080p or 4 K in 30 to 60 frames per second. Some devices have an inbuilt screen, where we can see the video being recorded and it is also helpful in changing various settings (Fig. 22.1).

There are also other external devices that connect to USB A or USB C port available in Windows or Macbook. These convert video signal output in HDMI or SDI to USB format for capture by computers. These can connect HDMI or SDI video source cable on one side and USB A or USB C port on the other.

When choosing a video capturing device, consider factors like the types of sources you need to capture, the quality of the video and audio you require, compatibility with your computer, and any additional features like pass-through, live streaming capabilities, or bundled software. Additionally, consider your budget, as

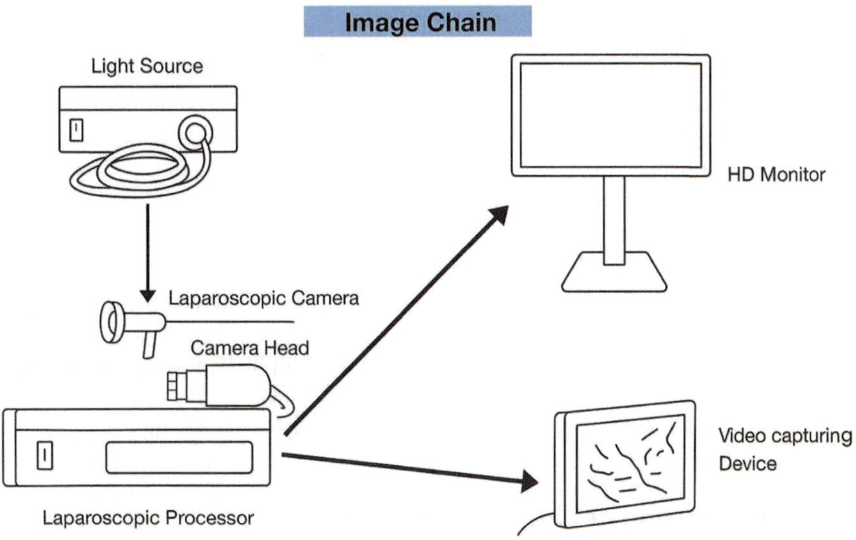

Fig. 22.1 External video capturing device connected to laparoscopic camera for video recording

video capture devices vary widely in price, from affordable consumer options to high-end professional solutions.

22.5.3 4 K/UHD, 3D Video Capturing

Blackmagic Video Assist 4 K, ATOMOS Shogun Inferno, etc., can capture videos in 4 K/UHD resolution and 3D videos in side-by-side pattern.

Apple users can record the videos in *ProRes* format in HD resolution with data rate of 70 to 100 Mbit/second. The file format is QuickTime.mov. Windows users can record videos in uncompressed AVI format, though file size might be huge.

22.5.4 Connecting a Recorder with a Laparoscopic Camera

To ensure seamless recording, follow these steps to connect an external recorder to a laparoscopic camera system:

1. *Identify Output Ports*: Check the laparoscopic camera system for available output options such as HDMI, SDI, DVI, or USB.
2. *Select the Right Cable*: Use an appropriate cable based on the output type:
   - HDMI cable for high-definition output.
   - SDI cable for professional-grade signal transmission with minimal latency.
   - DVI-to-HDMI adapter if only DVI output is available.

3. *Connect to the Recorder*:
   - Plug one end of the cable into the laparoscopic camera system's output port.
   - Connect the other end to the input port of the external medical-grade recorder.
4. *Set Recording Parameters*:
   - Configure the recorder to match the resolution and frame rate of the laparoscopic camera.
   - Adjust brightness and contrast settings if needed.
5. *Test the Connection*:
   - Preview the live feed on the recorder's display or a connected monitor.
   - Ensure smooth video transmission without lag or artifacts.
6. *Start Recording*:
   - Begin recording and periodically check the output to ensure quality and stability.
   - Use external storage options if the recorder has limited capacity.

22.6 Production of Videos After Editing

The finished edited videos can be produced in any of the following formats for presentation and storage.

1	4 K/UHD quality	Highest
2.	Full-HD quality	Intermediate
3.	HD/SD for Web	Lowest

22.6.1 Pitfalls in Post-production

Proper understanding of the video quality formats is essential in producing high-quality videos. One must be aware of the highest resolution in which the camera is able to transmit video signals and should try to capture in the same resolution to avoid any quality loss. Project should match such settings when editing, and video should be exported in a similar resolution. Exporting in lower resolution to save space will decrease the quality of final video and exporting in higher resolution will just increase the size of video without increasing quality.

22.7 Tips to Produce High-Quality Digital Video

The signal from the laparoscope has to pass through various stages to ultimately reach the monitor and the recording device. All the components in these stages should work in perfect condition and coherence to obtain a clear video signal.

22.7.1 Lens Fogging

We often find that the laparoscope gets fogged as soon as it is introduced into the abdominal cavity. This is due to the sudden change in the temperature at the tip of the laparoscope, from cold atmosphere into the warm and moist abdominal cavity. This often results in reduction of video clarity. This happens more frequently if the CO_2 insufflation is connected to the camera port. The continuous insufflation of cold CO_2 by the side of the laparoscope further increases the fogging of the lens. Hence, it is always better to connect the insufflation tubes to any of the ports other than that of the camera port. Use of warm saline (to heat up the lens) and heated gas can mitigate this problem.

22.7.2 Smudging of Lens

It is a habit of all the camera surgeons to clean the tip of the lens by gently rubbing the scope over organs such as the liver and the small bowel. Even though it is quick and effective at times, it is better avoided. A thin film of tissue fluid sticks on to the surface of the lens. This fluid subsequently dries up resulting in image deterioration.

It is always a better practice to clean the tip of the lens with warm saline kept at near body temperature by keeping it in a flask. The laparoscope should be carefully withdrawn from the port and the tip cleaned with a clean, white gauze piece dipped in warm saline. Before introducing the cleaned scope into the cannula, the port seal should be wiped of any blood-stained fluid. If the inside of the trocar is stained with blood, it should be cleaned with the help of a gauze piece before introducing the laparoscope.

22.7.3 Fumes from Haemostatic Devices

The field of vision may become hazy with the use of haemostatic devices like electrosurgery and ultrasonic shears. Intermittent use of such devices and intermittent letting out of the fumes during surgery can help in evacuation of the fumes. One may leave one of the 5 mm ports in a partially opened position to evacuate fumes. Use of coagulation mode may emit lesser fumes as compared to cutting mode.

22.7.4 Camera Head

At times the clarity of the picture remains the same even after cleaning the tip of the scope properly. This is usually the case when the lens in the camera head is not clean. It should be cleaned with a dry gauze before it is connected to the laparoscope.

22.7.5 Role of Camera Surgeon

The camera surgeon plays a vital role in the production of a good quality video. An experienced camera assistant is a valuable asset, especially when 30° scopes are used. It is better to use the services of an experienced camera surgeon or a staff nurse during the surgeries where we wish to record for a special purpose.

A panoramic view of the abdominal cavity should be shown in the initial phase, and an intermediate view should be shown for dissection purposes. A close-up view is ideal for inspection and division of tissues and endo suturing. The tip of the working instruments should always be in the centre of the monitor irrespective of close-up or panoramic view. A good camera surgeon can make difficult tasks easier, and an average camera surgeon can make easier things more difficult.

22.7.6 Recording and Editing Setup

Video editing can be performed effectively on both Windows and Mac systems, but there are some key differences in hardware specifications and software ecosystems between the two platforms as shown in Table 22.2.

Remember that the specific requirements may vary depending on your video editing software and the complexity of your projects. Always research the recommended system requirements for your chosen software and tailor your system accordingly.

Table 22.2 Recommended hardware and software specifications for video editing using macOS and Windows

Feature	macOS	Windows
Operating system	macOS Ventura or later	Windows 11
Processor (CPU)	Apple silicon M1 or better	Intel Core i5 or better
		AMD Ryzen 5 or better (for AMD-based PCs)
Graphics processing unit (GPU)	Integrated or dedicated GPU (varies by model)	Integrated or dedicated GPU (varies by model)
Memory (RAM)	16 GB or more	16 GB or more
Storage	SSD strongly recommended—minimum 500 GB size	SSD strongly recommended—minimum 500 GB size
Monitor	High-resolution display—Retina 24 inch or better	High-resolution display—4 K 24 inch or better
Video editing software	Adobe Premiere Pro, Final Cut Pro X, DaVinci Resolve	Adobe Premiere Pro, DaVinci Resolve, etc.
Input devices	Keyboard, mouse, graphics tablet	Keyboard, mouse, graphics tablet
Audio	Built-in speakers or external audio devices	Built-in speakers or external audio devices
External storage	USB, Thunderbolt, or network-attached storage	USB, Thunderbolt, or network-attached storage

22.7.7 Video Backup

External hard drives are commonly used as they are the cheapest solutions available for a large amount of storage. One should use them in pairs by making two identical drives for the sake of redundancy. Network-attached storage (NAS) is a great option for adding automatic redundancy to your backup. One can set NAS system to create perfect copies of hard drives on its own. Any crash of a hard disk can be detected by the system and can be replaced by the user without fear of data loss. SSDs can also be used independently or part of NAS setup. They are faster but more expensive and are better reserved for data transfer. Cloud storage is more secure but again more expensive and slower to operate when we are dealing with a huge amount of data in surgical videos.

22.7.8 Video Editing Software

Surgeons who want to edit surgical videos for educational purposes, presentations, or documentation can use various video editing software. The ideal software should offer precision editing, stabilization, annotation tools, and support for high-resolution videos. Here are some of the most popular video editing software options for surgeons:

1. *Adobe Premiere Pro*

Best for: Professional surgical video editing with advanced features.

- Offers timeline-based editing for precise cuts.
- Supports high-resolution 4 K/8 K videos, useful for detailed surgical recordings.
- Features stabilization tools to reduce camera shake.
- Allows annotations and text overlays for educational purposes.

2. *Final Cut Pro*

Best for: Mac users who need high-performance editing.

- Optimized for Apple devices with smooth playback and rendering.
- Magnetic timeline for efficient editing.
- Supports advanced colour grading for enhanced surgical visuals.
- Multicam editing for combining footage from different angles.

3. *DaVinci Resolve*

Best for: High-quality colour correction and free editing tools.

- Advanced colour grading enhances surgical videos for better visibility.
- Free version includes powerful editing features.
- AI-powered stabilization for handheld surgical recordings.
- Supports 4 K/8 K editing with professional effects.

4. *Camtasia*

Best for: Simple editing with screen recording for educational videos.

- Easy-to-use interface with drag-and-drop editing.
- Built-in screen recorder to capture live surgeries or demonstrations.

- Offers annotations, callouts, and voiceover options for educational purposes.

5. *iMovie*

Best for: Beginners using macOS for quick edits.
   - Simple and intuitive interface.
   - Basic transitions, titles, and audio enhancements.
   - Free for Mac users.
   - Good for quick edits but lacks advanced features.

6. *Filmora*

Best for: Budget-friendly editing with essential tools.
   - User-friendly interface with drag-and-drop functionality.
   - Supports 4 K editing and basic stabilization.
   - Good for quick video cuts and simple annotations.

7. *OpenShot (Free & Open-Source)*

Best for: Surgeons looking for free, basic editing tools.
   - Cross-platform (Windows, macOS, Linux).
   - Simple timeline-based editing.
   - Basic transitions, effects, and text overlays.

8. *VEGAS Pro*

Best for: Advanced video editing with AI-powered tools.
   - AI-assisted editing features for smooth cuts.
   - Motion tracking and stabilization.
   - 4 K video support for high-quality surgical visuals

22.7.9 Choosing the Right Software

- *For professional use*: Adobe Premiere Pro, DaVinci Resolve or Final Cut Pro.
- *For quick and simple edits*: iMovie or Camtasia.
- *For free editing*: OpenShot or DaVinci Resolve (free version).
- *For Windows users*: VEGAS Pro or Filmora.

Surgeons can choose software based on their expertise level, budget, and editing needs. Some offer free versions or trial periods, so you can explore and find the one that best suits your requirements. Keep in mind that the video editing software landscape is continuously evolving, with new features and improvements being added regularly.

22.7.10 Tips for Surgical Video Editing

Editing surgical videos requires precision and efficiency to convey critical information accurately. Here are some tips to help you edit surgical videos more quickly and effectively:

- *Organize Your Footage*:
  Properly label and organize your video clips and assets to quickly locate the footage you need. Pre-operative (investigation, patient pictures and reports, external pictures), videos during the surgery (e.g. ports, team setup, endoscopy, C-arm, ERCP, etc.) and post-operative pictures and videos (patient pictures and videos showing results, pathology slides and report) should be kept in a sequence.
- *Create a Clear Workflow*:
  Develop a step-by-step editing workflow to streamline the process. This might include importing footage, sorting clips, trimming, adding effects, and exporting.
- *Use Keyboard Shortcuts*:
  Learn and use keyboard shortcuts in your video editing software to perform common tasks quickly. This can significantly speed up your editing process.
- *Real-Time Playback*:
  Invest in a computer with sufficient processing power and a dedicated GPU to ensure real-time playback of your footage, reducing the need for constant rendering.
- *Auto Colour Correction*:
  Utilize auto colour correction tools to quickly correct white balance and exposure in your clips.
- *Keyboard Editing*:
  Use your keyboard for precise editing. Learn to navigate the timeline, cut, trim, and move clips using keyboard commands.
- *Audio Editing Shortcuts*:
  Use audio editing shortcuts to adjust levels, apply filters, and remove background noise efficiently.
- *Keep It Simple*:
  Avoid overcomplicating your edits with unnecessary effects or transitions. Keep the focus on the surgical content.
- *Regularly Save Your Work*:
  Save your work frequently to prevent loss of progress due to software crashes or technical issues.
- *Learn the Software*:
  Invest time in learning the ins and outs of your chosen editing software. The better you know the tool, the faster you can work.
- *Collaborate*:
  If possible, collaborate with others who specialize in video editing. They can offer fresh perspectives and help expedite the process.
- *Hardware Acceleration*:
  Ensure your computer hardware supports hardware acceleration in your editing software for smoother playback and rendering.
- *Render and Export Efficiently*:
  Optimize your export settings to balance video quality with file size. Use presets for common export formats.
- *Power Supply*:
  Ensure your system is connected to a stable power source during critical editing tasks to prevent unexpected shutdowns.

22.7.11 Data Privacy and Compliance

- *Anonymize Patient Data*: Remove any identifying details.
- *Follow Hospital and Legal Guidelines*: Adhere to HIPAA, GDPR, and medical ethics.
- *Use Encrypted Storage*: Ensure secure storage on medical-grade cloud platforms or encrypted drives.

22.7.12 Work Flow

Editing laparoscopic videos should focus on clarity, educational value, and conciseness.

General Recommendations:

Step 1: Importing and Organizing Footage
- Transfer files from the recording device to a computer.
- Sort videos based on date, procedure type, and relevance.
- Create backups before making edits.

Step 2: Trimming and Cutting
- Remove Unnecessary Footage: Cut out redundant sections to keep the video concise.
- Highlight Key Moments: Focus on crucial steps of the procedure
- Maintain Flow: Ensure smooth transitions between clips.

Step 3: Enhancing Video Quality
- Stabilization: Reduce camera shake using built-in software tools.
- Brightness and Contrast Adjustments: Improve visibility of anatomical structures.
- Colour Correction: Enhance colour balance for accurate representation of tissues.

Step 4: Annotation and Text Overlays
- Add Labels and Captions: Identify anatomical landmarks, instruments, and surgical steps.
- Use Callouts and Arrows: Direct viewer attention to key areas.
- Include Voice Narration: Explain procedures for educational purposes.

Step 5: Speed Adjustments
- Slow Motion: Emphasize intricate techniques.
- Fast Forward: Skip repetitive or lengthy parts while keeping the video informative.

Step 6: Adding Transitions and Effects

- Use simple transitions (fade-in, fade-out) to maintain a professional look.
- Avoid excessive effects that may distract from the surgical content.

Step 7: Exporting the Video

- Choose the right format (MP4, MOV) with high-quality settings.
- Use appropriate resolution (1080p or 4 K) for clarity.
- Compress files if necessary while maintaining quality.

22.8 Conclusion

Recording and editing laparoscopic surgery videos require proper planning, high-quality equipment, and meticulous editing techniques. Well-edited surgical videos enhance education, improve surgical training, and contribute to medical research. By following best practices, surgeons and medical professionals can create impactful videos that aid in skill development and knowledge sharing.

Selected Reading

1. Berci G, Schwaitzberg SD. The importance of understanding the basics of imaging in the era of high-tech endoscopy: part I. Logic, reality, and utopia. Surg Endosc. 2002;4:377–80.
2. Berci G, Schwaitzberg SD. The importance of understanding the basics of imaging in the era of high-tech endoscopy: part II. Logic, reality, and utopia. Surg Endosc. 2002;16:1518–22.
3. Schwaitzberg SD. Chapter 13: Imaging systems in minimally invasive surgery. Mastery of endoscopic and laparoscopic surgery. 2nd ed. USA: Lippincott Williams and Wilkins; 2005. p. 118–29.
4. SAGES Video protection guidelines. Society of American Gastrointestinal Endoscopic Surgeons (SAGES) Toolbox; 2004
5. Parthasarathi R, Gomes RM, Palanivelu PR, Senthilnathan P, Rajapandian S, Venkatachalam R, Palanivelu C. First virtual live conference in healthcare. J Laparoendosc Adv Surg Tech A. 2017;27(7):722–5.
6. Busshoff J, Datta RR, Bruns T, Kleinert R, Morgenstern B, Pfister D, Chiapponi C, Fuchs HF, Thomas M, Gietzelt C, Hedergott A, Möller D, Hellmich M, Bruns CJ, Stippel DL, Wahba R. Gender benefit in laparoscopic surgical performance using a 3D-display system: data from a randomized cross-over trial. Surg Endosc. 2022;36(6):4376–85.
7. Özsoy M, Kallidonis P, Kyriazis I, Panagopoulos V, Vasilas M, Sakellaropoulos GC, Liatsikos E. Novice surgeons: do they benefit from 3D laparoscopy? Lasers Med Sci. 2015;30(4):1325–33.
8. Wilhelm D, Reiser S, Kohn N, Witte M, Leiner U, Mühlbach L, Ruschin D, Reiner W, Feussner H. Comparative evaluation of HD 2D/3D laparoscopic monitors and benchmarking to a theoretically ideal 3D pseudodisplay: even well-experienced laparoscopists perform better with 3D. Surg Endosc. 2014;28(8):2387–97.

Laser

23

Kalyan Kar

23.1 Introduction

Minimal Access Surgery (MAS) has revolutionized modern medicine by enabling precise, less invasive procedures with reduced patient trauma, accelerated recovery times, and minimal scarring. Among the key technologies driving this advancement is the utilization of lasers. LASER (Light Amplification by Stimulated Emission of Radiation) emits focused light energy to target tissues with exceptional accuracy. In surgical applications, various types of medical lasers are utilized based on their wavelength and interaction with biological tissues. This chapter delves into the role of lasers in MAS, elucidating their types, applications, and details about their machine and fibres. Furthermore, we will address the maintenance, troubleshooting, and future developments of medical laser systems.

23.2 What Is a Laser?

A laser is a device that emits a highly focused beam of light with a specific wavelength. This coherent light can be precisely controlled to cut, coagulate, or vaporize tissue, making it ideal for surgical applications. Lasers are classified based on their active medium (which can be gas, solid-state, or semiconductor), wavelength, and other characteristics. Each type of laser possesses unique properties that render it suitable for specific medical procedures.

K. Kar (✉)
KKM Lap Laser Surgical Center, Kolkata, West Bengal, India

J. S. Ahluwalia (ed.), *User Manual for Minimally Invasive Surgical Equipment*,
https://doi.org/10.1007/978-981-95-9019-3_23

23.3 Types of Medical Lasers in Surgery

Medical lasers can be categorized based on their wavelength and energy output, enabling their utilization in various surgical specialties.

23.3.1 Commonly Used Medical Lasers

Type of laser	Wavelength (nm)	Applications
Diode laser	980, 1470	Proctology, varicose veins, gynaecology
CO_2 laser	10,600	Dermatology, ENT, gynaecology
Holmium:YAG	2100	Urology, orthopaedic surgery
Nd:YAG	1064	Ophthalmology, oncology
Erbium:YAG	2940	Dermatology, dentistry

23.4 Description of Laser Machine

A laser machine utilized in surgical applications comprises several fundamental components meticulously engineered for precision, safety, and user-friendliness. Constructed with a robust structural framework, it incorporates an intuitive user interface and sophisticated control mechanisms to enhance surgical outcomes.

Given the diverse designs of laser machines manufactured by various companies, this document offers a comprehensive overview of the machine's operational functionality.

23.4.1 Front Panel Controls

The front panel of the laser machine typically includes:

Power Button: Used to turn the machine on and off.

Emergency Stop Button: A safety feature to immediately halt laser operation in case of an emergency.

Key Switch: Prevents unauthorized access and ensures controlled operation.

Fibre Connector Port: Where the laser fibre is attached securely to transmit laser energy.

Touchscreen Interface: The primary control hub, providing an intuitive user experience.

23.4.2 Back Panel Controls

The back side of the laser machine typically houses:

Power Input Port: Where the machine is connected to the power supply.

Foot Pedal Connector: An input for the foot pedal, which allows hands-free operation of the laser.

USB & Data Ports: For software updates, data logging, and procedural records.

23.4.3 Touchscreen Interface and Controls

The touchscreen interface provides complete control over the laser machine's settings, including:

1. *Power Adjustment*: Allows the surgeon to select the appropriate wattage based on the procedure.
2. *Mode Selection*: Offers Continuous Wave (CW) and Pulsed Mode settings for tissue interaction control.
3. *Timer Settings*: Enables precise duration control for energy delivery.
4. *Pre-Set Programs*: Customizable settings for different surgical applications such as proctology, varicose veins, urology, etc.
5. *Activation Status Indicator*: Displays whether the laser is in standby or active mode.
6. *Fibre Calibration Option*: Ensures that the laser fibre is properly aligned and calibrated before use.
7. *Safety Notifications*: Displays alerts for overheating, fibre misalignment, or system errors.
8. *System Settings*: For software upgrade, system information, etc.

23.5 Mechanism of Action of Laser in Different Surgical Applications

The mechanism of action varies based on tissue composition, water content, and absorption properties.

23.5.1 Mechanism of Action in Proctology

1. *Selective Absorption*: Different tissues absorb laser energy based on their water and haemoglobin content. The 1470 nm laser is absorbed more by water, ensuring controlled tissue interaction, while the 980 nm laser is absorbed by both water and haemoglobin, providing deeper penetration.
2. *Photo-thermal Effect*: The laser beam generates heat upon absorption, leading to controlled coagulation and vaporization of targeted tissues and minimising bleeding.
3. *Minimally Invasive Approach*: The laser fibre can be inserted into the fistula tract or hemorrhoidal tissue, delivering precise energy to shrink and obliterate abnormal tissue while preserving surrounding structures.
4. *Reduced Postoperative Pain*: Laser procedures cause minimal collateral thermal damage, preserving nerve endings and resulting in enhanced patient comfort and accelerated recovery.

23.5.2 Mechanism of Action in Varicose Veins Treatment

1. *Endovenous Laser Ablation (EVLA)*: Laser energy is delivered inside the vein, causing thermal injury to the vein wall, leading to fibrosis and eventual closure of the vein.
2. *Wavelength Selection*: The 1470 nm laser is preferred due to its high-water absorption, allowing precise vein wall collapse without excessive heat diffusion.
3. *Minimized Side Effects*: Less post-operative pain and bruising compared to traditional vein-stripping procedures.

23.5.3 Mechanism of Action in Urology

1. *Lithotripsy*: High-energy laser pulses break down stones into small fragments that can pass through the urinary tract.
2. *Tissue Ablation*: Used in treating urethral strictures and bladder tumours by precisely removing abnormal tissue.
3. *Haemostasis*: Provides good coagulation, minimizing bleeding in delicate urinary structures.

23.6 Comparison of Different Lasers in Surgical Applications

23.6.1 Comparison of Lasers Used in Proctology

Feature	980 nm Laser	1470 nm Laser
Absorption	Moderate absorption in water and haemoglobin	Higher absorption in water
Depth of penetration	Deeper penetration	Superficial penetration
Thermal spread	Higher thermal spread	Lower thermal spread
Coagulation effect	Effective but deeper	Precise and controlled

23.6.2 Comparison of Lasers Used in Varicose Veins Treatment

Feature	980 nm Laser	1470 nm Laser
Vein wall closure	Moderate	Superior
Post-op pain	Slightly higher	Lower
Efficiency	Effective	More efficient

23.6.3 Comparison of Lasers Used in Urology

Feature	Holmium:YAG (2100 nm)	Nd:YAG (1064 nm)
Application	Stone fragmentation, strictures	Tumour ablation, coagulation
Tissue penetration	Shallow	Deep
Bleeding control	Moderate	High

23.7 Wattage Used in Different Surgical Specialties

Specialty	Typical wattage range
Proctology	8 W–15 W
Varicose veins	6 W–12 W
Urology	40 W–100 W

23.8 Mode Selection: Continuous Wave Versus Pulsed Mode

Continuous Wave Provides a continuous laser beam until the user ceases signal transmission by deactivating the activation switch. Suitable for situations requiring a continuous supply of energy, such as fissure in ano surgery.

Pulsed Mode Emits energy in pulses of time determined by the user, rather than a continuous beam. Suitable for delivering a fixed quantity of energy over a large area, while fibre positioning may need to be continuously adjusted. This approach prevents the delivery of excessive energy to a single area, such as fistula in ano, haemorrhoids, and varicose veins surgeries.

23.9 Fibre Optic Laser Fibres

Laser fibres are a fundamental component of laser proctology, serving as the conduits for transmitting laser energy to the target tissue while minimizing collateral damage. The selection of fibre types is contingent upon the specific surgical procedure being undertaken.

Fibre type	Description	Application
Radial fibre	Emits energy in a 360-degree pattern	Varicose vein treatment and fistula procedures
Bare fibre	Emits energy directly from the fibre tip	Fissure in ano and lithotripsy
Conical fibre	Its sharp tip helps in penetration of tissue	Haemorrhoids
Side-firing fibre	Emits energy at an angle	Prostate treatments

23.10 Foot Pedal Safety Mechanism

The foot pedal includes a safety interlock to prevent accidental activation.

Dual-action mechanism ensures intentional activation, reducing unintended laser emission.

23.11 Safety Precautions in Using Medical Lasers

When operating medical lasers, adherence to strict safety guidelines is essential to prevent accidents and ensure patient and operator protection.

1. *Personal Protective Equipment (PPE)*
   Always wear laser-specific safety goggles rated for the laser's wavelength.
   Ensure all staff members in the operating room use protective eyewear.
2. *Controlled Access*
   Restrict entry to the laser operating area to authorized personnel only.
   Display warning signs indicating laser usage to prevent accidental exposure.
3. *Patient Safety*
   Provide protective eyewear to the patient if necessary.
   Ensure proper tissue hydration to avoid burns from unintended energy absorption.
4. *Fire and Electrical Safety*
   Keep flammable materials away from the laser beam.

23.12 How to Calculate Energy Delivered by the LASER

$$E = P \times T$$

where

- E = Energy (Joules, J).
- P = Power of the laser (Watts, W).
- T = Time for which the laser operates (seconds, s).

Example Calculation:
Suppose a laser machine operates at 50 watts and is used for 10 seconds.

E = 50 times 10 = 500 J

So, the laser machine delivers 500 joules of energy in 10 seconds.

23.13 Maintenance

Maintaining laser machines and optical fibres utilized in surgical applications is paramount to ensure their optimal performance, safety, and longevity. Regular maintenance mitigates the likelihood of malfunctions, energy degradation, and adverse patient outcomes.

23.13.1 Laser Machines

A. Routine Inspection and Cleaning
   1. Exterior Cleaning
      Use a soft, lint-free cloth with a mild disinfectant to clean the laser unit's exterior.
      Avoid harsh chemicals that may damage the casing or touch screen.
   2. Cooling System Check
      If the laser has an internal cooling system (water- or air-cooled), ensure no leaks or blockages.
      Replace coolant (if applicable) as per the manufacturer's guidelines.
   3. Ventilation and Air Filters
      Dust accumulation can lead to overheating. Regularly check and clean air filters and exhaust vents.

B. Calibration and Energy Output Verification
   1. Power Output Testing
      Use an energy meter to ensure the laser emits the correct power levels.
      Any deviation from the standard should be addressed by a technician.
   2. Beam Alignment
      Misalignment can lead to inaccurate laser delivery. Perform regular alignment checks using alignment tools provided by the manufacturer.

C. Optical Components Maintenance
   1. Lens and Mirror Cleaning
      Use optical-grade lens wipes and ethanol-based solutions to clean lenses and mirrors.
      Avoid touching optical components with bare hands to prevent oil contamination.
   2. Fibre Connection Ports
      Inspect ports for dust, burns, or misalignment. Clean with compressed air if needed.

D. Software and Electrical System Maintenance.
   1. Software Updates
      Keep firmware/software updated to ensure bug fixes, security patches, and performance enhancements.
      Follow manufacturer guidelines for updates.

2. Electrical and Safety Checks
   Inspect cables, connectors, and foot pedals for any wear or damage.
   Test the emergency stop function and interlock systems regularly.

23.13.2 Laser Fibres

A. Handling and Storage
   1. Avoid Excessive Bending
      Laser fibres are delicate. Avoid tight coiling or kinking, which can damage the fibre core.
   2. Use Protective Caps
      When not in use, always keep the connector of fibre covered with a protective cap to prevent dust accumulation and inadvertent damage.
   3. Proper Storage Conditions
      Store in a dry, dust-free environment at room temperature.

B. Cleaning and Sterilization.
   1. Pre-Cleaning
      Use a lint-free cloth with isopropyl alcohol to wipe the fibre after each use.
      Avoid water immersion, as moisture can degrade optical performance.
   2. Sterilization Process
      Autoclaving: Many surgical laser fibres are autoclavable, but verify the manufacturer's instructions.
      Low temperature sterilization: Ethylene oxide (EtO) or plasma sterilization can be used.
   3. Check Fibre Integrity
      Inspect the fibre tip for burn marks, cracks, or discoloration before use.
      Perform a light transmission test (shining a low-power light through it) to check for breaks.
      Attach the fibre to the laser and verify that light exits evenly and at the expected power level.
      If damage is visible, discard or replace the fibre.

23.14 Troubleshooting

Problem	Possible cause	Solution	Preventive measures
Laser does not turn on	1. Power supply issue (unplugged or faulty cable) 2. Blown fuse or circuit breaker tripped 3. Faulty power switch or internal electrical issue	1. Check power connections and confirm proper voltage 2. Replace fuse/reset breaker 3. Contact technical support if internal failure suspected	1. Regularly inspect power connections 2. Keep a stock of spare fuses

(continued)

Problem	Possible cause	Solution	Preventive measures
Laser power is too low	1. Dirty or misaligned optical components 2. Aging or faulty laser diode 3. Fibre damage or contamination	1. Clean optics with appropriate materials 2. Replace laser diode if needed 3. Inspect fibre for bends or cracks	1. Regular cleaning of optical components 2. Avoid excessive laser operation at high power
Intermittent laser firing	1. Loose or damaged fibre connection 2. Faulty footswitch or handpiece trigger 3. Internal circuit malfunction	1. Secure and inspect fibre connections 2. Test and replace the footswitch/handpiece if faulty 3. Contact manufacturer for internal repairs	1. Properly secure fibre connectors 2. Regularly inspect footswitch/handpiece
Burning or charring at fibre tip	1. Excessive power settings 2. Carbonization of fibre tip 3. Improper cooling or irrigation	1. Reduce power settings 2. Clean or trim fibre tip 3. Ensure proper cooling or irrigation during procedures	1. Monitor fibre condition frequently 2. Use optimal power settings
Laser beam misalignment	1. Optical component misalignment 2. Fibre improperly seated 3. Internal mirror or lens issue	1. Align optical components 2. Reseat fibre correctly 3. Contact manufacturer for lens/mirror adjustments	1. Handle optics carefully 2. Perform periodic alignment checks
Error codes on laser display	1. System software issue 2. Safety interlock activated 3. Internal sensor failure	1. Reboot the system 2. Check interlock connections 3. Contact manufacturer for diagnostics	1. Keep software updated 2. Ensure interlock mechanisms are functional
Unusual noises from the machine	1. Faulty cooling fan 2. Loose internal components 3. Transformer or power supply issue	1. Inspect and replace cooling fan if needed 2. Tighten internal components if possible 3. Contact manufacturer for power supply inspection	1. Regular maintenance checks 2. Keep ventilation areas clear

23.15 Future Directions for Medical Lasers

Medical laser technology is evolving rapidly, with ongoing advancements in wavelength optimization, fibre delivery systems, and AI-assisted surgical precision. Future developments may include:

Smart Lasers: AI-driven adaptive power adjustments for enhanced safety and efficiency.

Multi-Wavelength Lasers: Combining multiple wavelengths to optimize tissue interaction.

Robot-Assisted Laser Surgery: Enhancing precision with robotic integration.

Laser technology continues to redefine surgical standards, improving patient outcomes through minimally invasive and highly efficient procedures.

Use laser-safe drapes and covers.

Ensure proper grounding of the machine to prevent electrical hazards.

Regular Maintenance and Calibration

Conduct periodic checks to ensure proper functioning of the laser system.

Follow manufacturer guidelines for cleaning and servicing.

Maintain accurate records of laser usage and servicing.

23.16 Conclusion

This LASER machine is a cutting-edge tool for proctology and other surgical fields, providing high precision with minimal invasiveness. Understanding its mechanism of action, user settings, and energy calculations ensures safe and effective treatment. Adhering to best practices and safety protocols enhances the machine's longevity and improves patient outcomes.

Part III

Laparoscopic Instruments

Veress Needle and Trocar

24

Jasmeet Singh Ahluwalia

24.1 Veress Needle

The Veress needle, less commonly spelled as "Veres," was invented in 1936, predating the widespread adoption of laparoscopy due to the limited development of video systems at the time [1]. János Veress, born in Kismajtény, Hungary, in 1903, held the position of head of the Department of Pulmonology and Internal Medicine at Kapuvár Hospital by 1932. During that era, tuberculosis was prevalent, and artificial creation of pneumothorax was considered a rudimentary form of treatment, albeit with the inherent risk of lung injury. Dr. Veress developed this needle to facilitate safe pneumothorax creation and published it in 1936 after nearly 1000 successful procedures [2].

24.1.1 Description

The Veress needle comprises two primary components: a sharp, beveled outer needle and an inner, blunt-tipped, and spring-loaded stylet with a side hole (Fig. 24.1). This unique design ensures that the inner spring-loaded stylet is retracted into the sharp outer cannula as the needle is advanced through the fascia. Upon entering the peritoneal cavity, the blunt inner stylet emerges due to the loss of resistance, safeguarding the underlying viscera. Typically, the external diameter is usually 2 mm or 14 gauge, while the length is usually 70–120 mm, although slight variations may occur depending on the manufacturer.

J. S. Ahluwalia (✉)
Department of Bariatric & Minimal Access Surgery, STAR Superspeciality Hospital, Jalandhar, Punjab, India

J. S. Ahluwalia (ed.), *User Manual for Minimally Invasive Surgical Equipment*,
https://doi.org/10.1007/978-981-95-9019-3_24

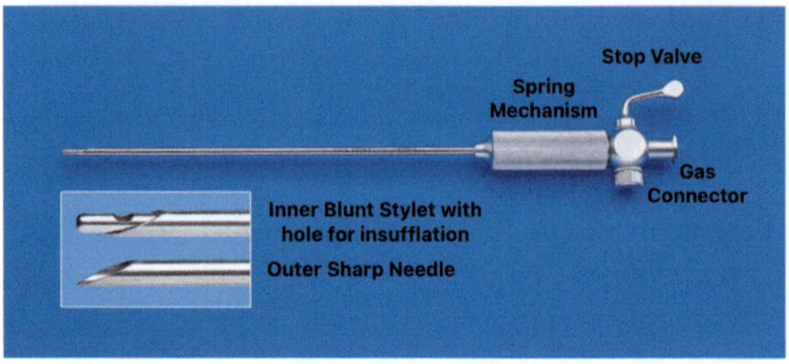

Fig. 24.1 Reusable Veress needle

24.1.2 Reusable Veress Needle

1. *Inner Stylet*: This blunt-tipped stylet has a hole at its tip. The blunt tip is designed to avoid injuring organs as the needle enters the peritoneal cavity. The hole at the tip allows carbon dioxide gas to be released, creating a pneumoperitoneum. This part immediately springs out once the needle enters the abdominal cavity due to the loss of resistance.
2. *Outer Sharp Needle*: This is beveled and sharp to help penetrate the fascia as it is introduced inside the abdominal cavity.
3. *Spring Mechanism*: A spring is concealed within this component, which exerts pressure on the inner stylet, ensuring that its tip remains exposed unless pressure is applied at the tip, as during the introduction of the needle into the abdomen or any other cavity. This component can be rotated to disassemble the Veress needle.
4. *Stop Valve*: This valve regulates the flow of gas into the needle. When positioned in the direction of the needle, it permits gas flow; conversely, when perpendicular to the needle, it obstructs the gas flow.
5. *Connector for Gas Pipe*: This end facilitates the connection of the gas pipe.

24.1.3 Disposable Veress Needle

The disposable needle is largely similar to its reusable counterpart, albeit constructed from a more delicate material, typically plastic (Fig. 24.2). Its spring mechanism is usually transparent, adorned with an indicator that indicates the precise position of the needle. As the needle penetrates the peritoneum and the inner stylet retracts, the position of the indicator becomes evident due to the change in its location and color. Unlike its reusable counterpart, these disposable needles cannot be disassembled.

24.1.4 How to Use

After making a small incision (approximately 2–3 millimeters) in the skin, the Veress needle should be held in a pencil grip fashion and introduced perpendicular to the abdominal wall. If using an umbilical access point, the needle should be

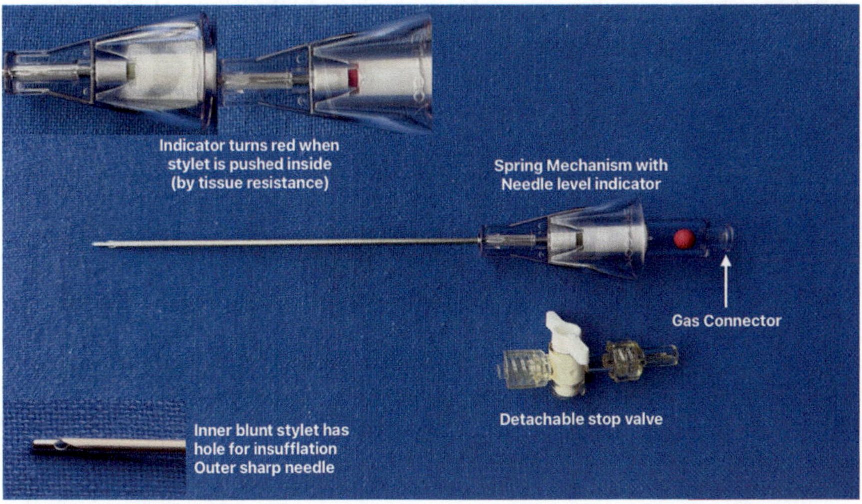

Fig. 24.2 Disposable Veress needle

introduced at a caudal angle to avoid the retroperitoneal major vessels. Alternative sites may be utilized if umbilical entry is not possible or is difficult. Palmer's point is favored by some surgeons, situated in the left upper quadrant, in the mid-clavicular line, 3 centimeters below the costal border.

24.1.5 Tests for Successful Placement

Successful placement of the Veress needle in the free peritoneum can be confirmed through several tests [3]:

Aspiration Test: It checks for fluid or material aspiration when a syringe draws from the needle. Ideally, nothing should aspirate out as the needle should lie freely inside abdominal cavity.

Injection Test: It involves injecting 5 milliliters of normal saline and observing only moderate resistance.

Recovery Test: It ensures no liquid is recovered on aspiration after injecting 5 milliliters of saline.

Saline Drop Test: It visualizes the liquid dropping into the peritoneal cavity after it is placed on the end meant for gas connection.

24.1.6 Troubleshooting

A lot of trouble can be avoided by following a routine check before every insertion of the Veress needle.

- Before using the needle, ensure that it is patent by inserting saline into it and verifying the proper flow of saline from its distal end without applying excessive force.
- Subsequently, seal the tip of the needle and apply moderate pressure to inspect for leaks. A leak in a disposable Veress needle necessitates replacement, while a reusable needle requires tightening the screw.
- Additionally, verify the proper functioning of the spring mechanism by pressing the needle onto a hard surface (for instance, the handle of a knife). The inner stylet should glide smoothly in and out as the needle is pushed and subsequently released. The red indicator of the disposable needle should also move accordingly.

Even after all these checks have been cleared, and still, there is a problem during surgery, one can look for the following reasons:

- Failure to Achieve Pneumoperitoneum:
  - Check for Obstruction: Make sure the needle is not obstructed by clotted blood, fat or any other tissue. Flush the needle with saline to clear any obstruction and ensure that it is patent.
  - Make sure the needle is inside the abdominal cavity by repeating saline test.
  - Look for Intra-Abdominal Pressure: If it is high (over 8 mm initially), the needle may be in the preperitoneal space or in subcutaneous fat. Reinsert the needle to position it correctly.
- Aspiration of Blood, Bowel Contents, or Urine: Indicates possible organ injury. Stop the procedure immediately and do not insufflate any further. Evaluate the patient for any signs of vascular or visceral injury (e.g., hypotension, tachycardia, hematuria, or signs of peritonitis). If the patient is stable, one can create pneumoperitoneum at an alternative site or with an open method and perform diagnostic laparoscopy. If patient is unstable for laparoscopy or the repair of injury is not possible laparoscopically, one may convert to open surgery.
- CO_2 Leakage: Ensure the tubing is properly connected to the Veress needle and the insufflator.
- Subcutaneous Emphysema: Occurs when carbon dioxide accumulates in the subcutaneous tissue rather than the peritoneal cavity, resulting in swelling of the abdominal wall. The Veress needle is likely not positioned within the peritoneal cavity. Withdraw the needle and reposition it correctly. Subcutaneous emphysema typically resolves spontaneously once the needle is correctly positioned. If subcutaneous emphysema persists, stop using the Veress needle and switch to the open technique for safe access to the peritoneal cavity.
- Gas Embolism: A rare but serious complication where CO_2 enters the bloodstream. It can present with sudden patient distress, such as hypotension, bradycardia, or difficulty breathing during insufflation. If suspected, stop insufflation immediately, place the patient in a left lateral decubitus and head-down position (Durant maneuver), and aspirate the right atrium if central venous access is available [4].

24.1.7 General Safety Measures

- Patient Positioning: Ensure that the patient is positioned in a suitable manner (flat or slightly Trendelenburg) to facilitate entry and minimize the risk of organ damage.
- Preoperative Imaging Assessment: For patients with a history of surgical procedures, adhesions, or other risk factors, preoperative imaging (e.g., computed tomography scan) is recommended to evaluate for potential complications.
- Limit Attempts: If multiple unsuccessful attempts to insert the Veress needle are made, switch to an open technique instead of continuing with blind insertion.

24.1.8 Cleaning

After each use, it is imperative to flush reusable Veress needles promptly to prevent tissue from drying out within them. Subsequently, the needle is opened and cleaned from within. It is crucial to note that the needle contains a spring that can be easily misplaced if not stored properly. Routine disinfection and sterilization procedures should be followed after this, as with other reusable laparoscopic instruments.

Disposable Veress needles should be discarded after single use in accordance with hospital policy.

24.2 Trocar

24.2.1 Introduction

The term "trocar" has its origin from the French word "trocart," meaning "to bore through." Ancient civilizations, including the Egyptians, Greeks, and Romans, used hollow reeds (crude metal tubes) to evacuate fluids from cavities. In the early nineteenth century, Reginald Southey invented the Southey tube [5], which probably laid the foundation of modern trocars. Although it is not certain when exactly trocars appeared in the medical field first, but they continued to exist and to develop over thousands of years.

Trocars are specialized instruments employed to establish external access to the abdominal cavity (or any other region of interest) during minimal access procedures. Their indispensable role in contemporary laparoscopy facilitates the insertion of surgical instruments, laparoscopic cameras, and prostheses while maintaining a gas seal to prevent intra-abdominal pressure loss. The selection of suitable tracers significantly contributes to the safety and efficiency of surgical interventions. An ideal trocar system should possess low insertion force, secure retention, and minimal tissue damage.

Most trocars comprise two primary components: the obturator and the cannula.

Obturator: The inner component that seals the hollow cannula as the trocar is inserted and also helps in the penetration of the trocar.

Cannula: The outer hollow sleeve through which instruments are introduced once the trocar is in place and the obturator has been removed.

Trocars can be categorized into various types based on numerous factors. For simplicity, we can classify them into disposable and reusable types.

24.2.2 Disposable Trocars

These are designed for single-use to ensure sterility and minimize the risk of cross-contamination (Fig. 24.3). They are typically constructed from medical-grade plastic to maintain cost-effectiveness. While there may be variations in shape and components among different manufacturers, a basic design is described here as a reference.

24.2.2.1 Cannula

It is a hollow tube through which a camera and surgical instruments can be inserted. These are available in various lengths ranging from 70 mm to 150 mm and diameters ranging from 5 mm to 15 mm (except special-purpose trocars). It has following parts:

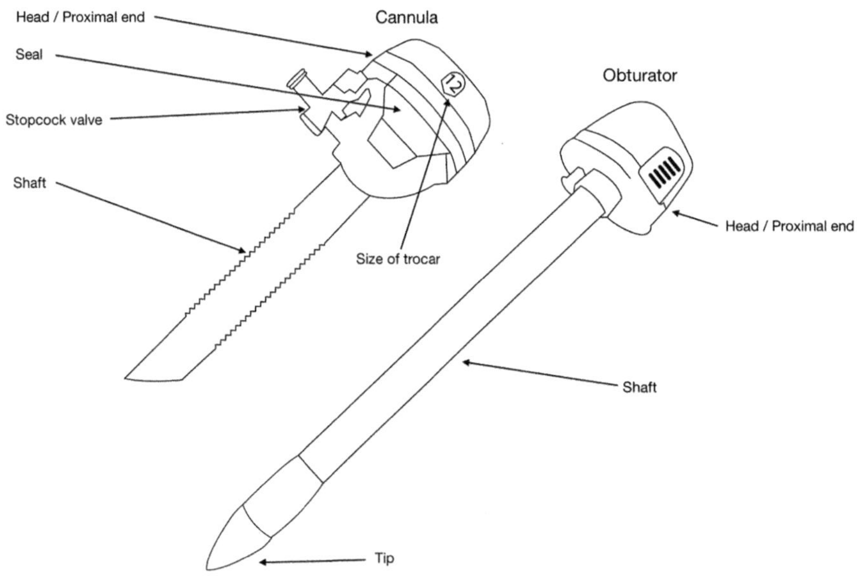

Fig. 24.3 Disposable trocar

(a) Head/Proximal End: This remains outside the body and allows insertion of the obturator, camera and instruments. This may or may not be openable and houses a gas seal. If it has an opening mechanism, this may be opened to allow passage of a large mesh or large specimen.
(b) Seal: Ensures a secure seal around the instruments to prevent gas leakage. Disposable trocar seals typically permit the passage of instruments of various sizes without the necessity of a reducer, unlike reusable trocars.
(c) Stopcock Valve and Leur Lock Connector: This is used to connect the insufflation pipe thereby facilitating the introduction of gas and controlling its flow.
(d) Shaft: This may be serrated to increase anchoring with the abdominal wall.

24.2.2.2 Obturator

It is designed to facilitate the initial entry of the cannula through the abdominal wall. It has the following parts:

(a) Head: This is the proximal portion of the obturator that is pushed by the surgeon's hand. Its broad shape ensures that a larger surface area maintains low pressure on the surgeon's hand.
(b) Shaft: The elongated and narrow component of the obturator that penetrates the cannula. It serves as a connecting link between the head and the tip, providing structural support and guiding the tip through the tissue layers.
(c) Tip: The distal, pointed end of the obturator possesses a relatively sharp edge to enhance the force applied, facilitating the passage of the trocar through the abdominal wall. Trocar tips can be of various types.

    (i) Bladed Tip: This tip features a sharp, cutting edge that facilitates the easy penetration of the abdominal wall. However, it may cause increased tissue trauma.
    (ii) Bladeless Tip: This tip has a conical or pyramidal shape designed to spread tissues without cutting. It reduces tissue trauma and the risk of injuring internal organs. While it may require a higher force to insert the trocar, the surgeon should exercise caution to avoid overshooting the abdominal wall and hitting the underlying viscera.
    (iii) Blunt Tip: This tip is suitable for cases involving previous incisions and may reduce the risk of injuring underlying organs. It can also be used in pediatric patients.
    (iv) Optical Tip: This tip incorporates an integrated optical system that enhances visualization during trocar insertion. The surgeon can insert the scope into the obturator (preferably a 0-degree scope) to view the surrounding tissues as the trocar is advanced into the abdomen. As soon as a breach in the peritoneum is detected, the surgeon will be able to observe and respond accordingly. Since the insertion is performed under visual observation, the use of such tracers is generally considered safer, especially in challenging situations. They can also be used to enter the preperitoneal space and the retromuscular space. Some obturators incorporate a

locking mechanism that secures the scope within the device, thereby preventing slippage during the trocar's rotation as it advances into the abdomen.

24.2.3 Reusable Trocars

These are robust and durable surgical instruments crafted from metal and intended for multiple reuses after sterilization (Fig. 24.4). Similar to disposable trocars, these instruments comprise several essential components that help in their proper functionality and ease of sterilization. While there may be variations in shape and components among different manufacturers, a fundamental design is described here as a reference.

24.2.3.1 Cannula

A hollow tube serves as a conduit for inserting cameras and surgical instruments. These trocars are available in various lengths, ranging from 70 mm to 150 mm, and diameters, from 5 mm to 15 mm (excluding specialized trocars). The trocar comprises several distinct components:

(a) Head/Proximal End: This external portion facilitates the insertion of an obturator, camera, and instruments. It is designed to be openable for proper cleaning after use.
(b) Seal: The seal ensures a secure connection around the instruments, preventing gas leakage. Reusable trocar seals typically permit the passage of only one size of instrument. Specialized reducers are necessary to accommodate instruments

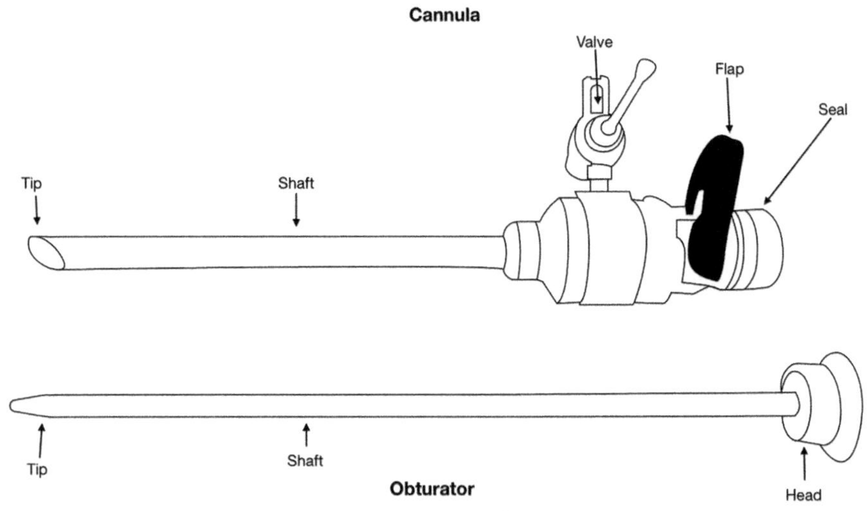

Fig. 24.4 Reusable trocar

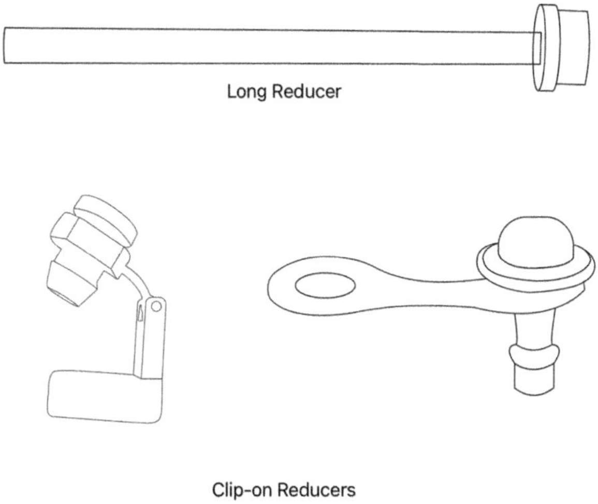

Fig. 24.5 Reducers for cannulas

or scopes of smaller sizes to avoid gas leakage (Fig. 24.5). It is crucial to match the exact dimensions of the reducer, cannula, and scope or instrument to prevent gas leakage.

(c) Stopcock Valve and Leur Lock: This component connects the insufflation pipe to introduce gas into the abdominal cavity and control its flow.
(d) Flap: Reusable cannulas may possess an external flap that can be pressed to open the internal gas seal mechanism. This can be used just prior to the insertion of a scope to prevent damage to the tip of the scope. It can also be pressed to facilitate the removal of specimens, needles, etc. Some cannulas incorporate magnetic flaps that automatically open and close as the scope or instrument is inserted or withdrawn. However, due to a lack of external control, it may be difficult to retrieve a specimen or needle through such cannulas.
(e) Shaft: Most reusable trocars feature a smooth shaft to facilitate easy insertion and cleaning after use. Threaded cannulas are also available for specific situations where cannula slippage poses a challenge.

A longer reducer provides enhanced security but may cause a gas leak when the instrument is withdrawn. Conversely, a clip-on reducer offers reduced security but does not pose the risk of gas leakage during instrument exchange.

24.2.4 Hassan's Trocar

This specialized trocar is employed in the open method to establish a pneumoperitoneum. It is named after Dr. Harrith Hasson, who pioneered this technique to minimize the risk of organ damage during the initial entry. These trocars are available in both disposable and reusable configurations. Some of their distinctive features include the following (Fig. 24.6):

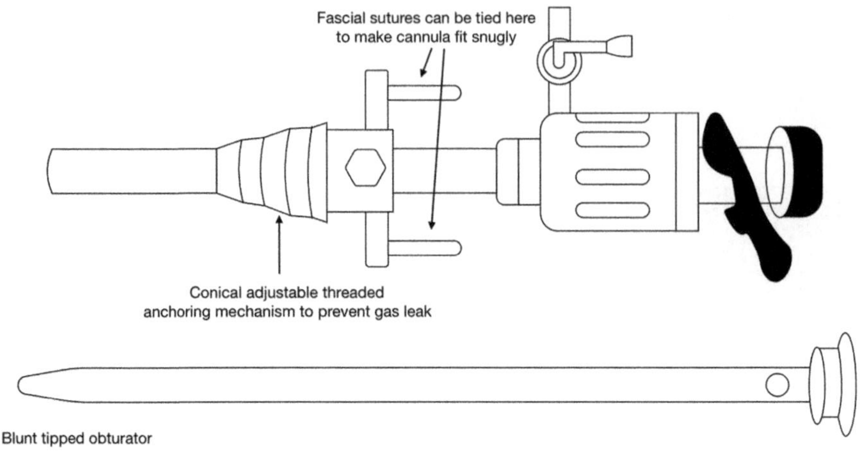

Fig. 24.6 Hasson's trocar

Fig. 24.7 Balloon-tipped trocar

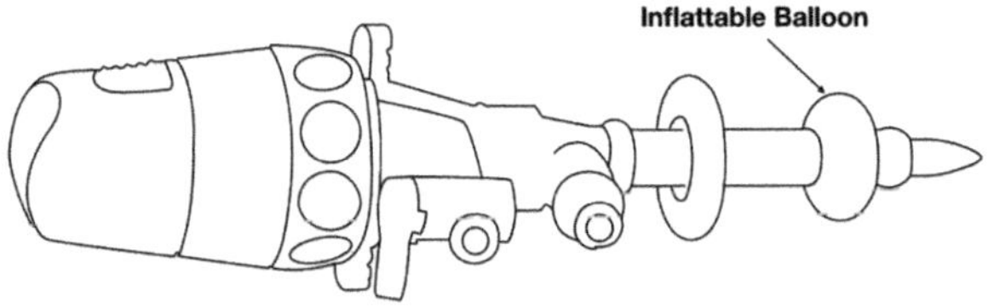

24.2.4.1 Obturator

This is just like a routine trocar with a blunt conical tip to avoid injury to underlying organs, as this is the first object to enter the abdomen in the open technique of creating pneumoperitoneum. A sharp tip is also not required, as the abdominal wall tissues are already opened before this trocar is inserted.

24.2.4.2 Cannula

This has a special conical, threaded, and adjustable anchoring mechanism over its shaft, with the tapering end of the cone facing distally. This helps to plug the gap between the abdominal opening and the cannula to prevent gas leak. Some cannulas also have special attachments to tie fascial sutures to make the cannula fit snugly into fascial opening.

24.2.5 Balloon-Tipped Trocars

These cannulas feature a balloon at the distal end of the trocar. Once the cannula is inserted into the abdominal cavity, the balloon can be inflated, thereby securing the trocar in place. This action minimizes the likelihood of the trocar dislodging during the procedure (Fig. 24.7).

24.2.6 Maintenance

Disposable trocars must be discarded in accordance with hospital policy after single use. Proper care and maintenance of reusable trocars are crucial to ensure their longevity, optimal performance, and patient safety. Some best practices for the same are:

1. Immediately after procedure:
   - Disassembly and Rinsing:
   - After complete disassembly, immediately rinse the trocar with distilled water to prevent the drying of blood or bodily fluids on its surfaces.
   - Manual Cleaning:
   - Soak the trocar components in an enzymatic detergent solution specifically formulated for surgical instruments for the recommended time. Use a soft-bristled brush to clean all surfaces, ensuring thorough coverage of lumens and crevices. Flush out lumens and internal channels with water.
   - Special Cleaning Devices:
   - If an ultrasonic cleaner is available, it may be utilized for enhanced cleaning of the trocar.
2. Inspection

   After cleaning, visually inspect each component for any damage, such as cracks, bends, or other signs of wear that could compromise the instrument's future functionality. Additionally, verify the proper functioning and smooth operation of all moving parts, including valve mechanisms and seals.
3. Sterilization

   Place the components of trocars within sterilization pouches or trays specifically designed for surgical instruments. Sterilize the trocars using an autoclave, ethylene oxide, hydrogen peroxide plasma, or any other suitable sterilization method in accordance with the hospital's sterilization protocol and the guidelines provided by the instrument manufacturer.
4. Storage

   Store sterilized trocars in a dry and cool environment to prevent corrosion and contamination.
5. Lubrication

   Medical-grade lubricants should be applied to moving parts if specified by the manufacturer to ensure smooth operation as well as to extend the instrument's lifespan.

24.2.6.1 Troubleshooting

Having intricate knowledge of trocars is critical to troubleshoot problems that may arise during any laparoscopic procedure.

Problem	Possible cause	Solution
Air leak	Damaged seal or valve Incorrect or loose assembly or of cannula Breakage of cannula	Replace seal or valve Properly assemble the cannula Replaced a broken cannula
Difficulty in the insertion of the trocar	Blunt or damaged tip of the obturator Relatively small skin incision Incorrect technique Insufficient pneumoperitoneum pressure	Replace the obturator Make an appropriate skin incision Ensure proper angle and force for entry Create adequate pneumoperitoneum pressure
Jammed valve for gas insufflation	Improper cleaning Improper drying Lack of lubrication Prolonged disuse	Clean the trocar properly Dry after every wash Lubricate regularly Avoid prolonged disuse
Loss of pneumoperitoneum	Leak from seals/valves Trocar and instrument size mismatch	Check for leaks in seals/valves Ensure proper match of trocar and instrument size
Bleeding at the trocar site	Bleeding from superficial or deep vessels	Direct pressure will usually suffice. Deeper vessels may at times require deep sutures
Subcutaneous emphysema	Gas escapes into the subcutaneous tissue	Reposition the trocar Ensure gas does not leak from the sheath. Tighten the seal around sheath
Intra-abdominal injury	Injury to internal organs such as the bowel or bladder	Stop procedure if injury is suspected Evaluate and repair injuries laparoscopically or convert to open surgery if needed

24.2.7 Future Directions

The development of laparoscopic trocars should prioritize several key areas to enhance their efficacy and safety. Emerging technologies in these areas include:

- Antimicrobial Properties: Trocar materials with antimicrobial properties can reduce the risk of surgical site infections.
- Lightweight and Durable Alloys: The use of lightweight and durable alloys can alleviate surgeon fatigue.
- Tissue Trauma Minimization: Refining tip designs and reducing diameter can minimize tissue trauma, improve cosmetic outcomes, and alleviate postoperative pain and incisional Hernia.
- Real-Time Feedback: Incorporating sensors can provide real-time feedback on tissue resistance.
- Improved Visualization: Embedding high-definition cameras and optical systems within the trocar can enhance visual acuity.

- Reusable Trocars: Developing more robust reusable trocars that can withstand multiple sterilization cycles without degradation addresses environmental concerns and reduces long-term costs.

References

1. Spaner SJ, Warnock GL. A brief history of endoscopy, laparoscopy, and laparoscopic surgery. J Laparoendosc Adv Surg Tech A. 1997;7:369–73.
2. Veres J. Uj légmellkészit t. Orv Hetil. 1936;80:536–7.
3. Skovsen AP. Veres needle. Br J Surg. 2023;110(1):22–3. https://doi.org/10.1093/bjs/znac362.
4. McCarthy CJ, Behravesh S, Naidu SG, Oklu R. Air embolism: practical tips for prevention and treatment. J Clin Med. 2016;5(11):93. https://doi.org/10.3390/jcm5110093. PMID: 27809224; PMCID: PMC5126790.
5. Southey R. Chronic parenchymatous nephritis of right kidney. Left kidney small and atrophied. Old scrofulous pyelitis. Trans Clin Soc Lond. 1877;X:152–6.

Dissecting and Grasping Forceps 25

Ankita Singh and Devender Singh

The advent of the laparoscopic era has brought with it the continuous need to understand and improve the technology for making patient care safer and more effective. The art of dissection and grasping of tissues and viscera during surgery has evolved from the use of open instruments to laparoscopic and robotic dissecting and grasping instruments. This chapter is aimed at describing various types of laparoscopic dissecting and grasping forceps available, their parts and make, maintenance, troubleshooting, and recent advances.

25.1 List of Instruments with Pictures of These Instruments [1]

Name of instrument	Picture	Features
DISSECTING and GRASPING FORCEPS: Unnamed		
(a) Atraumatic: for grasping	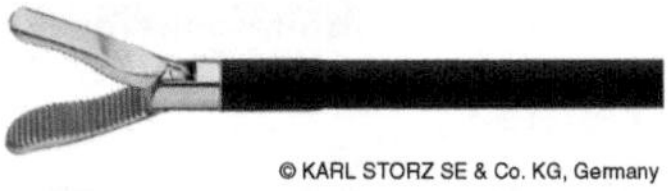	Non-toothed, broad, horizontal serrations, and double action jaws
(b) Atraumatic: for grasping	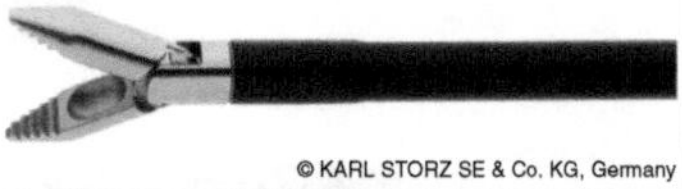	Non-toothed, short, slender with hollow jaws, and double action
(c) Conical (blunt; toothed): for effective mechanical hemostasis	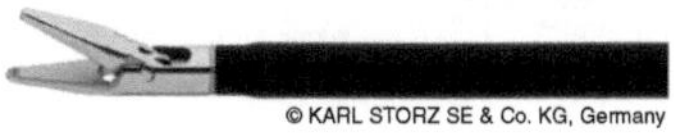	Non-toothed and toothed, conical, and single action jaws

(continued)

A. Singh (✉) · D. Singh
Department of Surgical Disciplines, All India Institute of Medical Sciences Delhi, New Delhi, India

J. S. Ahluwalia (ed.), *User Manual for Minimally Invasive Surgical Equipment*,
https://doi.org/10.1007/978-981-95-9019-3_25

Name of instrument	Picture	Features
(d) "Duck bill" jaws and blunt: for effective mechanical hemostasis	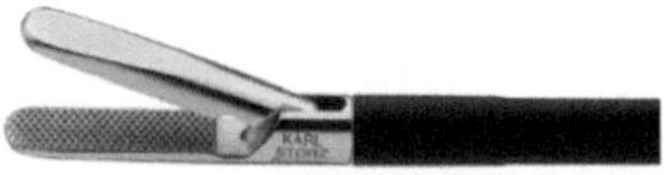 © KARL STORZ SE & Co. KG, Germany	Non-toothed, flat, rounded tip, crisscross serrations, and single action jaws
(e) "Dolphin nose"	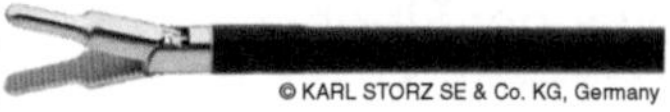 © KARL STORZ SE & Co. KG, Germany	Non-toothed, dolphin-nosed jaws, horizontal serrations, and double action
(f) Right-angled jaws	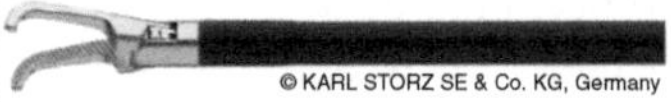 © KARL STORZ SE & Co. KG, Germany	Non-toothed, right-angled, horizontal serrations, and double-action jaws
(g) "Alligator" jaws	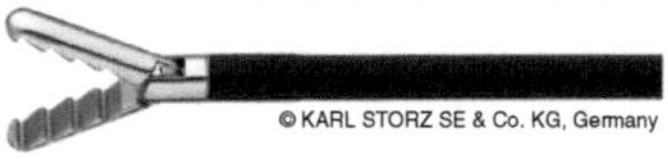 © KARL STORZ SE & Co. KG, Germany	Soft-toothed, double action jaws
(h) "Tiger" jaws	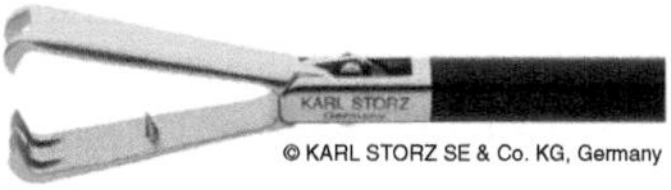 © KARL STORZ SE & Co. KG, Germany	Toothed (2x3), double-action jaws
Reddick -Olsen dissecting and grasping forceps and robust (stout)	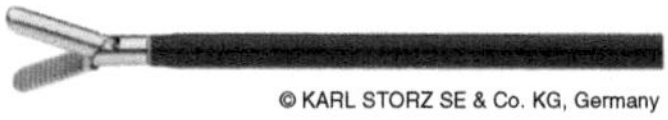 © KARL STORZ SE & Co. KG, Germany	Non-toothed, horizontal serrations, and double action jaws
Uyama dissecting and grasping forceps: for dissection	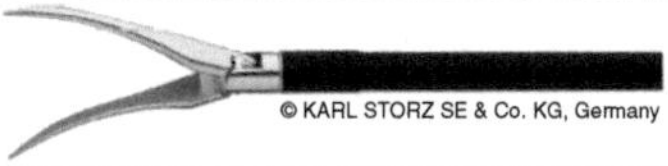 © KARL STORZ SE & Co. KG, Germany	Non-toothed, long and fine, and double action jaws with a reservoir
Noshiro dissecting and grasping forceps: For dissection	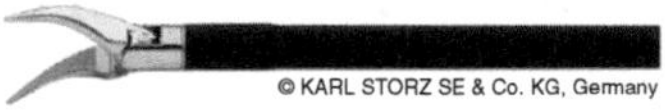 © KARL STORZ SE & Co. KG, Germany	Non-toothed, short and fine, and double action jaws
Mouret dissecting and grasping forceps	 © KARL STORZ SE & Co. KG, Germany	Atraumatic, slender, fenestrated, and single-action jaws
	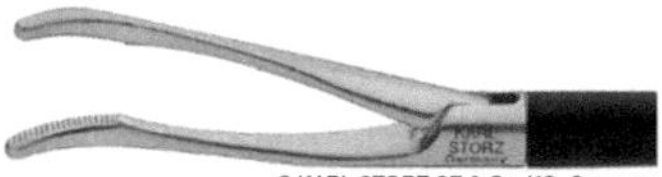 © KARL STORZ SE & Co. KG, Germany	Atraumatic, slender, curved, single-action jaws with large reservoir
Tan dissecting and grasping forceps	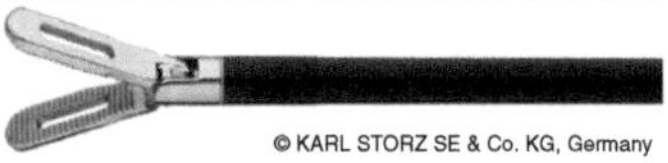 © KARL STORZ SE & Co. KG, Germany	Atraumatic, fenestrated, horizontal serrated, single-action jaws with rounded tips.
Inaki dissecting and grasping forceps	 © KARL STORZ SE & Co. KG, Germany	Atraumatic, slender, fenestrated, curved, and single-action jaws.
Grasping forceps (unnamed)		
(a) Atraumatic	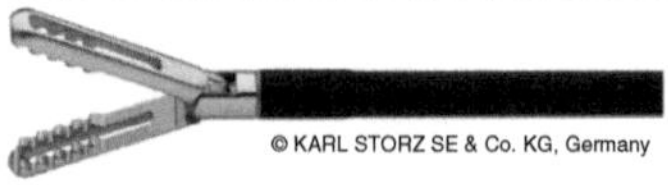 © KARL STORZ SE & Co. KG, Germany	Atraumatic, fenestrated, long, and double action jaws

(continued)

Name of instrument	Picture	Features
(b) Atraumatic	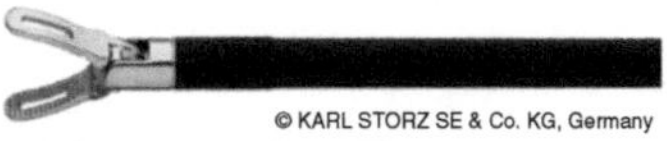 © KARL STORZ SE & Co. KG, Germany	Atraumatic, fenestrated, short, stout, and double action jaws
(c) Fine atraumatic	 © KARL STORZ SE & Co. KG, Germany	Atraumatic, fenestrated, fine, long, serrated, and double action jaws
(d) Atraumatic	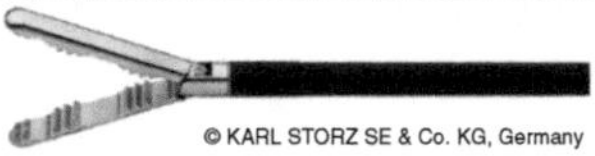 © KARL STORZ SE & Co. KG, Germany	Atraumatic, wavy serrations, and double action jaws
(e) Atraumatic	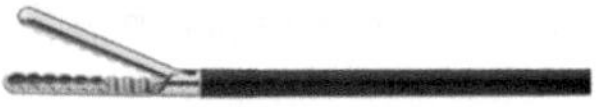 © KARL STORZ SE & Co. KG, Germany	Atraumatic, fenestrated, hollow, and single action jaws
(f) Atraumatic	 © KARL STORZ SE & Co. KG, Germany	Atraumatic, fenestrated, and double action jaws
(g) Multiple teeth :for atraumatic and accurate grasping	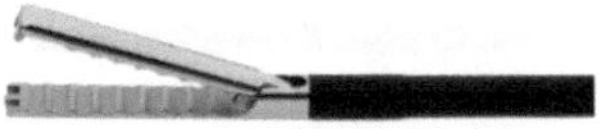 © KARL STORZ SE & Co. KG, Germany	Atraumatic, multiple teeth, spoon shaped, and single action jaws
(h) Multiple teeth: for atraumatic and accurate grasping	 © KARL STORZ SE & Co. KG, Germany	Atraumatic, fenestrated, multiple teeth, wide jaws, and double action
(i) Multiple teeth: for atraumatic and accurate grasping	 © KARL STORZ SE & Co. KG, Germany	Atraumatic, multiple teeth, width of jaws 3 mm, and single action
(j) "Cobra jaws"	 © KARL STORZ SE & Co. KG, Germany	Toothed (1 × 2), horizontal serrations, and single-action jaws
(k) "Tiger jaws: for grasping and removal of solid organs	 © KARL STORZ SE & Co. KG, Germany	Toothed (2 × 4), horizontal serrations,single-action jaws
Babcock grasping forceps		
(a) Atraumatic and fenestrated grasping forceps	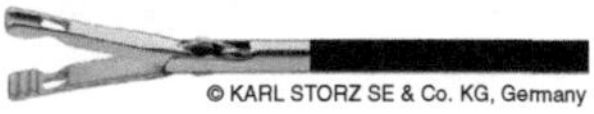 © KARL STORZ SE & Co. KG, Germany	Atraumatic, fenestrated, flat tip, and double action jaws
(b) Atraumatic and fenestrated grasping forceps.	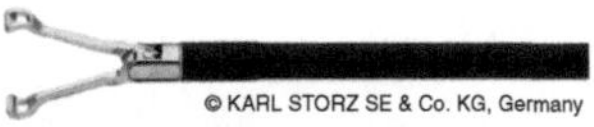 © KARL STORZ SE & Co. KG, Germany	Atraumatic, fenestrated, curved and serrated tip, and double action jaws
(c) Atraumatic and fenestrated grasping forceps	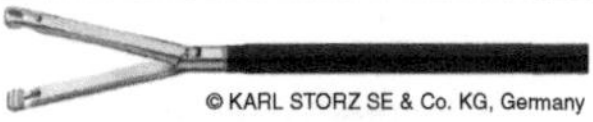 © KARL STORZ SE & Co. KG, Germany	Atraumatic, fenestrated, flat tip, long, and double action jaws
(d) Atraumatic, fenestrated, and toothed grasping forceps	 © KARL STORZ SE & Co. KG, Germany	Atraumatic, fenestrated, multiple teeth, and single action jaws

(continued)

Name of instrument	Picture	Features
(e) Atraumatic, jaws with multiple teeth, fenestrated, and long	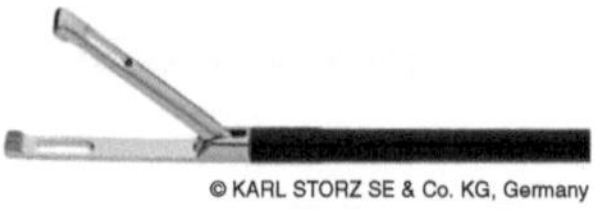	Atraumatic, fenestrated, multiple teeth, single-action jaws, and long
Reddick-Olsen grasping forceps	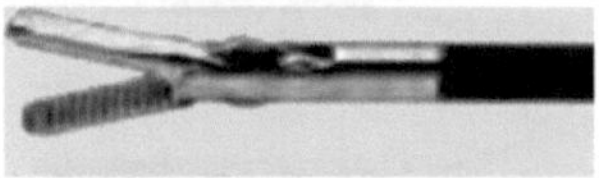	Atraumatic, horizontal serrations, and double action jaws
Mouret grasping forceps	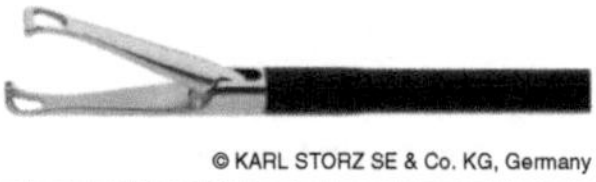	Atraumatic, fenestrated, slender, curved, and single-action jaws
DeBakey grasping forceps	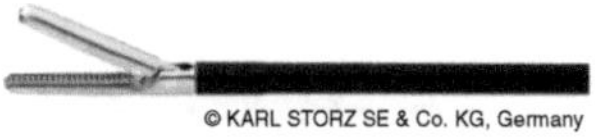	Atraumatic, long, fine DeBakey style longitudinal serrations and single-action jaws
	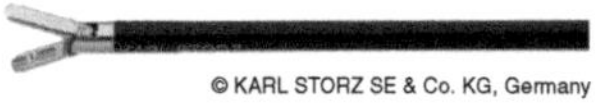	Atraumatic, stout, fine DeBakey style longitudinal serrations, and double action jaws
	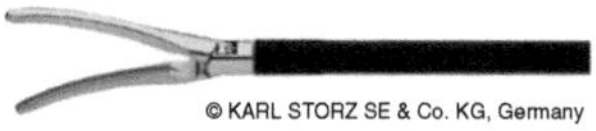	Atraumatic, curved, slender, fine DeBakey style longitudinal serrations, and double action jaws
Olsen clamp (endoscopic cholangiogram forceps)		Atraumatic, fenestrated, horizontally serrated, and double action jaws
Matkowitz grasping forceps	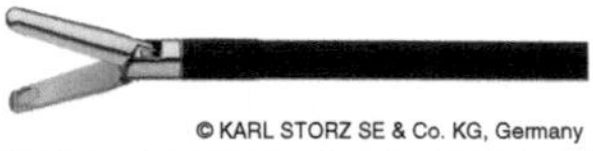	Atraumatic, broad, and double action jaws
Koh grasping forceps	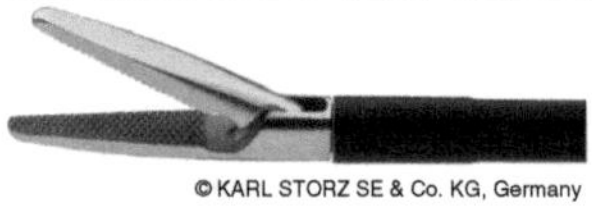	Atraumatic, slender, straight, single-action jaws (curved for ipsilateral suturing technique)
Schneider lymph node grasping forceps	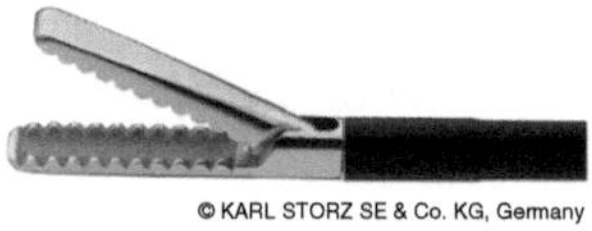	Atraumatic, serrated, and single-action jaws
Kelly dissecting and grasping forceps (Maryland dissector) (a) Normal (b) Long	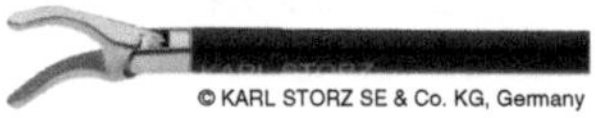 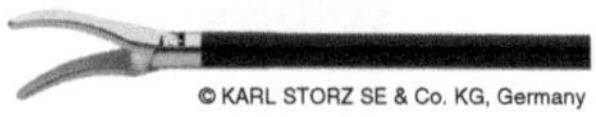	Curved, criss-cross serrated, and double action jaws
Claw forceps	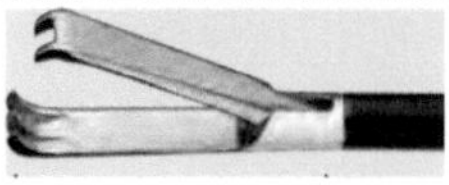	Toothed (2 × 3) and single-action jaws

(continued)

Name of instrument	Picture	Features
Bowel grasper		
(a) Fenestrated	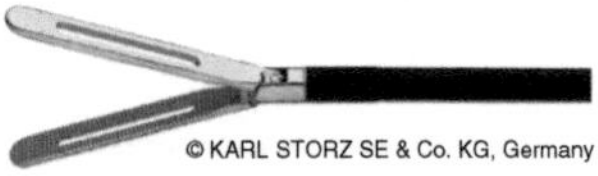 © KARL STORZ SE & Co. KG, Germany	Atraumatic, fenestrated, horizontally serrated, and double action jaws
(b) Fenestrated	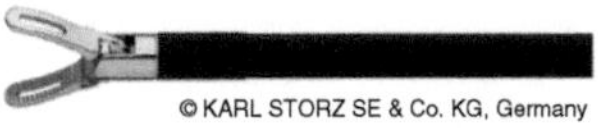 © KARL STORZ SE & Co. KG, Germany	Atraumatic, short, fenestrated, horizontally serrated, and double action jaws
(c) Two rows of atraumatic teeth	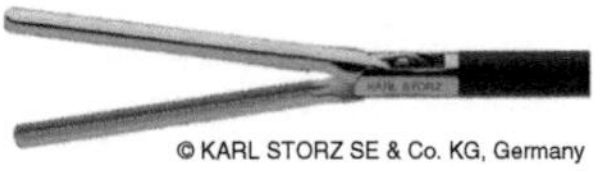 © KARL STORZ SE & Co. KG, Germany	Atraumatic, toothed (2 rows) and double action jaws
(d) Longitudinal serrations	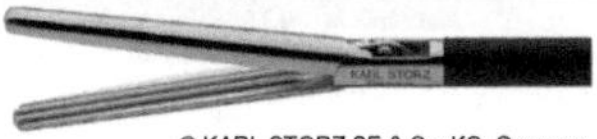 © KARL STORZ SE & Co. KG, Germany	Atraumatic, longitudinally serrated, and double action jaws
(e) Rothenberg Bowel grasper	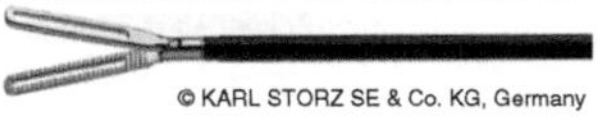 © KARL STORZ SE & Co. KG, Germany	Atraumatic, fenestrated, horizontally serrated, slender, and double action jaws
(f) Curved bowel grasper	 © KARL STORZ SE & Co. KG, Germany	Atraumatic, fenestrated, horizontally serrated, slender, curved, and double action jaws
Urethra grasping forceps	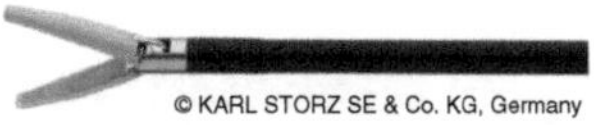 © KARL STORZ SE & Co. KG, Germany	Atraumatic, concave, inwardly curved, continuously toothed, and double action jaws
Berci multifunctional grasping forceps	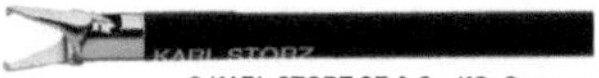 © KARL STORZ SE & Co. KG, Germany	Toothed (1 × 1), curved inwards and double action jaws
Mangeshikar grasping forceps		
(a) 2 × 1 teeth	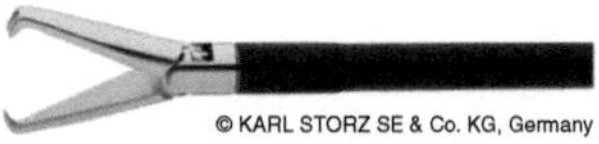 © KARL STORZ SE & Co. KG, Germany	Toothed (2 × 1), curved inwards, and double action jaws
(b) Serrated	 © KARL STORZ SE & Co. KG, Germany	Atraumatic, horizontally serrated, broad, and double action jaws
Grasping forceps: for stapler pressure plates	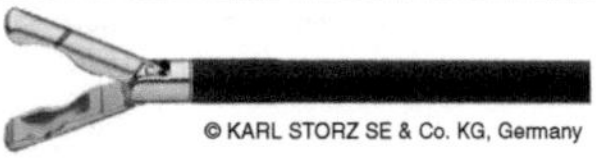 © KARL STORZ SE & Co. KG, Germany	Spoon-shaped, curved inwards, and double action jaws
Gallstone holding forceps: to retrieve spilled gall stones	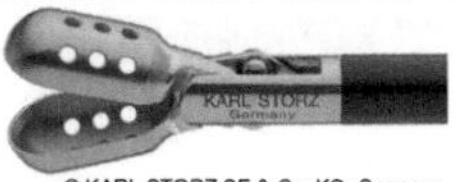 © KARL STORZ SE & Co. KG, Germany	Spoon-shaped, multiple fenestrations, and double action jaws
Tan pyloric spreader and grasping forceps	 © KARL STORZ SE & Co. KG, Germany	Fenestrated, inside and outside serrated, pointed tip, and double action jaws

(continued)

Name of instrument	Picture	Features
Pyloric spreader	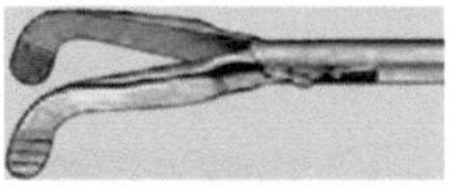	Atraumatic, right-angled, broad, flat tip, and double-action jaws
Geiger pyloric grasper	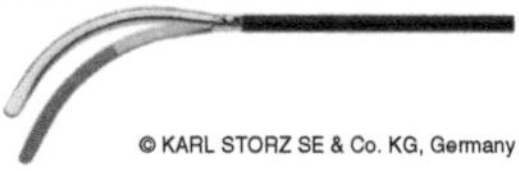	Atraumatic, curved, long, slender, flat, horizontally serrated, and double action jaws
Jet grasper	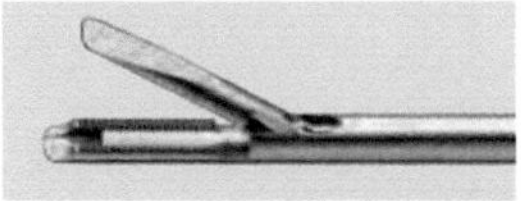	Atraumatic, duckbill, single-action jaws with an irrigation port
Adhesion forceps	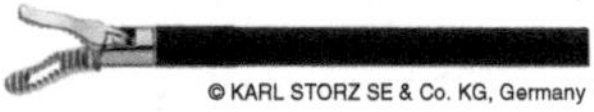	Horizontally serrated, one fenestrated jaw, and double-action jaws
Ovary grasping forceps (a)	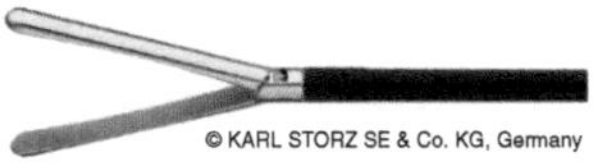	Atraumatic, long, flat, horizontally serrated, and double-action jaws
(b) (inward curved jaws)	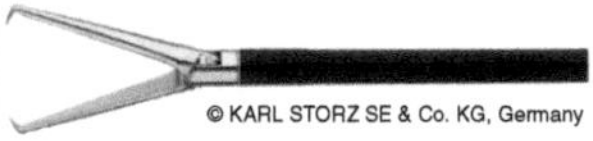	Toothed (1 × 1), curved, long, slender, and double-action jaws
Oviduct forceps	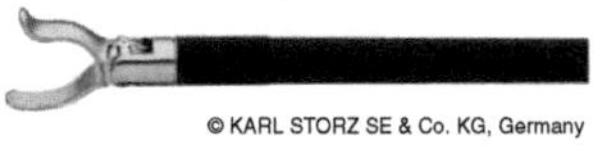	Atraumatic, curved, broad, and double-action jaws
Meso-ovarian forceps	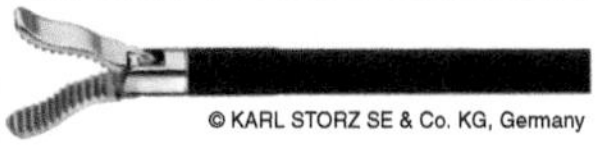	Horizontally serrated, curved, and double-action jaws
Swolin grasping forceps: protect against injury and allow fallopian tubes or similarly delicate structures to be handled gently	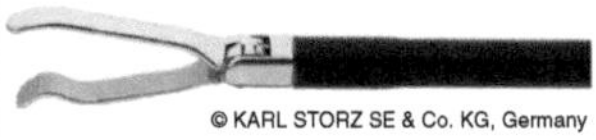	Atraumatic, blunt edges, flat, curved, and double-action jaws
Babcock clamp (a)	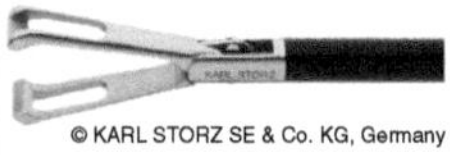	Atraumatic, fenestrated, curved inwards, horizontally serrated tip, and double-action jaws
(b)	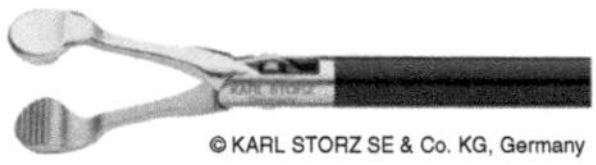	Atraumatic, curved inwards, horizontally serrated, flat and rounded tip, and double-action jaws
Sawalhe tenaculum forceps	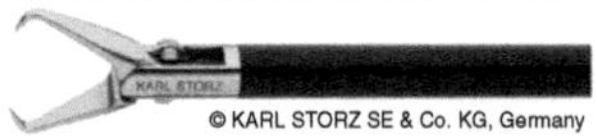	Toothed (1 × 1), curved, slender, and double-action jaws
Duval grasping forceps (with reinforced bayonet coupling)	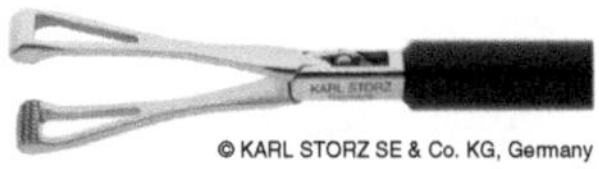	Atraumatic, fenestrated, triangular, horizontally serrated tip, and double-action jaws
Sponge holder (self-retaining)	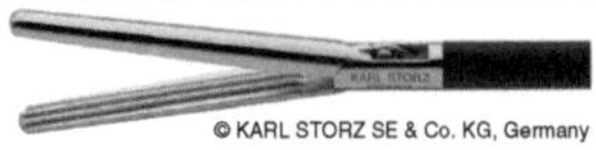	Atraumatic, longitudinally serrated, and double-action jaws

25.2 Detailed Description of Instruments

A dissecting and grasping forceps are handheld laparoscopic instrument that are used to either grasp or both grasp and dissect tissue during laparoscopic surgery. They are available as single use, i.e., disposable and reusable instruments. The reusable instruments are expensive but are cost effective in long run. They are manufactured with modular system which allows the user to individually assemble the desired instrument, which typically comprises of the following three or sometimes two components [1–4]:

- Handle
- Outer sheath : it is aninsulated tube
- Working insert : it contains the tip of the instrument
  - Grasping type
  - Grasping and Dissecting type

(Outer sheath and working insert:) or an outer sheath with a working insert

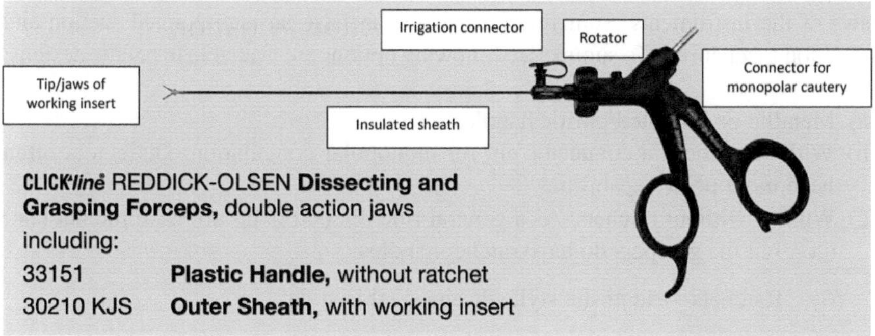

25.2.1 Parts of a Dissecting and Grasping Forceps

This two or three piece design of the instrument allows the surgeon a few advantages:

1. Ability to use instruments with different
   (a) Lengths: Which come in 20 cm, 30 cm, 36 cm, and 43 cm
   (b) Sizes: 2 mm, 3 mm, 3.5 mm, 5 mm, and 10 mm as required
2. Various choices of handle styles.
3. Ease of dismantling with easy maneuvering.
4. Autoclavable even in the assembled state.
5. In case of damage to a component, the entire assembly can still be used after replacement of only the defective component.

25.2.2 Handle

It usually comprises finger rings and allows the surgeon to control the movement of the instrument in its length, and the movement of the jaws through finger-in-ring grip. While those with a pistol handle allow gripping of instruments by palmer grip hand position, where the thumb of the surgeon lies outside the ring with the palm resting on the thumb ring. This grip requires less force; thus, it is more comfortable and effective.

Some of the handle designs allow firm grasping of the tissues, even for a longer time without application of constant force, possible by locking of the jaws. This locking mechanism is usually in the form of ratchet, which allows locking of jaws with different pressures and unlocking by disengagement of the ratchet. For grasping soft organs and soft tissues, the instruments without ratchets may be used to avoid any inadvertent injury due to the crushing effect. However, those with the atraumatic grasping jaws may not cause injury to tissues when locked.

Most of them have a connector pin for monopolar coagulation required for dissection and hemostasis. The handle may also contain a rotator wheel for rotating the tip or jaws of the instruments. Sometimes a handle can have an incorporated suction and irrigation mechanism. To summarize following options are available in handle designs:

(a) Metallic or insulated/plastic handles.
(b) With or without a connector pin for monopolar coagulation: Dissectors often have monopolar capabilities.
(c) With or without ratchets: As a general rule dissectors do not have ratchet handles, but the graspers do have ratchet handles.
    (i) Ratchets—Hemostat style, disengageable style.
(d) With or without large contact area at the finger rings.
(e) Axial handles.
(f) Rotating working insert by use of rotating wheel/rotator.

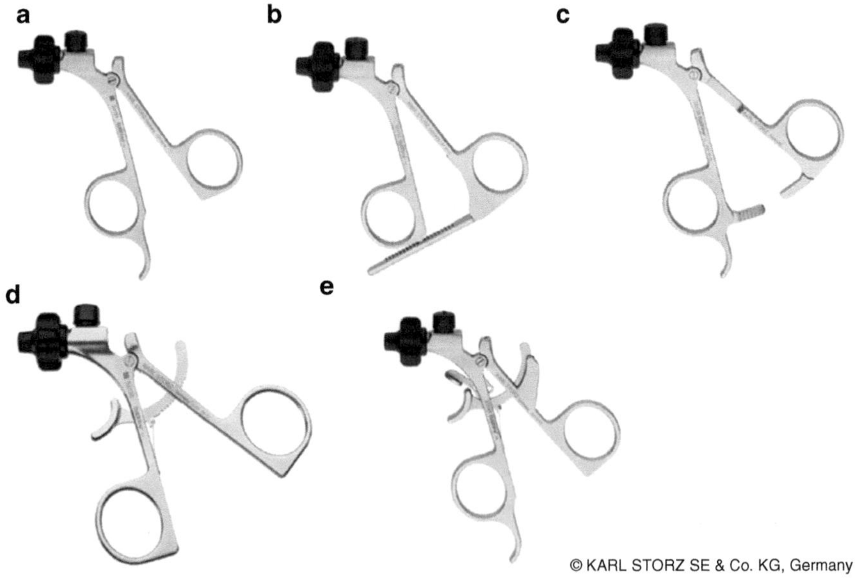

Types of handles : Metal handle (a) without ratchet; (b) with ratchet; (c) hemostat style ratchet; (d) with ratchet; and (e) with disengageable ratchet.

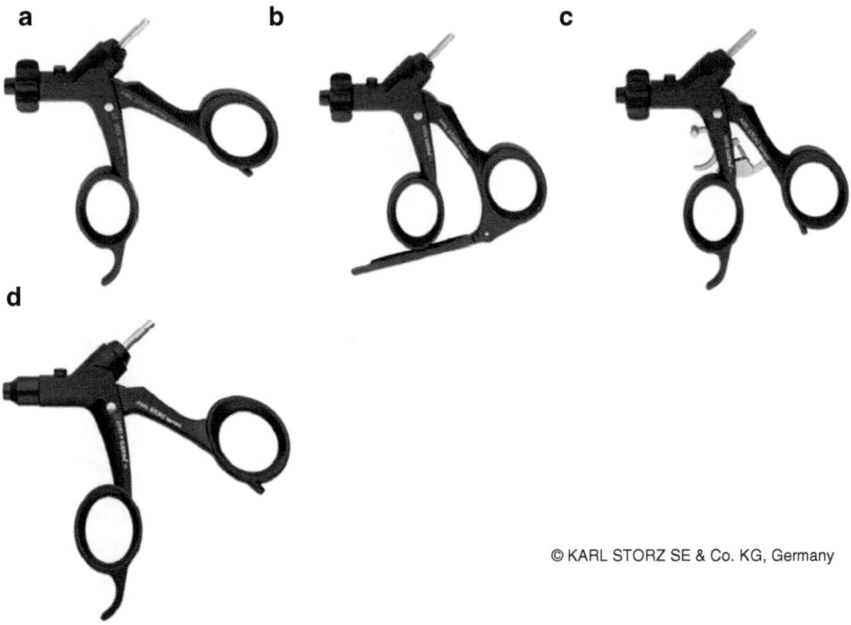

Types of handles: Plastic handle (a) without ratchet, with large contact area at the finger ring b) with ratchet, with large contact area at the finger ring (c) disengageable ratchet, with large contact area at the finger ring (d) nonrotating, without ratchet, with four locking positions.

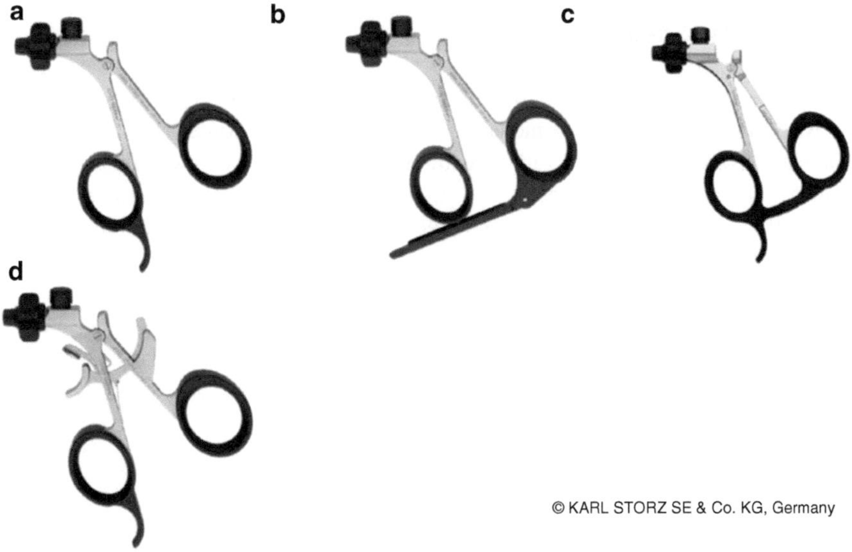

Types of handles: Metal handle with plastic finger rings (a) without ratchet, with large contact area at the finger ring (b) with ratchet, with large contact area at the finger ring (c) hemostat style rachet, with large contact area at the finger ring (d) disengageable ratchet, with large contact area at the finger ring.

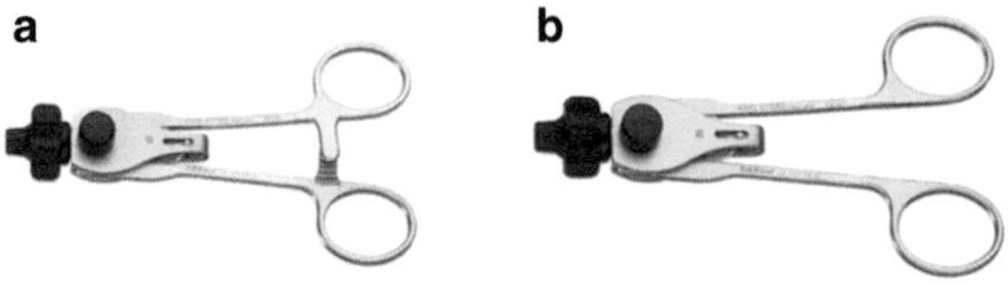

Types of handles: Metal handle, axial (a) hemostat style ratchet, with double action handle shanks (b) without rachet, with double action handle shanks.

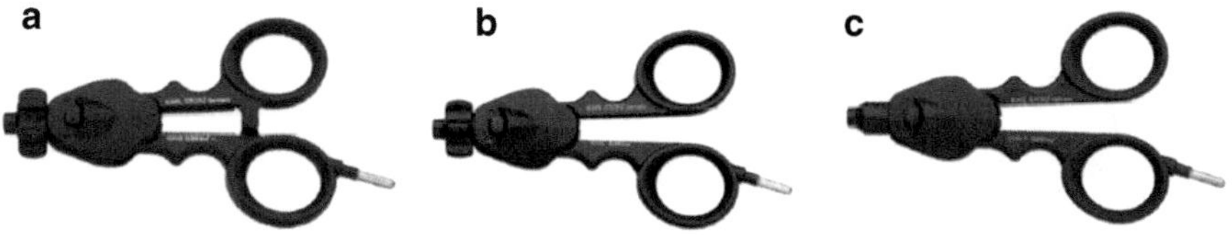

Types of handles : Plastic handle, axial (a) with ratchet, with double action handle shanks (b) without ratchet, with double action handle shanks (c) non rotating, without ratchet, with double action handle shanks, with four locking positions

25.2.3 Outer Sheath

It is a hollow tube made up of either plastic or silicon. This insulated sheath contains the working element and is detachable. These instruments come with an irrigation connector used for cleaning, with or without using a Luer-lock mechanism and are available in various sizes namely, 20 cm, 30 cm, 36 cm, and 43 cm. Any wear and tear in this sheath can leak current while using monopolar coagulation and can cause inadvertent injury.

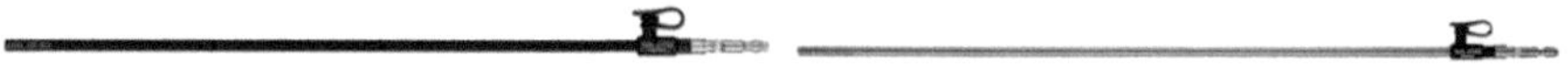

25.2.4 Working Insert

The tip of a working insert is available in variable designs. This tip is designed in the form of jaws, which are used for grasping, dissecting, and coagulating the tissues during surgery. The jaws of a grasping and dissecting instruments can be single action or double action. The single action jaws open less, as only one jaw is mobile while other is fixed but close with greater force, thus used when more pressure is required. However, most of the grasping and dissecting forceps have double action jaws which have wider opening [2, 4].

Single action jaws.

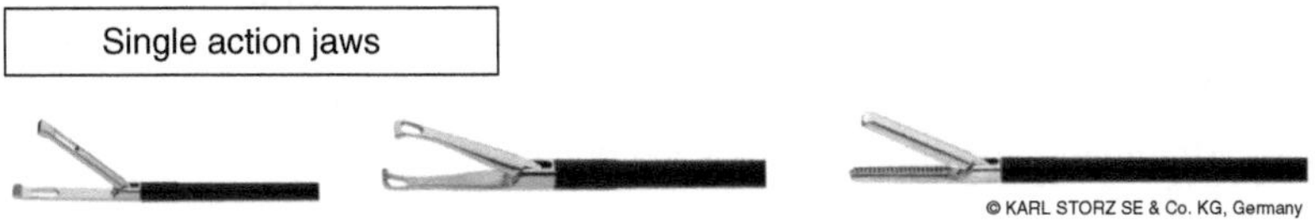

Double-action jaws.

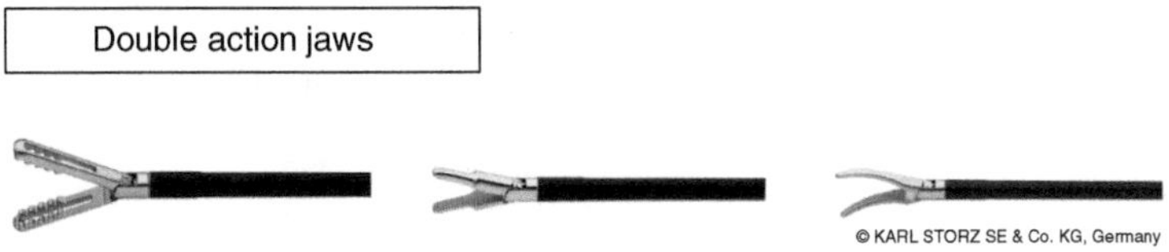

The working inserts for a grasping and dissecting forceps are available in different sizes, shapes, and designs, which can be used as per requirement.

25.2.5 The Grasping Forceps

They are used for grasping and dissecting tissues and organs, sponges, needle, and sutures during surgery.

The grasping instruments can be categorized as single and double action jaw graspers:

(a) Atraumatic and traumatic (toothed)
(b) With ratchet and without ratchet
(c) Locking toothed jawed and soft toothed jawed
(d) Curved and straight
(e) Serrated, fenestrated, and hollow

25.2.6 Babcock Grasping Forceps

It has straight fenestrated jaws with rounded and flared ends with a smooth, flattened tip.

Use: For atraumatic grasping and encircling tubular and delicate structures such as the appendix, bowel, fallopian tubes, and ureters.

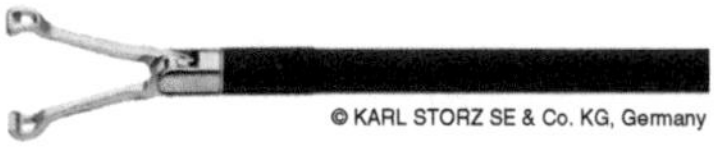

- Debakey Forceps
  It has fenestrated and elongated jaws with a blunt tip. There are two parallel rows of fine serrations that run along the entire length of the inner aspect of one of the jaws. While the other jaw has one row of longitudinal serrations in the center that allows interlocking when both jaws are closed, for a better grasp.
  Use: Atraumatic grasping of tissues and organs.

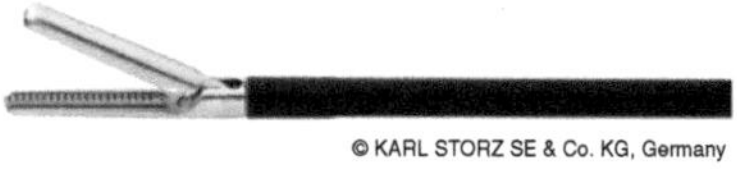

- Blunt Grasper
  It has straight jaws with a rounded tip, horizontal serrations that do not run throughout its length and has a proximal recess.
  Use: For grasping tissues and organs with minimal trauma.

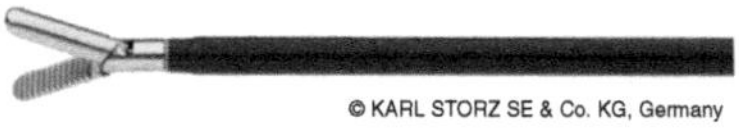

- Claw Grasper
  It has straight, wide, elongated spring-loaded jaws with 2 × 3 heavy interlocking teeth.
  Use: For grasping excised tissues and organs for retrieval from the abdominal cavity.

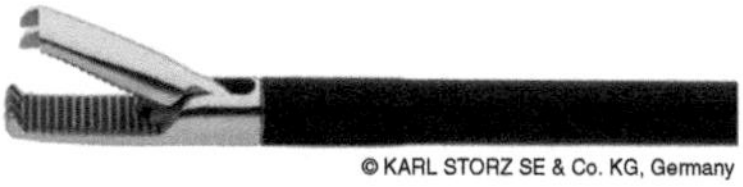

- Cobra Grasper
  It has straight jaws with horizontal serrations that run along the entire length of the inner aspect of the jaws. One jaw has a single tooth, and the other has two teeth that interlock when the jaws are closed.
  Use: For grasping and retracting dense tissues such as fascial layers.

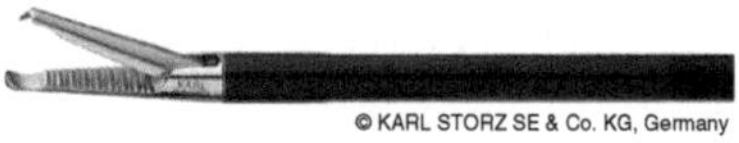

- Bowel Grasper
  It has straight, long, and fine jaws with rounded tips. There are two parallel rows of fine serrations that run along the entire length of the inner aspect of one of the

jaws. While the other jaw has one row of longitudinal serrations in the center that allows interlocking when both jaws are closed.
Use: For atraumatic grasping of delicate tissues.

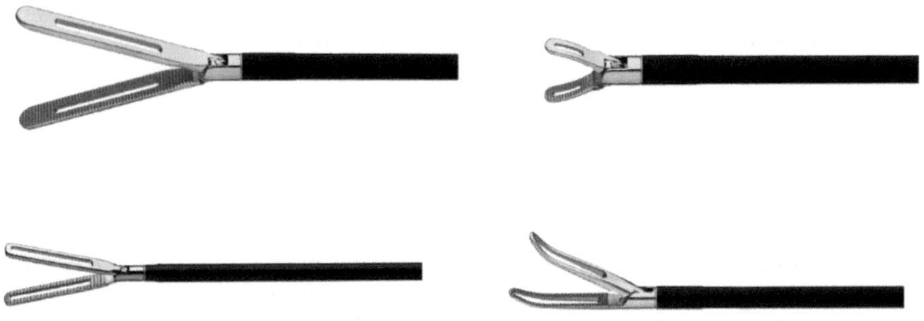

© KARL STORZ SE & Co. KG, Germany

- Olsen Clamp
  Also known as endoscopic cholangiogram forceps. It has a proximal port with distal rounded fenestrated jaws that have horizontal serrations that run along the entire length of the inner aspect of the jaws. The cholangiogram catheter is passed through the proximal port until the tip extends beyond the jaws. This catheter is held in place by closing the jaws of the forceps.
  Use: For grasping of cholangiogram catheter and negotiation into the common bile duct for injection of the contrast media for intraoperative cholangiography.

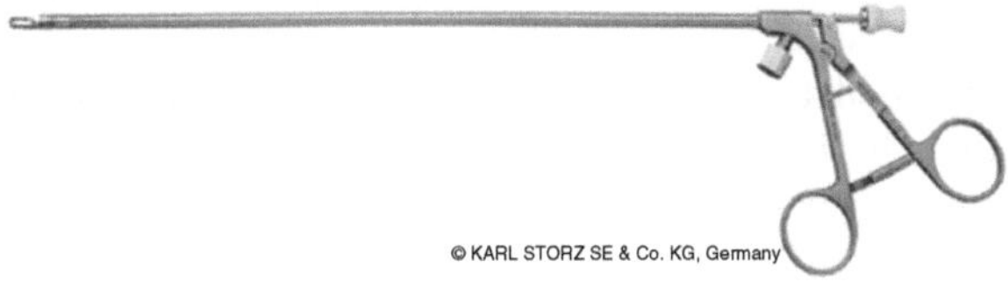

© KARL STORZ SE & Co. KG, Germany

- Jet Grasper
  It is a grasping instrument with an integrated jet for irrigation. This allows blunt dissection of adherent tissues or opening up of anatomical tissue planes. This instrument has duckbill-shaped jaws of size 5 mm with an irrigation port. This port is continuous with an irrigation channel that runs along the outer sheath of the working element. The special handle has a port for the connection of irrigation from a source. It is a rotating and dismantling instrument with a metal handle without a ratchet and without a connector pin for unipolar coagulation. For cleaning of the instrument, a luer-lock irrigation connector is provided.

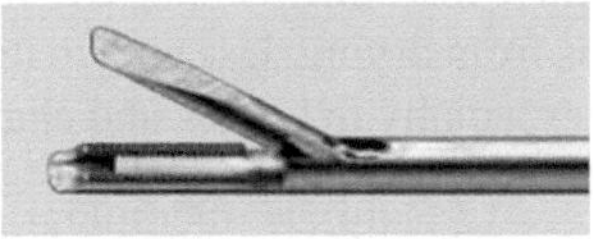

25.2.7 The Dissecting Forceps

- Maryland Dissector
  It has curved jaws that are fine-tapered and have horizontal serrations that run along the entire length of the inner aspect of the jaws.
  Use: For fine dissection and separation of thin tissues.

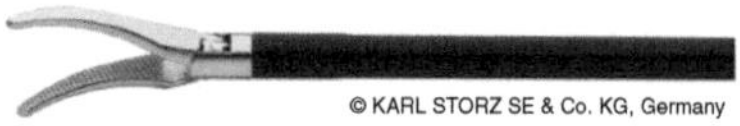

© KARL STORZ SE & Co. KG, Germany

- Right-Angle Forceps
  Also known as mixter. It has a curved, right-angled tip with cross-hatch serrations that run along the entire length of the inner aspect of the jaws. Often has a connector pin for monopolar coagulation at the handle end.
  Use: For dissecting through tissue planes and around tubular structures.

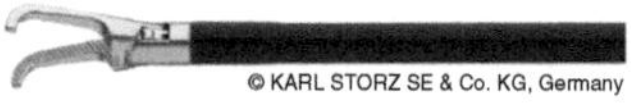

© KARL STORZ SE & Co. KG, Germany

- Dolphin Nose Dissector
  It has straight jaws that taper to a fine tip, with horizontal serrations on the inner aspect of the jaws.
  Use: For fine dissection and separation of thin tissues.

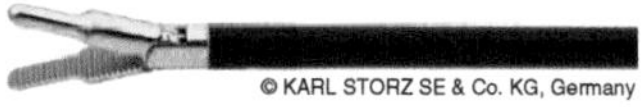

© KARL STORZ SE & Co. KG, Germany

- Conical Tip Dissector
  Also known as bullet nose dissector. It has conical or bullet-shaped tapered jaws with or without horizontal serrations on the inner aspect of jaws.
  Use: For blunt dissection and separation of tissue planes.

© KARL STORZ SE & Co. KG, Germany

25.3 Maintenance

Proper maintenance of laparoscopic hand instruments is critical to ensure their longevity, optimal performance, and patient safety. The following key practices help prevent damage and extend the life of these precision tools [3–5]:

1. *Immediate Cleaning*: Rinse instruments in sterile water immediately after use to prevent blood and debris from drying. Use enzymatic detergents and soft brushes for thorough cleaning, especially in hinges and channels.
2. *Avoiding Damage*: Handle instruments gently—avoid dropping, overbending shafts, or forcing movements that can stress delicate mechanisms. Insulated instruments should be checked for cracks or breaches to prevent electrosurgical burns.

3. *Lubrication*: Regularly apply instrument-grade, water-soluble lubricants to joints, box locks, and moving parts after cleaning. This reduces friction, prevents corrosion, and ensures smooth operation.
4. *Inspection*: Routinely inspect for signs of wear, rust, misalignment, or malfunction. Replace worn or damaged parts immediately to avoid intraoperative failure.
5. *Proper Storage*: Store instruments in designated trays with silicone holders to prevent movement and impact damage. Keep them in dry, well-ventilated areas to avoid moisture buildup and corrosion.
6. *Sterilization Precautions*: Ensure all instruments are completely dry before sterilization. Use manufacturer-recommended sterilization protocols, and avoid stacking heavy items on top of delicate instruments.

By following these precautions, surgical teams can maximize the functional lifespan of laparoscopic instruments and ensure safe, efficient procedures.

25.4 Thorough Inspection of Insulation

The majority of laparoscopic instruments have an outer insulation sheath. Damage to the protective insulation sheath may result from a combination of physical insult, mechanical degradation, harsh cleaning, temperature cycling from repeated sterilization. Failures of adequate insulation may result in inadvertent electrosurgical injuries from alternate pathways of the current. Small breaches in insulation are more dangerous than large breaches, as the current density is inversely proportional to the size of the breach. Also, small breaches are not visible to the naked eye and can be easily missed. Visual inspection of the insulation sheath is suggested before use, after use, and after the processing of the laparoscopic instruments. Interestingly, only 10% of insulation failures are detected visually. The use of an insulation break detector or high voltage porosity detector improves the identification of insulation failure. Regular maintenance of Laparoscopic instruments helps to circumvent large-scale repairs and premature replacement of these instruments [3, 6].

25.5 Troubleshooting—When the Instrument Does Not Work—What to Do to Make It Work/Any Alternatives

- Instrument is not opening: Ensure that the lock of the instrument in the handle is open and in a functional state. Ensure proper assembly of the instrument. Ensure there is no breakage at the joint.
- Instrument is not holding/gripping: Ensure a tight connection between the insert and outer insulation sheath. This can be checked by "pull test", gently pull the outer sheath over the insert; if there is a gap, tighten the assembly. The grip of the instrument should be checked before use by holding a lint-free towel with the laparoscopic grasper and pulling back. Other reasons include a damaged instrument that may need replacement.

- Insulation sheath is broken: Most instruments have the same outer insulation sheath, which can be replaced.
- Instrument is very tight in opening, closing, and rotation: Ensure that there is no rust at the joint, and the instrument can be sent for lubrication for adequate functioning. Replace if the problem persists.

25.6 Future Directions and Emerging Technologies in Laparoscopic Hand Instruments

The field of laparoscopic surgery is advancing rapidly, with innovations focused on improving precision, ergonomics, safety, and surgeon control. Future developments in laparoscopic hand instruments are expected to evolve in the following areas:

25.7 Integration with Digital and Smart Technologies

- *Smart Instruments*: Incorporation of sensors that provide real-time feedback on force application, tissue interaction, or thermal energy use.
- *RFID and Instrument Tracking*: Enables monitoring of usage, sterilization cycles, and wear patterns to optimize maintenance and inventory control.

25.8 Enhanced Ergonomics and User-Centered Design

- *Adaptive Handles*: Redesigned grips that reduce fatigue and enhance precision by conforming to natural hand movements.
- *Modular Instruments*: Customizable instruments with interchangeable components tailored to specific surgical tasks or preferences.

25.9 Robotic-Assisted Manual Instruments

- *Mechanically Enhanced Tools*: Instruments that provide wrist-like articulation without requiring a full robotic system.
- *Haptic Feedback Systems*: Development of tools capable of simulating tactile sensation to improve tissue handling and reduce unintentional trauma.

25.10 Advanced Materials and Surface Coatings

- *Lightweight Composites*: Use of durable yet light materials like carbon fiber and titanium alloys to reduce strain.
- *Nonstick and Antimicrobial Coatings*: Reduce tissue adhesion and enhance sterility, making cleaning and reprocessing more efficient.

25.11 Conclusion

Laparoscopic hand instruments are diverse, with a wide array of designs tailored to specific surgical tasks—grasping, dissecting, cutting, coagulating, and more. This variety allows surgeons to select instruments that best suit their technique, the procedure at hand, and patient-specific anatomy. A thorough understanding of the available options—along with their design features, strengths, and limitations—empowers surgeons to make informed choices that can enhance precision, reduce operative time, and improve overall outcomes. Equally important is the care and maintenance of these instruments. Regular cleaning, proper lubrication, careful handling, and correct storage are essential not only for preserving the instruments' function and longevity but also for maintaining surgical safety and efficiency. By combining technical knowledge of instrument types with diligent maintenance practices, surgeons, and surgical teams can optimize their operative performance, ensure consistent results, and uphold the highest standards of minimally invasive surgery.

References

1. Karl Storz SE & Co. KG. Chapter 4: Dissecting and grasping forceps: instrument handbook. In: Laparoscopy in surgery, gynecology, urology. 9th ed. Tuttlingen; 2022. p. 75–152.
2. Scott-Conner CEH. The SAGES manual: fundamentals of laparoscopy, thoracoscopy and GI endoscopy. 2nd ed. New York: Springer; 2006. https://doi.org/10.1007/0-387-30485-1.
3. Bhandarkar DS, Katara AN. Chapter 3: Sterilization and maintenance of instruments & equipments. In: Kriplani A, Bhatia P, Prasad A, Govil D, Garg HP, editors. Comprehensive laparoscopic surgery. New Delhi; 2007. p. 20–5.
4. Mishra RK. Laparoscopic equipment and instrument. In: Textbook of practical laparoscopic surgery. 3rd ed. New Delhi: Jaypee; 2013. p. 32–44.
5. Lomanto D, Chen WTL, Fuentes MB. Mastering endo-laparoscopic and thoracoscopic surgery: ELSA manual. Singapore: Springer Nature; 2023.
6. Yazdani A, Krause H. Laparoscopic instrument insulation failure: the hidden hazard. J Minim Invasive Gynecol. 2007;14(2):228–32.

Laparoscopic Scissors and Biopsy Forceps

26

Qurrat Al Ain Atif and Alpa Morawala

26.1 Laparoscopic Scissors [1]

In modern medicine, laparoscopic scissors play a crucial role as surgical instruments. These scissors are designed to allow surgeons to perform precise cutting and dissection with minimal tissue trauma. Laparoscopic scissors are available in various shapes, sizes, and materials to accommodate different surgical needs and preferences. They may feature different blade configurations, such as straight, curved, or angled, to facilitate access to specific anatomical structures and ensure optimal cutting efficiency.

26.1.1 Parts of Laparoscopic Scissors

Laparoscopic scissors are made up of several individual parts:

1. Handle: The handles are built ergonomically to provide the user with a firm and comfortable grip during the surgery. The handle may be straight or angled to allow for easier access to certain areas. Usually, the handle for scissors is non-ratcheted.
2. Shaft: The shaft is a long, thin section of the instrument that connects the handle to the working end.
3. Working End (Blades): This is the end of the instrument that does the cutting. It includes two blades, and either one or both of them move to cut the structure in between. Blades come in different shapes and sizes.
4. Rotation Knob: It gives a 360-degree rotation and can be color coded depending upon the manufacturer.

Q. A. A. Atif (✉) · A. Morawala
General Surgery, Barts Health NHS Trust, London, UK

J. S. Ahluwalia (ed.), *User Manual for Minimally Invasive Surgical Equipment*,
https://doi.org/10.1007/978-981-95-9019-3_26

5. Electrosurgical Attachment: This makes it possible to connect scissors to monopolar or bipolar diathermy.

The cutting force of scissors operates on the principle of levers, particularly class 1 levers, where the pivot (fulcrum) is between the effort and the load. The longer the handle or fulcrum, the less force is required for cutting. Although laparoscopic scissors may not strictly adhere to the law of levers due to their cylinder action, their design facilitates force amplification through lever action.

Scissors perform cutting through a combination of gripping, squeezing, and tearing actions. When the blades of scissors close, their sharp edges grind against each other, resulting in the cutting of any tissue caught between them.

26.1.1.1 Materials used in Laparoscopic Scissors [2, 3]

The blades of the laparoscopic scissors can be made from different materials, including stainless steel, titanium, and tungsten carbide. Handles are usually made from medical-grade plastic or polycarbonate.

Stainless Steel

Surgical grade stainless steel is the most commonly used material for blade of laparoscopic scissors as it is strong, durable, corrosion-resistant, and easy to sterilize.

Titanium

Titanium is another material used for making blades of laparoscopic scissors. It is lighter and more durable than stainless steel, and it provides better visibility during surgery.

Tungsten

Tungsten carbide is a hard and durable material that is resistant to wear and tear, making it suitable for the cutting edges of laparoscopic scissors.

26.1.1.2 Sizes of Laparoscopic Scissors

Laparoscopic scissors come in different sizes, diameters, and lengths. The size of the scissors will depend on the type of surgery and the tissue being operated on. The smaller the scissors, the less invasive the surgery, and the less scarring there will be.

26.1.1.3 Diameters

Laparoscopic scissors vary from 3 mm to 10 mm.

1. 3 mm: The smallest laparoscopic scissors available, they are ideal for small incisions and delicate tissue dissection.
2. 5 mm: This is the most commonly used size of laparoscopic scissors, suitable for a broad range of surgical procedures.
3. 10 mm: These are the largest laparoscopic scissors available, and they are reserved for heavy-duty tissue dissection.

26.1.1.4 Shaft Length

The length of laparoscopic scissors can vary from 34 to 37 cm. Some bariatric instruments are available in 45 cm length, whereas pediatric instruments come in 20–30 cm lengths.

26.1.1.5 Jaw Length

The jaw length for laparoscopic scissors usually varies from 9 mm to 18 mm.

26.1.2 Types of Laparoscopic Scissors

There are different types of laparoscopic scissors, and each type has a specific use. The types of laparoscopic scissors can be categorized based on:

1. Usability
2. Blade type
3. Specialized function

26.1.2.1 Usability

Laparoscopic scissors can be either single-use, reusable, or reposable.

Single-Use/Disposable: Available in sterilized packages [3, 4]. Disposable scissors help mitigate the risk of cross-contamination between patients. Overall cost per patient usually comes out to be higher due to their disposable nature.

Reusable: Can be sterilized and reused. The main drawbacks are the risk of cross-contamination and loss of sharpness over time. Their upfront cost might be higher, but per use cost comes out to be much less compared to disposable ones.

Reposable: Have a disposable scissor shaft and jaws, but a reusable handle to provide appropriate sharpness in every use. It also cuts the cost in comparison to disposable scissors (Fig. 26.1).

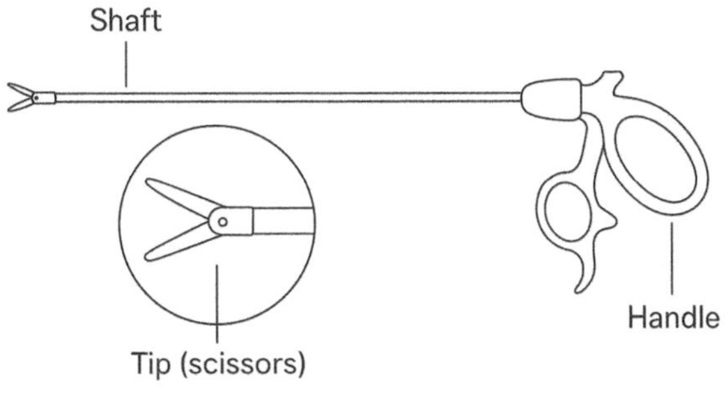

Fig. 26.1 Parts of scissors

26.1.2.2 Blade Type

Based on the type of blade, laparoscopic scissors can be straight, curved, hooked, serrated, micro-tip or articulated.

Types of Jaws Available

- *Straight Scissor Double Action*: Straight laparoscopic scissors: These instruments have blades that are straight and run parallel to the shaft of the device. They are used for cutting and dissecting tissues (Fig. 26.2).
- *Curved Metzenbaum Scissor Double Action*: These instruments have blades that are curved at an angle to the shaft of the device. They are most often used for the dissection and transection of soft tissues. The advantage is of better angulation and view.
- *Serrated Laparoscopic Scissors*: The serrated edges allow for adequate grasp and avoid slippage during cutting (Figs. 26.3 and 26.4).
- *Hook Scissor Single Action*: These scissors have a hook at the end of the blade, making them useful for cutting tissues that are difficult to reach or tubular structures like a duct or artery. They are also used for cutting sutures while doing laparoscopic suturing (Fig. 26.5).

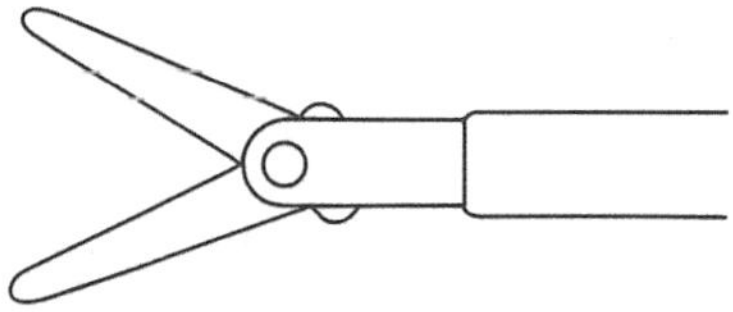

Fig. 26.2 Straight scissors

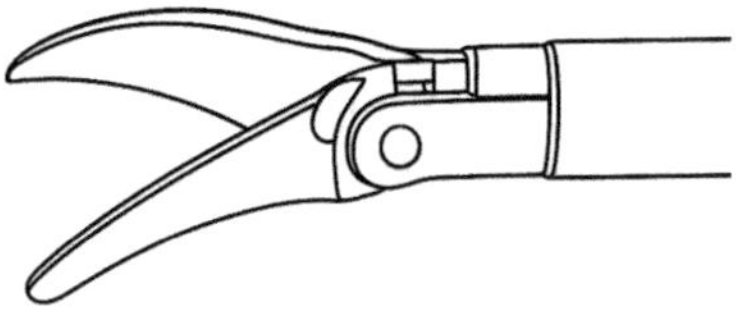

Fig. 26.3 Curved scissors

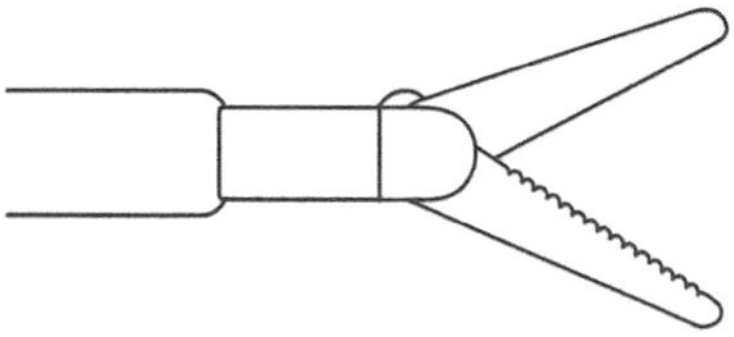

Fig. 26.4 Serrated scissors

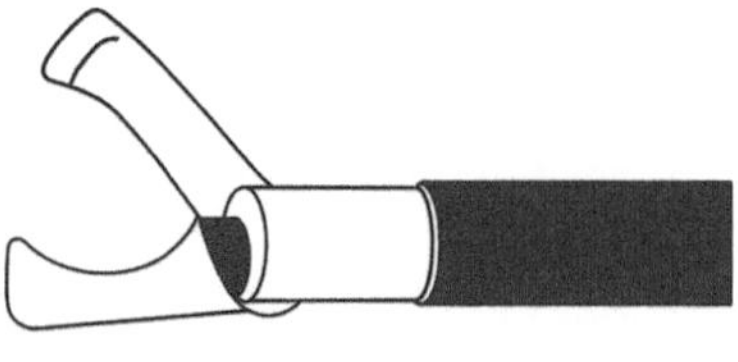

Fig. 26.5 Hook scissors

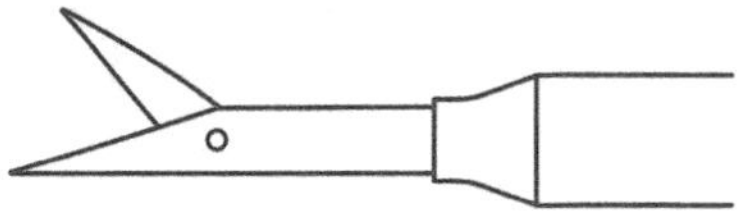

Fig. 26.6 Micro-tip scissors

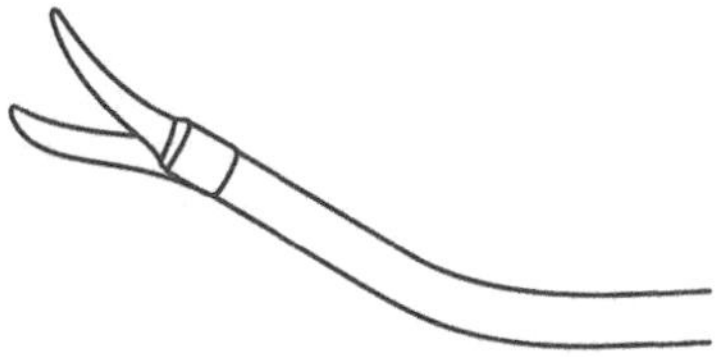

Fig. 26.7 Articulated scissors

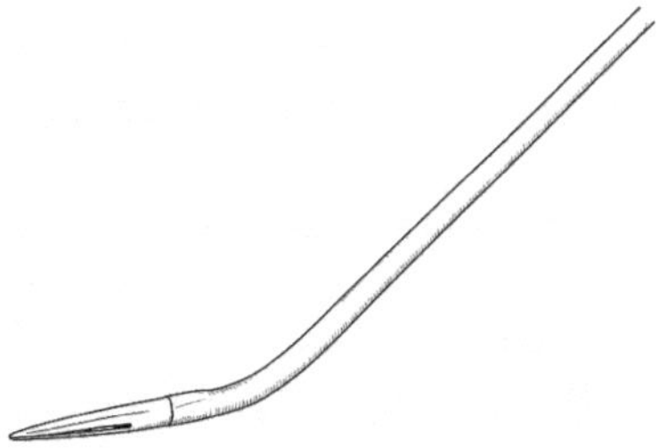

Fig. 26.8 Angled scissors

- *Micro-Tip Laparoscopic Scissors*: These have the advantage of making small nicks in ducts for cannulation, for example, performing intraoperative cholangiogram (Fig. 26.6).
- *Articulated Laparoscopic Scissors*: These are a newer version of laparoscopic scissors, which provide a wristed motion at the end. It provides flexibility and precision during laparoscopic surgery (Fig. 26.7).
- *Angled Scissors*: Angled laparoscopic scissors are designed to provide the surgeon with better access to hard-to-reach areas of the body. The angled design of the blade makes it easier for the surgeon to get around organs and other structures in the body (Fig. 26.8).

26.1.2.3 Usability (Specialized Function)

Ultrasonic Scissors

These scissors use high-frequency sound waves to cut through tissues instead of mechanical blades. The oscillation of blades produces frictional heat used to cut. They are detailed in a separate chapter.

Electrical Scissors

An electrosurgery unit can be attached to scissors to help in cutting while maintaining hemostasis.

26.1.3 An Overview of Working Mechanism of Laparoscopic Scissors

Laparoscopic scissors work by transmitting energy to their blades, which in turn cut through tissues. This energy can be mechanical, electrical, or ultrasonic.

1. Mechanical scissors use a lever and a fulcrum-like mechanism to cut through tissues.
2. Electrical scissors use high-frequency electrical energy to generate heat, which cuts through tissue. Monopolar or bipolar diathermy can be attached to the scissors.
3. Ultrasonic scissors use high-frequency sound waves to break down tissue molecules, which cut through the tissue.

26.1.4 Handling Laparoscopic Scissors

Laparoscopic scissors need to be handled with care during surgery. They should be held with the dominant hand. The other hand should be used to manipulate tissue around the scissors.

Best practices for handling laparoscopic scissors:

1. Sterilize the instrument before use to prevent infection.
2. Ensure that the instrument is properly assembled before use. The blades should be correctly aligned and adjusted to ensure optimal cutting performance.
3. Hold the instrument securely around the handle, but avoid gripping too tightly, as this can cause hand fatigue.
4. Slowly introduce the instrument into the cavity, keeping it under vision at all times, taking care not to damage any surrounding tissues.
5. Operate the laparoscopic scissors in a deliberate, controlled manner to avoid causing any unnecessary damage.

26.1.5 Uses of Laparoscopic Scissors

Laparoscopic scissors have many different uses in surgery. They can be used for tissue dissection, cutting through vessels and ducts, adhesiolysis, for suture cutting, etc.

26.1.6 Troubleshooting

In case the scissors are not cutting properly, look for the following reasons:

1. Make sure the instrument is properly assembled, and there is no loose point at the distal or proximal end.
2. A reusable pair of scissors will become blunt over time and may need replacement.
3. Since scissors are delicate instruments, they may break when used against hard objects and will need replacement.
4. If scissors are hard to operate, clean any debris and lubricate the joints.
5. If there is damage to the instrument while it is inside and the jaws are left open and the control to close them is lost, one may use an instrument from the other port to close the jaws to facilitate their removal.

26.1.7 Maintenance

Proper maintenance can prolong the life of reusable and reposable scissors.

1. After every use, clean them thoroughly after disassembling them and make sure all residue is removed.
2. Dry scissors properly before assembling them again.
3. Store them in a way that their tips are protected against damage when not in use.
4. Use of electro-cautery with scissors is believed to blunt its edges; this may be avoided wherever possible.
5. The insulating sheath must be checked before and after every use for any damage.
6. Gentle handling while using them can also enhance their life.

26.2 Laparoscopic Biopsy Forceps: Overview and Types

Biopsy forceps have revolutionized the way in which medical practitioners obtain tissue samples from various organs for histological analysis. Laparoscopic biopsy forceps are a type of surgical instrument designed to take tissue samples with minimal trauma and bleeding during laparoscopy.

Parts

Laparoscopic biopsy forceps typically consist of four components: a handle, a shaft, jaws, and a locking mechanism.

1. Handle: The handle is designed to fit comfortably in the surgeon's hand, with a textured surface to provide a secure grip. The handle can be plain or ratcheted.
2. Shaft: The shaft is a long, slender tube that connects the handle to the jaws of the biopsy forceps.
3. Jaws: The jaws are the most critical component of the instrument, designed to grasp and extract tissue from the targeted organ.
4. Rotation Knob: It provides a full 360-degree rotation.

Sizes

Laparoscopic biopsy forceps are available in various sizes, ranging from 2 mm to 12 mm in diameter. The length of the shaft varies from 34 cm to 37 cm, with bariatric instruments up to 45 cm and pediatric down to 20 cm.

26.2.1 Types of Laparoscopic Biopsy Forceps

There are three types of biopsy forceps based on the shape of the jaws:

1. Cup and spoon biopsy forceps
2. Punch biopsy forceps
3. Tooth biopsy forceps

Cup and Spoon Biopsy Forceps

These are commonly used to obtain tissue samples from organs such as the liver, pancreas, and kidneys (Fig. 26.9).

Punch Biopsy Forceps

Punch biopsy forceps are designed to remove a cylindrical sample of tissue from the body. These forceps have a sharp cutting edge that is used to remove the tissue sample (Fig. 26.10).

Tooth Biopsy Forceps

These forceps have a sharp tooth on each jaw (Fig. 26.11).

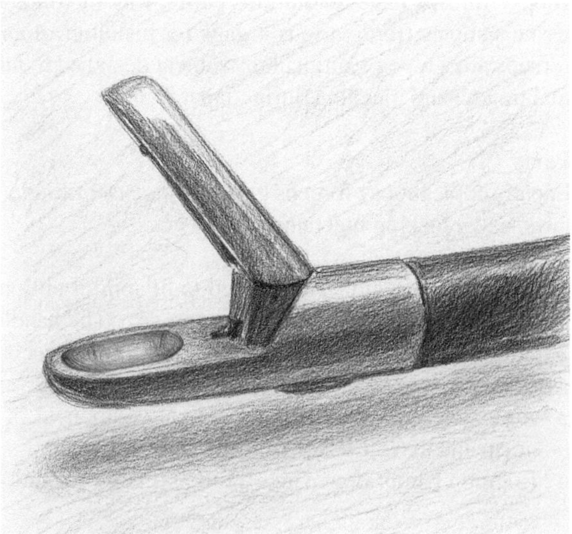

Fig. 26.9 Cup and spoon biopsy forceps

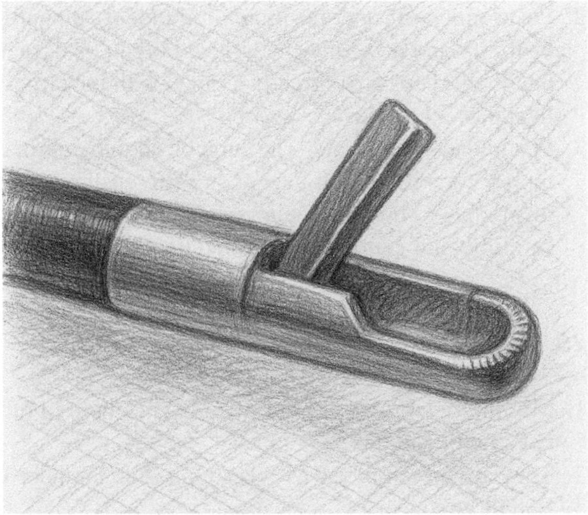

Fig. 26.10 Punch biopsy forceps

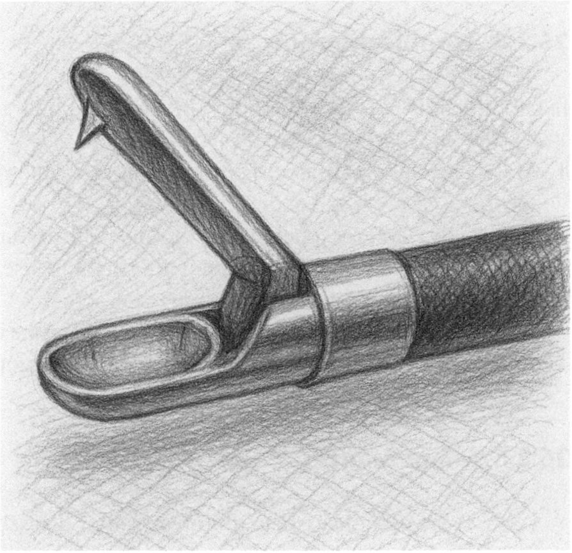

Fig. 26.11 Tooth biopsy forceps

26.2.2 Handling of Laparoscopic Biopsy Forceps

Proper handling of laparoscopic biopsy forceps is critical to ensure accurate extraction of tissue samples, maintain the longevity of the instrument, and reduce the risk of injury to the patient or surgeon.

1. Sterilization—Laparoscopic biopsy forceps should be thoroughly sterilized before and after every use. Proper sterilization procedures are essential in preventing infection and cross-contamination.

2. Positioning—Proper positioning of the instrument is essential to ensure optimal visibility and access to the targeted organ or tissue. The surgeon should ensure that the forceps are correctly aligned with the target to avoid crushing or damaging adjacent tissues.
3. Placing and Removal—The surgeon should approach the tissue sample with the biopsy forceps at a 90-degree angle to ensure successful extraction. The instrument's jaws should remain open until they have reached the target tissue, then carefully and gently close around the tissue to grasp it securely for excision.

26.2.3 Advantages of Laparoscopic Biopsy

1. Minimally invasive approach, and hence help in reducing the risk of postoperative complications.
2. They are more precise as everything is done under vision.
3. Enhance recovery of the patient.

26.2.4 Troubleshooting

In case the biopsy forceps do not work properly, look for the following reasons:

1. Make sure the instrument is properly assembled, and there is no loose point at the distal or proximal end.
2. If the jaws are not opening or closing and are stuck, they might have been jammed due to improper cleaning after the last use. Dip them in a warm saline or soapy solution to overcome jam.
3. In case of breakage, the instrument has to be replaced.
4. Always be ready with coagulation devices, as a biopsy can lead to bleeding.

26.2.5 Maintenance

1. After every use, clean them thoroughly after disassembling them and make sure all residue is removed.
2. Before every use, make sure the jaws are opening and closing properly.

References

1. Mishra R, Al-Galladi A. Laparoscopic equipment and instruments. In: Laparoscopic hernia repair. Jaypee Brothers Medical Publishers (P) Ltd; 2013. p. 42. Available from: https://www.jaypeedigital.com/book/9789350258729/chapter/ch3.
2. Mishra DRK. Technological advances in laparoscopic equipment and instruments. Available from: https://www.laparoscopyhospital.com/news/index.php?id=452&p=5&search=.

3. What tools are used in laparoscopic surgery | Laparoscopic.MD. Available from: https://www.laparoscopic.md/surgery/instruments.
4. Hangzhou Boer Medical Instruments Co., Ltd. A new era in minimally invasive surgery: embracing the convenience of disposable laparoscopic scissors. Available from: https://www.boermedicals.com/embracing-the-convenience-of-disposable-laparoscopic-scissors.html.

Coagulation Instruments

27

Romeo Kansakar

27.1 Introduction

Laparoscopic surgery, a cornerstone of contemporary minimally invasive surgery, hinges on the effective utilization of specialized tools for tissue dissection, incision, and coagulation. Among the diverse energy modalities employed, monopolar coagulation stands as a widely adopted technique for controlling bleeding and achieving hemostasis during surgical interventions. Monopolar energy possesses versatility and can be delivered through various laparoscopic instruments tailored to specific tasks, including tissue dissection, coagulation, and incision.

This chapter delves into the specific monopolar instruments employed in laparoscopic surgery, namely the hook electrode, spatula, ball-tip electrode, and needle electrode. These instruments, when powered by a monopolar electrosurgical generator, assume pivotal roles in executing precise tissue manipulation, incision, and coagulation during a broad spectrum of laparoscopic procedures. The description of electrosurgery is dealt with in a separate chapter.

27.2 Mechanism of Monopolar Coagulation

Monopolar coagulation entails the application of electrical current to tissue via an active electrode. The current traverses the patient's body from the active electrode to a return electrode (grounding pad) affixed to the patient's skin. The high-frequency alternating current generates localized heating at the point of contact between the active electrode and tissue, resulting in tissue coagulation, incision, or desiccation.

R. Kansakar (✉)
Department of Surgery, Greencity Hospital, Kathmandu, Nepal

J. S. Ahluwalia (ed.), *User Manual for Minimally Invasive Surgical Equipment*,
https://doi.org/10.1007/978-981-95-9019-3_27

In laparoscopic surgery, monopolar instruments are integrated into an electrosurgical unit (ESU), which provides controlled current for coagulation and incision. Monopolar energy strikes a harmonious balance between power, precision, and ease of use, rendering it suitable for a diverse range of laparoscopic procedures. However, meticulous control is paramount to prevent unintended thermal injury to surrounding tissues due to the dispersion of current through the body.

27.3 Basic Parts of Monopolar Coagulation Instruments

The majority of these instruments share fundamental design elements that are consistent across them. We will commence by describing these elements before delving into the specifics of individual instruments (Fig. 27.1).

- *Electrosurgical Cable Connector*: This component connects the instrument to the electrosurgical generator, facilitating the flow of monopolar energy to the active tip.
- *Handle*: The handle serves as the surgeon's primary grip and control mechanism for the instrument. Its ergonomic design facilitates ease of use and manipulation during surgical procedures.
- *Shaft*: The shaft transmits the electrosurgical energy generated by the generator to the instrument's tip. Some instruments have an incorporated button to activate the electrosurgical energy upon pressing. Insulation envelops the shaft, ensuring that electrical energy is confined to the active tip. This isolation prevents unintentional burns or injuries to the surrounding tissues.
- *Active Tip*: The tip is shaped differently in different instruments to give it a unique advantage. Usually, the name of the instrument is based on the shape of the tip (Fig. 27.2).

27.4 Hook

The hook electrode, a widely utilized monopolar instrument in laparoscopic surgery, bears a curved tip resembling a miniature hook. Its versatility enables precise tissue dissection, cutting, and coagulation.

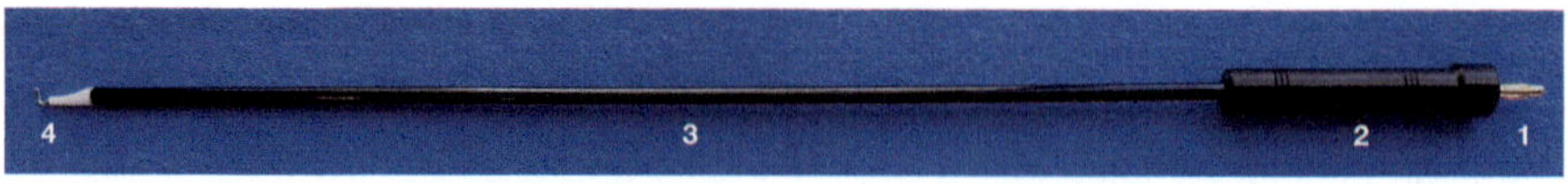

Fig. 27.1 Parts of the coagulation instrument

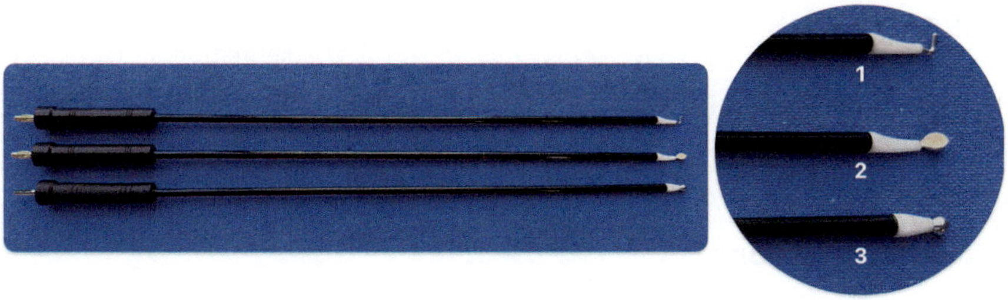

Fig. 27.2 Coagulation instruments: 1—Hook, 2—Spatula, and 3—Ball

27.4.1 Design

The hook electrode's fine, curved tip facilitates controlled cutting and coagulation, especially in delicate or intricate dissections.

27.4.2 Applications

- Tissue separation (e.g., cholecystectomy, dissecting the gallbladder from the liver bed).
- Dissection and coagulation of blood vessels.
- Coagulation of small bleeders within the surgical field.

27.4.3 Advantages

- The hook's design facilitates precise tissue manipulation, minimizing collateral damage to surrounding structures.
- Its compactness enables efficient utilization in confined spaces due to its controlled tip.

27.4.4 Limitations

- The hook's limited surface area may compromise its effectiveness in coagulating larger vessels or tissues with substantial bleeding.

27.5 Spatula

The spatula electrode, a flat, paddle-shaped instrument, serves both cutting and coagulation functions. Its broad surface area facilitates extensive tissue contact compared to the hook electrode.

27.5.1 Design

The spatula electrode possesses a wide, flat tip that can be blunt or slightly pointed, tailored to meet the specific surgical requirements.

27.5.2 Applications

- General tissue dissection.
- Coagulation of larger surfaces (e.g., extensive tissue planes or substantial vessels).

27.5.3 Advantages

- The broad surface area expedites and facilitates uniform coagulation of larger tissue areas.
- Its dual functionality enables efficient dissection and coagulation, optimizing surgical time.

27.5.4 Limitations

- The wide tip may pose challenges in achieving precise dissection in narrow or delicate areas.

27.6 Ball-Tip

The ball-tip electrode is a spherical electrode at its active end, primarily utilized for coagulation rather than cutting. It offers a concentrated point of contact, making it ideal for targeting specific bleeding sites.

27.6.1 Design

The ball-tip electrode comprises a small, rounded metal ball at the end of a slender shaft, ensuring precise application of monopolar energy.

27.6.2 Applications

The ball-tip electrode is employed for:

- Coagulation of small blood vessels or bleeding points.

- Focal coagulation of tissue to achieve hemostasis.

27.6.3 Advantages

- The spherical tip enables precise coagulation of small, specific areas without affecting adjacent tissues.
- It reduces the risk of unintended tissue damage due to the focused application of energy.

27.6.4 Limitations

- The ball-tip electrode is not suitable for cutting or extensive coagulation over large areas.

27.7 Needle

The needle electrode is a fine, pointed instrument designed for delicate tissue dissection and coagulation. It possesses high precision in both cutting and coagulation, particularly in procedures that require precise tissue handling.

27.7.1 Design

The needle electrode features a sharp, slender tip that can be effortlessly inserted into tissues for precise cutting and coagulation.

27.7.2 Applications

The needle electrode is utilized for:

- Fine dissection of tissues in procedures where precision is paramount.
- Coagulation of small vessels or specific bleeding points.

27.7.3 Advantages

- It provides high precision for delicate dissection and coagulation.
- It can be employed in confined or challenging areas where larger instruments may be impractical.

27.7.4 Limitations

- The needle electrode is not effective for coagulating larger areas or tissues.
- The fine tip can lead to higher energy concentration, potentially increasing the risk of deeper thermal injury.

27.8 Troubleshooting

Problem	Possible cause	Solution
No response from hook	Loose or faulty cable connection Damaged instrument cable Foot pedal or activation button malfunction	Check all connections Inspect and replace damaged cable Test the foot pedal or switch to manual activation
Unintended burns or tissue damage	Insulation damage High power setting	Repair insulation or change instrument Lower power settings
Electrical arcing or sparking	Power settings are too high Dirty or charred hook tip Damaged insulation on the instrument	Lower power settings Clean the hook tip Inspect and replace the instrument if the insulation is damaged
Insufficient cutting or coagulation	Power settings too low Tissue debris on hook tip Inadequate contact with tissue Presence of fluids or blood	Adjust power settings Clean the hook tip Ensure proper contact with tissue Suck out fluids
Instrument heating	Prolonged or continuous activation Insulation breakdown	Limit activation time and use in short bursts Replace the instrument if necessary
Instrument malfunction of energy flow	Loose connections Faulty electrosurgical unit	Ensure all connections are secure Repair or replace the unit
Return electrode burns	Poor grounding pad contact Incorrect pad placement on bony or uneven surface Damaged grounding pad	Reapply grounding pad securely to a flat, well vascularized area (e.g., thigh) Ensure proper pad placement with adequate contact Replace grounding pad

27.9 Maintenance

Proper maintenance of these instruments is of paramount importance to ensure optimal performance, patient safety, and instrument longevity. Regular care, inspection, and handling are essential to prevent complications during surgery and extend the instrument's lifespan. Below are the key steps and guidelines for maintaining these instruments.

27.9.1 Pre-operative Inspection

Prior to each utilization, a comprehensive inspection should be conducted to verify the instrument's functionality.

- Insulation Integrity: Visualize the entire shaft of the instrument for any break in the insulation to prevent any energy leakage and patient burns.
- Hook Tip: Ensure it is clean and not damaged.
- Cable Connector and Cable: Verify that the cable is undamaged and the connectors are functioning properly. Additionally, ensure a secure connection between the cable and the instrument connectors.

27.9.2 Intra-operative Care

- During surgical procedures, it is imperative to maintain the functionality of the hook electrode.

Preventive Measures

- Regular Cleaning: Maintain the cleanliness of the hook tip by using a sterile sponge or pad during surgery. This ensures the instrument's efficient energy transfer for cutting and coagulation purposes.
- Monitoring for Overheating: If the instrument experiences heat buildup or becomes hot to the touch, cease its use and allow it to cool down. Prolonged activation without adequate breaks can lead to excessive heat accumulation and melting of insulation material.
- Limited Activation: Employ the hook electrode in short bursts rather than continuous activation to mitigate the risk of overheating and tissue charring.

27.9.3 Post-operative Cleaning

- Proper cleaning after each procedure is paramount to maintaining the instrument's functionality and ensuring sterility for future use.
- Immediate Rinse: Immediately after use, rinse the hook electrode in cold, sterile water or an enzymatic solution to remove blood, tissue, and debris. This prevents the drying and hardening of organic material on the instrument.
- Manual Cleaning: Gently scrub the hook, shaft, and cable with a soft brush, paying particular attention to crevices around the hook tip and insulation.
- Ultrasonic Cleaning: If available, utilize an ultrasonic cleaner to ensure comprehensive cleaning, particularly for removing microscopic debris from the hook tip.
- Rinse and Dry: Rinse thoroughly with sterile or deionized water to remove all cleaning agents, and dry the instrument completely before sterilization.

27.9.4 Sterilization

- Proper sterilization is paramount to prevent infections and ensure the safety of the laparoscopic hook. In accordance with the institution's policy and the guidelines provided by the manufacturers, one may opt for autoclave, ethyl oxide, or plasma sterilization methods.

27.9.5 Storage

- Store instruments in a dry and secure environment.

27.9.6 Routine Maintenance and Replacement

- Periodically, the instrument should undergo more comprehensive inspection and maintenance by trained personnel.
- Regular Insulation Testing: Conduct electrical insulation tests using insulation testers or dielectric strength testers to identify any microcracks or deterioration in the insulation that may not be discernible to the naked eye.
- Replacement of Worn Parts: Replace the instrument or its components (such as the cable or hook tip if possible) when damage is detected.

27.10 Conclusion

Monopolar coagulation instruments are indispensable in laparoscopic surgery. These instruments facilitate precise tissue manipulation, coagulation, and cutting, facilitating hemostasis and tissue dissection. While monopolar energy offers numerous advantages, surgeons must exercise caution and be cognizant of its limitations and potential risks to ensure patient safety and successful surgical outcomes.

By acquiring proficiency in utilizing these instruments and comprehending their applications, limitations, and safety protocols, surgeons can elevate their laparoscopic techniques and enhance patient care.

Retractors and Extractors

28

Wei-Liang Loh

Safe and effective dissection during surgery requires adequate visualization and retraction to enable the surgeon to identify critical structures. Laparoscopic surgery at times necessitates operating within a narrow field with interfering organs and structures. To overcome this, specially crafted laparoscopic retractors have been engineered that allow for safe retraction of tissues in a variety of anatomical locations.

Laparoscopic retractors can be broadly categorized into rigid and articulating types. These, in turn, can be held by an assistant or held in a semifixed, adjustable position by clamp systems in order to provide stability and free up the assistant's hand for other duties.

28.1 Rigid Retractors

They come in many forms. Some of them are described below.

28.2 Nathanson Liver Retractor (Figs. 28.1 and 28.2)

The Nathanson liver retractor is one of the most commonly used retractors and is used mainly for the retraction of the liver lobes. It comes in a variety of sizes and slightly different curves, but the main design is similar. To deploy it, a skin incision is first made, followed by the use of a trocar to create a tract for the intra-abdominal portion of the Nathanson retractor to be inserted. In the case of left liver lobe

W.-L. Loh (✉)
Department of Hepatopancreatobiliary and Transplant Surgery, Singapore General Hospital, Singapore, Singapore

J. S. Ahluwalia (ed.), *User Manual for Minimally Invasive Surgical Equipment*,
https://doi.org/10.1007/978-981-95-9019-3_28

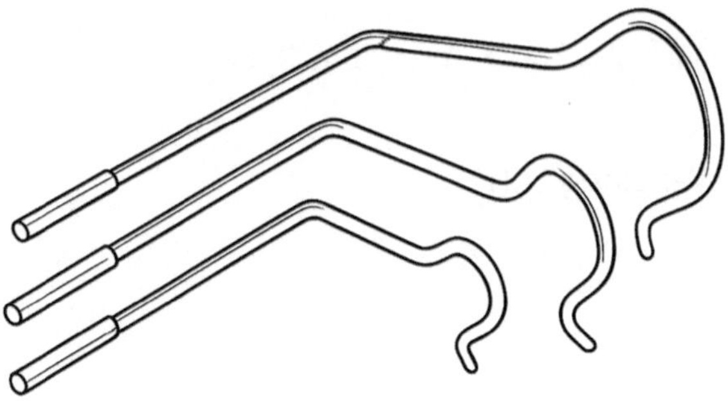

Fig. 28.1 Nathanson liver retractors, in a set of three different sizes

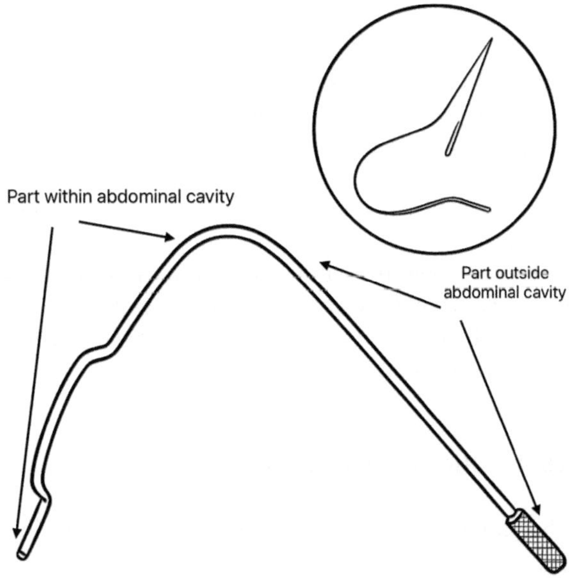

Fig. 28.2 Parts of a Nathanson liver retractor

retraction for upper gastrointestinal surgery, the skin incision is usually in the epigastrium.

The Nathanson retractor is then inserted through the pre-made tract, following the curve of the instrument. The intra-abdominal portion of the retractor is usually placed below the left lobe of the liver, then elevated and held in place with the assistance of a fixed clamp system. The clamp, if used, will be fixed along the shaft of the extra-abdominal portion of the retractor; this allows for steady retraction and frees the assistant up for other duties.

28.3 Adjustable/Articulating Retractors

Besides laparoscopic retractors with a fixed shape or configuration, there are plenty of laparoscopic retractors available on the market that are able to articulate and/or alter their shape in order to provide adequate retraction based on a particular organ or anatomical region.

These retractors usually have a knob at the base or a rotatable handle that allows for the alteration of their head's configuration, while the shaft remains rigid in shape.

Most of these types of retractors are used for liver and esophageal retraction, but they can be easily deployed for use in different situations at the discretion of the surgical team.

28.3.1 Fan and Kite Retractors

Fan retractors are a popular type of articulating retractor, and are commonly used for esophageal and/or liver surgery. Their blade numbers can vary, and some may have a fenestration at the tip for the passing of tape or sutures. A close cousin of the fan retractor is the kite retractor.

The fan and kite retractor tips are inserted collapsed into the abdominal cavity, deployed under vision to avoid inadvertent injury to viscera, then used for retraction and pivoting by the surgeon or assistant.

28.3.2 Gold Finger

The "Gold Finger" was initially used for esophageal surgery or gastric banding. It has a rigid shaft and an adjustable tip that can be deployed into a curved tip using a knob located at the base of the handle. In addition, it also has a groove or cleft at its tip, which facilitates the placement of a suture or tape to allow encirclement of organs or vessels. Its use has now been extended to a variety of laparoscopic procedures, such as hepatopancreatobiliary, colorectal, and gynecological surgeries.

Description:
Set of laparoscopic retractors with adjustable heads (Fig. 28.3).

1. Knobs (1) at the base of the retractor, which, when wound, alter the head's configuration. The head's configuration is initially straight and semiflexible, but gradually becomes more curved and rigid as the knob is wound.
2. Handle (2) of the laparoscopic retractor; this is for the assistant to hold during surgery.
3. Shaft (3) of the laparoscopic retractor; this portion remains rigid even when the head's shape and configuration change. This portion can also be held by a fixed-clamp system in order to reduce reliance on an assistant.
4. Head (4) of the laparoscopic retractor; different shapes and sizes exist commercially.

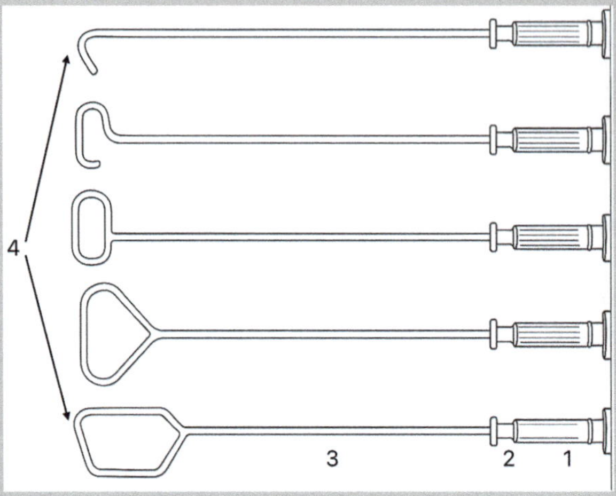

Fig. 28.3 A set of laparoscopic retractors with adjustable heads

Description:
Model of an undeployed fan retractor (Fig. 28.4).

1. This is the adjustable tip (1) of the fan retractor, and is deployed when within the abdominal cavity. The tip shape is variable, and can be straight or curved to different degrees, have a different number of blades, with some having a fenestration for passing sutures or tapes.
2. The shaft of the retractor (2) is rigid and allows for pivoting forces applied from the handle. It will be partly intracorporeal and extracorporeal during its use.
3. This handle (3) remains extracorporeal and is used by the assistant to exert retraction and pivoting forces.
4. The knob (4) for deploying the adjustable tip is usually located at the base of the handle. When turned, it deploys the tip into its functional form while it is intracorporeal (Fig. 28.5).

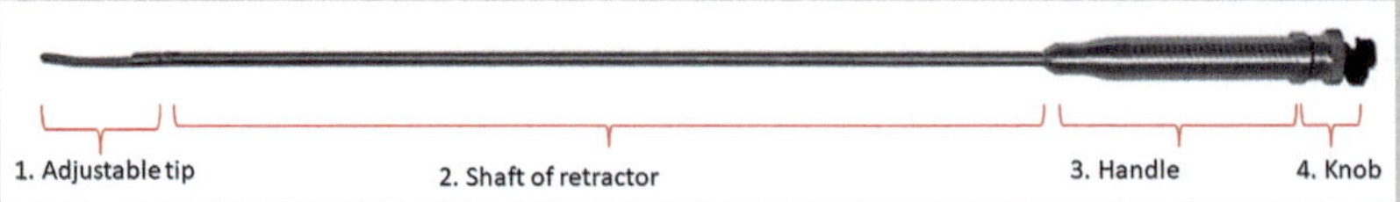

Fig. 28.4 Model of an undeployed fan retractor

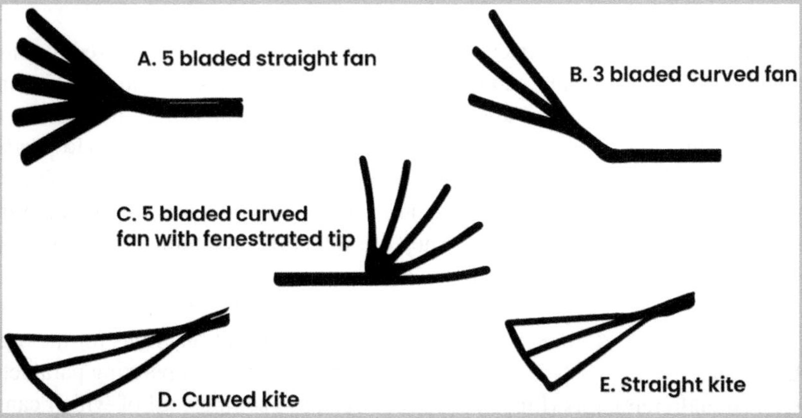

Fig. 28.5 Types of fan and kite tips

Description:
Gold finger (Fig. 28.6).

1. The knob (1) positioned at the base of the handle deploys the adjustable tip while intracorporal.
2. The handle (2) allows for steady retraction and remains extracorporeal.
3. The shaft (3) of the retractor is rigid and allows for pivoting forces applied from the handle. It will be partly intracorporeal and extracorporeal during its use.
4. The adjustable tip (4) of the Gold finger allows for a curvature of almost 180 degrees, facilitating the encirclement of organs and/or vessels.
5. The groove (5) at the tip is used to place a suture or tape, and allows the surgeon to sling the organ or vessel of interest.

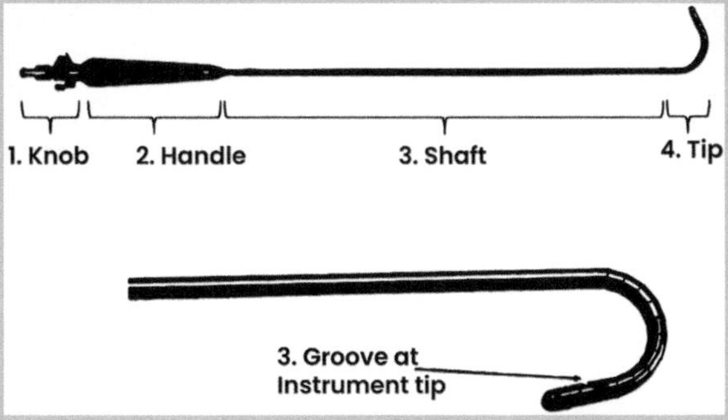

Fig. 28.6 Gold finger

28.3.3 Curved Endo Retractors

Curved endo retractors usually come in different sizes, and can be utilized for either retracting tissues or passing sutures and ties around vessels or critical structures. The curved tip is initially sheathed in its undeployed form within the shaft of the instrument, and upon deployment, extends outwards to form a curved tip. Depending on the model, the deployment is either via a slider on the handle or a knob at the base of the handle. The slider and knob are usually ridged in order to increase friction and aid in the tip's deployment. They usually come in 5 mm and 10 mm sizes.

Description:
Curved endo retractors (Fig. 28.7).

1. This curved retractor tip is initially sheathed within the shaft (2), and deployed when the retractor is intracorporeal by either pushing the slider (3) forward or by twisting the knob (4), depending on the model.
2. This rigid shaft houses the curved retractor tip and its deployment mechanism, and will be partially intracorporeal and extracorporeal during use.
3. This slider, seen in use on the 5 mm model, has ridges and peaks on its surface to increase friction and aid in its use by means of a finger or thumb.
4. This knob, seen in use on the 10 mm model, has ridges to increase friction and aid in its use with a thumb and finger.

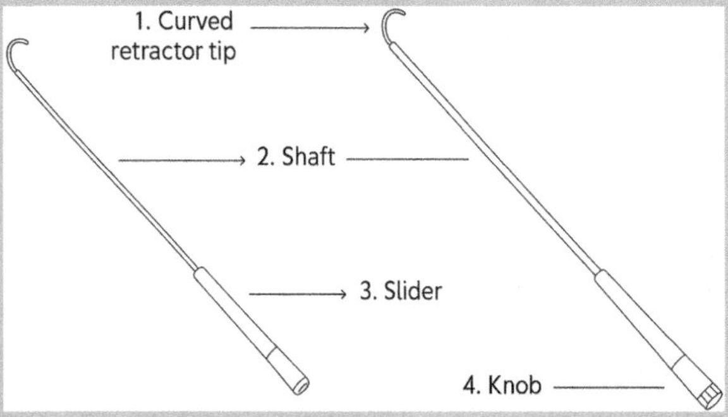

Fig. 28.7 Curved endo retractors (5 mm size on left, 10 mm size on right)

Description:
Paddle retractor (Fig. 28.8).

1. This paddle retractor is deployed via means of twisting the knob (4) at the base of the handle.
2. The rigid shaft houses the paddle retractor in its undeployed form; it is partially intracorporeal and extracorporeal during use.
3. This handle is four-sided and thick to aid in the manoeuvring of the retractor.
4. The knob meant for the paddle deployment is situated at the base of the handle and ridged for extra friction

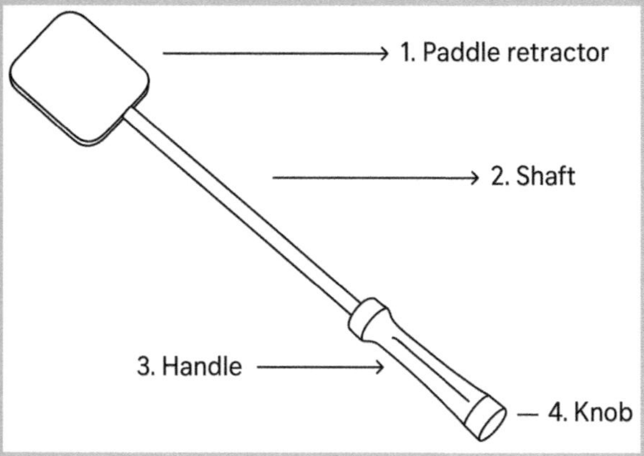

Fig. 28.8 Paddle retractor

28.3.4 Paddle Retractors

Paddle retractors are useful for nontraumatic retraction of a large surface area, and are used for liver and abdominal surgery frequently. The paddle is composed of a fabric that is pulled across a metal frame and a central bar in its deployed form. In its undeployed form, the metal frame and central bar collapse and fold with the fabric, to allow the entire composite structure to fit within a 12 mm shaft. The deployment is by way of a knob at the base of the handle, patterned with ridges to increase friction and surface area.

Description:
Peanut retractor/dissector (Fig. 28.9).

1. The peanut tip is covered in a soft, cloth-like fabric to allow gentle traction and dissection.
2. The shaft and handle are 5 mm in diameter and allow for pivoting forces to be applied to aid in traction and dissection.

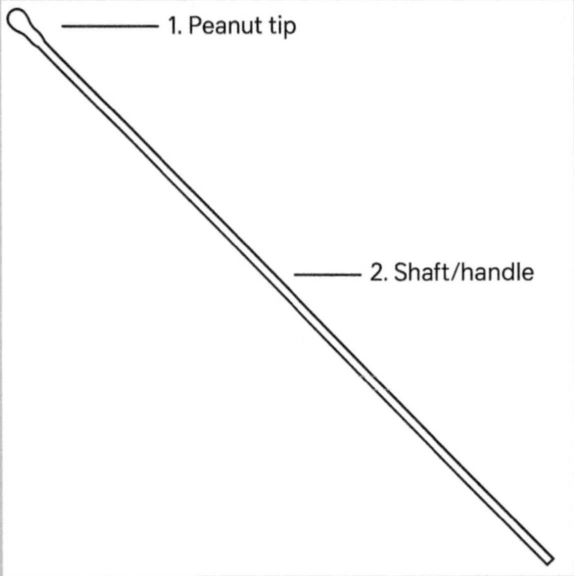

Fig. 28.9 Peanut retractor/dissector

28.3.5 Peanut Retractor/Dissector

The peanut retractor or dissector, is an instrument with a peanut-shaped soft tip. It is used mainly for dissection near critical structures, but can also be utilized as a retractor in tight, critical spaces where fine control is paramount.

Description:
General set-up of a fixed clamp system (Fig. 28.10a, b).

1. This clamp (1) is the initial starting point of the entire system; the indicated lever adjusts the jaws of the clamp and fixes it on to the side bars of the surgical table.
2. These knobs (2) allow the height adjustment of the vertical bars, the next step in the setup of the system

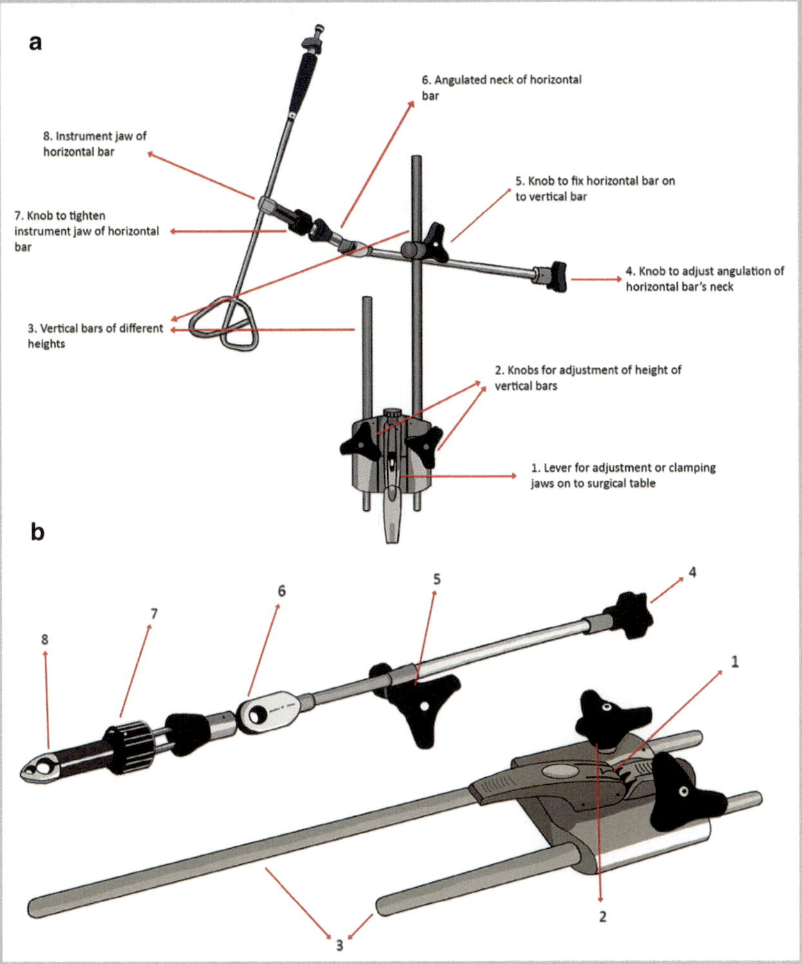

Fig. 28.10 (**a**) General setup of a fixed clamp system. (**b**) Components of a fixed clamp system, disassembled (numbered as per Fig. 28.3a)

(continued)

3. These vertical bars (3) are of different heights, to allow up to two instruments to be fixed using a single system. Their different heights allow for the fixing of their horizontal bars at different levels so as to minimize instrument clashing.
4. This knob (4), located at the back end of the horizontal bar, allows adjustment of its angulated neck.
5. This knob (5) is attached to the shaft of the horizontal bar, is fitted on to the vertical bar from its top end, and allows the fixation of the horizontal bar on to the vertical bar.
6. This is the angulated neck of the horizontal bar (6), and gives it more degrees of freedom when fixating a laparoscopic instrument or laparoscope.
7. This knob (7), close to the instrument jaws of the horizontal clamp, allows for the tightening of the jaws on to the intended laparoscopic instrument or laparoscope.
8. These jaws (8) are usually padded and grasp the laparoscopic instrument or laparoscope in a fixed, stable position.

28.4 Clamp Systems

A fixed clamp system, as alluded to earlier, is a useful tool in ensuring steady and fixed retraction in laparoscopic surgery. It consists of multiple components that is first fixed to the surgical bed, followed by vertical and horizontal bars, and finally instrument clamps on the horizontal bar to hold laparoscopic instruments in a fixed position.

Description:
Example of fixed clamp system (Fig. 28.11a, b).

1. Adjustable jaws (1) used for fixing the vertical bar to the surgical table.
2. Knob (2) on the top end of the vertical bar to close the jaws (1) for secure fixation to the surgical table.
3. Shaft (3) of horizontal bar.
4. Lever (4) attached to the vertical bar, used to secure the horizontal bar at an appropriate height.

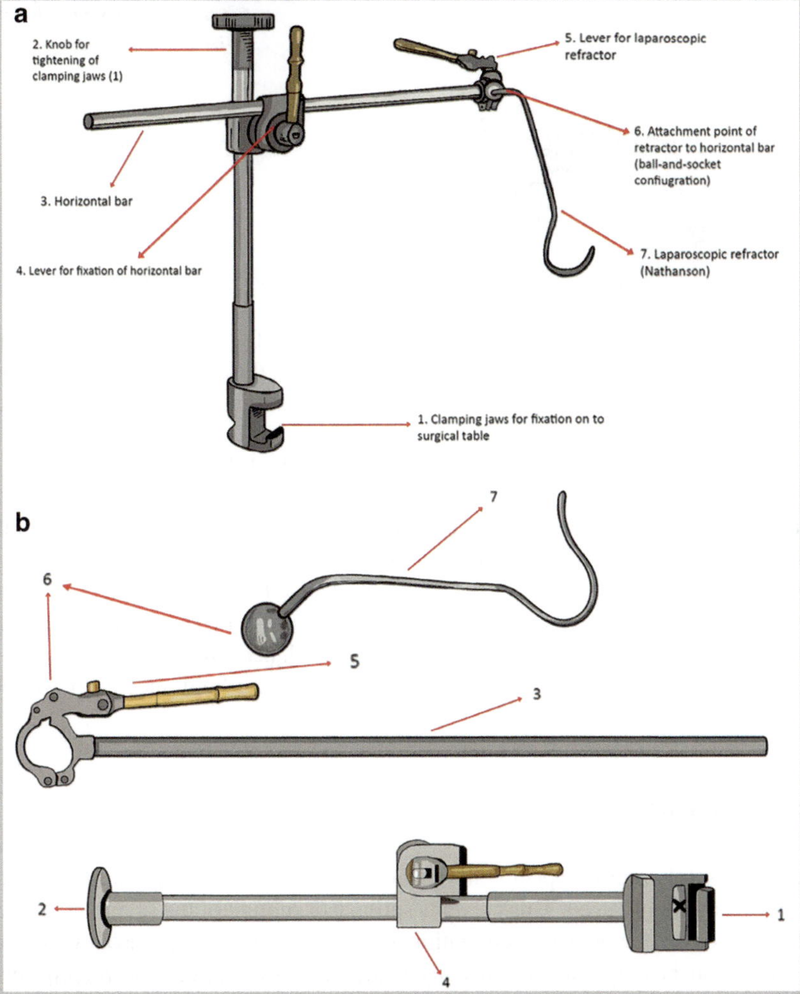

Fig. 28.11 (**a**) General setup of a fixed clamp system. (**b**) Components of fixed clamp system, disassembled (labeled as per figure **a**)

(continued)

5. Lever (5) attached to the patient end of the horizontal bar, for fixation of the laparoscopic retractor
6. Attachment point between the horizontal bar and the laparoscopic retractor. In this particular example, a ball-and-socket configuration can be appreciated.
7. Laparoscopic retractor, a Nathanson-type retractor in this particular example.

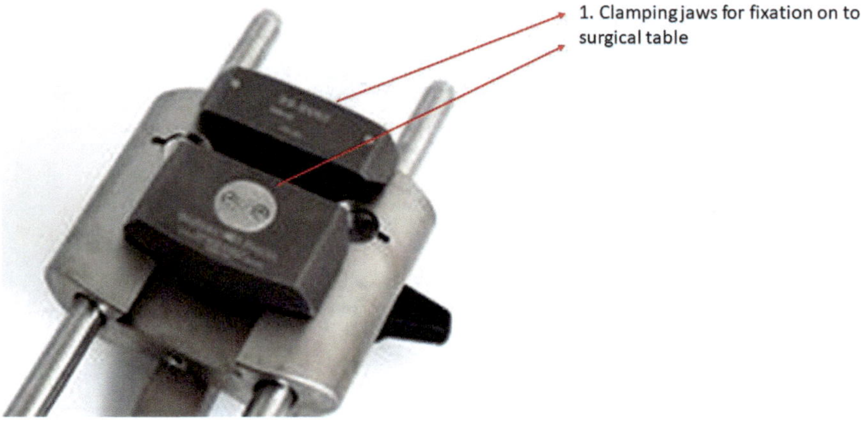

Fig. 28.12 Inner facing side of the table clamp portion of a fixed clamp system

In addition, there are more elaborate fixed-clamp systems, such as a flexible dual-arm fixed-clamp system, which allows the simultaneous securement of up to two laparoscopic instruments or a camera during surgery. This has the potential of freeing up the assistant to concentrate on more critical tasks or reducing the reliance on assistants during surgery. However, this has to be balanced against having too much hardware in the surgical field, which may possibly cause hindrance to the surgical team (Fig. 28.12).

28.5 Extractors

In order to safely remove specimen(s) from the abdomen, an extractor bag or pouch system is commonly used. This prevents spillage or rupture of the specimen, thereby reducing the risk of wound contamination or tumor seeding in the case of malignancy.

These pouches and bags are usually made of plastic, nylon, or synthetic polymers, which have variable amounts of stretch and resistance to tearing. Despite minor differences in their deployment, closure, and retrieval, most retrieval systems are largely similar in their method of usage.

Description:
Flexible dual-arm fixed-clamp system (Fig. 28.13).

1. Clamp (1) for attachment to the side of the surgical table.
2. Knob (2) for tightening of clamp (1) on to surgical table.
3. Vertical bar (3) of the fixed-clamp system.
4. Lever (4) to lock the horizontal bar in place.
5. Horizontal bar (5) of the fixed-clamp system.
6. Clamps and knobs (6) for securing the base of flexible arms on to horizontal bar. It allows for the flexible arms to be distanced appropriately to prevent the clashing of equipment.
7. Knobs (7) to lock flexible arms in position.
8. Flexible arms (8); these arms, while flexible, are also semirigid and allow for the stable position of laparoscopic instruments/camera once fixed in place.
9. Instrument clamps (9) of the flexible arms; these are padded to prevent trauma to the laparoscopic instruments/camera.
10. Laparoscopic instrument/camera (10), which can be secured using this clamp system.

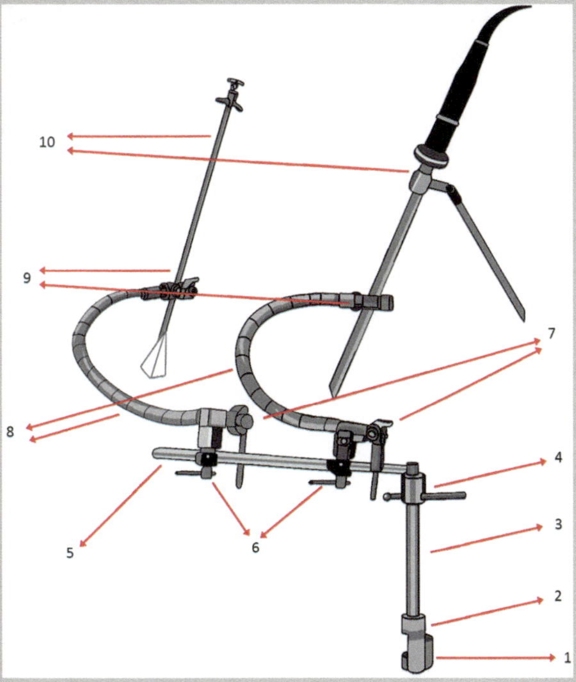

Fig. 28.13 Example of a flexible dual-arm fixed-clamp system

Description:
Example of a pouch retrieval system (Fig. 28.14).

1. Pouch for specimen retrieval. This pouch is collapsed within the plastic sheath (3) during insertion into the abdomen via a port.
2. Opening of pouch. The opening of the pouch is usually ringed by a semi-rigid metal ring that keeps the opening from collapsing. This ring closes and is removed after the specimen is pouched.
3. Plastic sheath. This sheath houses the collapsed pouch during entry into the abdomen. In addition, it houses the strings and pulley mechanism that collapses and deploys the pouch.
4. Plastic flanges. These flanges are meant for the operator's fingers to apply counter-traction as the pouch is deployed by pushing in (6).
5. String for pouch closure. Pulling on this string closes the pouch (1) and collapses the metal ring at the opening of the pouch.
6. Handle: This handle deploys the bag when pushed in and collapses the bag into the sheath (3) when withdrawn.

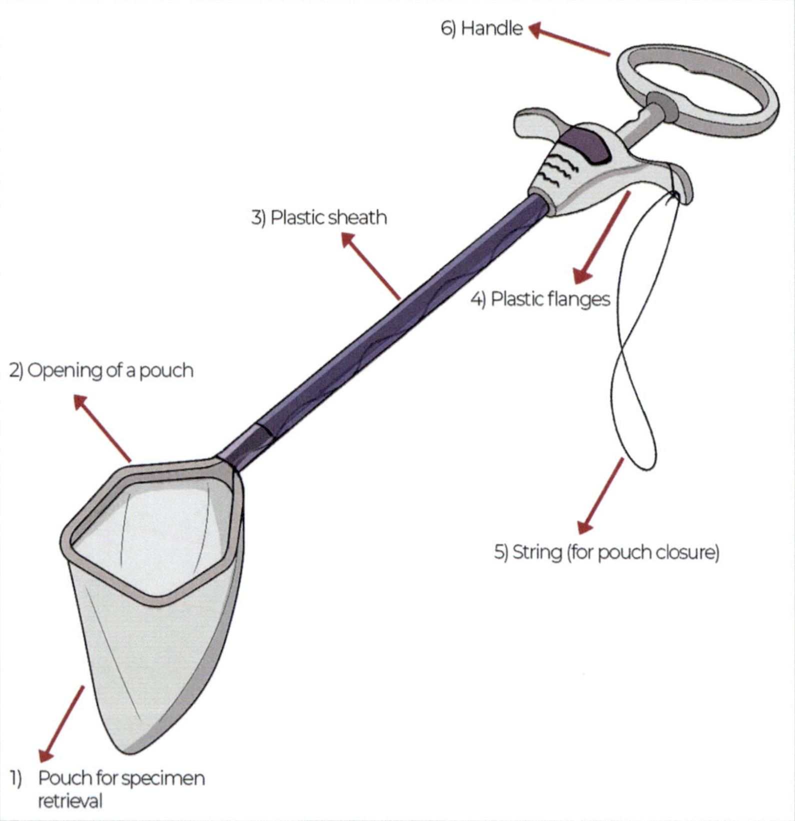

Fig. 28.14 Example of a pouch retrieval system

Description:
Example of a pouch retrieval system (Fig. 28.15).

This pouch is similar to the one showcased in Fig. 28.14. However, the tip of the string is not readily visible in the deployed state.

1. String around the opening of the pouch. This string allows the opening and closure of the pouch's opening by pushing in and withdrawing the handle.
2. Location of tip of string: Once the bag is closed by withdrawing on the handle, the tip of the string appears at this location, and is then grasped and removed from the plastic sheath casing and the rest of the retrieval system.

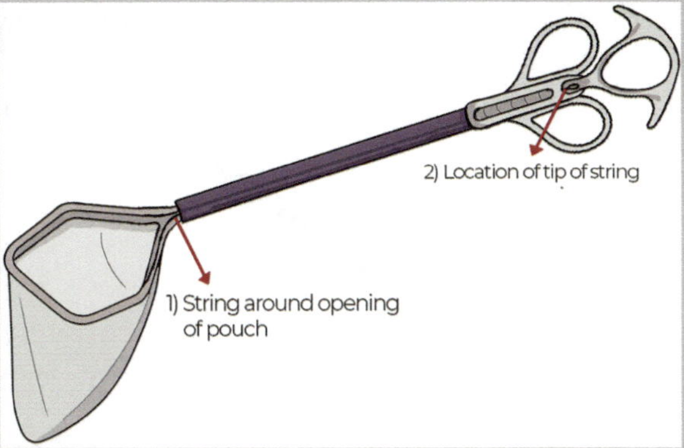

Fig. 28.15 Example of a pouch retrieval system

28.5.1 Pouch Retrieval Systems

Most laparoscopic extractors fall into this category; a bag is first introduced into the abdomen via a port collapsed and sheathed in a plastic trocar, whereby it is deployed or opened intracorporeally, receives the specimen(s), and is then closed.

Once the pouch has been fully closed, the sheath, ring, handles, and levers are removed from the pouch and string. The string attached to the pouch can then be used to extract the pouch. The pouch containing the specimen(s) is brought to the skin surface through the port or via a separate incision for specimen extraction. These pouches can also be utilized in natural orifice specimen extraction (NOSE) procedures, usually transrectally or transvaginally.

These pouches come in varying sizes, from a diameter of 5 mm, 10 mm, 12 mm, 15 mm, and up to 25 mm. Similarly, their capacity ranges from 200 ml to 4 l, allowing the retrieval of specimens of different sizes and volumes.

Description:

Example of a pouch retrieval system (Fig. 28.16).

This pouch is similar to the ones showcased in Figs. 28.14 and 28.15. The pouch is initially sheathed and is deployed by pushing in on (1).

1. Handle with a ring attached to a string. This handle is pushed in to deploy the pouch within the abdomen. Once the specimen has been received, the ring, which is attached to the string pulley system, is withdrawn, hence closing the pouch's opening. The string is then removed from the rest of the plastic sheath and pouch retrieval system.

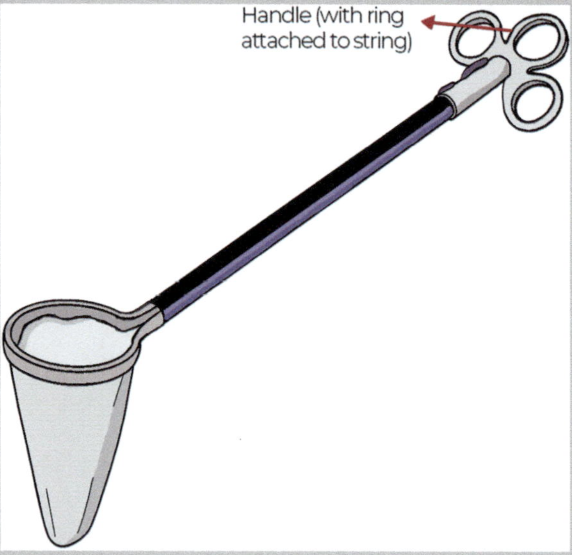

Fig. 28.16 Example of a pouch retrieval system

There are other, less commonly used systems, such as isolated pouches with no strings or handles attached. These can be inserted straight via a port or via a plastic trocar that helps to deliver the pouch into the abdomen. Other pouches come with only a string that enables the closure of its opening; these can either come as they are or be removed from the plastic casing and housing of the previously demonstrated pouch retrieval systems.

Description:
Example of a pouch insertion system (Fig. 28.17).

1. Plastic trocar. This trocar enables the operator to deliver the folded pouch into the abdomen. The pouch is first folded and inserted into the trocar, and the trocar is then inserted into a laparoscopic port, and the pouch is pushed into the abdominal cavity.
2. Pouch, unfolded. This pouch is to be folded and inserted into the trocar (1) before being delivered into the abdomen.

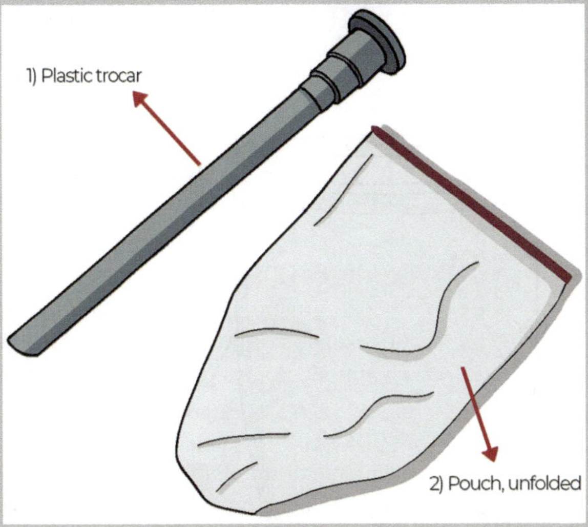

Fig. 28.17 Example of a pouch insertion system

Description:
Example of a pouch insertion system (Fig. 28.18).

1. Pouch: This type of pouches either come packaged in this form or can be extracted from a commercial pouch system as previously described.
2. Pouch opening. The opening is ringed by a string, and the opening can be tightened or closed by pulling on the string.
3. String: Pulling on the string with counter-pressure on the knot at the opening of the pouch allows for closure of the pouch opening. The tip of the string can either be left intracorporeally or extracorporeally, based on the operator's discretion.

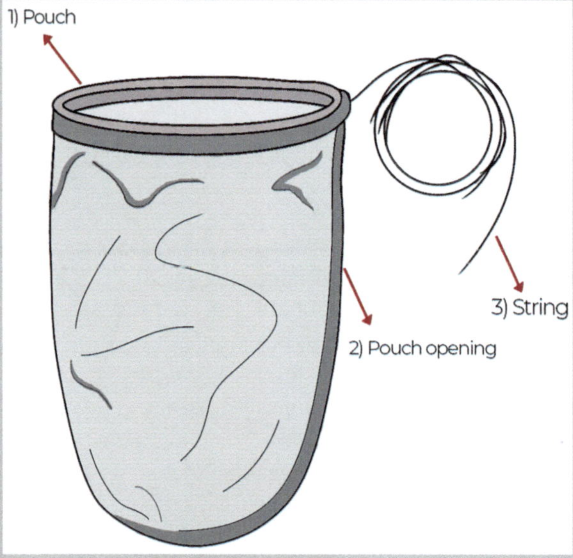

Fig. 28.18 Example of an isolated pouch

28.6 Conclusion

Retractors and extractors are indispensable tools in both open and minimally invasive surgery, playing a crucial role in enhancing visibility, access, and tissue manipulation. While retractors facilitate exposure of the surgical field by displacing tissues safely and effectively, extractors assist in the careful removal of specimens, foreign bodies, or calculi with minimal trauma. The proper selection, handling, and understanding of these instruments are vital for surgical precision, efficiency, and patient safety. As surgical techniques continue to evolve, so too do the designs and capabilities of retractors and extractors—underscoring the need for ongoing familiarity with emerging technologies and their practical applications. Mastery of these tools reflects not just technical skill, but thoughtful surgical judgment.

Tissue Approximation Instruments

29

Mohammad Alqasem Aladaileh and Ancuta Muntean

Throughout history, knots have served various purposes, from primitive uses like trapping animals and crafting weapons to more contemporary applications. In the realm of laparoscopic surgery, the knots employed today are essentially evolved versions of those utilized by seamen, fishermen, weavers, and hangmen. In literature on laparoscopic surgery, the learning curve for mastering the technique is often described as steep. This is because laparoscopy represents not just a novel approach but an entirely distinct method of operating, particularly in terms of tissue approximation. The visualization, instruments, and tactile elements involved in laparoscopy differ significantly from traditional methods. The art of laparoscopic suturing and knotting is a skill that demands extensive practice. Aspiring surgeons dedicate countless nights repetitively tying knots until achieving perfection, illustrating the arduous nature of the learning process. There exist several methods for laparoscopic tissue approximation, with the most commonly employed ones being [1]:

- Laparoscopic extracorporeal and intracorporeal knots
- Laparoscopic loops
- Laparoscopic clips
- Laparoscopic staplers (please refer to a separate chapter on them)

M. A. Aladaileh (✉)
Department of Surgery and Anesthesia, Yarmouk University, Irbid, Jordan

A. Muntean
Paediatric Surgery Department, King's College Hospital, London, UK

J. S. Ahluwalia (ed.), *User Manual for Minimally Invasive Surgical Equipment*,
https://doi.org/10.1007/978-981-95-9019-3_29

29.1 Needle Holder

A laparoscopic needle holder is a surgical instrument designed to facilitate minimally invasive surgical operations by securely holding the suturing needle. These needle holders possess elongated shafts to access deep internal structures through the trocar. Their serrated jaws provide a firm grip on the needle, enabling delicate handling during suture passage through tissue. Most models incorporate a ratcheting mechanism to lock the needle in position, enhancing stability during suturing. Additionally, ergonomic needle holders are available to reduce hand fatigue during extended surgical procedures. Some ergonomic holders incorporate a rotary mechanism, allowing surgeons to adjust the needle's angle without interrupting their work [2].

Here are the descriptions for the main parts of laparoscopic needle holders (Fig. 29.1):

1. Handle

The handle of the laparoscopic needle holder is designed to facilitate manipulation in the surgeon's hand. Handles can be equipped with various combinations of thumb rings, finger grips, and palm-held structures, tailored to meet the surgeon's specific requirements for precise movements. Additionally, some handles offer the option of rotation, allowing for adjustment of the instrument's angle without altering the surgeon's hand position.

Types of Handles

1. *Scissor-Style (Ring) Handle*: This surgical instrument bears a resemblance to traditional scissors, featuring two finger loops for thumb and finger insertion. Consequently, many surgeons find transitioning to this design more convenient than open surgeries. It provides excellent control and precision, facilitating the manipulation of the needle holder with ease. However, a significant challenge

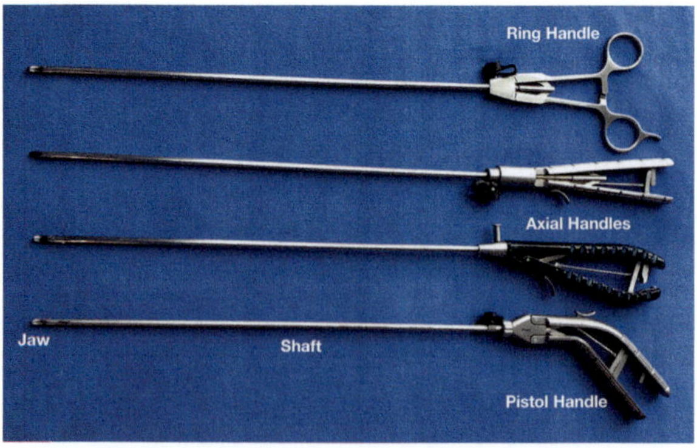

Fig. 29.1 Needle holders

arises from the potential for hand fatigue during extended surgeries due to sustained finger tension.

2. *Axial Handle (In-Line)*: The handle and the instrument shaft are in a straight line, offering an axial or pen-like grip. The entire palm can be used for gripping, making it more ergonomic to decrease fatigue. Being in-line with the tip, movements of the hand reflect well at the tip. This provides high precision, ideal for delicate procedures where small, controlled movements are necessary. May not offer as much comfort as a pistol grip and may not provide same level of fine control as ring handles under certain situations.
3. *Pistol Grip Handle*: Designed to resemble a pistol, the surgeon's handle is fully grasped, similar to holding a firearm. This ergonomic design provides a more relaxed grip and reduces wrist fatigue. It enables comfortable suturing in challenging areas and during extended use. It may not only provide the same level of precise control as ring handles in certain situations but also it may require some adjustment for the surgeon to adopt its angled position.
4. *Rotating Handle with Locking Mechanism*: Typically integrated into other handle designs, the rotating mechanism allows the needle holder's jaws to rotate 360 degrees without moving the surgeon's hand. This provides increased manoeuvrability and precise control over needle orientation.

2. Shaft

The shaft is a cylindrical component of the laparoscopic needle holder, situated between the handle and the jaws of the instrument. It is typically constructed from stainless steel or a comparable material that resists deformation in harsh environments, such as corrosion or sterilization. The shaft's slender design enables its use in small puncture sites or ports ranging from 5 to 10 mm in minimally invasive surgical procedures. Additionally, shafts incorporate an internal mechanism that transmits the surgeon's hand movements to the jaws, facilitating holding and locking of the needle.

3. Jaws

The jaws of a laparoscopic needle holder are also a crucial part of the instrument, designed to grasp and manipulate the surgical needle during suturing. They come in straight and curved designs to provide optimal control, precision, and needle stability. Here are the key features:

1. *Straight Jaws*: These are straight with no curvature, allowing for direct manipulation of the needle. This allows for more straightforward control of the needle and is best for general suturing where angulation is not required, as they are easier to control for simple suturing tasks. Same needle holder can be used for left or right-handed surgeon.

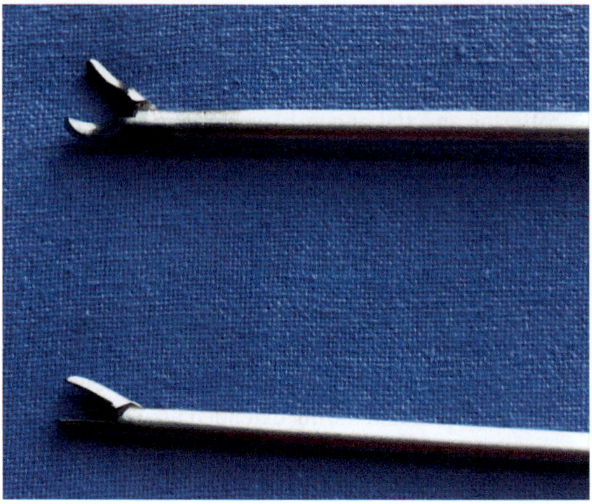

Fig. 29.2 Curved (above) and straight (below) jaws

2. *Curved Jaws*: The jaws are curved inward, allowing for better positioning and control of the needle and facilitates suturing in areas that are difficult to reach with straight jaws, such as tight or angled spaces. They also may provide better needle angulation and make it easier to rotate suture around the jaw. Curvature helps in knotting as well. But they may require more practice to master compared to straight jaws.

The inside of the jaws is usually serrated and may be made of tungsten carbide to enhance grip on the needle and longevity. For delicate needles, one may opt for smooth jaws.

Depending on individual procedural characteristics, tissue type, and needle size, a particular type of tip of the instrument can be chosen to ensure the best results in suturing (see Fig. 29.2).

29.2 Knot Pusher

A laparoscopic knot pusher is a specialized instrument employed in minimally invasive surgical procedures to facilitate knot tying and secure sutures within the abdominal cavity. Its primary function is to reduce the physical effort required for knotting, thereby enhancing the efficiency and comfort of the surgical process [3] (Fig. 29.3).

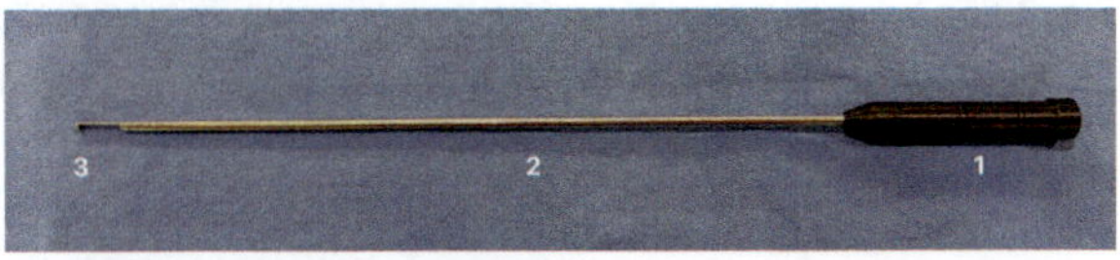

Fig. 29.3 Parts of a laparoscopic knot pusher (1—Handle, 2—Shaft, and 3—Tip)

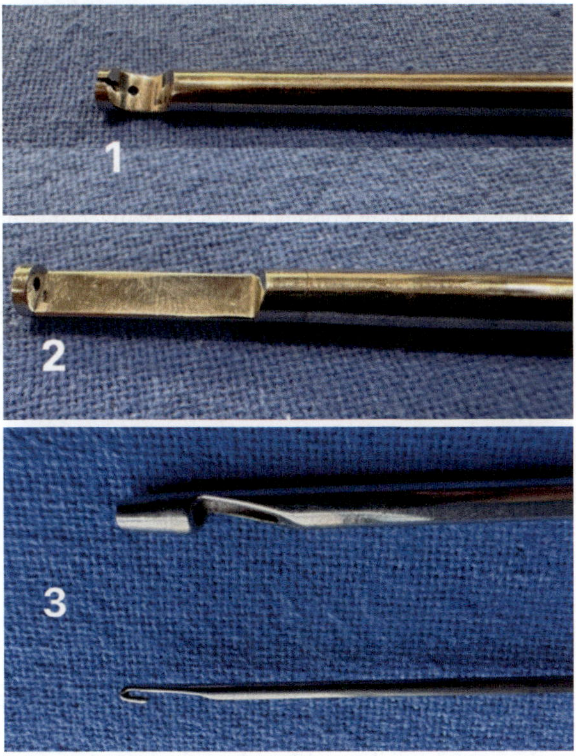

Fig. 29.4 Types of tips of knot pusher: 1—Grooved, 2—Closed-loop, and 3—Hooked

1. Handle

   The portion of the surgical instrument that the surgeon typically holds is meticulously designed to offer a secure and comfortable grip.
2. Shaft

   The elongated and slender portion of the instrument that enables it to penetrate the abdominal cavity while maintaining external control.
3. Tip

   The terminal end of the knot pusher, which interacts with the suture to secure the knot, is designed to accommodate the specific type of knots the instrument is intended to manipulate. The design of the tip may be grooved, closed loop, or hooked (Fig. 29.4).

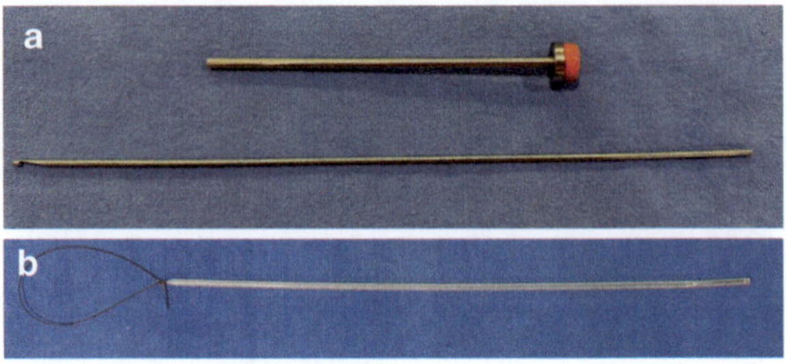

Fig. 29.5 Loop applicators: (**a**) Reusable and (**b**) Single-use preformed loop

29.3 Loop Applicator

A laparoscopic loop applicator is a specialized instrument used to apply pre-tied suture loops (often called ligature loops or endo-loops) around tissues, vessels, or structures during minimally invasive surgeries. The main advantage is that a ligature can be placed without requiring a knot to be manually tied by the surgeon. These loops are preloaded on the applicator and can be tightened around the targeted structure by advancing the applicator shaft. Loop applicators are commonly used in procedures such as appendectomies, cholecystectomies, and vessel ligations, where it is necessary to securely tie off tissues without direct manipulation [4].

Key Features

Single-Use vs. Reusable Options: Loop applicators are commonly available as single-use sterile instruments with a pretied suture loop at their distal end. However, reusable versions exist that can be loaded with new loops for repeated use.

Tightening Mechanism: The suture loop can be tightened by pulling the suture outwards and pushing the tip toward the target. One must maintain control so that the loop gets tightened exactly at the target area.

Loop Sizes and Materials: The loop material selection depends on the tissue type, and options include absorbable sutures (such as polydioxanone) and nonabsorbable materials (such as polypropylene) in various diameters (Fig. 29.5).

29.4 Endostitch

The laparoscopic Endo Stitch (trademark of Medtronic) device is a specialized suturing instrument meticulously engineered to streamline the suturing process during minimally invasive or laparoscopic surgeries. In contrast to conventional suturing techniques that necessitate intricate hand movements within confined spaces, the Endo Stitch device automates the needle manipulation, facilitating suturing in restricted areas with enhanced speed and precision [5] (Fig. 29.6).

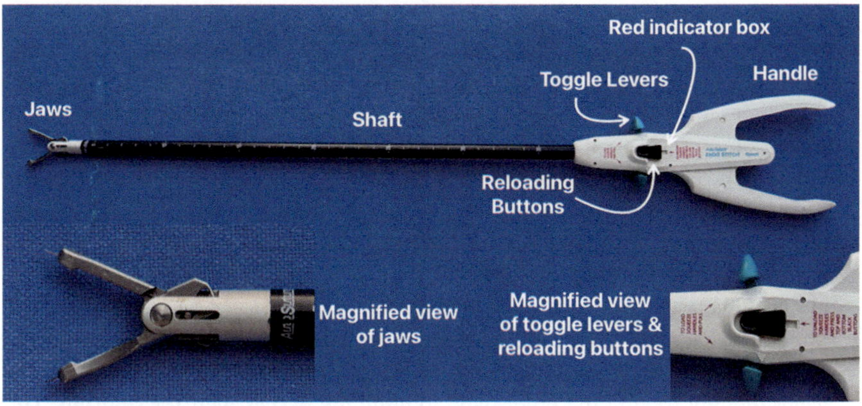

Fig. 29.6 Parts of Endo Stitch

Parts of Endo Stitch

1. Handle: The handle incorporates a trigger mechanism that enables the surgeon to control the needle's movement, allowing it to reciprocate between the jaws. Pressing the toggle lever transfers the needle from one jaw to the other, facilitating stitch placement. Toggle levers can be operated only when the jaws are closed by pressing the handle.
2. Shaft: The shaft, a long and narrow tube, serves as a conduit for the suture and needle mechanism to function effectively within the limited confines of the device. It has a scale marked on it to help the surgeon to cut the suture to the desired length.
3. Jaws: The jaws hold and pass the needle between each other. The needle is passed through the tissue and trigger mechanism is activated to pass the needle to the other jaw. Similarly, passing of needle from one jaw to the other helps in framing of knots. They work in tandem to complete the stitch. The jaws are designed to grip the needle and suture material without excessive force, helping reduce tissue trauma.
4. Needle and Suture Cartridge: This is a preloaded cartridge that contains both the suture and the needle. This sterile cartridge is loaded into the device before the procedure.

Needle Passing Mechanism This is an intricate mechanism in the jaws that automatically passes the needle back and forth. Each jaw has grooves or indentations to hold the needle securely during the pass.

Suture Material The cartridge is available with various types and lengths of sutures (absorbable or nonabsorbable) depending on the specific surgical requirements. Even barbed sutures have been made available recently.

Advantages of Endo Stitch

- Improved Ergonomics: The device is likely to reduce strain on the surgeon's hand and wrist, as compared to other designs of needle holders which use traditional sutures and needles.
- Reduced Procedure Time: The ease of certain suturing processes, like passing of a needle from one jaw to the other by Endo Stitch device, can help in decreasing the duration of surgical procedures. The needle always remains in contact with the instrument, and there is no need for frequent grasping of the needle or adjusting its angle.
- Single Handed Operation: The device is designed to allow the surgeon to pass the needle through tissue and also to grasp the needle after passage by using one hand, thereby freeing the other hand to align the tissues well for suturing. This may enhance comfort, speed, and precision.

Loading the Needle Start by keeping the jaws open with the metal bars fully extended. The teal toggle levers should be forward, and the red indicator boxes fully exposed. Insert the jaws into the single-use loading unit and press down at the apex to seat them. With one hand, completely squeeze the handles while the other pulls both toggle levers back from the jaws until a click confirms the needle is loaded. The red indicator boxes are covered by a black button. Gently press the tab at the top of the loading unit to release the jaws. Unreel the suture from the spool and, if desired, manually cut it to length using the scale on the shaft. Before use, test the needle's seating by passing it back and forth between the jaws. If it doesn't pass smoothly, unload and reload the needle [5].

Unloading the Needle Align the toggle levers with the arrows on the handles' bodies by squeezing them together. Then simultaneously press the two black reloading buttons on the instrument's front and rear. Slide the buttons forward to reveal the red indicator boxes. Place the instrument's jaws over a suitable needle disposal site, release the handles and remove the needle. The instrument is now ready for reloading [5].

29.5 Clip Applicator

A laparoscopic clip applicator is used to secure clips onto blood vessels, ducts, or other tubular structures. These clips serve as a means of controlling bleeding or closing off structures by exerting a pinching force, thereby facilitating hemostasis or sealing during surgical interventions (Fig. 29.7).

Parts of Clip Applicator

1. Handle: The handle is used to control the positioning of the clip applicator and to apply clips by squeezing them together.

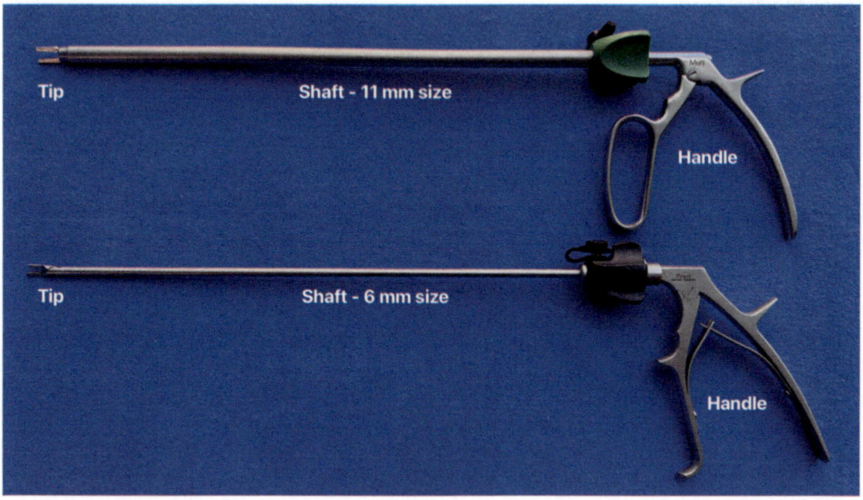

Fig. 29.7 Clip applicators (reusable)

2. Shaft: The slender, elongated, tube-like shaft facilitates access to internal structures through small incisions or ports.
3. Jaws: The jaws at the applicator's tip securely hold and align the clip around the target structure. Activation of the handle triggers the jaws to close, thereby pinching them onto the target structure.

Clip Loading Most disposable applicators are preloaded with multiple clips, which remain securely held until required. Upon each clip application, the device automatically advances to the next clip. Most reusable applicators can load a single clip at a time, and a new clip has to be loaded after each application. They can be directly loaded to the clip applicator tip just by pushing the jaws against the cartridge of clips.

Types of Clips

- Titanium Clips: These clips are commonly utilized due to their exceptional strength and compatibility with body tissues. They do not have any locking mechanism as they hold their position once pressed.
- Polymer Clips: These may be absorbable or nonabsorbable. They usually have a locking mechanism that holds them in position once locked, as polymers otherwise cannot hold. Locking mechanism also makes them preferred choice for larger vessels which may not be properly occluded with titanium clips. These clips can also be employed for improved visibility during imaging procedures and to minimize interference with MRI scans [6–8].

Troubleshooting

Problem	Possible cause	Troubleshooting steps
Clip misfire (clip not deploying properly)	Misaligned jaws Improper clip loading Faulty applicator	Check jaw alignment and remove any obstruction Ensure clips are loaded and aligned properly Replace applicator if needed
Incomplete or partial clip closure	Insufficient closing force Worn mechanism Oversized clip for structure	Apply adequate closing pressure Replace the instrument Use appropriately sized clips
Applicator fails to release the clip after closure	Debris on the jaws Defective applicator	Clean the jaws Replace instrument
Loss of clip retention in the jaws	Debris on the jaws Defective applicator Clip not compatible with applicator due to size or design	Clean the jaws Replace instrument Ensure compatibility

29.6 Troubleshooting

Issues may arise due to improper maintenance, wear and tear, or handling errors. Below are some common problems and solutions for troubleshooting a laparoscopic needle holder:

1. Jaws Not Closing Properly: Remove any tissue or debris between the jaws or at joints. If the jaws are misaligned or the locking mechanism is not working properly, instrument may need professional repair or replacement.
2. Needle Slippage: Make sure the needle holder is fully locked before passing suture from tissue and needle is properly aligned for the job. But if this is because of worn-out jaws or improper alignment of the jaws, it will need repair or replacement.
3. Difficulty Locking/Unlocking the Needle Holder: Make sure there is no debris in the ratchet mechanism. Thoroughly clean and lubricate the ratchet mechanism to ensure smooth operation. A worn-out or damaged ratchet mechanism will need repair or replacement.
4. Inability to Hold Fine Needles: Inspect the jaws for wear or damage. Try using smooth or atraumatic jaws designed for delicate needles and fine sutures.
5. Instrument Too Stiff: Poor cleaning is the usual culprit leading to the buildup of debris or dried biological material. Others could be a lack of lubrication in the hinge or moving parts. Rule out rust or corrosion as well. Clean the needle holder thoroughly, paying attention to the hinge and moving parts and lubricate well. Inspect for corrosion or rust, which may require replacement if severe.

29.7 Maintenance

Needle holders are typically more expensive than other laparoscopic hand instruments. Regular maintenance is crucial in extending their lifespan and ensuring optimal performance.

1. Cleaning: Always clean the needle holder immediately after use to remove any blood, tissue, or debris that may interfere with its function.
2. Sterilization: Follow manufacturer guidelines and hospital protocols for sterilization to avoid damage caused by excessive heat or improper chemicals.
3. Inspection: Before and after every procedure, check the instrument for signs of wear, misalignment, or damage to ensure it is in good working condition.
4. Servicing: If issues persist, send the instrument to a professional for servicing or repair to ensure it is functioning optimally.

29.8 Popular Styles of Laparoscopic Knot Pushers

1. Grooved or Slotted Knot Pusher

   The grooved knot pusher features a small groove, slot, or notch at its tip, where the suture remains securely positioned when the surgeon advances the knot. Its simplicity and ease of use for both extracorporeal and intracorporeal knots are notable advantages. However, the surgeon must exercise caution to prevent the suture from dislodging from the groove as the knot is directed toward the target.
2. Closed-Loop Knot Pusher

   This type of knot pusher has a loop or ring at the end of it, through which the suture is passed, and it pushes the knot along the line of the thread. The closed-loop configured design provides for secure suture grip while advancing the knot. But it can only be used for extracorporeal suturing.
3. Hooked Knot Pusher

   It has a small hook at the tip that helps in feeding the suture across the knot pusher and may also guide the knot down. The hook securely holds the knot, allowing it to be pushed down without slipping. Both extracorporeal and intracorporeal knot tying, especially in tight or hard-to-reach spaces, are possible.

29.9 Troubleshooting Knot Pusher

Problems while using a knot pusher can involve a range of mechanical and technique-related issues. Here are some common problems and their solutions:

1. Knot Hard to Slide: Make sure there is no blood or tissue clogging the mechanism. The suture should not be too thick to slide. The knot should be properly tied and amenable to slide.

2. Knot Slipping Off the Pusher: Make sure the technique of handling of the suture is proper, and the knot is not too thin for the pusher. Always hold slight tension on the suture with one hand while using the knot pusher with the other to maintain control.
3. Knot Not Securing Tightly: Make sure the knot has been fashioned properly to be used with a knot pusher, and the pusher fully engages the knot.

References

1. Laparoscopic tissue approximation techniques. 2009. Available from: https://www.laparoscopyhospital.com/~rkmishra/fewbookpdf/laparoscopic-tissue-approximation-techniques.pdf.
2. Chu CC, von Fraunhofer JA, Greisler HP, editors. Wound closure biomaterials and devices. Boca Raton: CRC Press; 2018.
3. Baumgarten KM, Wright RW. Arthroscopic knot tying: an instruction manual. Philadelphia: Lippincott Williams & Wilkins; 2005.
4. Schollmeyer T, Mettler L, Ruther D, Alkatout I, editors. Practical manual for laparoscopic & hysteroscopic gynecological surgery. London: JP Medical Ltd.; 2013.
5. Covidien Endo-Surgery. EndoStitch user manual [Internet]. ManualsLib. [cited 2025 Nov 27]. Available from: https://www.manualslib.com/manual/1958590/Covidien-Endo-Stitch.html.
6. Soper NJ, Scott-Conner CE, editors. The SAGES manual: basic laparoscopy and endoscopy, vol. 1. New York: Springer Science & Business Media; 2012.
7. Jain SK, Stoker DL, Tanwar R. Basic surgical skills and techniques. London: JP Medical Ltd.; 2018.
8. Smith AD, editor. Smith's textbook of endourology. PMPH-USA; 2007.

30 Video-Assisted Thoracoscopic Surgery Equipment

Narendran Balasubbiah

30.1 Introduction to Video-Assisted Thoracoscopic Surgery (VATS)

Video-assisted thoracoscopic surgery (VATS) refers to the performance of thoracic surgery using endoscopes or small incisions, typically with no rib spreading, and almost always with scopes for visualization (Fig. 30.1). The common early procedures were pleural-based to evaluate fluid, perform pleural biopsies, or deal with simple lung issues like spontaneous pneumothoraces. Thoracoscopy took on the term video-assisted thoracic surgery, VATS, as many procedures were hybrid types, using small thoracotomies with scope assistance. This procedure evolved from mini-thoracotomies with rib spreading, to eventually the elimination of the rib spreading and using the projected picture (no longer looking through the open incision into the thoracic cavity) to guide the entire procedure. After many years of experience, it became established that oncologic principles were followed, including adequate nodal dissection, and VATS lobectomy became accepted. These complex procedures would not have evolved without the advances in instruments to perform VATS.

The specific instruments that are used in a particular VATS procedure will vary depending on the type of surgery being performed. For example, a VATS lung lobectomy will require different instruments than a VATS mediastinal tumor excision. VATS instruments are designed to be angled at the tip, small and lightweight, so that they can be easily inserted through small incisions on the chest wall, enabling surgeons to perform surgery with precision and accuracy. VATS instruments have revolutionized the way thoracic surgery is performed. They allow surgeons to

N. Balasubbiah (✉)
Hospital Raja Permaisuri Bainun, Ipoh, Malaysia

Department of Surgery, Thoracic Unit, Kuala Lumpur General Hospital, Kuala Lumpur, Malaysia

J. S. Ahluwalia (ed.), *User Manual for Minimally Invasive Surgical Equipment*,
https://doi.org/10.1007/978-981-95-9019-3_30

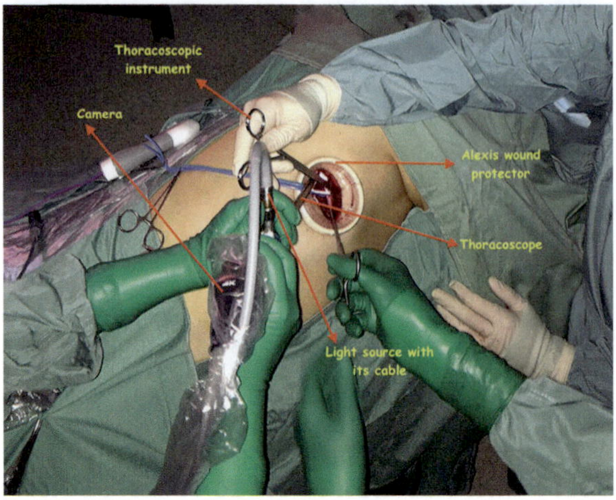

Fig. 30.1 Uniportal VATS surgery with the instruments and wound protector used during surgery

perform minimally invasive surgery, which can lead to shorter recovery times, less pain, and improved cosmesis for patients.

Here is a list of instruments that are commonly used in VATS:

- Trocars and obturators (Thoracoport).
- Thoracoscope.
- Camera.
- Light source.
- Video monitor.
- Surgical instruments, such as forceps, scissors, and staplers.
- Needle holders.
- Irrigation and suction devices.
- Vessel sealing device (described in other chapters).
- Electrocautery unit (described in other chapters) (Fig. 30.1).

30.2 Thoracoport (Fig. 30.2)

Thoracoport consists of an outer hollow cannula and an inner obturator. They are then used to insert the other instruments into the chest cavity after removal of the obturator from the inner cannula.

- Obturators are usually sharp (current newer generations come with blunt tip) pointed blades that are used to create small incisions in the chest wall.
- Cannulas are hollow tubes which functions to hold the other instruments in place. Cannulas come in a variety of sizes, depending on the size of the instruments that will be inserted through them.

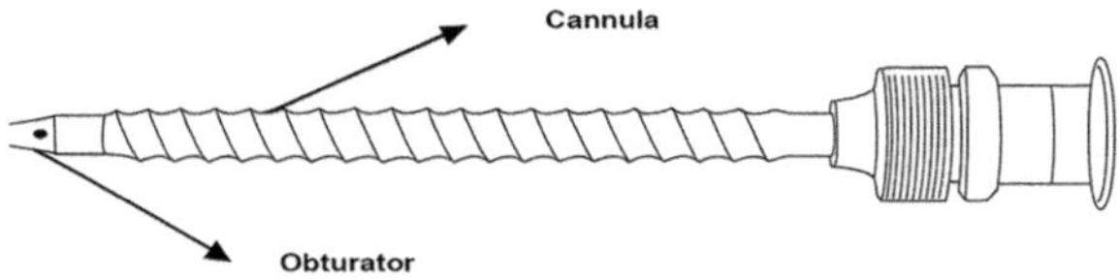

Fig. 30.2 Thoracoport with the obturator and cannula used in VATS. (Picture selfcreated)

- Use of a thoracoscopic port helps reduce the possibility of nerve damage occurring from instruments traumatizing the intercostal space and helps protect thoracoscopic equipment passed into the thoracic cavity.
- The major difference between the laparoscopic port and the thoracoport is the length of the cannula and the trocar. The length of the thoracoport is shorter, measuring 3–5 cm and the luminal diameter is larger. In patient with thick chest wall, longer ports can be used replacing the standard thoracoport if the instrument size can enter through it into the thoracic cavity.

30.2.1 Maintenance

- Correct sized thoracoport is used for the instrument that is required to pass through it into the thorax. If the instrument Is larger than the port, it will be tight and the cannula will get damaged.
- Thoracoport cannula is always inserted with the trocar to prevent its leading edge getting damaged by tissues. Even in the case where the cannula slips out from the thoracic cavity, the cannula is reinserted back with the trocar to prevent damaging the cannula as well as the intercostal neurovascular bundle which can get caught into the cannula lumen.

30.2.2 Trouble Shooting

- If the cannula keeps slipping out, the incision made could be too large. Use a purse string around the port to tighten it.
- To prevent cannula slipping during insertion and removal of instruments, use a threaded cannula which has traction on the soft tissue at insertion site.
- If more instruments or a larger sized instruments need to go into the thorax to work, convert the port access to a larger size or use wound protector.

30.3 Thoracoscope

- It is a thin, tube-like scope that is inserted into the chest cavity through a thoracoport or wound protector. The thoracoscope allows the surgeon to see inside the chest cavity on a video monitor. It comes mainly in 2 diameter size, 5 millimeters, and 10 millimeters scope. The front lens is situated at two types of angles commonly; zero degree and the 30 degrees. The 30-degree camera angle is the preferred choice in VATS (Fig. 30.3).

30.3.1 Maintenance

- The thoracoscope should be handled gently and the tip whereby the lens is situated must never be placed on any sharp or hard objects. If the need arises to place the thoracoscope on the operation tray, gauze piece must be placed covering the tip so that it does not get damaged or scratched.
- The telescope must always be passed from the nurse to the surgeon, and vice versa with both hands to avoid accidentally dropping it.

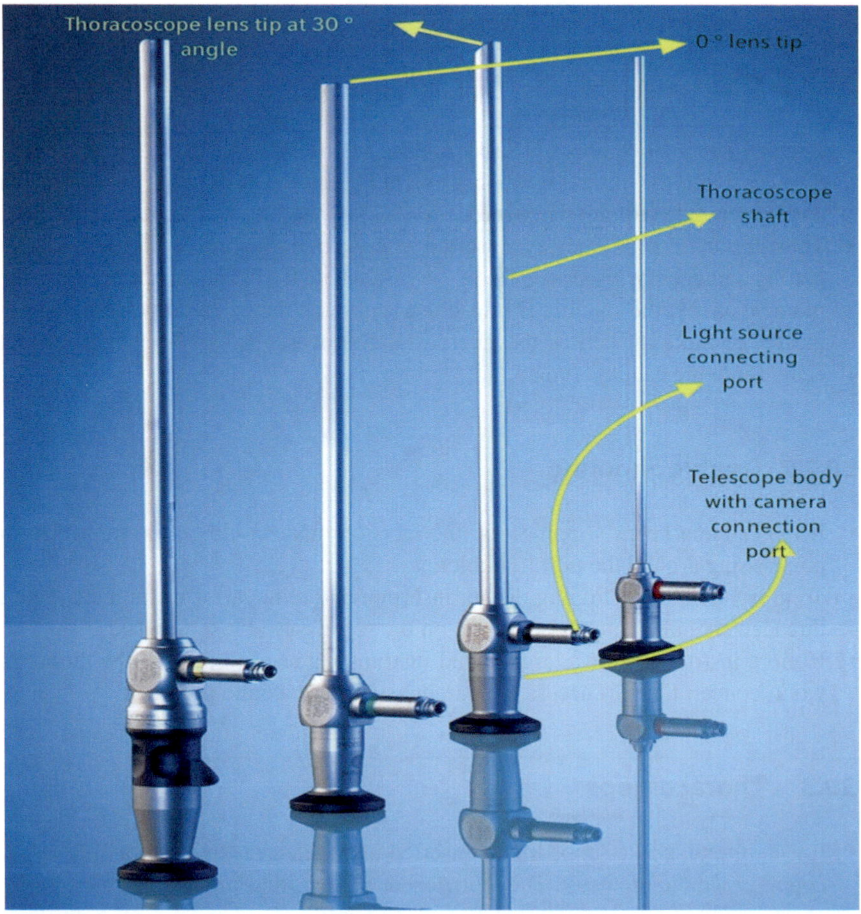

Fig. 30.3 Thirty-degree angled telescope or thoracoscope in VATS. (Image with permission from Karl Storz)

- The thoracoscope once sterilized, must be kept in the operating room temperature to avoid condensation on both the camera port and the lens tip.

30.3.2 Trouble Shooting

- The lens tip will get cloudy due to condensation whenever there is drastic temperature change between the outside environment which is cold and the thoracic cavity. Besides the smoke and mist formation in the thoracic cavity is another issue causing the surgeon to lose clear operating visualization. There are two main techniques to counter this issue:
  - Prepare a flask with hot water and immerse the lens tip into it for a short moment about 5 seconds. Wipe the tip dry with a gauze then wipe the lens with antifog solution.
  - (*Tips*: If antifog solution is not available, use chlorhexidine in 70% alcohol and pour it into a gallipot. Place a gauze piece into the gallipot and rub the lens tip of the thoracoscope and gently wipe the access solution distorting the image with dry gauze. This step is done right after hot water flask immersion).
  - Another technique is smoke ventilation technique. There is a simple, easy and cost-effective surgical smoke ventilation technique for uniportal video-assisted thoracoscopic surgery (uVATS) using a suction catheter to reduce the problem of lens tip condensation as described below (Fig. 30.4).

30.4 VATS Instruments (Figs. 30.5 and 30.6)

The instruments take their name based on the working tip jaw. The parts of VATS instruments is labeled in the diagram 12.

The difference between the laparoscopic and the VATS instruments are:

1. The fulcrum (moving joint of the instrument) of the VATS instrument is positioned further away from the working tip compared to laparoscopic instruments, where the fulcrum is situated closer to the tip.
2. The instrument is curved near to the distal fulcrum joint. This is to facilitate the working of the instrument within thoracic cavity to reduce fighting and scissoring disturbance (Figs. 30.7, 30.8, 30.9, 30.10, 30.11 and Table 30.1).

30.5 VATS Sucker

This is quite a versatile instrument. Besides using as a suction device of fluids in the surgical field, it is used for retraction, blunt dissection, compression for hemostasis, squeezing the lung for deflation, guiding and maneuvering stapler application, localization of nodules on the lung subpleural surface, finding planes of dissection,

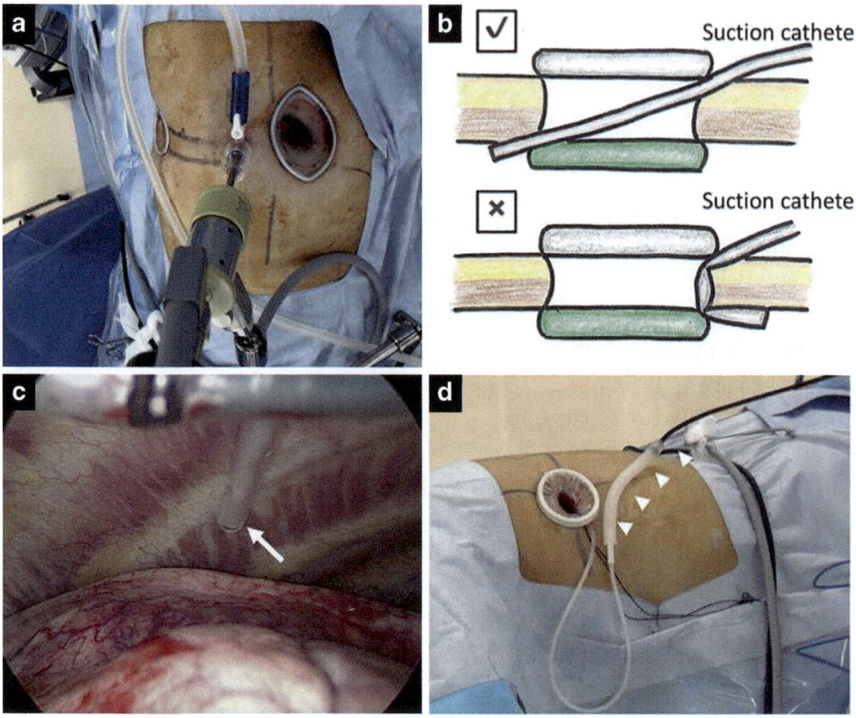

Fig. 30.4 Simple surgical smoke ventilation method. (**a**) Method to ventilate mist and smoke during conventional multiportal video-assisted thoracoscopic surgery. The suction tube is connected to the camera port. (**b**) A cross-section schema. The top schema is the correct method. The suction catheter is inserted straight. The suction catheter is kinked in the lower schema. (**c**) The head of the suction catheter is seen from the side of the wound retractor in the thoracic cavity (white arrow). (**d**) When the suction cannula is not used in the surgical field, the suction catheter is connected to the suction cannula via the connection tube (white arrowheads). The suction cannula may be connected to the suction tube directly. (Image used with permission (Mizukami et al. [1]))

removing tissues (e.g., lymph node), flipping the lungs along the hilar axis to visualize hilar structures, protection of important structures during fine dissection of blood vessels (e.g., to protect the brachiocephalic vein during VATS thymectomy), and many more (Figs. 30.12 and 30.13).

The different types of VATS sucker heads can be used for various function based on the surgery requirement. The normal head is versatile and used for dissection, compression, squeezing, flipping, protection, holding, and so on.

The conical sucker head is commonly used for complex dissections especially surrounding blood vessels like the pulmonary artery during lobectomies and fine suction to avoid the lung tissue from being sucked into its lumen.

The rough ball head is used for mechanical abrasion pleurodesis procedures after VATS bullectomy. It helps to abrade the pleura and at the same time suck the slow oozing which occurs during this procedure.

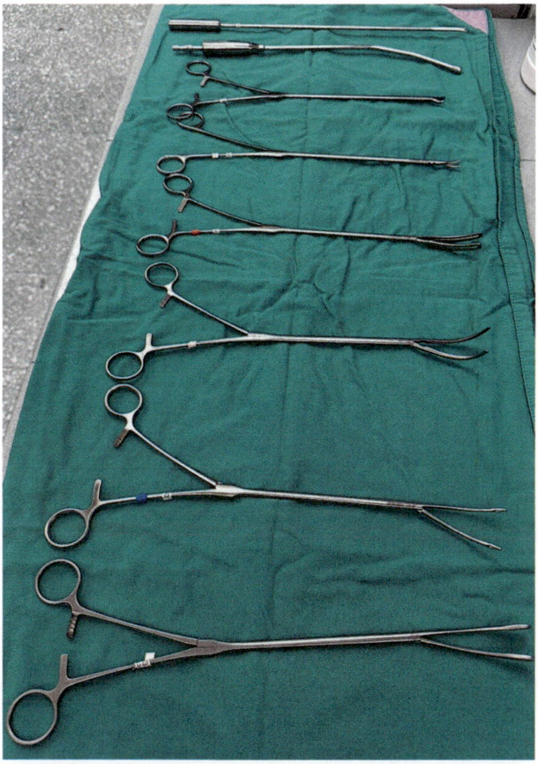

Fig. 30.5 Common VATS instruments required to perform lung resection surgery

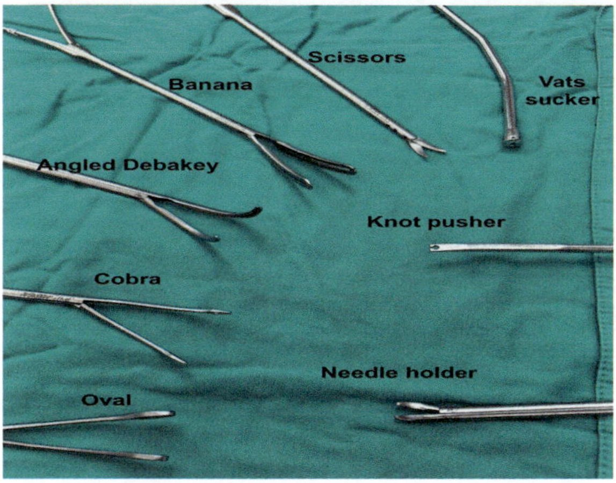

Fig. 30.6 Names of VATS instruments based on working jaw

The hollow head meanwhile has the best suction ability giving it an advantage to keep an oozy surgical field clear for visualization.

One of the modifications which can come with VATS sucker is the option of suction and coagulation in the same instrument thus speeding up surgery (Fig. 30.14).

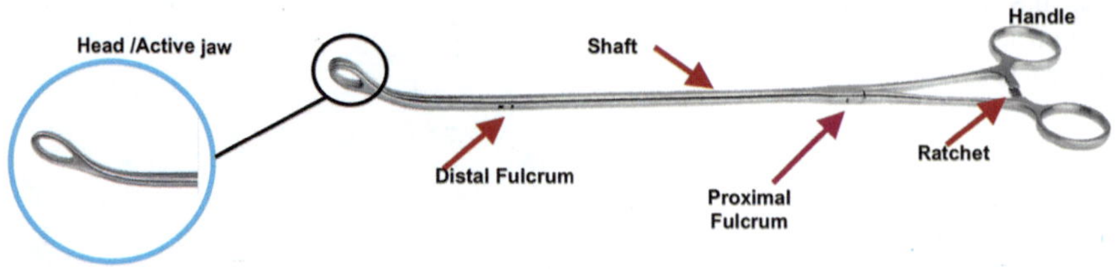

Fig. 30.7 Oval lung grasping forceps with its parts labeled. (Images with permission from RYU Medical)

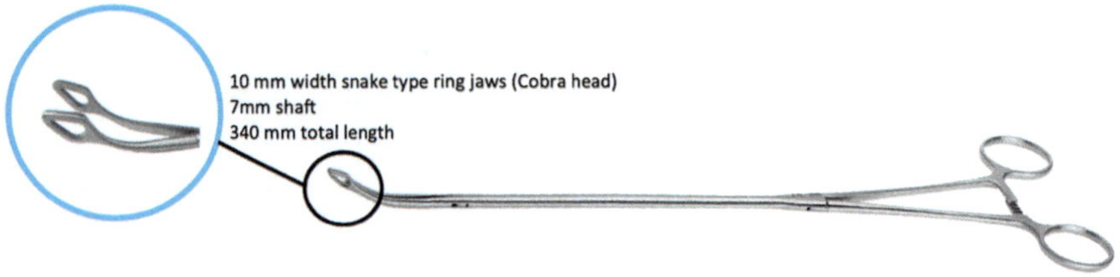

Fig. 30.8 Snake or cobra head VATS forceps. (Images with permission from RYU Medical)

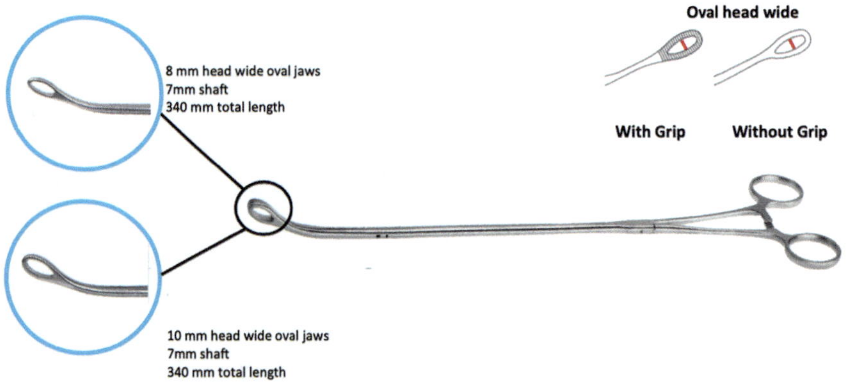

Fig. 30.9 Ring/oval jaw/lung grasping forceps. (Images with permission from RYU Medical)

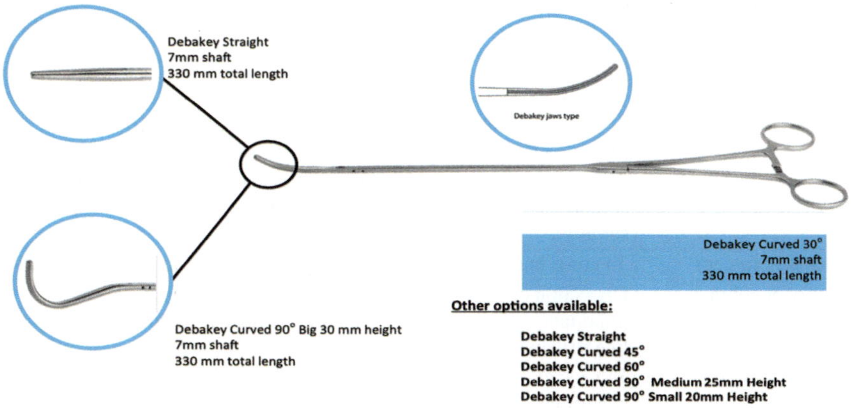

Fig. 30.10 Debakey straight and curved VATS forceps with multiple options. (Images with permission from RYU Medical)

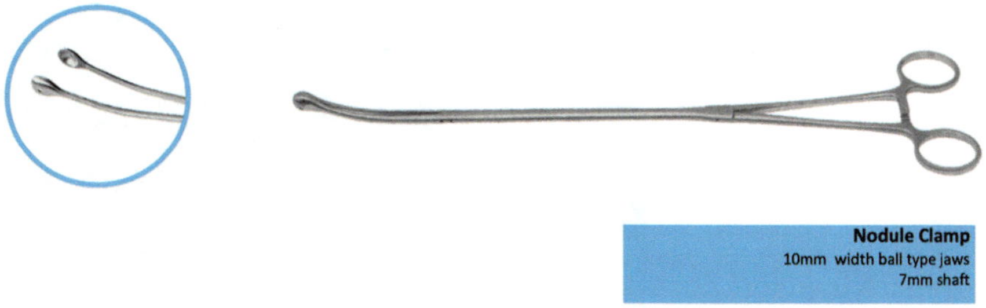

Fig. 30.11 VATS nodule or lymph node clamp. (Images with permission from RYU Medical)

Table 30.1 The different instruments are used as per table above

Thoracoscopic/VATS instruments	Usage
Ring, oval, or lung grasping forceps	1. To grasp lung, pericardial fat and muscles. 2. Can be modified to make tonsil swabs for point precision lung retraction by wrapping a half inch raytex gauze around its working jaw. 3. Tonsil swab can be used to mop up wet surgical field or even for compression haemostasis (exactly like swab sticks used in laparotomy surgery).
Debakey forceps	To grasp fine tissue, blood vessels, dissect tissues, and open up planes.
Snake or cobra forceps	Dissection close to neurovascular structures, opening planes near important structures, grasping the lung at specific points and catching fine structures such as sutures.
VATS suction	To suck and clear all debris and fluids. To dissect tissues, release adhesions, and create plane of dissection.
Ellis's forceps	To grasp tough tissues, e.g., tumor, fascia, and bone.

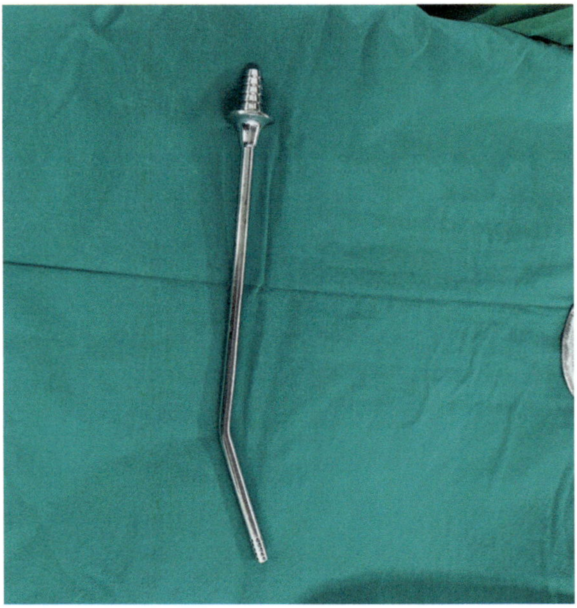

Fig. 30.12 VATS sucker with normal head. (Picture with permission from Ryu Medical)

30.5.1 Maintenance of VATS Instruments

- After usage, clean the instrument from all gross contaminants first before sending for sterilization. This will prevent the fulcrum edges from getting stuck with blood and becoming harder to open the jaws.
- To clean the instrument promptly during the operation to prevent tissues from getting stuck at the ratchet and fulcrum edges.
- To use the correct instruments for the proper tissue dissection, holding, and retraction. For example, the snake VATS forceps usually gets loose if tough tis-

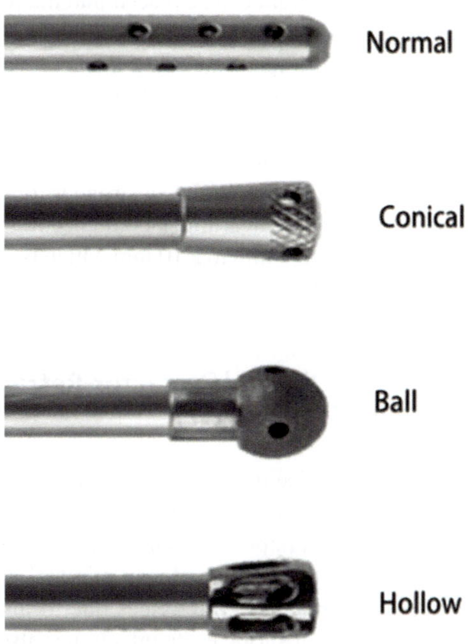

Fig. 30.13 VATS sucker with the different types of heads. (Images with permission from RYU Medical)

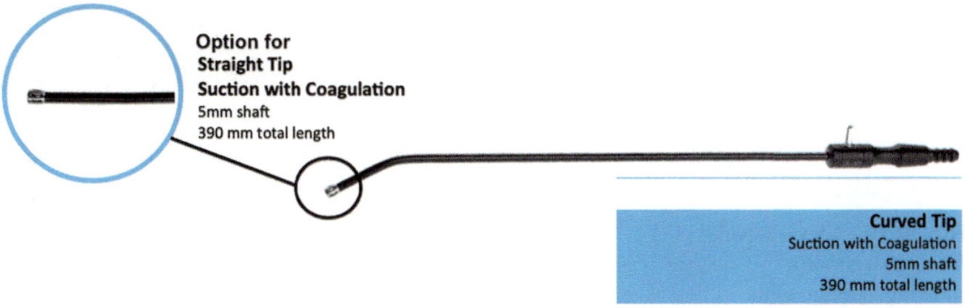

Fig. 30.14 VATS suction with diathermy function. The suction aperture is at the sides to prevent tissue adhesion. (Images with permission from RYU Medical)

sue like bone or calcified tissues are grasped. The Ellis or the oval head with grip forceps should be used instead.

- Regularly, lubricate the fulcrum to keep the working jaw and the handle movements smooth.

30.5.2 Trouble Shooting

- If the instrument gets hard and the jaw does not open well, must inspect for any rusting where stainless steel coating could be worn off. If there is no rusting some lubricant fluid can be placed into the fulcrum. If there is rusting, the instrument must be changed.

- The VATS instruments are small diameter at 7–10 mm, and it is sharp enough to cause major injuries. Hence, during introduction of VATS instruments into the thoracic cavity, retract the camera and get panoramic view to prevent injuries to surrounding structures.
- If instruments usage requires a stronger force due to a hard tumor, risk of bending the shaft of the instrument could occur. In this instance, use a larger diameter instrument from 7 mm to a 10 mm which is sturdier and can withstand higher the energy exerted.

30.6 Alexis Wound Protector-Retractor (AWPR) (Figs. 30.15, 30.16, and 30.17)

- AWPR is a device used in covering the surface of the wound in surgeries which requires an organ or a specimen to be removed via a small opening. In VATS, this equipment is an important tool functioning as a utility port. It functions both as a wound protector and retractor in minimal access thoracoscopic surgery. It also reduces the trauma to the tissues due to insertion and removal of instruments. The incidence of surgical site infection is also reduced. The outer hoop is slightly larger than the inner hoop to facilitate maximum exposure inside the thoracic cavity.

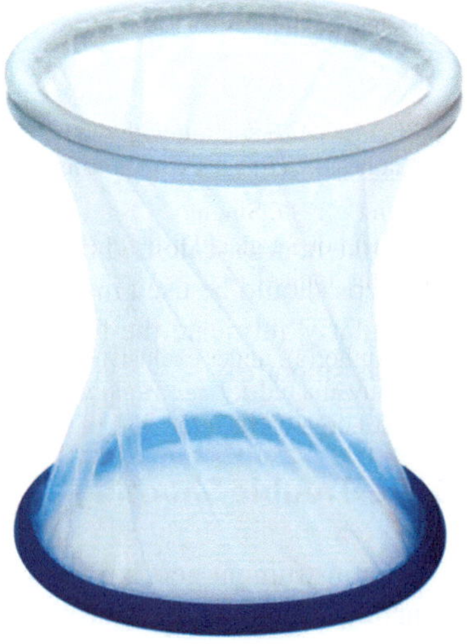

Fig. 30.15 Alexis wound protector-retractor showing. (Image with permission from RYU Medical)

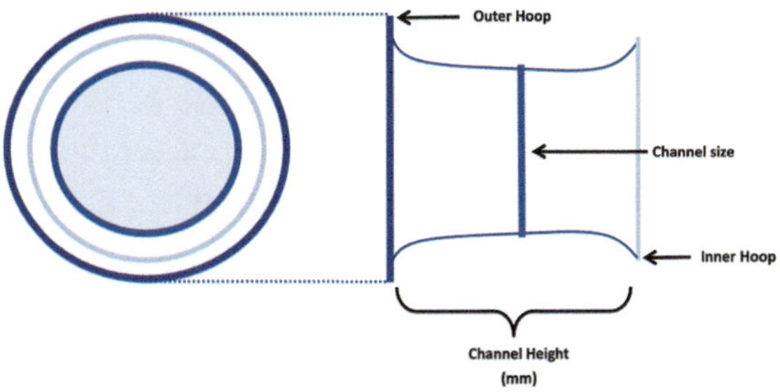

Fig. 30.16 Alexis wound protector-retractor. (Image with permission from RYU Medical)

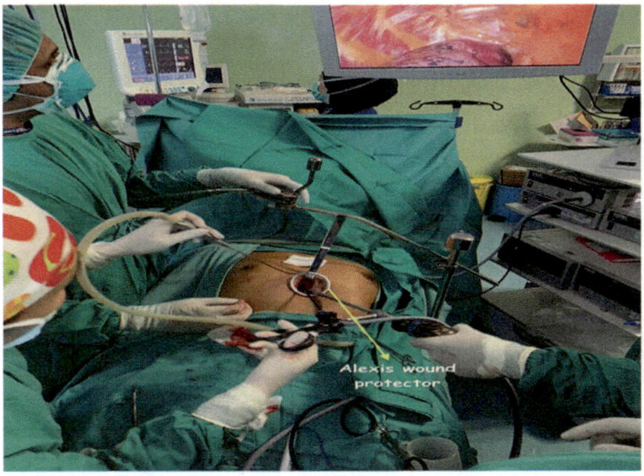

Fig. 30.17 Subxiphoid thoracoscopic VATS with wound protector-retractor. (Picture self performing surgery at Hospital Kuala Lumpur)

30.6.1 Maintenance

- Introduce instruments through the lumen to the target site without touching the sides of the wound protector to avoid tear or puncture to the soft plastic cover.
- Avoid sharp objects coming close to it as it can easily puncture the soft plastic cover.
- The skin incision site should be as close to the intercostal space where the working area is intended. If there is an angulation, the soft plastic covering the wound can easily slip and get damaged.

30.6.2 Trouble Shooting

- Use appropriate size for the wound to avoid slipping and movement of the protector. *Tips*: For uniportal VATS, inner channel size "XS" or 2–4 cm sized AWPR is ideal.
- If there is a sharp bony surface or rib fracture at the insertion site, smoothen it with a bone file before placing the AWPR to avoid tear to the plastic cover.
- Avoid reusing the protector as small puncture holes are difficult to be visualized rendering it ineffective to reduce surgical site infection. In cases where it is

reused, check thoroughly the soft plastic cover to look for puncture defects. If present avoid using it.

30.7 Diathermy Energy Device

Monopolar and bipolar diathermy devices used in thoracoscopic surgeries can be used in VATS to cut and coagulate tissues. These are described in detail in separate chapter (Fig. 30.18).

Hook is for sharp dissection and cutting of tissues. Meanwhile the ball and spatula is used for blunt dissection and hemostasis.

30.7.1 Trouble Shooting

- To reduce time wastage for the exchange of device during entry and removal, suction-irrigation instruments come with hook or spade tip which could retract into the shaft when not in use. It is useful especially when the surgical field is oozy or bleeding requiring the need for speed to localize the bleeding point followed by prompt haemostasis before the field gets wet. Another method is having the suction and diathermy function capability in the same device as shown in Fig. 30.14.
- The instrument does not work due to debris collecting from charred tissues getting stuck to the working tip. Regular and prompt cleaning of the instrument is required to keep it at optimum function during surgery.

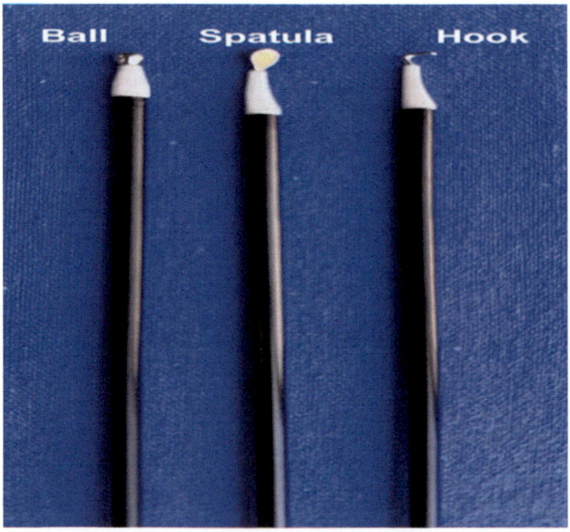

Fig. 30.18 Monopolar diathermy device working tips (Image from with permission from Ryu Medical)

30.8 Conclusion

VATS instruments are specially designed to reach deep areas in the thorax and perform surgery. Maintenance of these instruments are mainly by using the correct instrument to grasp the intended tissues and to not exert too much pressure during usage to prevent damage and loosening of the ratchets and fulcrum joints.

Reference

1. Mizukami Y, Maki R, Adachi H. Simple smoke ventilation method for uniportal video-assisted thoracoscopic surgery. Interact Cardiovasc Thorac Surg. 2022;35(2):ivac061.

Suction and Irrigation Instruments

31

Ioannis Gerogiannis, Georgios Bointas, and Sheza Arif Toor

Over the last 3 decades, we have seen a shift toward laparoscopic surgery, particularly in abdominal and pelvic surgery. This has led to innovation and improvement in the equipment and instruments used to perform these procedures. High-quality research has provided us with more user-friendly, advanced, and sophisticated equipment that allows for better and safer outcomes. Surgery can be likened to a battlefield that needs to be well organized and equipped, with each member of the team being well versed in the equipment available and its literature. This ensures that the team works like a well-oiled machine. A good knowledge of the mechanism of action, material, expiry date, and function of instruments is essential. Lack of information can affect the course of the procedure and put the patient's health at risk. Each instrument should be inspected regularly. Scissors, graspers, suction and irrigation devices, trocars, and trocar sleeves should be checked for loose or broken tips.

A good laparoscopic view is crucial to successful surgery, and this often requires the field to be clear and free of fluid or tissue debris. Suction and irrigation improve visual clarity, increase precision, and prevent complications. Irrigation can be used to remove debris, blood, fluid, identify the source of bleeding, and sometimes hydro-dissect and identify tissue planes. Suction is often used to remove irrigation fluid, intraperitoneal air and smoke. A central vacuum system or an additional suction pump can be used to achieve suction. Various laparoscopic suction devices have been designed to remove irrigation fluid or intraperitoneal air and smoke. Combined suction/irrigation devices are also available. A larger 10 mm suction-irrigation instrument is ideal for removing large blood clots or other surgical debris, such as gallstones, during laparoscopic cholecystectomy.

I. Gerogiannis (✉) · G. Bointas · S. A. Toor
General and Emergency Surgery, Kingston and Richmond NHS Trust, London, UK

J. S. Ahluwalia (ed.), *User Manual for Minimally Invasive Surgical Equipment*,
https://doi.org/10.1007/978-981-95-9019-3_31

31.1 Suction and Irrigation Device

Suction: Broadly speaking, a suction device consists of a long, slender tube with a suction tip at the end. The suction device is connected to a vacuum system that creates a negative pressure, allowing it to aspirate fluids and debris from the surgical area. *Irrigation System*: The irrigation system complements the aspirator by providing a controlled flow of sterile fluid to the surgical site.

31.2 Types of Grips Available for Suction Irrigation

31.2.1 Trumpet Grip

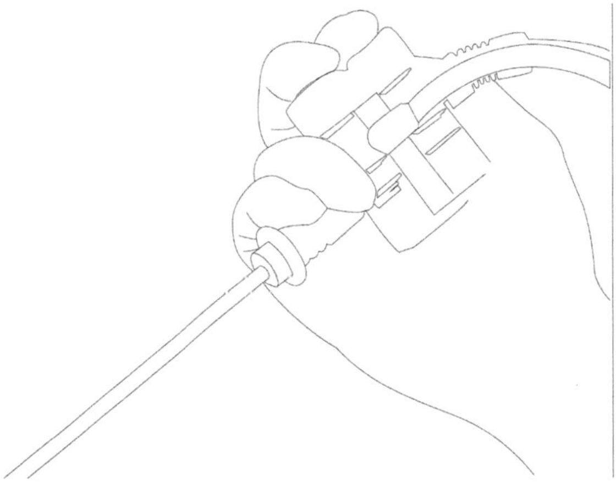

31.2.2 Pistol Grip

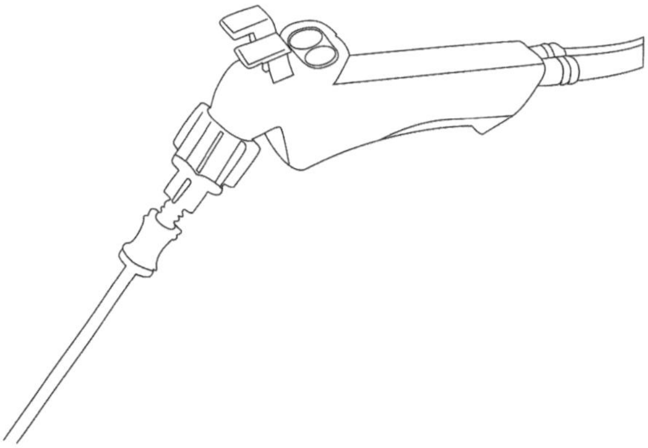

The trumpet valve handpiece offers suction/irrigation, smoke evacuation, and instrument interchangeability. It is ergonomically designed to fit the surgeon's preferred handling style, and some trumpet valve instruments can be easily reversed for left-handed use.

31.3 Types of Handles Available

Suction irrigation set comes with quick disconnect tips, irrigation, suction probes, and even diathermy tips. Types of irrigation and suction probes include the following:

1. 5 mm irrigation probe tip with irrigation holes (straight).
2. 10 mm irrigation probe tip with irrigation holes (straight).

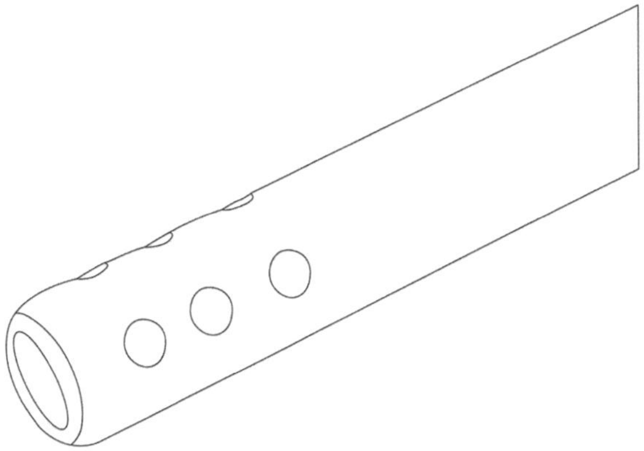

3. 10 mm pool suction cannula (round ended).

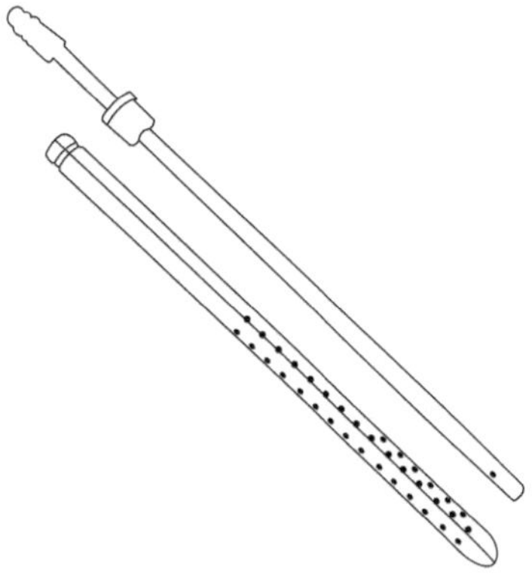

4. 5 mm pool suction cannula (round ended)
5. 10 mm stone extractor.

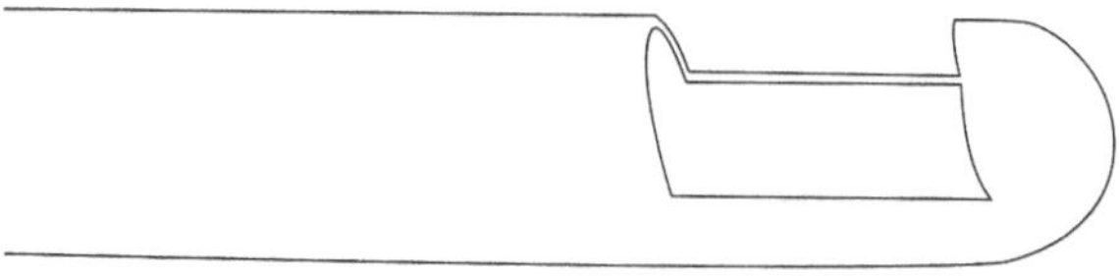

6. Additional specialty probe tips are available from some companies, including insulated and nonconductive tips for use with electrosurgery. These include the following:

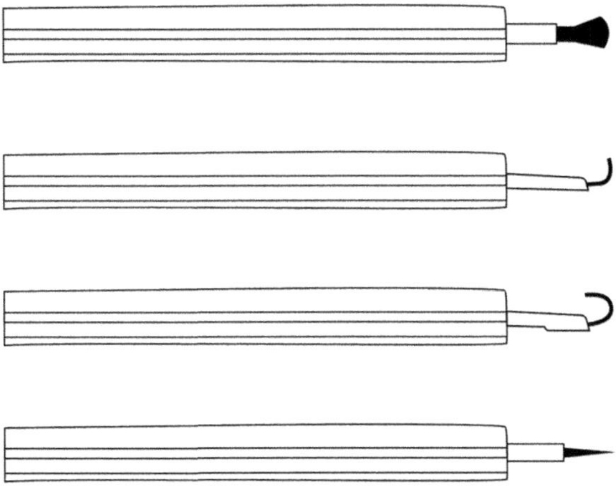

- Spatula.
- L Hook.
- J Hook.
- Needle.

The smallest applicable diameter is 3 mm, and the lengths of these vary from 28 cm, 33 cm, and 46 cm, with some variation between different companies.

31.4 When to Use a Laparoscopic Irrigator with Smoke Evacuation

It is used when controlled irrigation or aspiration of fluids and smoke from the surgical site is required. It may also be used for resection of filmy adhesions (i.e., hydrodissection) and peritoneal lavage. The fluids used should have a specific gravity of less than 1.

Recent advancements have made it possible to attach an electrosurgical device that allows cutting, coagulation, and dissection using monopolar or bipolar energy.

When fitted with the appropriate adapter and probe tip, the device can be used to introduce a laser fiber or laparoscopic surgical instrument into the peritoneal cavity during a laparoscopic procedure.

31.5 Contraindications of Laparoscopic Suction and Irrigation

1. Some laparoscopic suction and irrigation devices should not be used for hysteroscopy or for cavity distention.
2. If laparoscopy is contraindicated, then naturally the use of this instrument is contraindicated.
3. The use of electrosurgical instruments and electrode inserts with a non-insulated metal tip is contraindicated.

31.6 How to Assemble and Disassemble Them

1. *Inspect All Parts*
   - Check for damage, especially O-rings, valves, and lumens.
   - Make sure all parts are clean and dry.
2. *Insert the Internal Rod*
   - Carefully slide the internal suction/irrigation rod back into the cannula if it is a double cannula system.
3. *Attach the Cannula to the Handle*
   - Align the cannula and lock or screw it into place on the handpiece.
4. *Assemble the Handle*
   - Reinsert valves, seals, and O-rings in the correct orientation.
   - Close and secure the handle using any clips or screws provided.
5. *Reconnect Tubing*
   - Attach the suction and irrigation tubing to the designated ports.
   - Ensure connections are tight and secure.
6. *Function Test*
   - Run sterile water through both suction and irrigation to confirm flow.
   - Check for any leakage or blockages.

31.7 Disassembly of Laparoscopic Suction-Irrigation Instrument

(Usually done after the procedure for cleaning and sterilization)

1. *Disconnect Tubing*
   - Detach the suction and irrigation tubing from the handle/valve section.
2. *Remove the Cannula (Outer Tube)*
   - Unscrew or slide out the outer cannula from the handpiece. Some models use a locking mechanism that needs to be released first.
3. *Separate the Inner Components*
   - Pull out the internal tube or rod that runs through the cannula.
   - Be careful with the delicate tips.
4. *Disassemble the Handle (If applicable)*
   - Open the handle using release clips or screws.
   - Remove valves, levers, and other small parts like O-rings (note their orientation!).
5. *Flush and Clean*
   - Use a cleaning brush and an enzymatic solution to clean all lumens and parts.
   - Follow with high-pressure flushing if recommended.

31.8 Proper Use of the Equipment Is Very Important

1. Like all laparoscopic sets, if the package is damaged, unsealed, or open already—Please DO NOT use it.
2. The user should be aware of the instrument, and the scrub nurse and theatre team should be aware of the mechanism of action, function, and durability of instruments, as well as any alternative options available.
3. One should ask the surgeon if he or she wants the irrigation and suction system in place before the start of surgery or in case a need arises during the procedure, as some procedures may not warrant the use of suction and irrigation.
4. Make sure that the pump has fluid in it and is not running dry because the motor can run continuously when fluid is not present in it. Therefore, long surgery without fluid in the system should be avoided as it can damage the system.
5. Avoid using bottled irrigants, as air can be pulled into the irrigation from the bottle.
6. Attach the pump to the I.V. pole before spiking the irrigation bag, since the spike will not securely support the pump while in use.
7. Adhesions, anatomical anomalies, or other conditions may prevent clear visualization of internal anatomy. Do not perform laparoscopic procedures if the internal anatomy cannot be positively identified.
8. Make sure that single-use irrigation and suction devices are disposed of and not sent for autoclaving or re-sterilizing. This kind of information is available in the user's manual issued by the companies.

31.9 Maintenance to Prolong Life

Regular checking of equipment, early detection of faults in part or all of the equipment and early reporting of faulty equipment are essential. Reported defects should be investigated to ensure good quality and long life of the equipment.

Laparoscopic instruments are more susceptible to deposition of bioburden (microorganisms and debris) in their crevices, making them difficult to clean, adequately sterilize and maintain. Due to their delicate design, gentle methods should be used to sterilize them. As the complexity of procedures increases, so does the incidence of resistant strains of bacteria, mycobacteria, fungi, and viruses. Sterilization is the absolute elimination or destruction of microbial life forms. It can be achieved using steam, gas, or chemicals. Disinfection, on the other hand, is the relative removal of pathogenic organisms other than spores.

31.10 Cleaning and Sterilization

Optimal processing includes the following steps:

1. Dismantling: Dismantle the instrument as detailed above.
2. Decontamination: This process is used to reduce the bioburden on reusable medical devices. It begins in the theatre. Nurses should wipe off visible blood tissue and body fluids in instruments with a damp sterile sponge. All soiled or contaminated instruments should then be placed in a container with a disinfectant solution, such as 0.5% chlorine, and left to soak for 10 minutes.
3. Cleaning and Rinsing: Users must ensure that there are no residues, proteinaceous material, or organic residues left on the surface of the instrument. This is particularly important where the instrument has several small moving parts and crevices; the accumulation of residue can eventually lead to corrosive damage and pathogenic colonization (bioburden). Many hospitals adopt the technique of washing their instruments in soap scrubs.
4. Drying: Instruments should be dried at the end of the cleaning and rinsing cycle before being packed for sterilization. This is ideally achieved by using an air gun to blow any water droplets off the surface of the instruments or by using an oven. However, the latter may only be available in CSSD units.
5. Sterilization: There are three sterilization processes available to us—steam, ethylene oxide, and peracetic acid. One can choose according to compatibility and availability.
6. Storage. Always store sterilized instruments in a secure and dry environment.

31.11 Troubleshooting

No suction or irrigation flow	Tubing is kinked or disconnected	Inspect and straighten or reconnect tubing
	Clogged instrument lumen or tip	Flush the lumen with sterile saline or use a cleaning brush
	Obstruction in suction/ irrigation port	Detach and clean ports; ensure proper alignment during assembly
	Suction or irrigation source not activated	Verify source is turned on and functioning
Leakage from handle	O-rings are damaged, misplaced, or missing	Inspect, reposition, or replace O-rings
	Improper handle assembly	Disassemble and reassemble per manufacturer's instructions
	Cracks in handle housing	Replace handle unit; do not use damaged components
Reduced suction/ irrigation pressure	Partial blockage in tubing or lumen	Perform high-pressure flushing or manual cleaning
	Air leaks due to loose connections	Tighten all tubing and port connections
	Filter (if present) is clogged	Clean or replace the filter
Instrument tip not visible or functioning	Fogging or fluid accumulation at tip	Warm tip or use antifog solution; ensure irrigation is active
	Tip damaged or clogged	Replace or clean tip as needed
Difficulty assembling instrument	Parts misaligned or forced incorrectly	Review assembly steps; do not force components
	Debris in connectors or threads	Clean thoroughly and try again
	Worn or incompatible components	Replace worn parts; ensure component compatibility

31.12 Future Directions

Since the dawn of the laparoscopic era, surgeons have continually sought to develop new instruments and devices to facilitate abdominal surgery and achieve the best possible outcomes for their patients. Particularly in the field of laparoscopic suction devices, efforts have been made to minimize the risk of injury to the omentum, small, and large bowel and to increase intraoperative safety. After a brief literature review, we found that Nishida et al. from Japan published their invention in 2015. Essentially, they used a cigarette-shaped silicone drain, which they cut to a length of 4 cm. This was then placed over the aspirator to cover the side holes, leaving 1.0 to 1.5 cm free from the end of the instrument. It was secured over the side holes with 1–0 silk. Finally, the free tip was divided vertically into four equal pieces like the arms of an octopus. This device could prevent the irregular adsorption of fatty tissue (greater and lesser omentum or epiploic appendages) and could aspirate saline, fresh, and coagulated blood almost continuously.

Another publication by Ozer et al. in 2008 reported on a new suction device (sponge tip suction tube; STST) that allows surgeons to more easily aspirate intra-abdominal fluid. The authors tested the efficacy of the STST in a simulated intra-abdominal space, such as a large transparent plastic bag containing fresh sheep intestine and omentum, with 2000 cc of physiological saline and 14 mm Hg of air pressure. While aspiration of all the fluid was difficult and time-consuming when using the conventional aspirator, all the saline was easily and quickly aspirated when using the STST.

We also identified a recent publication of a new technique for laparoscopic aspiration, the Straw Pressure Gradient and Gravity (SPGG) technique, by Gerges et al. According to the authors, this is a safe, cost-effective, and environmental friendly technique compared to conventional aspiration devices. The technique involves the use of a sterile, disposable 12–16 French aspiration catheter after positioning the patient according to the intended aspiration. The catheter is inserted through the laparoscopic port closest to the specimen and guided using laparoscopic forceps. The extracorporeal end must be clamped to prevent fluid spillage, and the catheter tip is placed in the collection. After releasing the clamp, the pressure gradient successfully drains the fluid into a pot placed at a lower level than the intra-abdominal collection. Minimal irrigation can be performed via the gas vent using a syringe. The SPGG is softer than rigid traditional suction devices and atraumatic. It can be used for aspiration, irrigation, and collection of fluid for sampling and as a drain for intraoperative indications. It is an easy-to-learn technique and a cost-effective device, as it is cheaper than the average disposable suction system and has multiple uses that can significantly reduce the annual cost of laparoscopy. It can also reduce the number of consumables and reduce the environmental impact of laparoscopic procedures.

Bibliography

1. SAGES. (Society of American Gastrointestinal and Endoscopic Surgeons) Laparoscopy Preparation and Troubleshooting Guide.
2. Ahmed U, Al Aswad F. A practical tip to prevent intraoperative blockage of suction tubing. J Surg Tech Case Rep. 2014;6(1):43–4. https://doi.org/10.4103/2006-8808.135165.
3. Bard Laparoscopic irrigation Systems. Bard Davol Inc. Bard, Davol, Advantage, Aspir-Vac, Endo-Pool, Hydro-Surg, Nezhat-Dorsey, SmokEvac and X-Stream are trademarks and/or registered trademarks of C. R. Bard, Inc. All other trademarks are the property of their respective owners. © Copyright 2015, C. R. Bard, Inc. All Rights Reserved.
4. World Laparoscopy Hospital 2023 (website) Sterilization and Upkeep of Laparoscopic Instruments & Equipment – Available at: https://www.laparoscopyhospital.com/sterilization-maintanance-laparoscopic-instrument.html
5. Nishida T, Ikuta H, Yoshida S, Yokoyama K. A new device to prevent irregular adsorption of fatty tissue while using an irrigation-suction instrument for laparoscopic surgery: divided silicone drain tip. Surg Laparosc Endosc Percutan Tech. 2015;25(3):e104–5. https://doi.org/10.1097/SLE.0000000000000145.

6. Ozer MT, Uzar AI, Eryilmaz M, Altinel O, Demirbas S, Arslan I, Tufan CT. A novel laparoscopic suction device for applying precise aspiration during laparoscopic surgery: sponge-tip suction tube. J Laparoendosc Adv Surg Tech A. 2008;18(5):747–50. https://doi.org/10.1089/lap.2008.0022.
7. Gerges F, Nour E, Gerogiannis IN. The straw pressure gradient and gravity (SPGG) technique: a safe and cost-effective technique for laparoscopic suction. Cureus. 2023;15(4):e37779. https://doi.org/10.7759/cureus.37779.

Mini-Laparoscopy Instruments 32

Gustavo Carvalho and Jasmeet Singh Ahluwalia

Mini-laparoscopy instruments refer to those laparoscopic instruments that have shaft diameters ranging from 1.9 to 3.5 mm and trocar sizes ranging from 2.2 to 4.2 mm [1, 2]. The term mini-laparoscopic surgery is generally applied to procedures performed using such instruments. In addition, most surgeons include procedures performed using one additional 5 or 10 mm trocar (primarily for imaging and/or for specimen extraction) as long as this site is hidden (usually at umbilicus) provided all other sites utilize mini-sized instruments only. "Hybrid-Mini" term is used where more than one non-mini trocar is used. Many different terminologies have been used like "minilaparoscopy," "mini-laparoscopy," "mini laparoscopy," "micro-laparoscopy," and "needlescopic surgery", leading to great confusion. Several scientific groups and professional medical societies have published consensus statements on terminology, with most settling on the term "mini-laparoscopy" [3].

Even though mini-laparoscopy was pioneered over 20 years ago [4–9], it could not become popular mainly due to limitations of first-generation instruments as they were not as functional and durable as 5 mm instruments. With availability of newer generation mini instruments that have improved rotation and strength with better ergonomics, more complex procedures are being undertaken with their help.

Mini-laparoscopy is just an evolution of technology in laparoscopy preserving its core strengths like triangular port placement and simplicity in application [10]. Learning curve is minimal while moving from conventional laparoscopy to mini-laparoscopy. Not much extra equipment is required making it cost-effective

G. Carvalho (✉)
Department of Surgery, University of Pernambuco – UPE, University Hospital Oswaldo Cruz, Recife, Pernambuco, Brazil

J. S. Ahluwalia
Department of Bariatric & Minimal Access Surgery, STAR Superspeciality Hospital, Jalandhar, Punjab, India

J. S. Ahluwalia (ed.), *User Manual for Minimally Invasive Surgical Equipment*,
https://doi.org/10.1007/978-981-95-9019-3_32

especially when reusable instruments and trocars are widely available. Operative times are almost similar.

So far mini-laparoscopy is being primarily reported in cholecystectomy though many studies have reported appendicectomy, hysterectomy, inguinal hernia repair, fundoplication, renal surgery, sympathectomy, etc. While comparing results of elective mini-laparoscopic vs laparoscopic elective cholecystectomy, it was observed to result in slightly longer operative times (3–5 min), slightly less early postoperative pain in first 24 h and better initial cosmetic results, with no other apparent significant differences when compared to laparoscopic cholecystectomy [1].

The development of a very low-friction trocar system might further enhance outcomes of mini laparoscopy. So far the mini trocars available were just miniaturized versions of traditional laparoscopic trocars. These have two seals to contain CO_2 loss: a rubber cap and an internal mechanical valve. Low friction trocars are valveless systems made to allow precise passage of instruments thereby minimizing gas loss through them [11, 12]. These trocars are longer with thinner walls and have minimal gap between the trocar and the instruments (Fig. 32.1). This arrangement accounts for minimal friction between trocar and instrument (0.13 N vs 4.3 N) and minimal CO_2 loss (<0.1 L/min). The minimizes tissue damage during trocar insertion (Fig. 32.2) [8, 9]. Studies have shown that the abdominal wall tissue injury caused by different trocar sizes is proportional to the square of radius of the trocar (Table 32.1, Figs. 32.3 and 32.4).

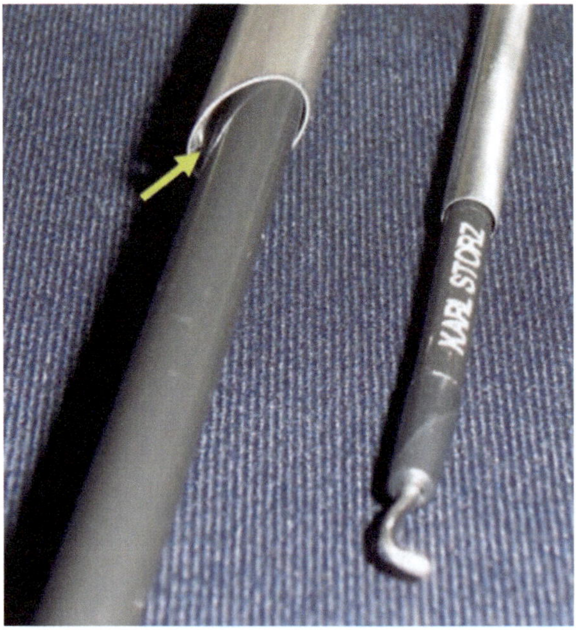

Fig. 32.1 Low-friction trocar system vs normal trocar system

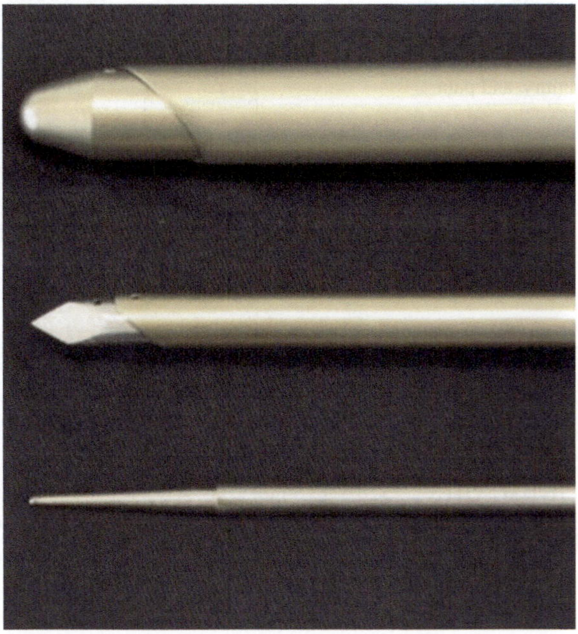

Fig. 32.2 Comparison of 10 mm, 5 mm and mini-laparoscopic trocars. Note long tapering conical blunt-tip obturator of low-friction mini-laparoscopy trocar

Table 32.1 Surgical access technique and parietal injury

Technique	Incisions	Parietal injury volume ($\pi \cdot r^2 \cdot h$)
Notes	Pure—no skin incision	~0
Hybrid Notes	(3.5 mm × 2)	612
Hybrid Notes	(6 mm × 1)	900
LESS (single port)	(28 mm)	19,600
LESS (single port)	(36 mm)	32,419
Mini-laparoscopy	(11 mm × 1 + 3.5 mm × 3)	3945
Std laparoscopy	(11 mm × 2 + 6 mm × 2)	7854

It has been studied that 10 mm trocar generates approximately five times more tissue damage than a 5 mm trocar and about 25 times more damage than a 2 mm trocar. Studies have shown improved precision, especially during dynamic and delicate tasks, lowered muscle effort and higher efficacy ($p < 0.001$) [13–16].

32.1 Instruments

Most instruments are available in lengths of 20 and 36 cm and for use with trocar sizes 3.5 mm and 3.9 mm (Fig. 32.5).

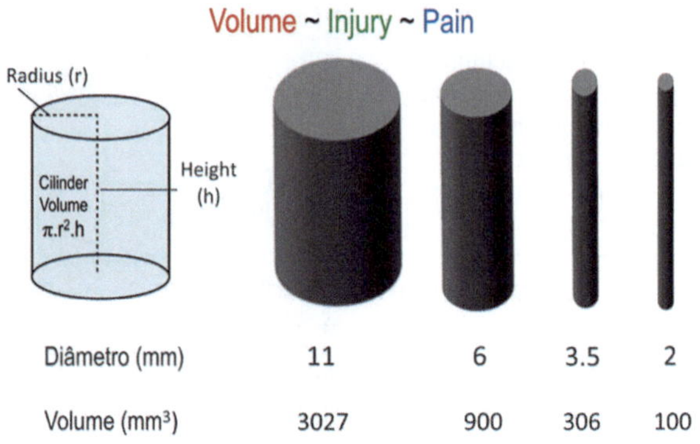

Fig. 32.3 Diagram illustrating the relationship between cylinder volume, injury, and pain

Technique	Incisions	Parietal injury volume ($\pi \cdot r^2 \cdot h$)
NOTES	Pure—no skin incision	~0
Hybrid NOTES	(3.5 mm × 2)	612
Hybrid NOTES	(6 mm × 1)	900
LESS (single port)	(28 mm)	19,600
LESS (single port)	(36 mm)	32,419
Mini-laparoscopy	(11 mm × 1 + 3.5 mm × 3)	3945
Std laparoscopy	(11 mm × 2 + 6 mm × 2)	7854

Fig. 32.4 Trocar sizes: Standard (11 mm and 6 mm), mini (3.9 mm), and low friction mini (3.5 mm) (Karl Storz Endoscopy; www.karlstorz.com)

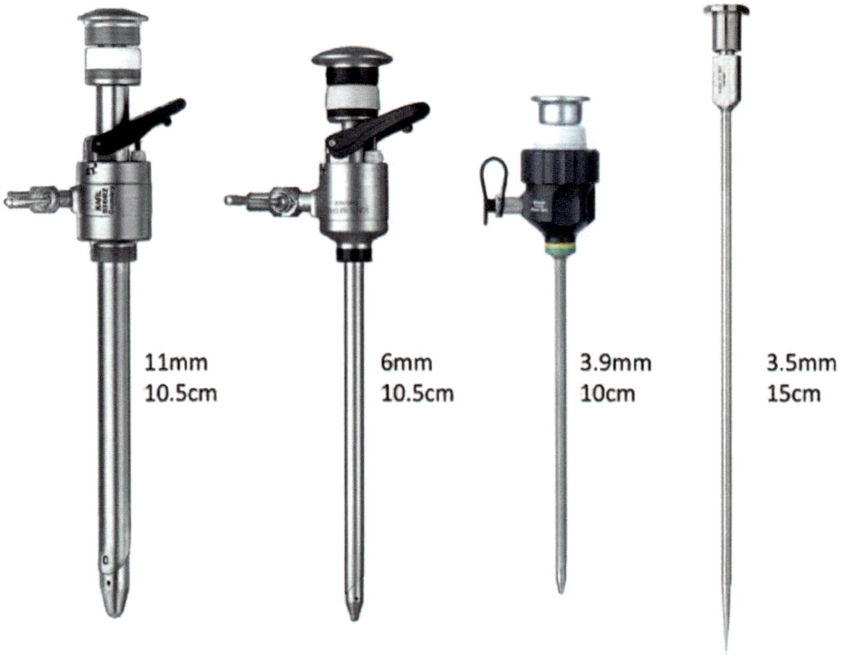

Fig. 32.5 Miniaturised version of routing trocar and cannula

Some commonly used instruments:

Instrument Type	Notes
Grasping Forceps (e.g., fenestrated, atraumatic)	For grasping and dissection
METZENBAUM Scissors (curved, serrated)	Double action jaws with irrigation
Micro Hook Scissors	Fine tip for precise dissection
KELLY Dissecting and Grasping Forceps	Available in straight and right-angled versions
Right angled dissecting and Grasping Forceps	For dissection around structures and for grasping
MANHES Grasping Forceps	2 × 4 teeth, single action jaws
REDDICK-OLSEN Dissecting and Grasping Forceps	Robust design with irrigation connection
KOH Ultramicro Needle Holder	With tungsten carbide inserts and ratchet
Bipolar Coagulating Forceps	Includes MANHES variant with 1 mm jaw width
CADIERE Coagulating and Dissecting Electrode	L-shaped, tapered distal tip with cm-marking
Palpation Probe	With cm-marking for depth assessment
Suction and Irrigation	For suction of fluid and for irrigation
Trocar with conical tip	3.5 mm diameter and 10 cm length

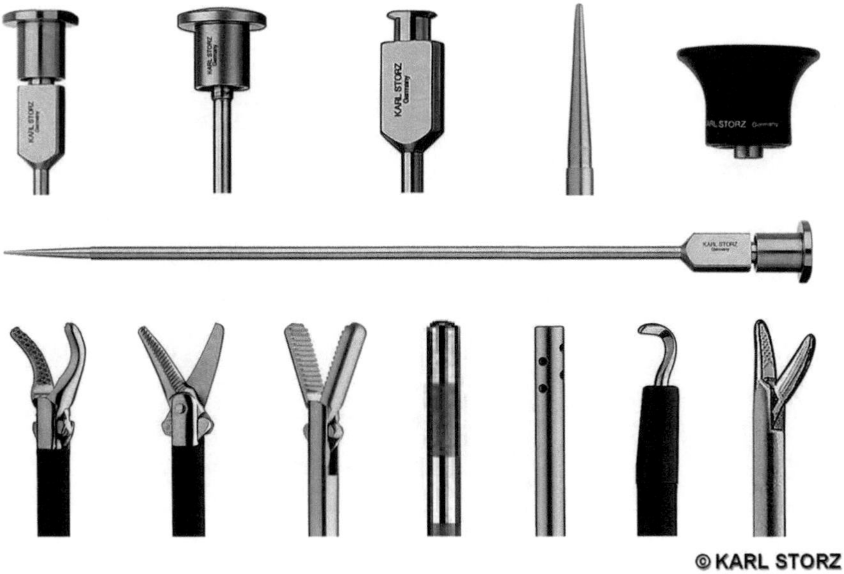

Fig. 32.6 Carvalho trocar and cannula along some common mini-laparoscopic instruments

32.2 Carvalho Trocar and Cannula

Carvalho along with Karl Storz developed special trocars and cannulas for mini-laparoscopy to further decrease tissue trauma and for facilitation of use of these thin instruments (Fig. 32.6). These are available in 3 mm and 3.5 mm sizes to suite the nature of instruments user intends to use with them.

Special Features

- Available for instruments in sizes 3 mm and 3.5 mm.
- Trocar features a long and flat tapered design to decrease tissue trauma and for ease of insertion.
- LUER-Lock connects trocar to cannula preventing dislocation of the trocar during insertion.
- LUER-Lock connector at the proximal end of the cannula allows use solely as an insufflation port if so desired.
- Flat trocar head allows placement on the instrument tray.
- Labeling on trocar sleeve and trocar for identification of compatible instrument size.
- Note that there is no separate insufflation channel on these instruments and we need to use a different cannula for insufflation of abdomen during the procedure. Since most mini-laparoscopic procedures are done in a hybrid way using at least one other instrument, one can use insufflation port of that cannula. Alternatively, one can use a miniaturized version of routine cannula as one of the ports to carry out insufflation (Fig. 32.7).

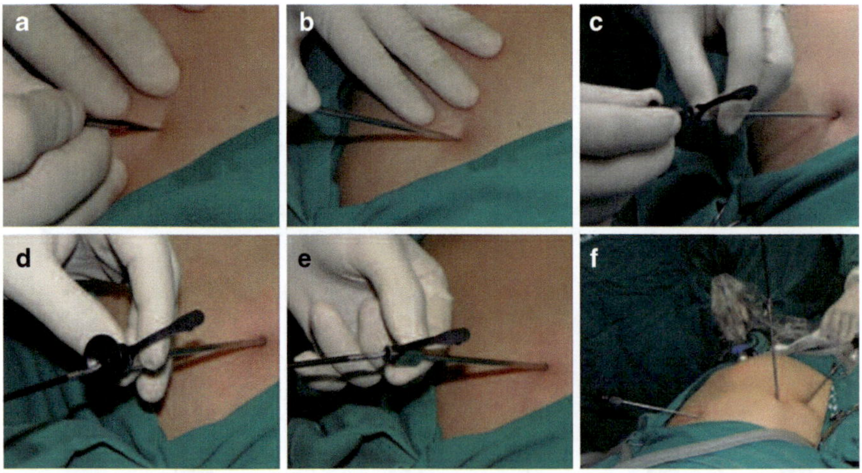

Fig. 32.7 Mini trocar insertion (Low-friction mini trocar with dilating tip, funnel cap and Luer lock—(**a**) A pinpoint skin incision is made with a scalpel. (**b**) Skin incision dilation and insertion of the trocar. (**c**, **d**) The provided funnel cap facilitates forceps insertion. (**e**) The trocar can alternatively be used without the cap, but this makes forceps exchange more difficult. (**f**) Mini trocars and forceps in action during a routine cholecystectomy

32.3 How to Insert (Fig. 32.7)

The following (Fig. 32.7) explains the insertion of low friction mini troca.

32.4 Scars in Comparison to Other Instruments

Figure 32.8 compares the incisions to be made for using different types of trocars.

Maintenance and Troubleshooting Please refer to the Chaps. 24 and 25. Please note that mini-laparoscopy instruments are much more delicate and often more expensive than routine laparoscopic instruments, hence they must be handled very delicately.

Future Directions Even though mini-laparoscopic instruments have come up much better than what they were in past, they still remain delicate or at least not as strong as their 5 mm counterparts. Optics that go through these ports are also not able to reproduce image comparable to larger scopes. Higher cost and higher breakdowns still remain a problem that has been only partially solved so far. We expect research to continue in making instruments and ports thinner and their make more sturdier in times to come.

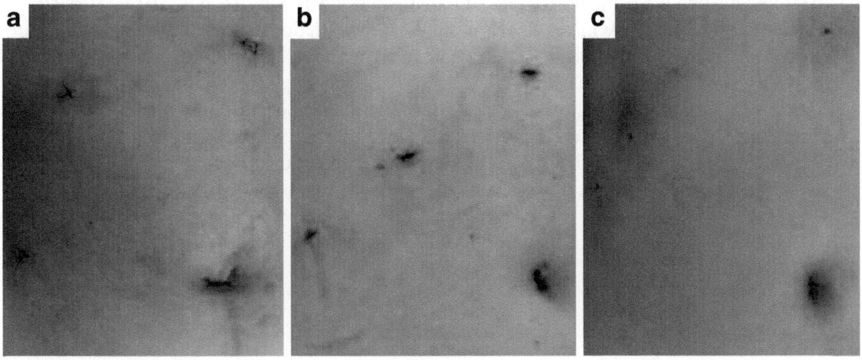

Fig. 32.8 Different wounds generated by different trocar types at the end of the procedure. (**a**) Standard laparoscopy. (**b**) Standard 3.8 mm Mini. (**c**) Low-Friction 3.5 mm Mini

References

1. Carvalho GL, Parqueting EM, Redan JA, Shadduck PP. The science behind mini-laparoscopic cholecystectomy. Surg Technol Int. 2016;XXIX:93–8.
2. Carvalho G, Redan JA, Shadduck P. Morphing into mini. Surg Technol Int. 2015;27:15.
3. Georgiou AN, Rassweiler J, Hermann TR, et al. Evolution and simplified terminology of natural orifice transluminal endoscopic surgery (NOTES), laparoendoscopic single-site surgery (LESS), and mini-laparoscopy (ML). World J Urol. 2012;30:573–80.
4. Ngoi SS, Goh P, Kok K, Kum CK, Cheah WK. Needlescopic or minisite cholecystectomy. Surg Endosc. 1999;13:303–5.
5. Reardon PR, Kamelgard JI, Applebaum BA, Brunicardi FC. Mini-laparoscopic cholecystectomy: validating a new approach. J Laparoendosc Adv Surg Tech A. 1999;9(3):227–32.
6. Reardon PR, Kamelgard JI, Applebaum B, et al. Feasibility of laparoscopic cholecystectomy with miniaturized instrumentation in 50 consecutive cases. World J Surg. 1999;23:128–31.
7. Tanaka J, Andoh H, Koyama K. Minimally invasive needlescopic cholecystectomy. Surg Today Jpn J Surg. 1998;28:111–3.
8. Uranues S, Peng Z, Kronberger L, et al. Laparoscopic cholecystectomy using 2-mm instruments. J Laparoendosc Adv Surg Tech A. 1998;8:255–9.
9. Yan RH, Lee WJ, Yu SC. Mini-laparoscopic cholecystectomy: a cosmetically better, almost scarless procedure. J Laparoendosc Adv Surg Tech A. 1997;7:205–11.
10. Brinkmann L, Lorenz D. Minilaparoscopic surgery: alternative or supplement to single-port surgery? Chirurg. 2011;82(5):419–24.
11. Carvalho GL, Lima DL, Sales AC, Silva JSN, Fernandes Jr FAM. A new very low friction trocar to increase surgical precision and improve aesthetics in minilaparoscopy. http://www.endoscopy-sages.com/2011/resource/posters.php?id36229. Accessed 11 Oct 2012.
12. Carvalho GL, Loureiro MP, Bonin EA, Claus CP, Silva FW, Cury AM, et al. Minilaparoscopic technique for inguinal hernia repair combining transabdominal pre-peritoneal and totally extraperitoneal approaches. JSLS. 2012;16(4):569–75.
13. Carvalho GL, Cavazzola LT, Rao P. Minilaparoscopic surgery-not just a pretty face! What can be found beyond the esthetics reasons? J Laparoendosc Adv Surg Tech A. 2013;23(8):710–3.
14. Carvalho GL, Melani AG, Veo CAR, et al. New low friction adapter for using minilaparoscopic instruments with transanal endoscopic microsurgery (TEO) improves visualization and dexterity. Surg Endosc. 2013;27:S164.
15. Firme WA, Carvalho GL, Lima DL, et al. Low-friction minilaparoscopy outperforms regular 5-mm and 3-mm instruments for precise tasks. JSLS. 2015;19(3):e2015.00067.
16. Passos GO Jr, Lima DL, Silva FW, et al. Surgeons' perceptions in relation to the minilaparoscopic instruments in surgical knots construction. Surg Endosc. 2014;28:S333.

Hepatopancreatobiliary Surgery: Special Instruments

33

Aali J. Sheen and Saurabh Jamdar

The most important aspect of any operation remains patient safety. Therefore, it is imperative that a surgeon must feel that he/she is comfortable using their chosen instruments that are in their surgical armamentarium. Most instruments are selected based on historical use in a department and/or by trial use in a "wet" or "dry" surgical laboratory. Good hemostasis will remain one of the main reasons cited for the choice of any instrumentation used, with the preferred instrument also vindicated by notable successful patient outcomes.

In this chapter, a comprehensive description of special instruments used in laparoscopic hepatopancreatobiliary (HPB) surgery is depicted. These instruments have other applications as well. HPB surgery often requires the surgeon to negotiate both difficult and unforgiving parenchyma immersed in swathes of large and medium-sized blood vessels. Damage to these structures can give rise to unrelenting and potentially fatal bleeding and leaks, hence employing safe and reliable dissection tools remain of paramount importance to surgeons for delivering successful operations.

33.1 LOTUS Ultrasonic Scalpel

The LOTUS device is a torsional ultrasonic scalpel that simultaneously seals, coagulates, and cuts tissue. In comparison to other ultrasonic dissectors on the market that rely on a longitudinal modality of energy delivery, operating between a frequency window of 35.4 to 36.6 kHz, the LOTUS ultrasonic scalpel's patented

A. J. Sheen (✉)
Department of HPB Surgery, Manchester Foundation NHS Trust, Manchester, UK

S. Jamdar
Department of HPB & General Surgery, Manchester University Foundation NHS Trust, Manchester, UK

J. S. Ahluwalia (ed.), *User Manual for Minimally Invasive Surgical Equipment*,
https://doi.org/10.1007/978-981-95-9019-3_33

torsional modality of energy gives an enhanced safety aspect to the device. The LOTUS system's strengths lie in reduced stray energy dissipation at the tip of the device, especially when compared to conventional longitudinal instruments. Unintentional distal energy output can thus be minimized. This allows the vessels to be sealed quickly and reliably with a smaller tissue thermal spread footprint.

This device is available in two variations, the first variant is the LOTUS dissecting shears which has indications to be used in general, plastic, gynecologic, urologic, thoracic, and other open and laparoscopic procedures in adult patients (Fig. 33.1). The second variant is the LOTUS liver resector (Fig. 33.2). Both the dissecting shears and liver resector use the same modality of torsional energy to coagulate, seal and cut tissue; the fundamental difference between the two models is the profile of the distal tip of the waveguide.

The distal tip of the dissecting shears (Fig. 33.3) has a finer profile compared to the liver resector (Fig. 33.4); the tip is also curved, with two energy focusing facets running the length of the tip. These facets are designed to focus the energy into targeted tissue and reduce stray energy (Fig. 33.3).

This is in comparison to the liver resector that has been specifically designed for parenchymal tissue. With a larger, flat contact surface area, the distal tip of the liver resector creates a more robust hemostatic effect.

The dissecting shears are available in three lengths: 176 mm, 349 mm, and 434 mm (Fig. 33.5) and the liver resector is available in two lengths, shorter for open surgery and longer for laparoscopy (Fig. 33.6). All shafts have identical diameters and are designed to fit comfortably into a 5 mm trocar port.

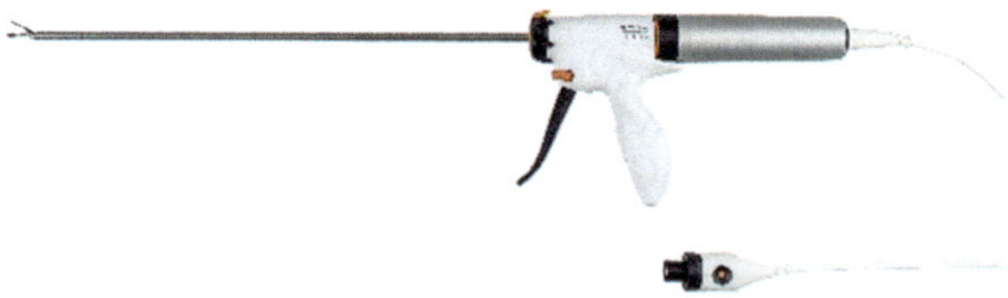

Fig. 33.1 LOTUS laparoscopic dissecting shear

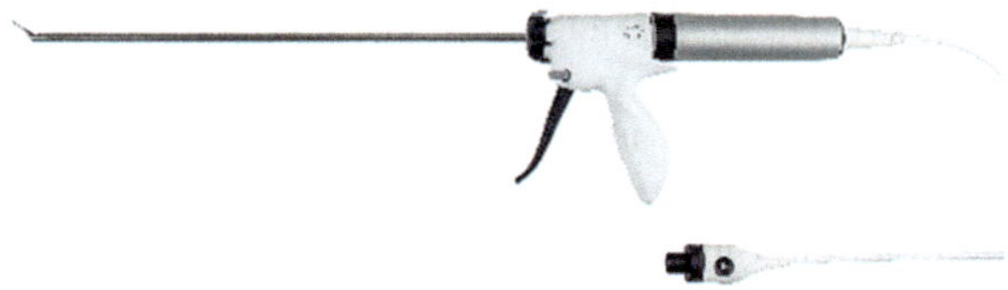

Fig. 33.2 LOTUS laparoscopic liver resector

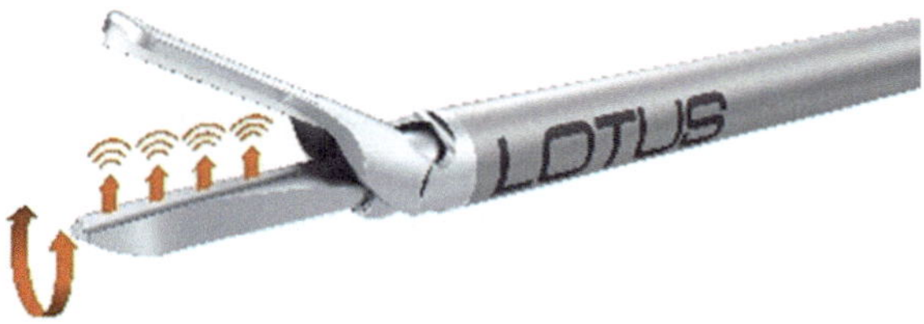

Fig. 33.3 Distal tip of dissecting shears

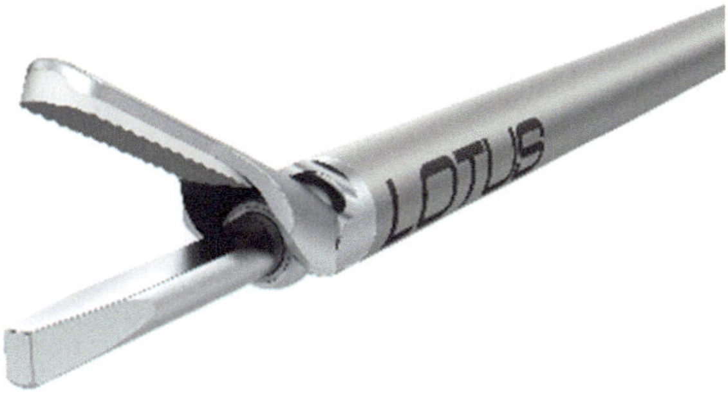

Fig. 33.4 Distal tip of liver resector

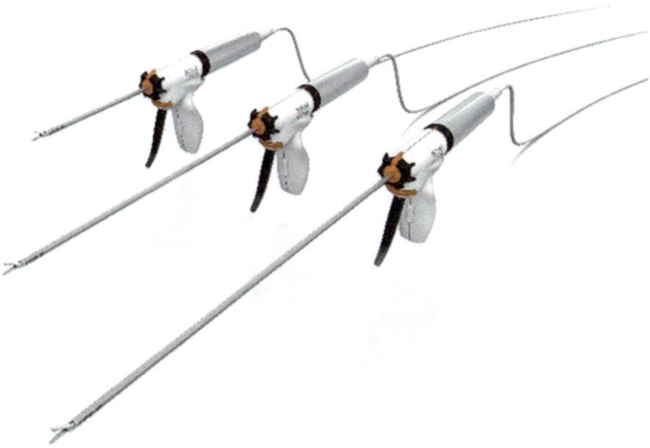

Fig. 33.5 Dissecting shears

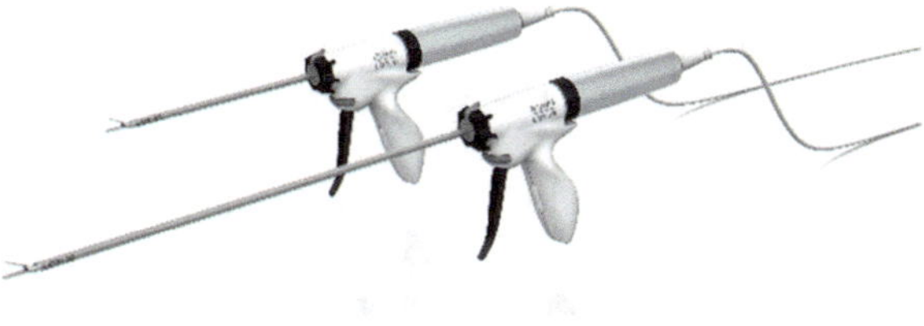

Fig. 33.6 Liver resector

33.1.1 Instrument Operation Instructional Guide

The ultrasound transducer is reusable, whereas the handpiece is a single-use system (Fig. 33.7).

The handpiece is designed (Fig. 33.8) with a circular control anteriorly to allow rotation of the end blade. In addition, the black grip handle is the main driving mechanism that controls the ultrasonic power. The grip handle also has a small white button, which will change the setting to low or high depending on the speed the surgeon wishes to use.

There is no immediate rule as to what setting the surgeon should use, as any such decision will normally be made on experience and the type of tissue being dissected. For liver parenchymal dissection, the lower setting is generally used. A further

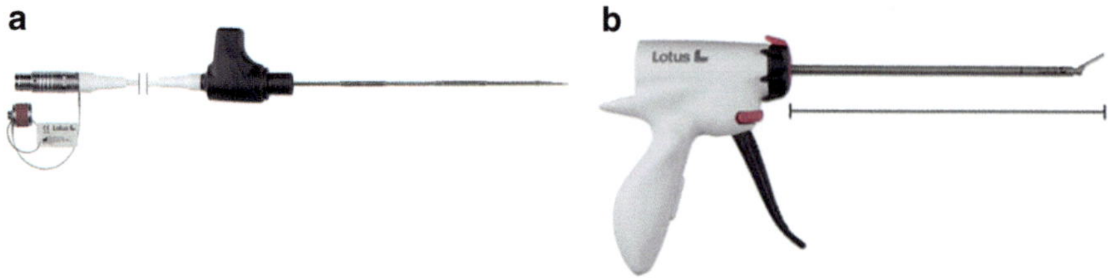

Fig. 33.7 Lotus transducer and handpiece are shown in (**a**) and (**b**), respectively

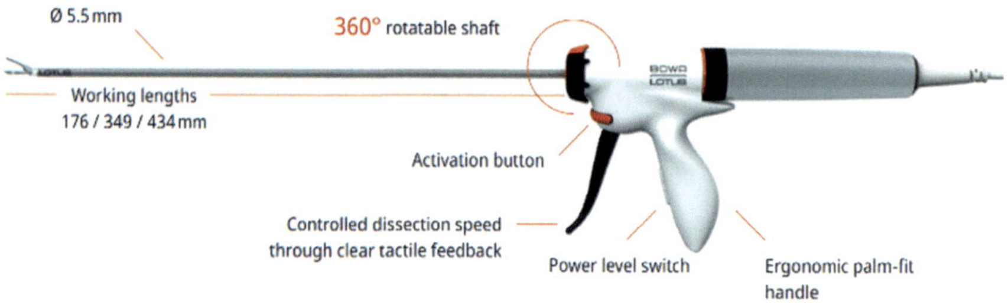

Fig. 33.8 LOTUS handpiece

ultra-low setting is also available, which is managed through a switch on the back of the console.

The reusable transducer is made from medical grade titanium and has a lifetime of 250 min of activation time, or approximately 50 cases.

The LOTUS ultrasonic scalpel is powered by a generator referred to as the LG4 (Fig. 33.9). The LOTUS transducer is plugged into the transducer socket on the front of the LG4 (a).

This screen of the LG4 momentarily illuminates with all the symbols being displayed when the LG4 is first switched on. There is a speaker in which the volume is controlled on the rear of the generator (b). The LG4 gives audible feedback in addition to visual feedback to the users, this audible feedback is in the form of beeps and tones to alert the operator to the power level they are using, a change in the system or if an error message appears on the screen.

The dissecting blade has a conical shape, and this allows the gradual hemostatic dissection of liver parenchyma. This design feature is important, especially when medium to large-sized blood vessels can be inadvertently damaged by the ultrasonic waves. The careful dissecting out of such blood vessels is possible with this device, in part because of the direction of ultrasonic waves from blade to blade, so there is no dissipation of heat and damage to other surrounding viscera and the frequency of the ultrasound allows a slow but steady parenchymal dissection. This also allows sealing of blood vessels up to 5 mm in diameter safely, with no additional clips required to secure the vessels.

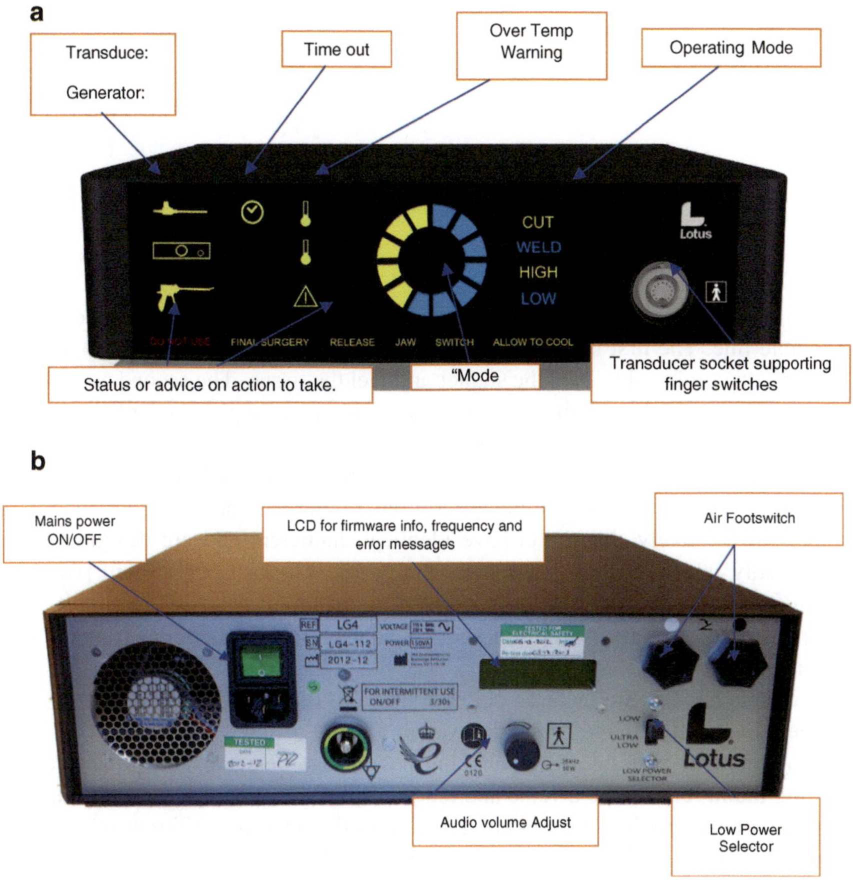

Fig. 33.9 LOTUS ultrasonic scalpel generator—front view (**a**) Rear view of generator (**b**)

33.1.2 Storage

The disposable handpieces are supplied pre-sterilized and are designed for single use and should be stored at room temperature.

33.2 AEON Endostapler

The AEON surgical stapler, like other surgical staplers, is used to simultaneously cut and staple tissue when resecting, transecting, or creating anastomoses. The product is used across surgical specialties, including general, abdominal, gynecologic, pediatric, thoracic, bariatric, colorectal, urological, and of course, hepatopancreatobiliary surgery. The instrument may be employed in both open and minimally invasive laparoscopic surgery (Fig. 33.10).

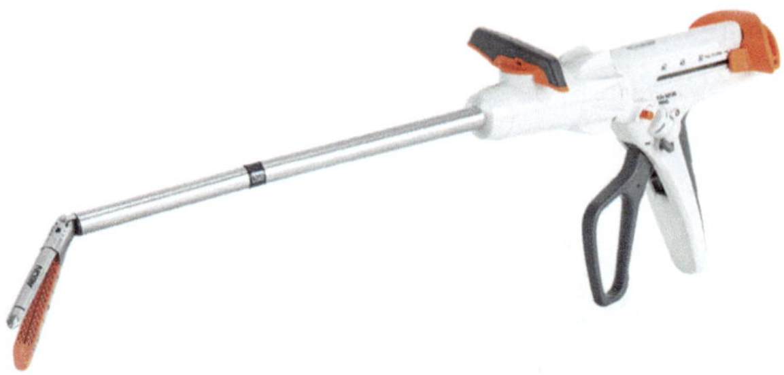

Fig. 33.10 AEON endostapler

The surgical stapler is comprised of two components that work together to deploy the staple line. The first is the handle, which is ergonomically designed so that the surgeon can comfortably hold the stapler and feel the tissue. The second component is the reload, which contains the single-use titanium staples and blade, and is designed for the creation of the staple line.

The AEON handle is available in three shaft-length configurations: 60 mm, 160 mm, and 260 mm. The manufacturer refers to these as short, medium, and long handles, respectively. All shafts have identical diameters and are designed to fit comfortably into a 12 mm trocar port (except black reload, which will require a 15 mm port 0. Practically, the long and medium handles are more commonly used in laparoscopic surgery, while the short handle is preferred for open abdominal surgery.

The three handles are pictured below (Figs. 33.11, 33.12, and 33.13).

The AEON reloads are presently available in 30 different configurations, with the manufacturer continuously launching new reload designs. The expansive and growing menu reflects the diverse and unique clinical scenarios in which a surgical stapler is employed. The factors contributing to the need for different reload configurations include varying tissue and vascular thickness, tissue health, tissue type, surgeon visibility limitations, proximity of the target transection area to delicate structures, and size of target stapling area.

Reload Colors: AEON reloads are available in five colors. Each color denotes a different size for the staples deployed from the reload. The shortest staple height is in the grey reload, which is most commonly used for vascular transection. The tallest staple height is in the black reload, which is used for the thickest tissue, such as stomach.

Each cartridge color, with recommended use in hepatobiliary surgery, is described below:

- Black: Designed for thick tissue and is most applicable for gastrointestinal (pylorus) tissue or otherwise fibrotic or dense tissue.
- Purple: Gastrointestinal tissue, as well as some pancreas transections.
- Orange: Medium thickness gastrointestinal tissue and most pancreas transections.
- White: Thin tissue, vascular use.
- Grey: Vascular use, especially smaller diameter blood vessels.

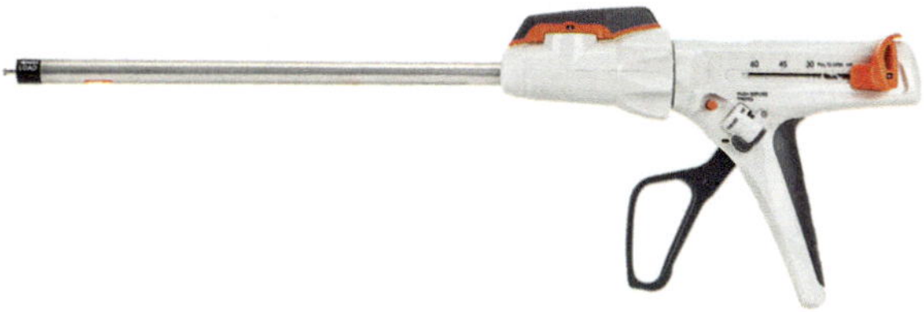

Fig. 33.11 AEON long handle and shaft length 260 mm

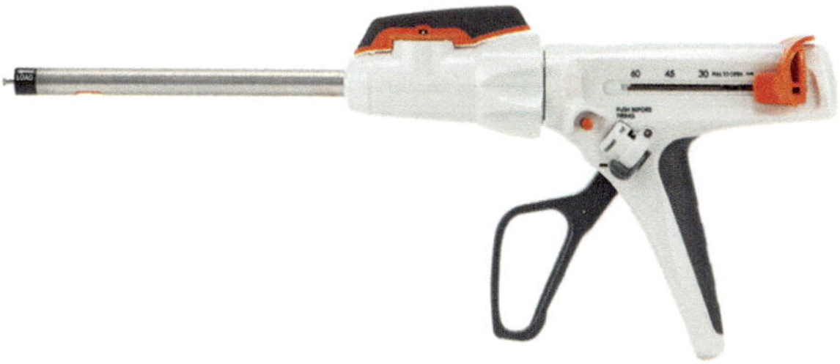

Fig. 33.12 AEON medium handle and shaft length 160 mm

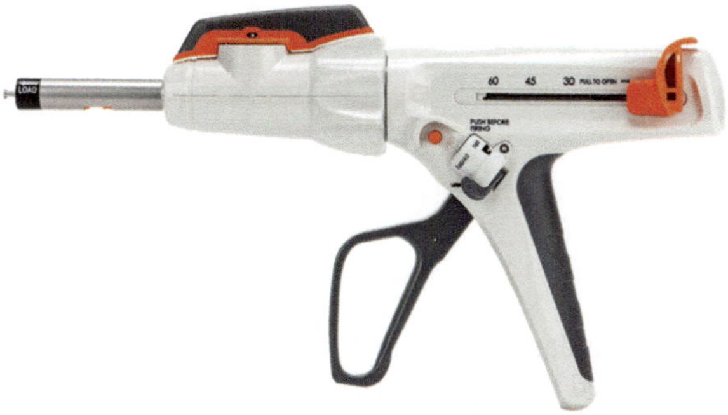

Fig. 33.13 AEON short handle and shaft length 60 mm

The cartridge and handle shaft diameter allows most of its configurations to easily fit down a 12 mm port, with its differing handle lengths allowing its function intraoperatively to accommodate the relative depths subjectively experienced in surgery based on varying organ anatomy as well as patient's body habitus. The one exception is the black cartridge with a 5.0 mm open staple height, which requires a 15 mm port.

The open and closed staple heights for each cartridge color are pictured below in Fig. 33.14.

Reload Anvils: AEON reloads are available with three different anvils. The anvil, in overly simplified terms, is the metal plate sitting opposite the colored staple cartridge. When staples are deployed from the cartridge and pierce the target tissue, the staples come into contact with the anvil, where precisely formed metal drives the staples to curve and form a "B" shape.

AEON staple formation is identical across anvil types. The products are differentiated in anvil tip geometry with three anvil tips available: Regular, Short, and Curved, pictured in Fig. 33.15.

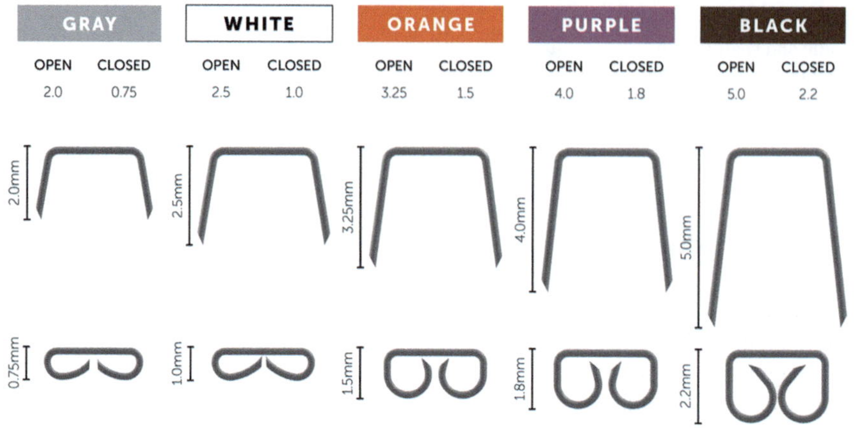

Fig. 33.14 AEON open and closed staple heights

Fig. 33.15 AEON anvil tips

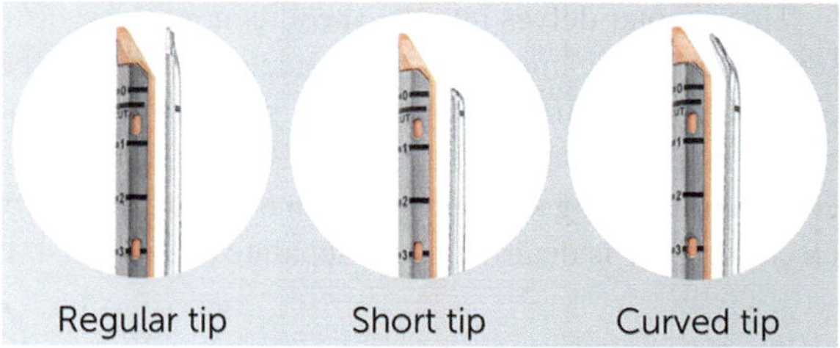

The regular tip anvil is designed with the same length as the stapler cartridge. The pointed tip may be used for guiding and dissecting when transecting.

The short tip anvil is shorter than the regular tip, and the tip is intentionally squared off to reduce the risk of tissue trauma caused by unintentionally blunting tissue with the anvil during navigation. The short tip is ideal for use where there may be danger of damaging distally placed blood vessels. Examples include a liver parenchymal transection where mid transection of a middle hepatic vein tributary may not be visible. The short tip is also a great fit where smaller "bites" are required, such as dissecting mesentery, especially when taking down the duodenojejunal (DJ) flexure in Whipple pancreaticoduodenectomy.

The curved tip anvil is curved, as the name indicates. The most obvious application is in enabling safe skeletonization of a large blood vessel. This is especially warranted in safe ligation of the portal and hepatic veins, where clear visualization as well as encirclement of the blood vessel in its entirety is critical.

Reload Lengths: Finally, reloads are available in three lengths and are denoted by the staple line length. These are 60 mm, 45 mm, and 30 mm. Reload length selection is usually a function of the target area size for dissection. A portal vein transection, for example, likely warrants a 30 mm reload. By contrast, an antrum resection requires multiple 60 mm cartridges. And finally, a 45 mm reload may be most appropriate for a duodenojejunostomy.

Fig. 33.16 Subset of five unique reload configurations

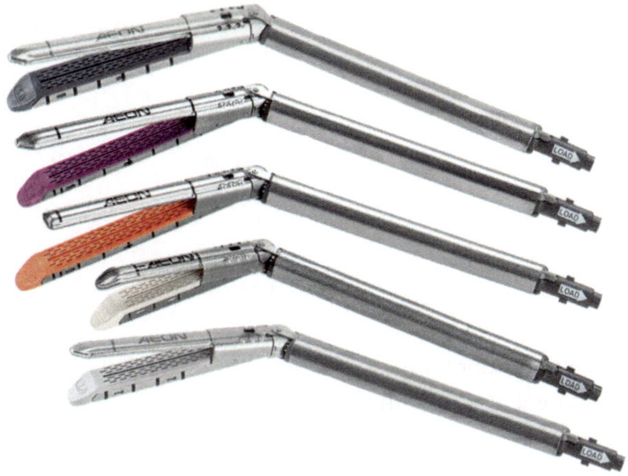

While reloads are available in five colors, three anvil types, and three cartridge lengths, not every feasible combination is available from the manufacturer due to the limited or nonexistent clinical need for certain configuration. Figure 33.16 shows a sample of the differing reload configurations.

Some aspects enhance the functionality of this device as a vascular and endoscopic stapler. The core innovation is described by the manufacturer as S3 engineering, pictured in Fig. 33.17 and described below.

I-Beam Design: The component of the reload that houses the transection blade contains an I-shaped profile that draws the cartridge from one side of the transection line, and the anvil from the opposite side together to precisely close the jaws to the correct distance as the staples are being deployed and as the tissue is being transected. This design translates into what is described as localized compression. The tissue is compressed gradually and precisely as the staple line is formed. The said design feature differs from some other vascular staplers, which more aggressively clamp or crush the tissue together when the jaws are initially clamped down.

The surgeon's technique remains a critical determining factor in staple line quality. The surgeon should take care to:

(a) Choose the appropriate reload configuration, and particularly the appropriate staple height/cartridge color. Choosing a staple height that is excessively large for the target tissue can result in leaking or bleeding as the tissue, ducts, and/or vasculature are not sufficiently compressed when stapling and transecting. Conversely, choosing a staple height that is unreasonably small for the target tissue can result in ischemia and ultimately lead to leaks or bleeding. The surgeon must be mindful to remember that the tissue must vascularize around the "B" formed staples after transection, and perfusion at the staple line is key to achieving this optimal long-term clinical outcome. The importance of choosing the correct staple size cannot be overstated. It is for this reason that AEON offers a spectrum of staple height reload configurations.

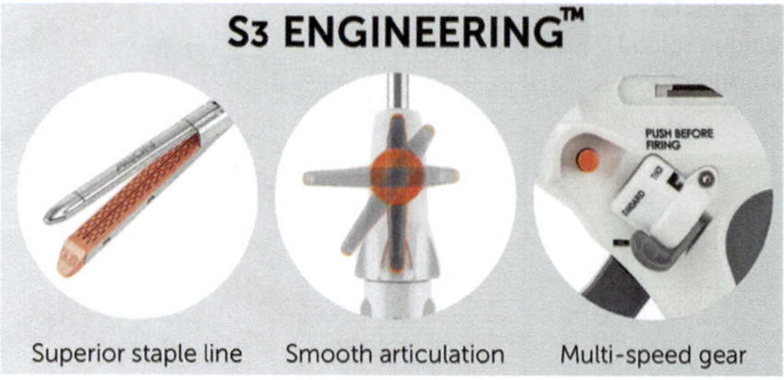

Fig. 33.17 S3 engineering

(b) Pre-compress the tissue prior to firing. When stapling on tissue, squeezing the target tissue with the stapler jaws releases extracellular fluid and compresses target tissue, thus allowing for a more solid tissue substrate for stapling and transection. A growing body of literature [1] suggests pre-compressing tissue for a minimum of 15 s prior to firing improves staple formation and the staple line.
(c) Fire in a slow and controlled manner. Deploying a staple line hastily can result in detrimental movement of the staple when clamped down on the tissue, which can cause tissue tearing or bleeding, and may also negatively contribute to staple formation quality and cut line quality. Surgeon should always take care to fire the surgical stapler in a slow and controlled manner (Fig. 33.18).

AEON's multispeed gear can be found on the side of the instrument and is used to reduce the force required to fire the instrument. A greater force may be required for large blood vessels or thicker tissue. When thicker tissue is encountered, the surgeon can move the gear switch from standard to thick. A unique feature of this function is that it may be changed at any point during the transection/firing process. Of note, the use of thick mode is not confined to thick tissue. Many surgeons prefer to use the gear for all stapler firings as the gear allows for slower, more controlled firing of the stapler, which results in improved staple formation and a better staple line.

The unique functionality that the AEON instrument offers is that the articulation is smooth and continuous, allowing for the surgeon to angulate the stapler jaws to precisely the desired position up to 45°. This unique feature is differentiated from some other surgical staplers which have a finite number of preset articulation positions that limit the surgeon's ability to place the reload at the precisely desired position. AEON's smooth articulation allows for easy negotiation of the instrument regardless of port placement, and to safely dissect out deeply placed vessels or undertake GI anastomoses (Fig. 33.19).

33.2.1 Clinical Applications in Hepatopancreatobiliary Surgery

The AEON instrument is used in a number of hepatopancreatobiliary surgery categories, and is ideal in both minimally invasive laparoscopic and open surgical cases.

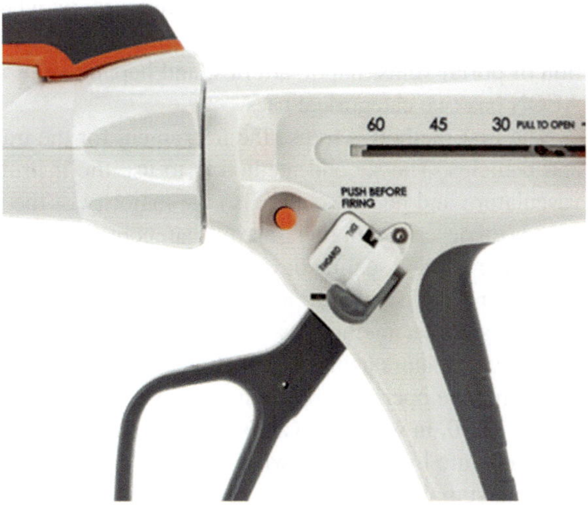

Fig. 33.18 Multispeed gear system

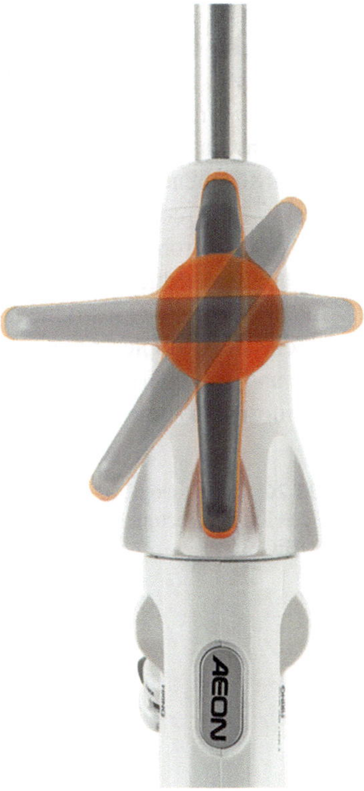

Fig. 33.19 Smooth articulation

The most common application is in liver surgery, where it has been used successfully for parenchymal transection, ligation of major Glissonean pedicles, and ligation of portal veins, haptic arteries, and hepatic veins. In hepatectomy procedures, AEON has two categorical uses.

The first method is to use the instrument for the transection only of vasculature and pedicles. The second method is to use the instrument for transection of both vasculature and pedicles, and also the majority of the parenchyma. Many methods have been described in literature for parenchyma dissection [1], including the use of ultrasonic energy, sealing devices, the "crunching method", radiofrequency sealers, and water jet dissection to name a few. What sets AEON surgical instrument apart from these other methods is operating time. Transection of both parenchyma and hepatic vasculature using AEON allows for hepatectomy procedures to be expedited and to reduce operating room time. The said transection method is pictured below in Fig. 33.20, in which AEON is used for an extended left hepatectomy.

A separate liver surgery where the instrument may be employed is for liver cyst wall marsupialization. AEON delivers a hemostatic transection of the cyst wall, thereby providing a clean separation from the liver parenchyma. The potential advantages of using AEON for cyst wall marsupialization is that surgery time may be reduced, and the risk of bile leaks may also be reduced. The said method is pictured below in Fig. 33.21.

In pancreatic surgery, the AEON endostapler is the ideal instrument for resection of the pancreas parenchyma in distal or lateral pancreatectomy procedures. The AEON instrument has shown validity with exceptionally good performance in HPB surgery, with a reduction in one case series of pancreatic fistula rates by two-thirds [2]. This is corroborated by bariatric clinical studies where AEON's staple lines were shown to reduce bleeding as compared to others (Fig. 33.22) [3, 4].

Finally, the AEON instrument may be used in pancreaticoduodenectomy surgery (both classic Whipple and pylorus-preserving) for transection of the small bowel, gastric and mesenteric ligation, and in gastrojejunostomy and duodenojejunostomy anastomoses. In some cases, the AEON endostapler can be used to safely dissect the

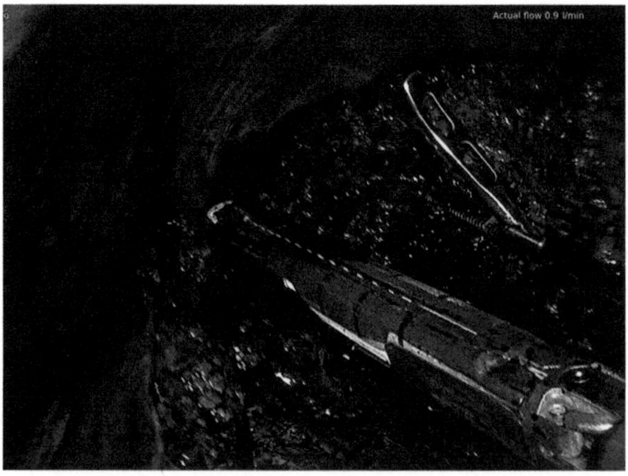

Fig. 33.20 Laparoscopic extended left hepatectomy using AEON

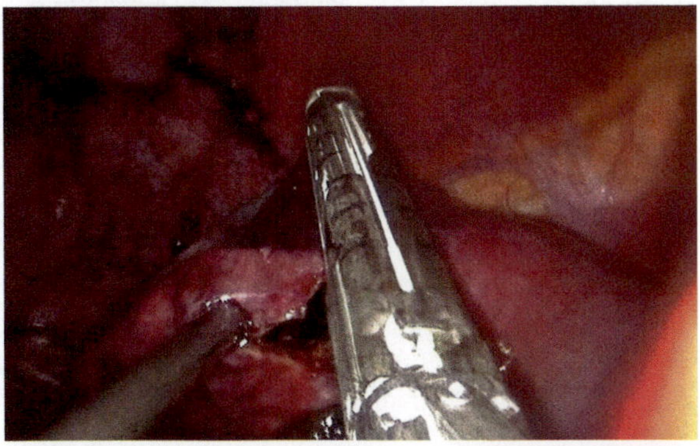

Fig. 33.21 Liver cyst wall marsupialization using AEON

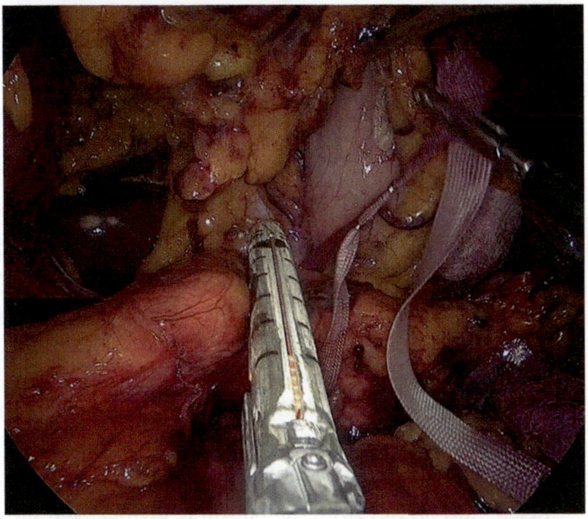

Fig. 33.22 Laparoscopic distal pancreatectomy pancreas resection using AEON (orange cartridge)

uncinate and head of the pancreas from the superior mesenteric artery, with excellent control and ligation of the superior and inferior pancreatoduodenal arteries. This has a potential benefit of reducing time in theatre as well as improved hemostasis (Fig. 33.23).

33.2.2 Instrument Operation and Troubleshooting Instructional Guide (Fig. 33.24)

To load a reload onto the handle, identify the "Load" arrow pictured on the reload and the "Load" arrow pictured on the handle. Align the two arrows, and press the two components together and rotate. Confirmation of proper fastening of the reload to the handle is achieved by three means:

Fig. 33.23 Open Whipple procedure, gastrojejunostomy using AEON

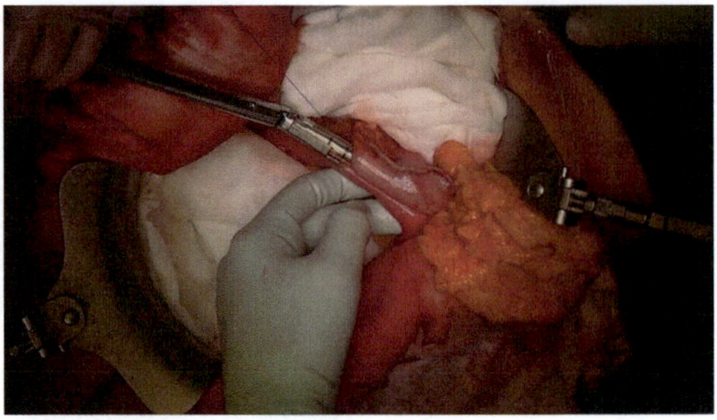

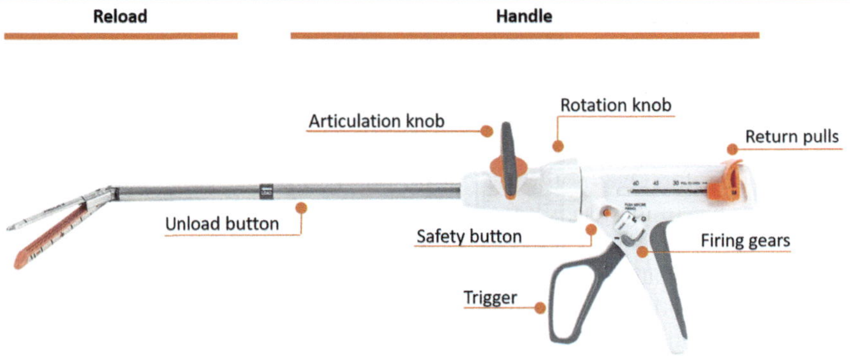

Fig. 33.24 AEON instrument components

1. An audible "click" is heard.
2. The unload button on the underside of the handle shaft will have clicked into place, and no red from the button is visible. See Fig. 33.25.

Note: If the scrub nurse is attempting to load the reload but the reload will not click into place, the handle is likely in a slightly articulated position. When loading the reload onto the handle, the articulation should be in a neutral position. The scrub nurse should straighten the articulation and load the reload again.

3. Perform a system check by squeezing the handle trigger, and thereafter by pulling on the return pulls. The jaws of the reload should close when the handle is squeezed, and should open when the return pulls are pulled. See Fig. 33.26.

Once the instrument is loaded, the surgeon must next position the reload onto the target tissue. In minimally invasive laparoscopic surgery, the surgeon will need to close the jaws of the reload in order to insert the instrument into the abdomen through the 12 mm or 15 mm trocar ports. Once inside the abdomen, the surgeon

Fig. 33.25 Loading reload onto the handle

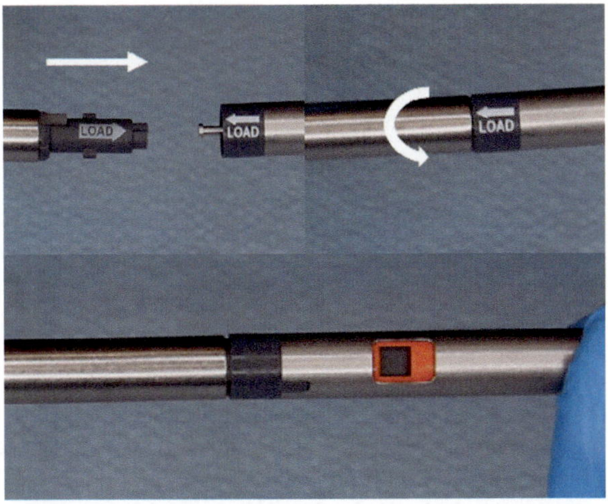

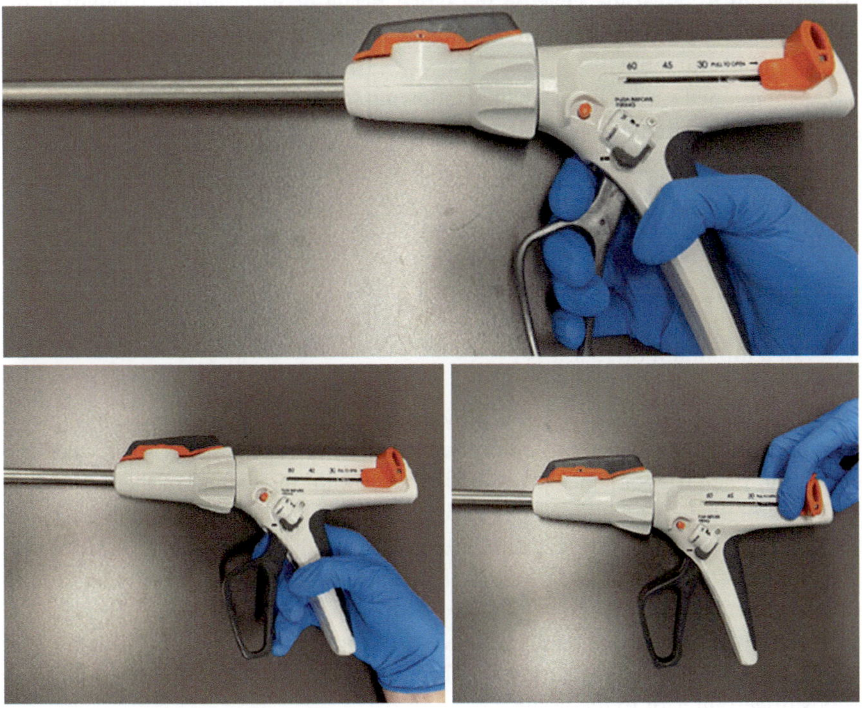

Fig. 33.26 Performing system check

may open the jaws and navigate the reload to the desired position using the rotation and articulation knobs.

The AEON instrument includes a grasping mode, that is the surgeon to use the instrument as a grasper to reposition tissue. This is achieved by using the trigger not

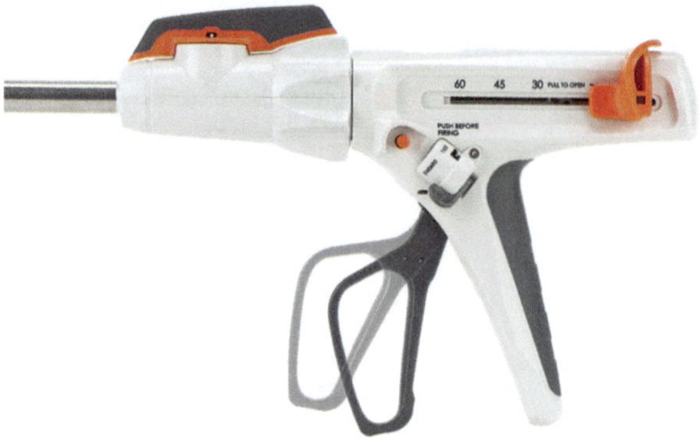

Fig. 33.27 AEON grasping mode

only to close the jaws, but also to push the trigger forward to unclamp the jaws. See Fig. 33.27 below.

Once the desired reload and tissue positions have been achieved, the trigger may be squeezed to close the jaws on the target tissue or vasculature. Thereafter, the safety button is pressed. The said button may be pressed from either the right or left side of the instrument.

As mentioned earlier in the chapter, allowing for sufficient pre-compression time is critical to optimizing the staple line. The author employs the following step-by-step process to achieve this goal:

1. Clamp down on target tissue.
2. Press safety button.
3. Move firing gear from standard to thick mode.
4. Squeeze the trigger once.
5. Wait a minimum of 15 s.

At this point, the surgeon may deploy the staple line. This is achieved by squeezing the trigger in a slow and controlled manner, releasing the trigger, and then repeating. Each trigger squeeze results in the forward movement of the knife blade and the simultaneous deployment and formation of staples across a finite distance. Continue squeezing the trigger until the entirety of the reload has been deployed. The progression and position of the knife blade can be visualized either by observing the return pulls, which travel forward with each trigger pull, or by observing the metallic tab on the reload itself, which is an exposed portion of the I-Beam, as it travels the reload distally. The travel of the I-Beam may be observed only if the anvil is positioned inferior to the tissue.

Note: If the surgeon is attempting to squeeze the trigger to begin firing but the trigger is stuck and not moving, the reload safety lockout mechanism may be engaged, which indicates the reload was already fired, even slightly. The surgeon should cease squeezing the trigger, and the reload should be replaced.

When firing the surgical instrument, the surgeon should be mindful of three important considerations:

1. While staple deployment and tissue transection occur simultaneously, the AEON instrument is designed to intentionally deploy staples distal to the knife blade, that is, ahead of the cut line. This design feature ensures that tissue or vasculature is sealed before it is transected.
2. If the surgeon experiences exceptionally strong resistance during firing, this may indicate that either an obstruction has been encountered, such as a surgical clip, or the staple size selected may not be appropriate for the target tissue, and a larger size should be selected. While firing the full length of each reload is best practice, the surgeon has the option to safely retract the reload using the return pulls even if the entirety of the staple line has not been deployed in this scenario.
3. While resistance measures may be subjective, an additional resistance measure that is objective is that a loud "crack" may be heard in the handle. The said sound is the activation of a mechanical fuse in the AEON handle that has been cleverly designed to limit the force a surgeon may exert on the reload progression to prevent potential downstream difficulties arising from firing into excessively thick tissue or an obstruction.

Note: Several mitigations are available to the surgeon in this scenario. First, the surgeon may pause the firing to allow additional time for tissue pre-compression, which may reduce tissue thickness and allow for subsequent staple line deployment. Second, the surgeon may change the gear to thick mode to reduce the firing force and speed of staple line deployment. Finally, the surgeon may retract the reload and replace it with a larger staple size reload.

After completing the staple line, the surgeon will need to retract the reload by pulling on the return pulls. Said action will drive the I-beam to return proximally and will release/open the stapler jaws, at which point the reload and handle can be removed and handed to the scrub nurse.

Note: If the surgeon is experiencing high force or resistance when retracting, the surgeon should use both hands to pull evenly on both sides of the return pulls. If clinically appropriate, the surgeon may reduce the reload articulation angle.

The surgeon should take care to inspect the staple line for staple formation and cut line quality after each firing, and any observed bleeding or leaking.

Once the instrument has been fired and retracted, the used single-use reload may be unloaded. To unload, the following steps should be taken:

1. Ensure the reload is fully retracted and the jaws are open.
2. Ensure the handle is not articulated, that is, the articulation knob should be centred.
3. Use one hand to pull down on the unload button, and use the other hand to gently twist the reload. Doing so should not require significant force. The reload should spring from the handle housing after twisting to unfasten. See Fig. 33.28.

Note: If the scrub nurse is attempting to unload the reload but is unable to detach the reload from the handle, ensure that (a) the reload jaws are open, (b) the

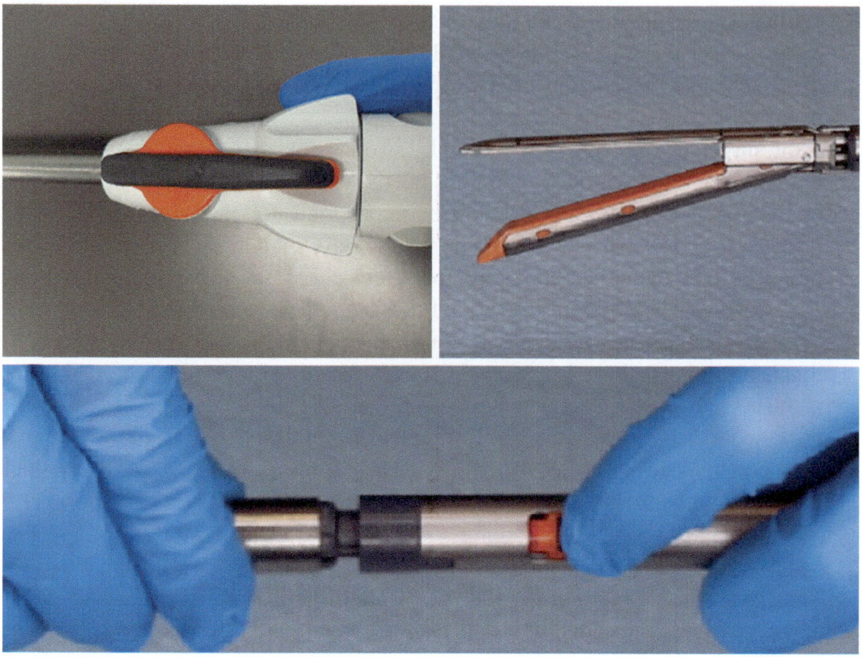

Fig. 33.28 Unloading reload from handle

articulation is in a straight or neutral position, and (c) the orange unload button is held down completely when twisting the reload from the handle.

33.2.3 Storage

The AEON endovascular stapler and reloads may be stored at room temperature.

AEON handles and reloads are supplied sterile. Each AEON reload can be used only once. Once the staples have been deployed, the reload cannot be used again and may be discarded in appropriately sanctioned biohazardous waste. The AEON handle may be used with up to 25 reloads and should be used in a single case. After completion of the case, the AEON handle should also be discarded in appropriately sanctioned biohazardous waste.

33.2.4 Cavitron Ultrasonic Surgical Aspirator(CUSA)

In the 1980s, the cavitron ultrasonic surgical aspirator (CUSA) was introduced for liver transection. CUSA is useful as a surgical device for excavation because it has multiple functions in one device, like fracturing the liver parenchyma, sucking blood, exposing, and handling the bridging blood vessels and bile ducts. The basis

Fig. 33.29 CUSA-PARTS

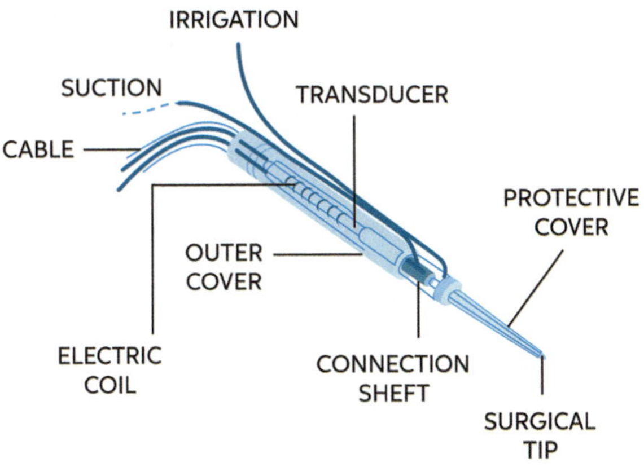

of the CUSA device is that it generates ultrasonic waves in the range of 23 kHz to produce tissue cavitations. This mechanical energy is delivered through a hollow 3 mm tip that vibrates at 23,000 cycles per second. The energy device is embedded with an irrigator and aspirator to dispose of the tissue debris. The coagulation effect was caused by protein denaturation, which occurs as a result of the destruction of hydrogen bonds in proteins.

The CUSA contains three main parts:

A. Piezoelectric Transducer: Ultrasonic waves are generated using the piezoelectric transducer. This is a crystal that transforms electrical oscillations into mechanical vibrations. The transducer consists of a stack of alloy plates constructed from nickel. A coil mounted around the plates produces a magnetic field that induces a mechanical motion of around 300 microns.
B. Connecting Body: The transducer vibrations are physically transferred to the surgical level. It also amplifies the transducer's vibratory shift.
C. Surgical Tip: Completes the motion amplification and makes contact with the surface. Therefore, the tip is comparatively long in accordance with its diameter, and this allows sufficient acceleration of motion (Fig. 33.29).

33.2.5 The Mechanism of Function

Electric current travels into a coil in the handpiece, which generates a magnetic effect. The magnetic field excites a nickel alloy transducer that extends and contracts to create an oscillating wave in the longitudinal axis at a frequency of 25 to 35 khz. From the alloy, the piezoelectric crystals allow the tip of the handle to oscillate. The electromagnetic movements of ultrasound are magnified over the length of the handpiece.

The oscillating tip that has come into touch with the tissue induces tissue displacement by creating ultrasound cavitation at the cell level, with low pressure outside the cell contributing to cell destruction. The high-frequency vibration produces heat, which is cooled by recirculation in the tip of the probe. This device maintains the tip temperature at around 40 °C.

For reference, we are going to describe SONOCA 300. During start-up it conducts an automatic self-test to confirm the availability of all functions for the user's convenience. When the handpiece is connected it offers initial operating parameters including ultrasonic power, aspiration, and irrigation settings, all of which can be adjusted later as needed (Figs. 33.30 and 33.31).

The orange and blue foot switches control the fracturing and water-dripping functions, respectively. The blue button on the handpiece is responsible for applying electrocautery. Initially, CUSA settings begin with aspiration and irrigation at 50% and 5 cc/min, and the amplitude at 80% without activating the Tissue Select mode. These settings are modified according to the tissue's texture and response to cutting (Fig. 33.32).

CUSA effectively accomplishes liver parenchymal fragmentation with ultrasonic energy and aspiration, typically in 1–2 mm diameter fragments. This exposes blood

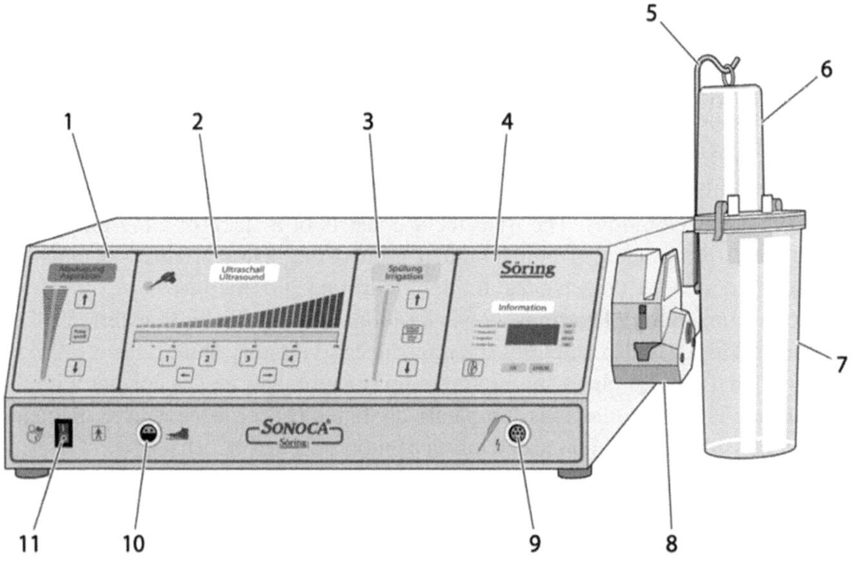

Fig. 33.30 Front view of Sonoca 300

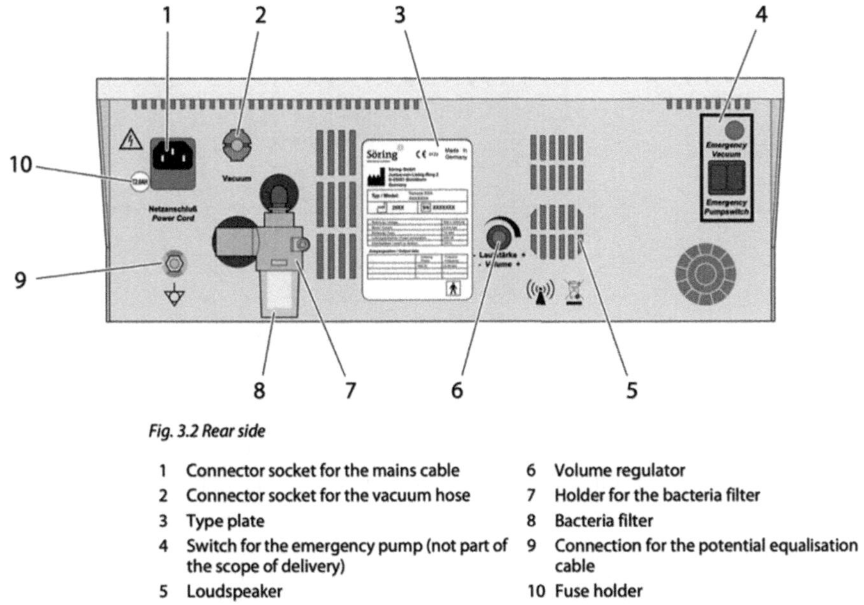

Fig. 33.31 Back view of Sonoca 300

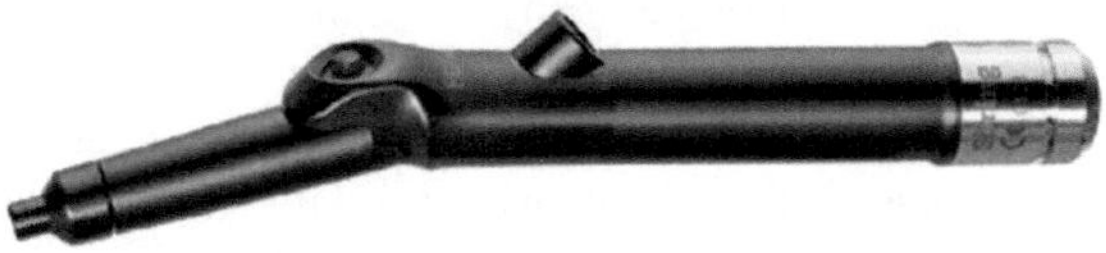

Fig. 33.32 Hand piece for Sonoca 300

vessels and biliary radicles, which can be subsequently clipped or ligated. In cases of significant hemorrhage hindering selective coagulation or ligation of smaller structures, inflow occlusion like the Pringle manoeuvre is applied as and when necessary.

For CUSAs with stanching function, adequate pressure on smaller blood vessels is maintained with the flank of the cylindrical tip to stop blood flow. The electrocoagulation mode is activated to coagulate the blood vessel followed by the activation of the fragmentation/ultrasound mode with irrigation. This allows the smooth removal of the tip from the area without adhering to the coagulated vessel.

33.2.6 Information on Cavitation

The sound field emitted is characterized by powerful high- and low-pressure phases. Cavitation bubbles oscillate nonlinearly with the sound field, sometimes over many vibration periods, until they implode during compression. Near interfaces, the bubbles implode aspherically, forming a water jet with considerable velocity (Fig. 33.33).

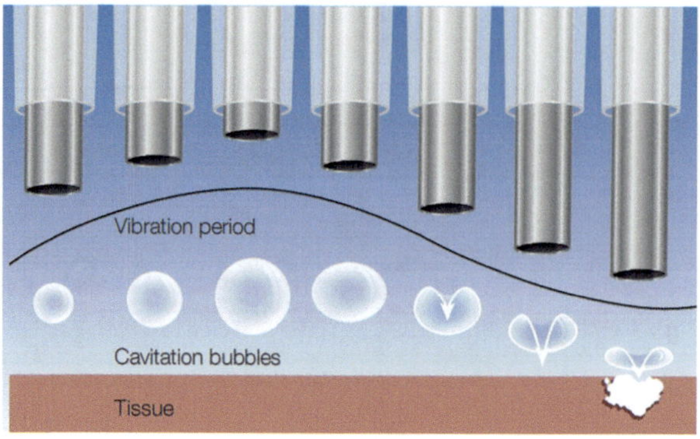

Fig. 33.33 Cavitation: The sound field emitted is in high- and low-pressure phases. Cavitation bubbles oscillate nonlinearly with the sound field until they implode during compression

The sonotrode vibrates back and forth with an amplitude of approx. 50–230 μm. When it enters into contact with enough tissue, the sonotrode tip hits the tissue at up to 6 m/s during this oscillation and mechanically breaks the cell bond (also known as the "jackhammer effect"). The mechanical tissue effect increases as the contact force increases.

In addition, the sonotrode vibration emits a sound field, causing alternating high- and low-pressure phases in the environment. Cavitation bubbles may form during the low-pressure phases. Imploding cavitation bubbles generate powerful pressure pulses as well as shock waves, which can lead to tissue removal (Fig. 33.34).

The direction of parenchymal transection varies depending on the surgeon's preference, including caudo-ventral, caudo-cranial, or cranio-caudal approaches. Knowledge of intersegmental planes is crucial for bloodless dissection, often following major hepatic veins where no Glissonean pedicle runs.

In laparoscopy, CUSA is inserted after the liver capsule has been breached using ultrasonic shears or something similar. The device is used to divide the parenchyma, with attention paid to the vector of CUSA movement to prevent uncontrollable bleeding as described by Honda et al. [5]. Thin vessels left by CUSA are handled using the energy device of choice of the surgeon or by clipping and cutting. When extending the cutting plane, the liver's surface portion is divided widely before proceeding closely around the hepatic vein. Any major hepatic vein injury if occurs can be repaired with fine polypropylene suture. The hepatic pedicle tissue and major hepatic veins can be transacted using a laparoscopic linear stapler. Studies have shown that CUSA is safe and effective in laparoscopic hepatectomy for HCC patients even with cirrhosis [6–8].

33.3 Troubleshooting

Common troubleshooting steps are presented in Table 33.1.

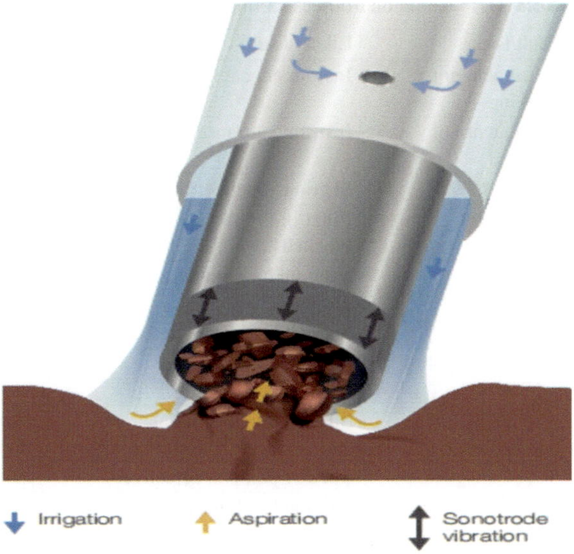

Fig. 33.34 Direction of irrigation, aspiration, and vibration

33.4 Water Jet Scalpel

Water jet scalpel (WJS) dissociates the liver parenchyma with the jet stream, and fine vessels can be selectively preserved without thermal damage. When the jet stream of WJS is applied to the edge of the vessel, the dorsal side of the vessel is dissected. This is because the Coanda effect causes the water flow to wrap around the dorsal side of the vessel. WJS is superior to other devices in that it does not cause thermal damage.

A pressure of 30–40 bar and a nozzle diameter of 0.1 mm are very effective to dissect normal liver tissue. In case of cirrhotic liver parenchyma the pressure needed for dissection is 10 bar higher (Figs. 33.35 and 33.36) [9].

33.5 Main Components of the Erbe Waterjet System

33.5.1 ERBEJET 2 Control Unit

This is the central module of the system. It regulates the water pressure, flow rate, and dissection mode. The unit interfaces with the surgeon via a touchscreen or rotary knob interface, allowing real-time adjustments to parameters. Preset programs are available for specific procedures or tissue types. The interface allows integration with other Erbe devices for combined hybrid dissection and coagulation workflows.

Table 33.1 Common troubleshooting steps

Fault/issue	Likely cause	Suggested solution
Instrument not working	Instrument cable is damaged.	Replace with a new cable.
Instrument not detected	Instrument transducer is faulty.	Use a different instrument.
Suction not functioning	Suction container lid is open.	Close the lid securely.
	Filter of the suction container is blocked.	Replace the filter or disposable liner.
	Vacuum hose not attached properly.	Reconnect the vacuum hose correctly.
	Suction hose is twisted or bent.	Straighten or reposition the hose.
	Instrument is blocked.	Rinse the instrument; if needed, use another.
	Suction pump is off.	Switch on the suction pump from the operator control panel.
	Suction pump is defective.	Switch over to a surgical aspirator.
	Suction level incorrectly set.	Adjust the suction setting properly; if required, disconnect and reconnect the instrument cable.
Error tone with ultrasonic treatment	Sonotrode tip pressure on tissue is too high.	Stop ultrasonic treatment and reapply the tip correctly.
OK display flashes during ultrasonic treatment	Instrument is overloaded.	Stop ultrasonic treatment.
Rinsing not working	No rinsing liquid left in the bottle.	Connect a new rinsing bottle.
	Rinsing spike is not positioned correctly in the bottle.	Insert the spike properly and check the drop chamber.
	Rinsing hose is not inserted correctly into the hose pump.	Reopen the pump and place the hose correctly.
	Vacuum present in the rinsing bottle due to the closed ventilation flap of the drop chamber.	Open the ventilation flap or relieve the vacuum using a syringe needle.
	Rinsing adjustment incorrect.	Correct the rinsing setting.

33.5.2 Water Reservoir and Pump System

A dedicated sterile saline container supplies the fluid medium. An internal high-pressure pump delivers the saline through the tubing system to the applicator at adjustable pressures (typically 15–60 bar, depending on tissue and surgical indication). The fluid is directed in a highly focused jet to achieve precise tissue separation.

33.5.3 Applicator Handpiece

The handheld dissection probe, or applicator, is ergonomically designed for both open and laparoscopic procedures. Available in various sizes and tip configurations

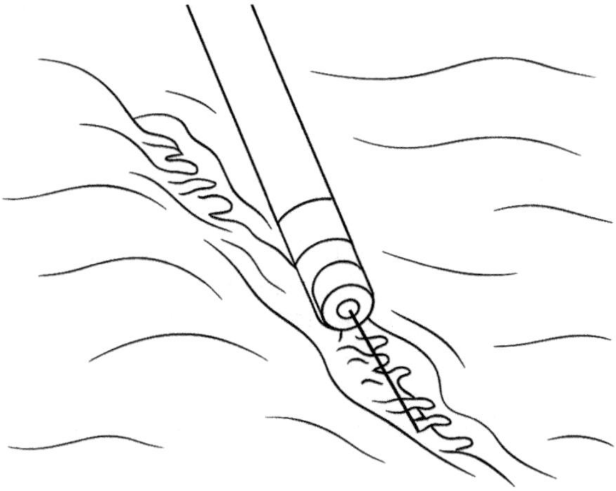

Fig. 33.35 The waterjet function of the applicator reveals vessels which may be selectively coagulated using electrosurgery

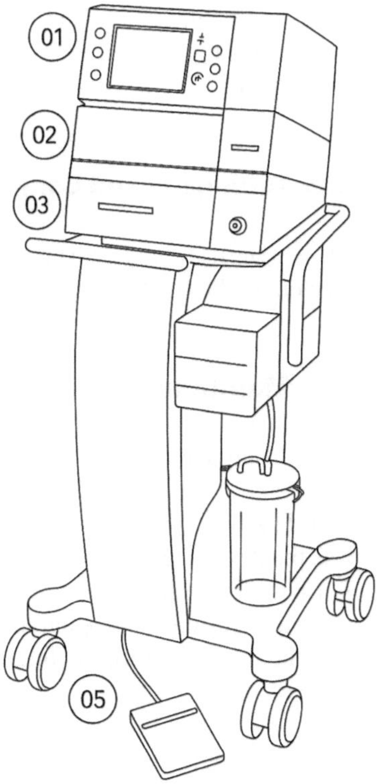

Fig. 33.36 Erbe Jet 2 is an example of a water jet scalpel. 01—Electrosurgical unit providing cutting and coagulation modes. 02—APC for hemostasis. 03—Waterjet module. 04—Suction module to permit good visibility of the target site and may be activated individually or synchronously with the waterjet. 05—Activation of the waterjet and change of program via footswitch

(straight, angled, and curved) for different anatomical challenges. The nozzle at the tip precisely emits the waterjet stream. Some versions include integrated electrosurgical capability, allowing coagulation to be performed through the same applicator.

33.5.4 Footswitch Pedal (Multifunctional)

Allows hands-free activation of the waterjet and switching between different modes (e.g., dissection, standby, and flush). May also be used to control synchronized suction if connected to the ESM 2 module.

33.5.5 ESM 2 Suction Module (Optional but Often Integrated)

This suction module connects directly to the ERBEJET 2 system. Allows synchronized or manual suction of fluid, debris, or blood from the operative field. Enhances visibility during dissection and minimizes fluid accumulation. It can be set to activate automatically when the waterjet is in use, ensuring continuous cleaning of the operative field.

33.5.6 Tubing Set and Connectors

Single-use sterile tubing delivers saline from the reservoir to the applicator. Includes connectors to the control unit, ensuring a closed sterile system.

33.6 Maintenance

After each surgical case, the following steps should be taken:

System Flush

- Use the designated flushing program on the control unit.
- Flush the entire fluid pathway with sterile water or designated cleaning solution to remove residual saline and prevent crystallization or biofilm formation.
- Run the flush cycle for the full duration recommended by the manufacturer.

Disposal of Single-Use Items

- Discard the disposable applicator, tubing set, and fluid reservoir according to hospital biohazard protocols.
- Never attempt to reuse disposable components, as this compromises sterility and functionality.

Surface Cleaning

- Wipe the exterior surfaces of the control unit, footswitch, and suction module with a soft cloth moistened with hospital-grade disinfectant.
- Avoid using abrasive materials or excessive moisture, especially near electrical ports and touchscreens.

Check for Leaks or Residue

- Inspect all connectors, tubing ports, and external modules for signs of fluid leaks, corrosion, or residual fluid buildup.
- Clean and dry affected areas immediately.

33.7 Troubleshooting

Common troubleshooting steps are presented in Table 33.2.

Table 33.2 Common troubleshooting steps

Issue	Possible cause	Recommended action
No water jet was emitted	Empty saline container Tubing not connected properly Blocked nozzle	Check and refill saline container Ensure all tubing connections are secure Replace applicator or nozzle if blockage persists
Weak or inconsistent water jet	Low pressure setting Air in the tubing Partially blocked nozzle	Increase pressure via control unit Prime tubing to eliminate air bubbles Flush nozzle or replace applicator
Footswitch unresponsive	Loose or damaged footswitch cable Footswitch not assigned to function System not in ready mode	Reconnect or replace the footswitch Assign the correct function from the control panel Confirm system is powered and in standby/ready
Water leaks from tubing or connections	Improperly seated tubing Damaged tubing or connectors	Disconnect and reconnect tubing firmly Replace tubing set if damaged
No suction during dissection	ESM 2 module not activated Suction tubing disconnected or clogged Suction canister full	Activate ESM 2 via the control unit Reconnect or flush suction tubing Empty or replace suction canister
Applicator not recognized by the system	Faulty applicator cable or connector Wrong applicator type Software error	Try reconnecting or replacing the applicator Ensure compatibility of applicator with system Restart the system and reinitialize

(continued)

Table 33.2 (continued)

Issue	Possible cause	Recommended action
System alarm or error message	System self-check failure Incorrect settings or connections Internal hardware/ software issue	Follow on-screen error instructions Check all external modules and settings Contact Erbe technical support if unresolved
No integration with electrosurgical unit (e.g., VIO 300D)	Communication cable not connected Mode mismatch Incompatible software versions	Check the connection cable between devices Verify integrated modes are correctly set Update system firmware if needed
Foggy camera due to water jet mist	Excessive water usage Inadequate suction or heat	Reduce water pressure if not needed Improve suction near the dissection zone Use antifog solution on the laparoscope
Inadequate dissection performance	Low pressure Incorrect applicator tip Fibrotic liver or hard parenchyma	Increase jet pressure Try a different applicator shape Use alternative dissection modality (e.g., CUSA and bipolar) if needed

33.8 Conclusion

Laparoscopic liver resection has evolved significantly with the development of specialized instruments that enhance precision, safety, and efficiency. Devices such as advanced energy platforms, waterjet dissectors, articulating instruments, and tailored vascular staplers have transformed what was once a technically formidable procedure into a reproducible and minimally invasive approach. These tools allow for selective parenchymal dissection, controlled hemostasis, and preservation of vital structures, all within the constraints of a laparoscopic environment. As technology continues to advance, the integration of these specialized instruments will play an increasingly pivotal role in expanding the indications and improving outcomes of laparoscopic liver surgery. Surgeons must remain adept with these tools and informed about emerging innovations to offer the highest standard of care.

Acknowledgments The authors would like to thank Dr. Adam Park from BOWA-LOTUS and Mr. Paul Rabinovich from Lexington Medical for their help and expertize with this chapter.

References

1. Aragon RJ, Solomon NL. Techniques of hepatic resection. J Gastrointest Oncol. 2012;3(1):28.
2. Sheen, et al. Preliminary experience in laparoscopic distal pancreatectomy using the AEON vascular stapler; PSGBI 2022 annual scientific meeting, 30 Nov 2022, Leeds.
3. Redmann JG, Lavin TE, French MS, Broussard TD, Lapointe-Gagner M. Improving hemostasis in sleeve gastrectomy with alternative stapler. JSLS. 2020;24(4):e2020–00073.
4. Raftopoulos Y, Rajkumar S, Davidson E, Papasavas P. Prospective randomized comparison of linear endostaplers during laparoscopic sleeve gastrectomy. Obes Surg. 2022;32(10):3472–80.
5. Honda G, Kurata M, Okuda Y, Kobayashi S, Tadano S, Yamaguchi T, Matsumoto H, Nakano D, Takahashi K. Totally laparoscopic hepatectomy exposing the major vessels. J Hepatobiliary Pancreat Sci. 2013;20(4):435–40. https://doi.org/10.1007/s00534-012-0586-7.
6. Liu F, Wei YG, Li HY, Wang WT, Wen TF, Hong W, Yang JY, Ming Qing X, Li B. LigaSure versus CUSA for parenchymal transection during laparoscopic hepatectomy in hepatocellular carcinoma patients with cirrhosis: a propensity score-matched analysis. Surg Endosc. 2018;32(5):2454–65. https://doi.org/10.1007/S00464-017-5947-5.
7. Yoon YI, Kim KH, Kang SH, et al. Pure laparoscopic versus open right hepatectomy for hepatocellular carcinoma in patients with cirrhosis: a propensity score matched analysis. Ann Surg. 2017;265:856–63.
8. Cheung TT, Dai WC, Tsang SH, et al. Pure laparoscopic hepatectomy versus open hepatectomy for hepatocellular carcinoma in 110 patients with liver cirrhosis: a propensity analysis at a single center. Ann Surg. 2016;264:612–20.
9. Rau HG, Duessel AP, Wurzbacher S. The use of water-jet dissection in open and laparoscopic liver resection. HPB (Oxford). 2008;10(4):275–80. https://doi.org/10.1080/13651820802167706. PMID: 18773110; PMCID: PMC2518306.

Pediatric Surgery Laparoscopic Equipment

34

Gali Divya

34.1 Introduction

Pediatric laparoscopy was first described by Kelling in 1923, but its use has increased over last three decades [1]. With miniaturization of endoscopic instruments, laparoscopic and thoracoscopic surgeries are being done even in neonates, apart from toddlers and older children. With the limited working space in the chest and abdomen, it is slightly more difficult in children when compared to adults, but it is feasible.

34.1.1 Preparation Before Starting the Procedure

Nasogastric or orogastric tube insertion can decompress the stomach, which can help in gaining extra working space in children. No need for catherization in older children if they can empty their bladder before surgery. But it is needed where dissection in the pelvis is required, e.g., extravesical ureteric reimplantation, laparoscopy-assisted pull-through procedures in cases of Hirschsprung disease or Anorectal malformations. Enemas are not usually needed.

The laparoscope should be made ready before the insertion of the first trocar. Higher intra-abdominal pressures with high flow rates and rapid insufflation may cause cardiovascular events, so insufflator settings must be matched with the age and body size of the patient. The normal range of intra-abdominal pressure maintained during surgery is 8–10 mm of Hg with flow rates of 4–6 L/min. Needles for intracorporeal suturing can be inserted directly through the abdominal wall, and they can be removed at the end along with the trocar, and the trocar can be reinserted if necessary.

G. Divya (✉)
Pediatric Surgery, All India Institute of Medical Sciences, New Delhi, India

J. S. Ahluwalia (ed.), *User Manual for Minimally Invasive Surgical Equipment*,
https://doi.org/10.1007/978-981-95-9019-3_34

As in adult laparoscopy, the pneumoperitoneum can be created either by Verres needle or by the open port Hasson's technique. After the first port insertion, it's always better to check the position of the port with the laparoscope prior to insufflation. The connecting tubes should be flushed with CO_2 before intra-abdominal insufflation. After establishing the pneumoperitoneum Endotracheal (ET) tube needs to be rechecked because pneumoperitoneum may cause elevation of the diaphragm and downward shift of the ET tube with risk of unilateral intubation.

34.1.2 Procedures That Can Be Done by the Minimal Invasive Technique

34.1.2.1 Thoracoscopic Procedures [2]

Esophageal atresia, congenital diaphragmatic hernia, foregut duplication cyst excision or mediastinal cysts excision, excision of posterior mediastinal neuroblastoma, segmentectomy, lobectomy or pneumonectomy, sympathectomy, thymectomy etc.

34.1.2.2 Abdominal Procedures [2]

Cardiomyotomy for achalasia, fundoplication, diaphragmatic repair for eventration of diaphragm/diaphragmatic hernia, splenectomy, pyloromyotomy for pyloric stenosis, Kasai portoenterostomy for biliary atresia, excision of choledochal cyst and hepatico-enterostomy, Kimura's duodeno-duodenostomy for duodenal atresia, Ladd's procedure for malrotation, adhesiolysis, appendicectomy, cholecystectomy, intussusception, laparoscopic-assisted pull-through for Hirschsprung disease and anorectal malformations, excision of mesenteric cyst or intestinal duplication cyst, etc.

34.1.2.3 Urological Procedures [2]

Undescended testes, inguinal hernia, varicocele, pyeloplasty, ureteric reimplantation both extra vesical and pneumovesicoscopic, nephroureterectomy, etc.

34.2 Equipment

Standard equipment like monitor, video equipment, light source and insufflator are the same as in adult patients [3].

34.3 Ports

A port is a path of entry and exit. Most commonly used ports in the practice of pediatric laparoscopic surgery are 3 mm, 5 mm and 10 mm (Fig. 34.1) depending on the age of the child. 12 mm, 13 mm, and 15 mm ports are also available. The two parts of the port are the trocar and the cannula. Trocar has two parts, which include tip and the head. Tip of the trocars have different shapes like conical, pyramidal and

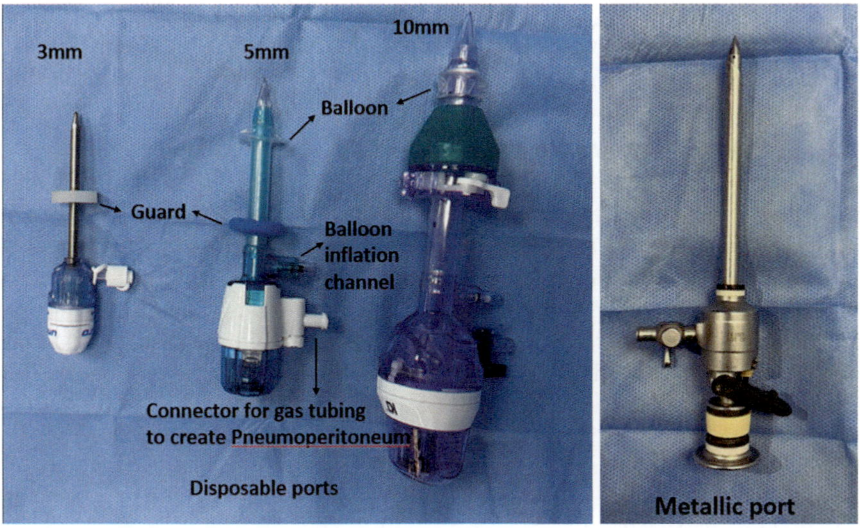

Fig. 34.1 Different types of ports

Fig. 34.2 3 mm ports of different lengths (8 cm and 13 cm) which can be used based on the contour of the abdominal wall of the child

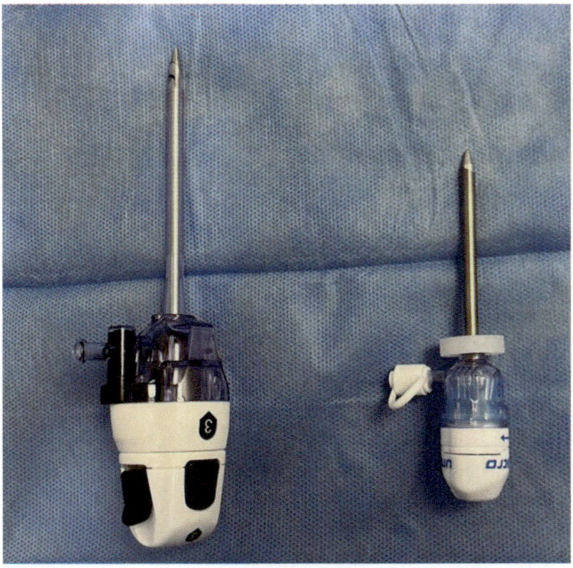

blunt-tipped trocars. Safety trocars are also available. Cannula has two parts—the cylindrical shaft and the valve. Metallic reusable ports, disposable ports, and balloon ports are available. The balloon ports have a balloon at the tip for self-retaining mechanism so that the ports do not get displaced after their placement. The balloon can be inflated with 5–10 ml of air. Trocars without self-retaining mechanism can be fixed with a suture to prevent displacement. And the length of these ports also differs, which are available with 8 cm, 13 cm (Fig. 34.2), 20 cm, and even longer lengths which can be chosen based on the contour of the abdominal wall of the child (Fig. 34.3).

34.3.1 Parts of Laparoscopic Instruments

All laparoscopic instruments have three parts which include the sheath, insert, and handle (Fig. 34.4). 3 mm and 5 mm instruments are most commonly used in pediatric surgery. And the usual length of the 5 mm and 10 mm instruments is 28 cm, 36 cm, and longer length instruments with 45 cm are also available. 3 mm instruments usually are 20 cm in length. The instruments used in pediatric laparoscopic surgery are finer, more delicate and break easily, hence these should be handled carefully.

Most commonly used instruments in pediatric laparoscopy are as follows:

1. *Maryland dissector*
2. *Right-angle Maryland*
3. *Laparoscopic scissors*
4. *Atraumatic grasper*
5. *Toothed grasper*
6. *Needle holder*
7. *Hook and spatula*

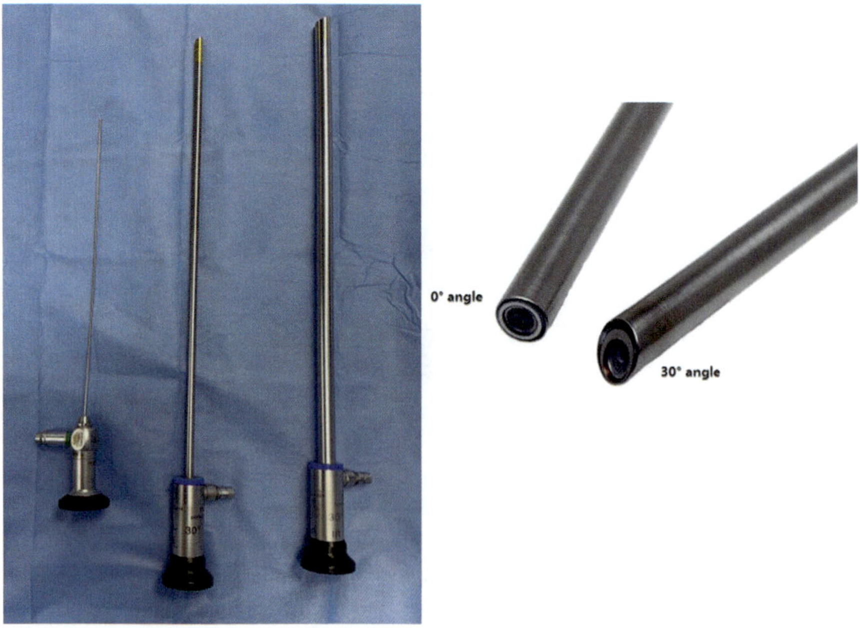

Fig. 34.3 3 mm, 5 mm, and 10 cm telescopes

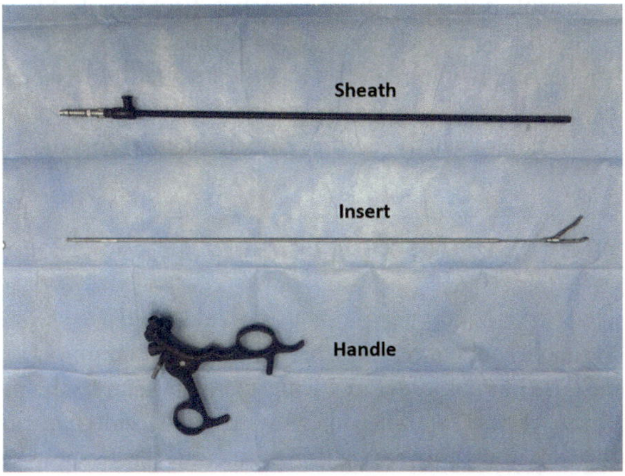

Fig. 34.4 Parts of laparoscopic instruments

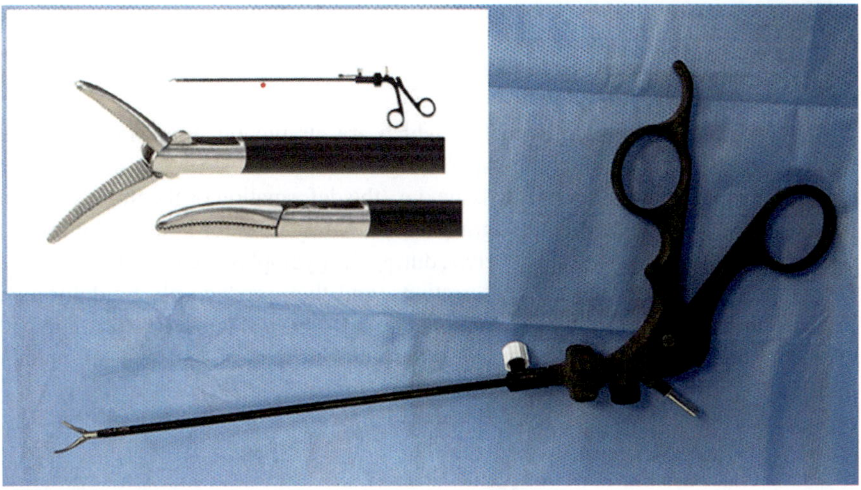

Fig. 34.5 Maryland dissector

8. *Clip applicator—metal & hemolock*
9. *Harmonic scalpel*
10. *Suction and irrigation cannula*

1. *Maryland Dissector and Right-Angle Maryland*

The Maryland dissector (Fig. 34.5) is most commonly used for blunt dissection. It has long, curved jaws with fine- tapered tip. It is a replica of artery forceps in open surgery. It can also be used for stripping the peritoneum, for creating a window in between the structures and also for hemostasis. This instrument is having double action jaws. The shaft can be rotated for 360° by the rotating wheel. It does not have a ratchet. Right-angle Maryland (Fig. 34.6) is also used for dissection; the advantage is that the tip will be in the field of dissection, so that inadvertent injury to the surrounding tissues is less likely. Devices like monopolar cautery can be connected to this instrument. Bipolar Maryland is also available, which can prevent lateral spread of the current.

34.4 Laparoscopic Scissors

These are mainly used to cut or divide the tissues. Straight and curved scissors are available, but curved scissors are the most commonly used type. Hook scissors are designed to cut structures from the distal end to the proximal, minimizing the risk of inadvertent injury to other structures. Monopolar cautery can be attached with the scissors and can be used for dissecting the tissues. Micro-scissors have fine jaws that can be used to divide the bowel adhesions (Fig. 34.7).

34.5 Laparoscopic Graspers

Three types of graspers are available, which are atraumatic, semi-traumatic and traumatic graspers. Atraumatic graspers (Fig. 34.8) have fine serrations, and they produce elastic deformation of the tissue, i.e., the deformation or the impression on the tissue is reversible. Atraumatic graspers are mainly used for holding the viscera like bowel, gall bladder, and renal pelvis, during the pyeloplasty, etc. Semi-traumatic and traumatic graspers have deep serrations, and they produce plastic deformity, i.e., the impression formed by the instruments on the tissues is irreversible. Toothed grasper (Fig. 34.9) or traumatic graspers have claw-like jaws, and they are mainly used during specimen removal or for holding tough structures.

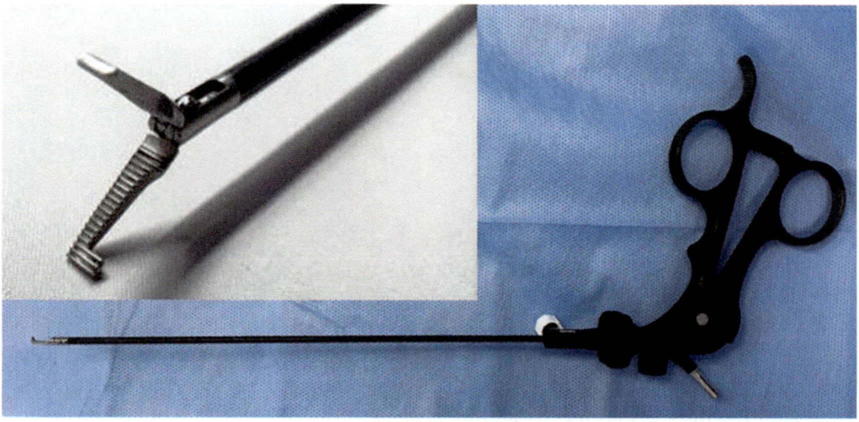

Fig. 34.6 Right-angle Maryland

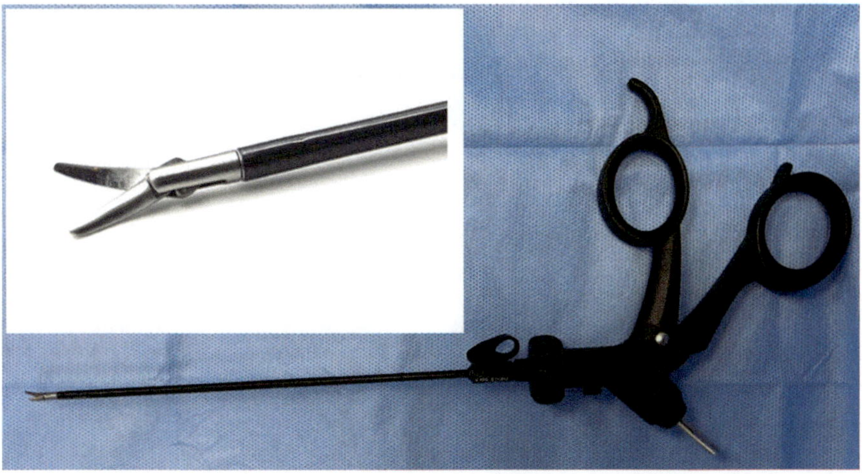

Fig. 34.7 Laparoscopic scissors

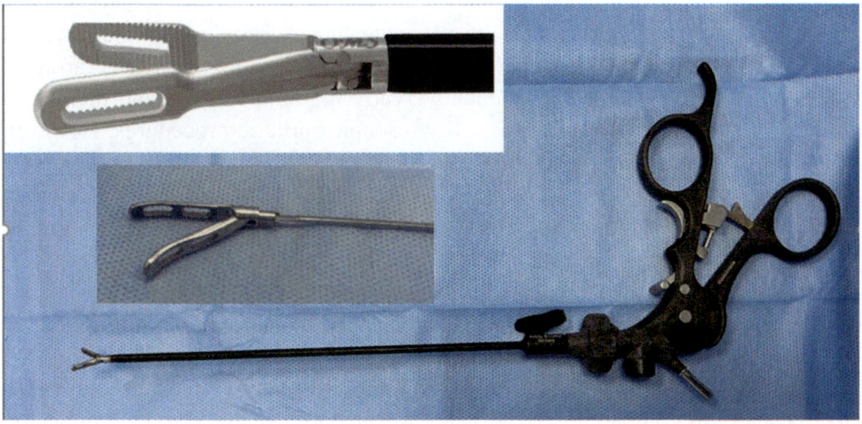

Fig. 34.8 Atraumatic grasper

34.6 Needle Holder

Both curved and straight needle holders are available. They usually have single-action jaws (as against most other hand instruments), i.e., only one jaw is moveable and the other jaw is fixed. For ergonomic purposes, it is preferred to keep the mobile jaw in an upward direction. Curved needle holders are different for the right hand and left hand. All needle holders have a locking mechanism. Self-aligning needle holders have a specific type of jaws to facilitate the automatic alignment of the needle as the jaws are closed (Fig. 34.10).

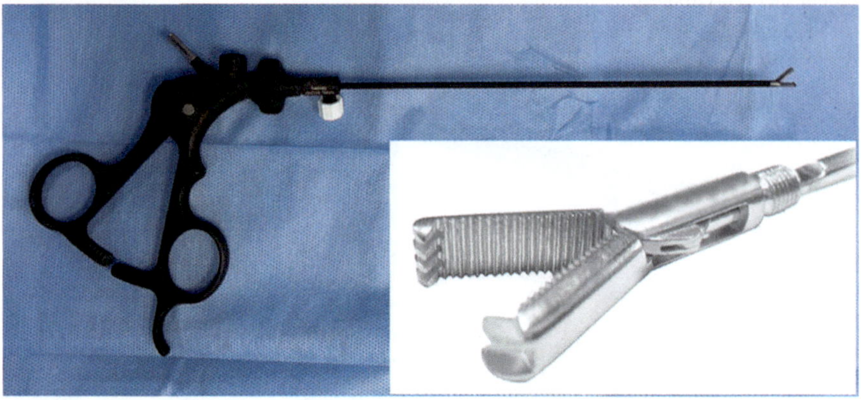

Fig. 34.9 Toothed grasper

Fig. 34.10 Needle holder

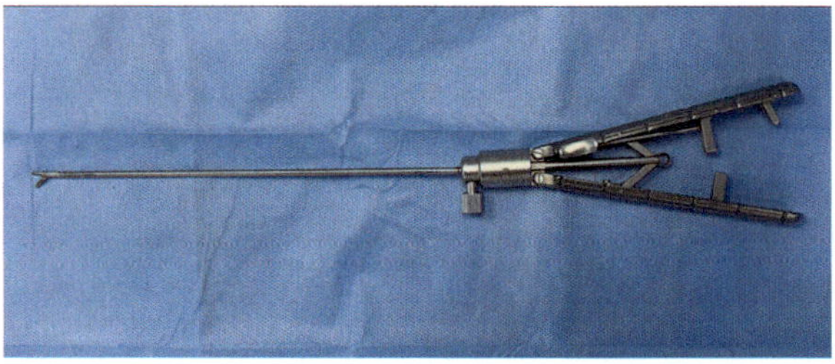

34.7 Hook and the Spatula

Hook and spatula are also available in smaller sizes for laparoscopic pediatric surgical use, and they can be connected to electrocautery and used mainly for dissection and hemostatis. Since they have a very small metal tip exposed and the rest of the shaft is covered with nonconducting sheath, these instruments are safer to use with electrocautery as compared to other hand instruments like the Maryland dissector. Shape of hook has unique advantage that allows it to pick tissue from its tip, take tissues away from important structure before their division (Fig. 34.11).

34.8 Clip Applicator

Clips are mainly applied before dividing a vessel or duct. Nitinol and titanium clips are used mainly. They are inert metals, and they have less tendency to get infected. Different-sized jaws are used based on the diameter of the vessel. Different cartridges are available, large, medium large, medium, and small. Color coding for large is yellow, which can be used for up to 8 mm structures, medium large is green in color, which can be used for the structures with diameter up to 6 mm, like cystic artery, cystic duct, and appendicular artery. Medium size cartridges are color coded with white and small is usually coded as blue and is used for small vessels with a

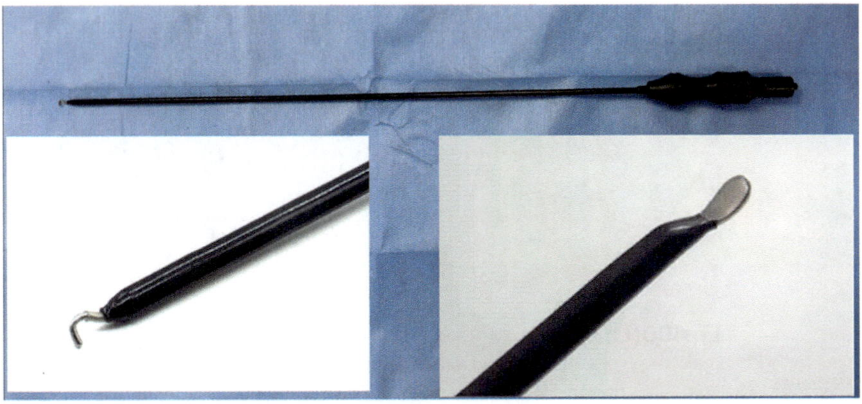

Fig. 34.11 Hook and spatula

Fig. 34.12 (**a**) Laparoscopic clip applicator for metal clips; (**b**) Laparoscopic clip applicator with hemolock clip

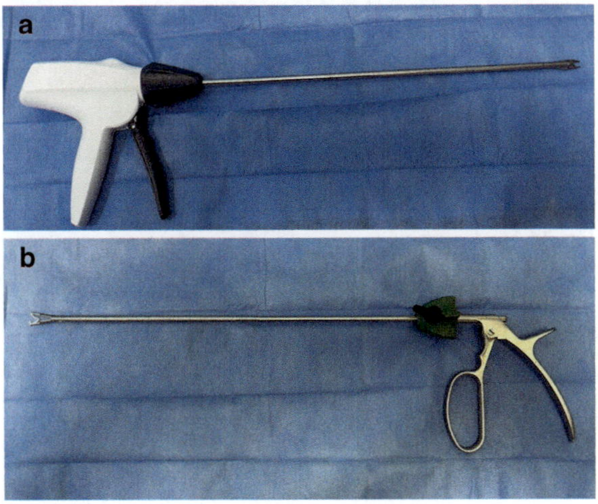

diameter of 3 mm. Dumbbell formation with constriction in the center and swelling on either side indicates the proper clip application with blockage of flow in the vessel or duct. If the second clip needs to be applied, it should be at least 3 mm away from the first one (Figs. 34.12, 34.13, and 34.14).

34.9 Endoscopes Used in Pediatric Surgical Practices

1. Cystourethroscope
2. Resectoscope
3. Ureteroscope
4. Nephroscope
5. Bronchoscope
6. Esophagoscope

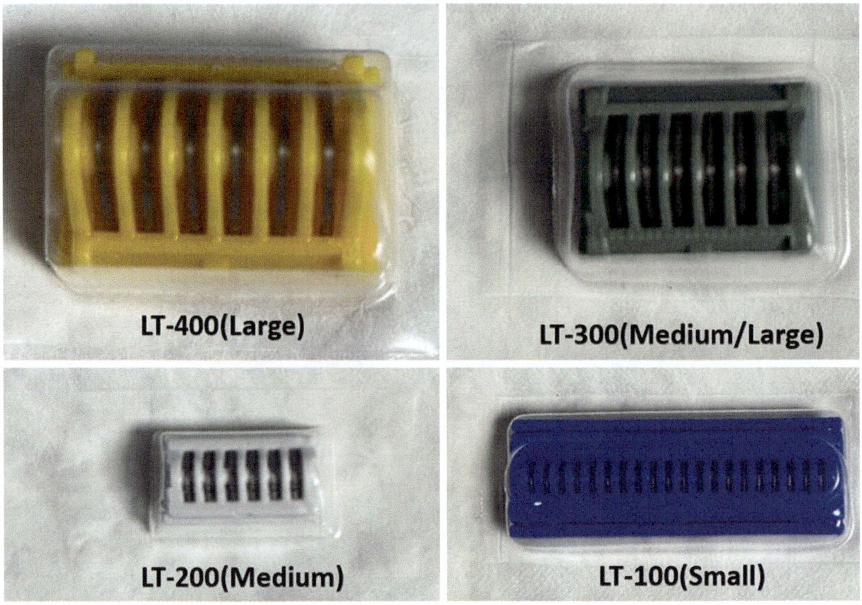

Fig. 34.13 Different size cartridges with color coding

Fig. 34.14 Harmonic scalpel (This is the same as that is used in adult laparoscopic surgery)

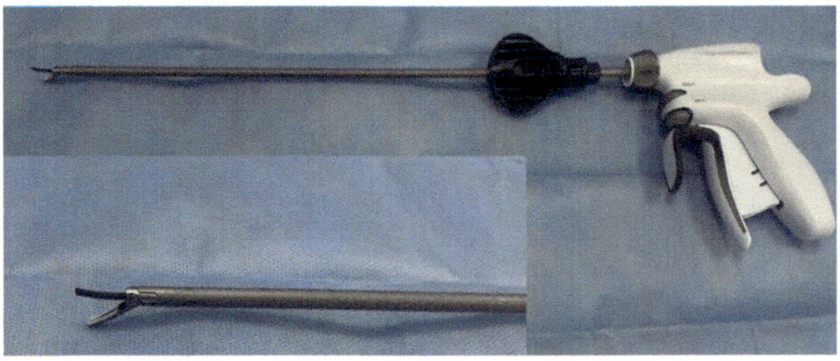

34.10 Cystourethroscope and Resectoscope

Cystourethroscopes (Fig. 34.15) are used both for diagnostic and therapeutic purposes. Posterior urethral valves, urethral strictures, false tracts in the urethra, any bladder pathology, configuration of the ureteric orifices can be diagnosed [4]. Through the working channel, guide wire, DJ Stents and forceps can be inserted. Resectoscopes (Fig. 34.16) are mainly used for posterior urethral valve fulguration or ablation. These valves can be ablated by using different energy devices like cold knife, bugbee (which is a monopolar electrode producing short bursts of current), electrocautery, or Holmium:YAG laser (Figs. 34.17 and 34.18).

Ureteroscopes are used for diagnosing ureteral strictures, removal of DJ stents that have migrated into the ureter and for removal of the stones in the ureter, etc.

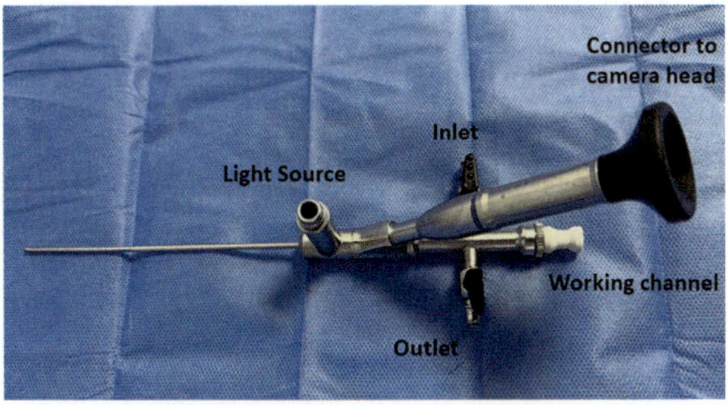

Fig. 34.15 Cystourethroscope

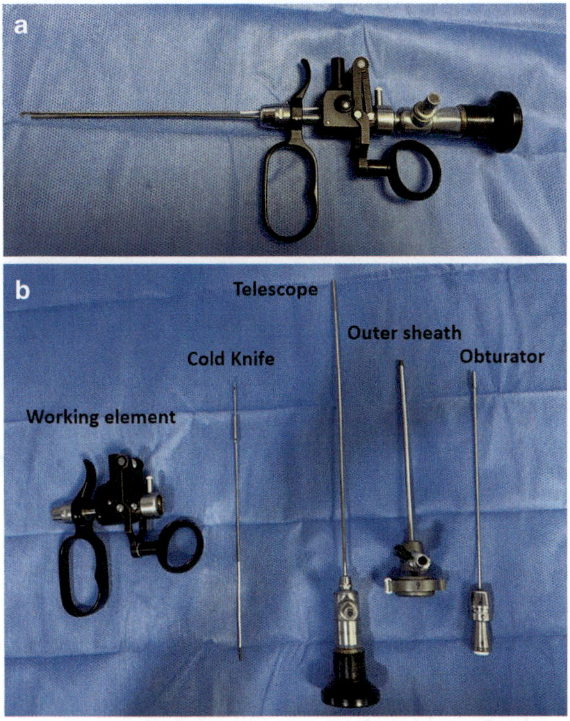

Fig. 34.16 (**a**) Resectoscope and (**b**) parts of a resectoscope

34.11 Bronchoscope and Esophagoscope

Different size bronchoscopes ranging from 2.5, 3, 3.5, 4, 4.5, 5, 5.5 to 6 mm are available for use in infants, toddlers, and older children. They are available in different lengths like 25 cm, 30 cm, and 40 cm. These are used for both diagnostic and therapeutic purposes [5]. Tracheo-esophageal fistula, intraluminal mass, or narrowing of the airway because of external compression can be diagnosed. Biopsy of the mass, foreign body removal can be done by bronchoscopy. Different types of optical forceps with bronchoscopes are used for foreign body removal. Esophagoscopes are

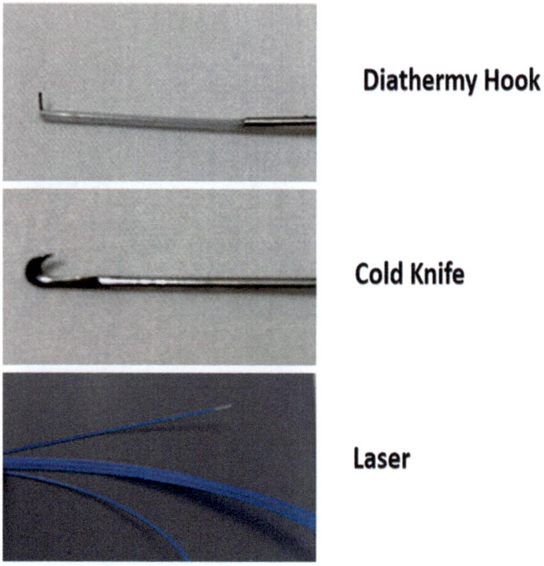

Fig. 34.17 Different energy devices used for ablation of posterior urethral valves

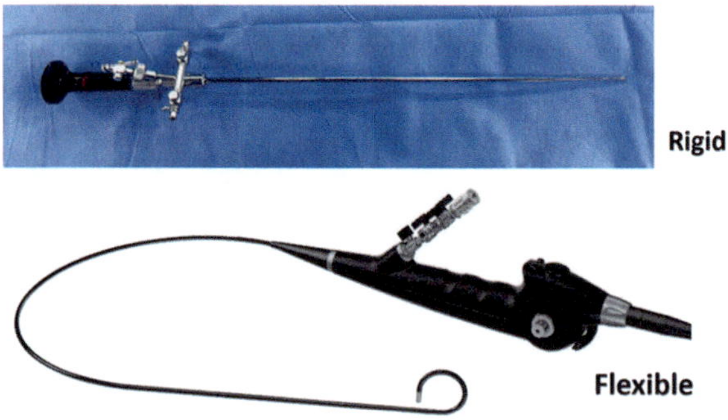

Fig. 34.18 Rigid and flexible ureteroscopes

also used for diagnosis and removal of foreign bodies or any intraluminal mass. As the esophagus is a collapsed structure, it needs to be insufflated with air during esophagoscopy (Figs. 34.19, 34.20, 34.21, and 34.22).

34.12 Care of the Instruments

All the instruments need to be disassembled after usage, and all the parts need to be cleaned separately. All of the parts need to be handled carefully, especially the sheath. Repeated handling of the sheath with Cheatle's forceps may cause wear of the insulating coat on it. Cleaning with a detergent or enzymatic cleaners should be done to remove all the foreign material, like blood, mucus, and any other proteinaceous material from the instruments. Lumen should be thoroughly cleaned. Soft-bristled brushes, suction devices, or ultrasonic cleaners can be used for this purpose.

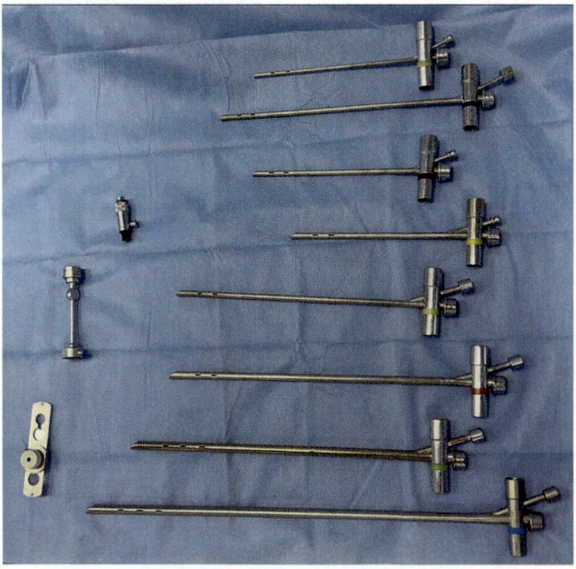

Fig. 34.19 Different sizes and lengths of pediatric rigid bronchoscopes

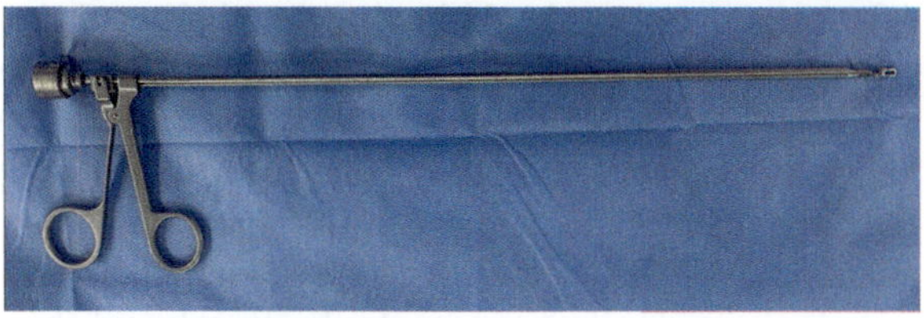

Fig. 34.20 Optical forceps for foreign body removal

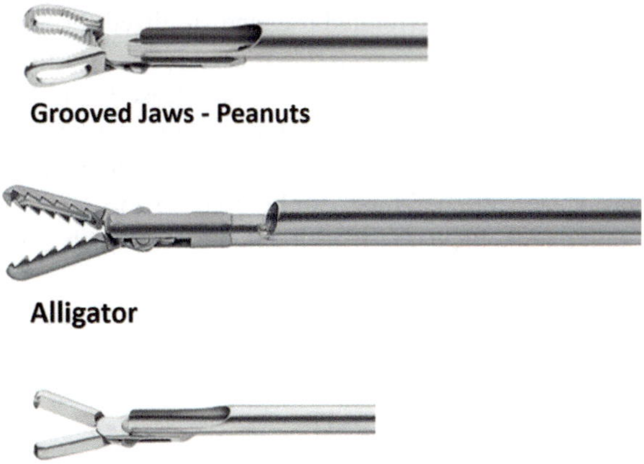

Fig. 34.21 Different types of optical forceps for different types of foreign bodies

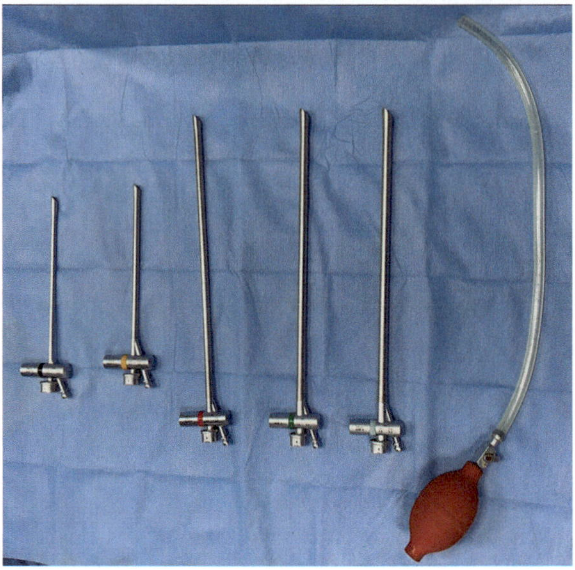

Fig. 34.22 Esophagoscope

After cleaning, they should be rinsed with filtered tap water or distilled deionized water. Then they should be air-dried before disinfection or sterilization. The most commonly used disinfectant is 2% glutaraldehyde. Centre for Disease Control and Prevention, Atlanta, recommends that endoscopic equipment should be exposed to chemical disinfectant for at least 20 minutes at a minimum concentration of 1% glutaraldehyde. Different methods of sterilization for laparoscopic instruments include steam sterilization, gas sterilization, liquid chemical immersion sterilization and plasma sterilization techniques. Steam sterilization can be done by placing the instruments in a perforated tray and sterilized for 3 min at 131 °C or for 15 min at 121 °C. Ethylene oxide (ETO) is used for gas sterilization, the disadvantage is that it requires long sterilization time of at least 3–6 h. Peracetic acid is the most commonly used agent for chemical immersion sterilization. Plasma sterilization is specially useful for instruments that are heat or moisture-sensitive. Hydrogen peroxide gas or peracetic acid gas can be used for this, as both of them emit nontoxic and noninflammable gases. This method is also much quicker than ETO [6, 7].

34.13 Troubleshooting in Pediatric Laparoscopic Surgery

34.13.1 Before Surgery

1. Written and informed consent should be obtained from the patient attendant after explaining all the possible complications. This is very important in the present era of medicolegal concerns. Consent for conversion to open surgery should also be taken in prior based on the probability, especially in previously operated cases

where bowel adhesions may cause difficulty in performing the laparoscopic surgery.

2. It's always better for the entire surgical team, anesthesia team and scrub nurse to discuss about all the concerns a day before surgery, so that the surgical team is ready to handle the intraoperative complications, anesthesia team will be ready to tackle the cardiorespiratory changes, and scrub nurse will be ready with all the required instruments including the electrosurgical equipment.
3. A surgeon should ideally check all the instruments before starting the procedure and should be well versed with troubleshooting.
4. Position of the child should be checked, so that the area of interest is better visualized. Excessive padding below the patient should be avoided because it may bring the major vessels into the reach of trocars, by which vascular injury can occur.

34.13.2 During the Surgery

1. Leakage of CO_2 from valves or from the port sites is one of the most commonly encountered problems. This will cause excessive consumption of CO_2 with high flow rates and make the peritoneal surfaces and bowel wall dry. Port site leakage can be prevented with the use of balloon ports or a suture to narrow down the port site incision. All the valves should be checked for any suspicion of gas leak and should be closed properly.
2. Repeated fogging and blurred vision are another frequently encountered problem. Briefly touching the peritoneum or mesentery may help, but it should be gentle. Placing the telescope in hot water for few seconds is the best option.
3. The working area should be at the center of the screen. If there is bleeding or any inadvertent injury to any other organ, don't move the camera or change the area of interest and then tackle it. Any injury to major vessels like the aorta, IVC or iliac vessels, leave the ports, leave insufflation and convert to open and then do the necessary procedure. Keeping the ports and insufflation will give some tamponade effect while converting into an open procedure.
4. If there is any problem with any of instruments, sheath, insert, and handle are interchangeable and can be changed accordingly.

34.13.3 After Surgery

Apart from the procedure-related complications, shoulder pain due to retained CO_2 gas in the peritoneal cavity is also common. Postoperative fever, nausea, vomiting are also seen in some patients.

34.13.4 Recent Advances

Gasless laparoscopy is a newer technique that eliminates the risk of pneumoperitoneum by using mechanical retraction. It will be helpful in children with cardiac and pulmonary diseases [1, 8]. The disadvantage of this technique is reduced visibility, and its application to pediatric patients is uncertain. Microlaparoscopy is a newer technique in pediatric surgical practice with the introduction of 2 mm instruments [9]. But the disadvantage with this technique is fragility of the instruments and difficulty in grasping the structures. Congenital diaphragmatic hernia repair, pyeloplasty, and laparoscopy-assisted pull-through for Hirschsprung disease can be done by using the microlaparoscopy technique [10]. Advanced energy sources like Ligasure, Enseal, 5 mm clips and staplers, new generation videoscopes with three-dimensional view increase the safety and efficacy of the procedure [11–14]. Robotic surgery has been safely practiced in India and DaVinci (Intuitive Surgical, since 2001) and Senhance (Transenterix, since 2020) robotic systems are currently available and certified for robotic surgery in children [15]. Deployable minirobots inserted into the abdominal and thoracic cavity to perform surgical procedures by remote control are being tried in animal models [16]. Artificial intelligence and augmented reality help the operating surgeon by giving real time feedback to find the delicate structures after analyzing thousands of such procedures [17].

References

1. Gupta R, Singh S. Challenges in paediatric laparoscopic surgeries. Indian J Anaesth. 2009;53(5):560–6. PMID: 20640106; PMCID: PMC2900088.
2. Hammer G, Hall S, Davis PJ. Anesthesia for general abdominal, thoracic, urologic, and bariatric surgery. In: Etsuro KM, Peter JD, editors. Smith's anesthesia for infants and children. 7th ed. Pennsylvania: Mosby Elsevier; 2006. p. 686–8.
3. Schier F, Turial S. Equipment, children, anesthesia, gas embolism. In: Laparoscopy in children; 2013. p. 1–9. https://doi.org/10.1007/978-3-642-37638-2_1.
4. Kramer SA. Cystourethroscopy in children. Endoscopy. 1984;16(2):64–6. https://doi.org/10.1055/s-2007-1018535.
5. Soyer T. The role bronchoscopy in the diagnosis of airway disease in children. J Thorac Dis. 2016;8(11):3420–6. https://doi.org/10.21037/jtd.2016.11.87. PMID: 28066622; PMCID: PMC5179461.
6. Ball KA. Care and maintenance of endoscopic instruments. In: Endoscopic surgery. Mosby; 1997.
7. Froelich MR, Young EC. Care of endoscopic instrumentation. Todays OR Nurse. 1993;15(3):21–6.
8. Tobias JD, Holcomb GW, Brock JW, et al. Cardiorespiratory changes in children during laparoscopy. J Pediatr Surg. 1995;30:33–6.
9. O'Donovan PJ, McGurgan P. Microlaparoscopy. Semin Laparosc Surg. 1999;6:51–7.
10. Turial S, Schwind M, Kohl M, Goldinger B, Schier F. Feasibility of microlaparoscopy for surgical procedures of advanced complexity in children. J Laparoendosc Adv Surg Tech A. 2009;19(Suppl. 1):S103–5.
11. Cuaresma R, Benavides M, Buela E, Bignon H, Martínez-Ferro M. Laparoscopic appendectomies in pediatric patients using Hem-o-lock clips. Cir Pediatr. 2009;22:103–5.

12. Lv B, Zhang X, Li J, Leng S, Li S, Zeng Y, Wang B, Yuan J, Fan J, Xing S, et al. Absorbable polymeric surgical clips for appendicular stump closure: a randomized control trial of laparoscopic appendectomy with lapro-clips. Oncotarget. 2016;7:41265–73.
13. Harrell AG, Kercher KW, Heniford BT. Energy sources in laparoscopy. Semin Laparosc Surg. 2004;11:201–9.
14. Highlights I KARL STORZ Endoskope. Available online: https://www.karlstorz.com/de/en/highlights-tp.htm#mod-9323.
15. Fernandez N, Barco-Castillo C, ElGhazzaoui A, Farhat W. Effective intracorporeal space in robot-assisted multiquadrant surgery in a pediatric inanimate model. J Robot Surg. 2021;15(1):25–30.
16. Forgione A. In vivo microrobots for natural orifice transluminal surgery. Current status and future perspectives. Surg Oncol. 2009;18:121–9.
17. Cercenelli L, Carbone M, Condino S, Cutolo F, Marcelli E, Tarsitano A, Marchetti C, Ferrari V, Badiali G. The wearable VOSTARS system for augmented reality-guided surgery: preclinical phantom evaluation for high-precision maxillofacial tasks. J Clin Med. 2020;9:3562.

Cholangiography and Choledochoscopy Instruments

35

Ernest Castro-Gutiérrez

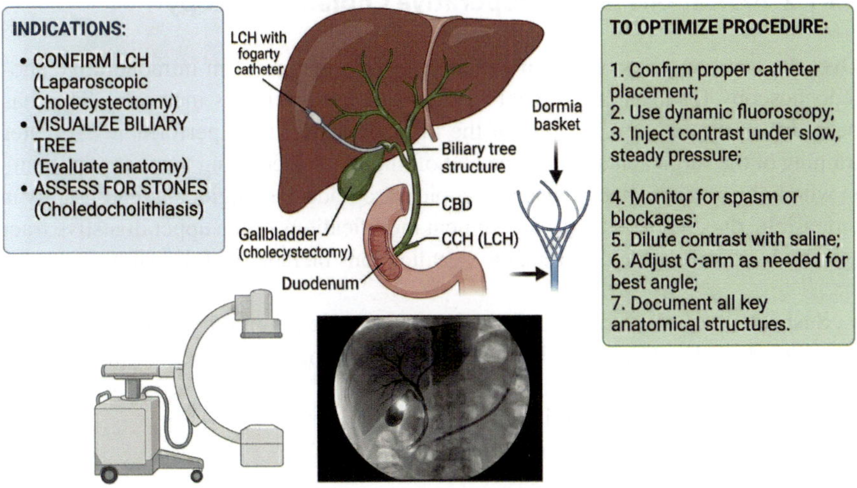

The anatomy of the biliary tract presents one of the greatest proportions of anatomical variability in the human organism. It is essential to understand it during interventions that involve action in this territory. Different surgical tools are currently available to help identify the biliary tract anatomy, to be able to detect injuries or pathologies of the same, and to treat them. The best known are cholangiography and choledochoscopy. To be able to carry them out, suitable material and specific technical skills are necessary, which will be described throughout this chapter.

E. Castro-Gutiérrez (✉)
Hepatic-Biliary-Pancreatic Unit, Department of General and Digestive Surgery, Hospital Universitari de Girona, Department of Medicine, Facultat de Medicina, Universitat de Girona, Girona Biomedical Research Institute (IDIBGI), Girona, Spain
e-mail: ecastro.girona.ics@gencat.cat

J. S. Ahluwalia (ed.), *User Manual for Minimally Invasive Surgical Equipment*,
https://doi.org/10.1007/978-981-95-9019-3_35

35.1 Indications [1–7]

35.1.1 Laparoscopic Cholangiography Indications

Laparoscopic cholangiography (IOC) is indicated during laparoscopic cholecystectomy (LC) for several reasons, primarily to delineate biliary anatomy, identify potential bile duct stones, and prevent bile duct injuries. Specifically, IOC is often performed when there's a clinical suspicion of common bile duct stones, a dilated common bile duct, uncertainty about biliary anatomy, or concerns about biliary injury. Other indications include a history of pancreatitis (particularly gallstone pancreatitis), elevated liver function tests, or a large common bile duct.

35.1.2 Indications for Intraoperative Choledochoscopy

Over the last few years, the notification of groups that perform intraoperative choledochoscopy for the management of choledocholithiasis has increased. This has been driven by the improvement of the instruments for their performance, greater training of the surgical teams and the fact of finding an increasing number of patients in whom the performance of an endoscopic retrograde cholangiopancreatography is unfeasible, due to post-surgery anatomical modifications of the upper digestive tract (gastric bypass, duodenal switch, etc.). Indications include the following:

- Suspected or known common bile duct stones: Helping in the identification and removal of the stones that have migrated from the gallbladder to the common bile duct.
- Evaluation of suspected biliary malignancies.
- Evaluation of biliary strictures.

If it is performed by an expert, it is possible to do an evaluation of the intrahepatic duct.

35.2 Instruments Required for Cholangiography and Choledochoscopy [6–11]

At the outset, in order to properly perform a laparoscopic cholangiography, minimally invasive surgery materials are needed.

35.2.1 Specific Material for Cholangiography

Olsen clamp, it is a special clamp that presses the catheterized cystic duct, avoiding the reflux of the radiological contrast (Fig. 35.1). Not all groups use it, given that it involves the loss of one of the working ports.

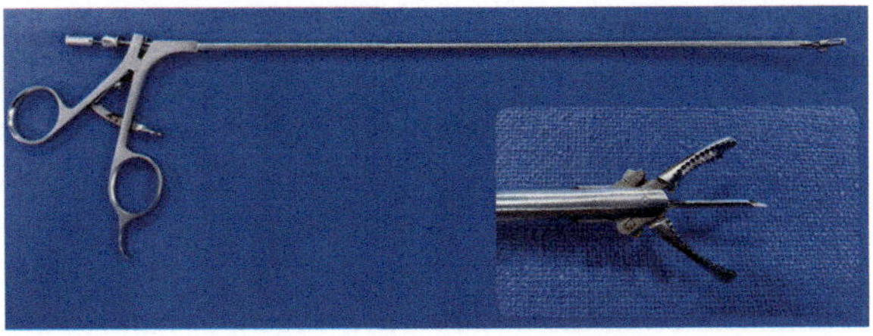

Fig. 35.1
Cholangiography clamp

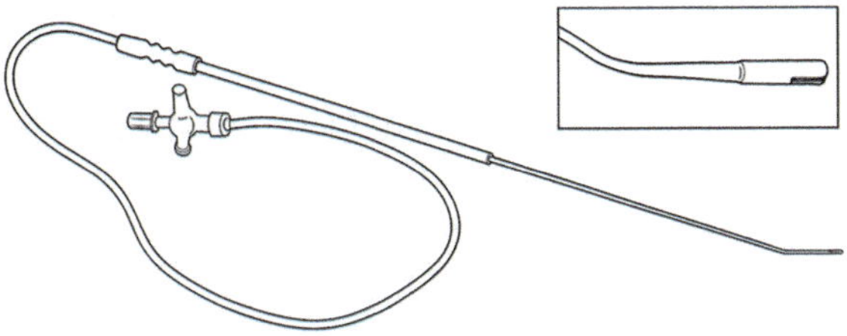

Fig. 35.2
Cholangiography catheter

Teams that do not use Olsen clamps usually insert the cholangiography catheter through a plastic peripheral venipuncture catheter, positioned so that the tip of the cholangiography catheter ends up facing the incision made in the cystic duct.

Cholangiography catheter consists of three parts; the proximal end has a cone connection where a syringe loaded with the contrast medium can be inserted (Fig. 35.2). The central part is a tubular system of flexible material. The distal end is usually made of metal or a stiffer plastic material than the central element, which allows its manipulation with laparoscopy forceps, its introduction into the cystic duct and its fixation with a titanium clip.

Endoclips will be required for occlusion of the cystic duct before the introduction of the cholangiography catheter. Once this step is taken, the rigid section should be held in place to prevent reflux and contrast leakage from the cystic duct. We must bear in mind that for this function, titanium clips are more useful, while plastic clips with a safety tab make their subsequent removal very complicated, despite having shown greater safety at the time of definitive clipping of the cystic duct.

Radiopaque contrast is required.

Some examples:

- An iso-osmolality-based iodine contrast agent: Lopamidol.
- A nonionic iodine contrast agents: Iohexol or Ioversol (has a rate of adverse reactions of 1%).

Radiolucent operating table to make sure the C arm can be used.

Padded Apron and Cervical Protection: Since the emission of ionizing radiation will be necessary, the essential operating room staff during the performance of the cholangiography must be protected from it.

Portable C-Arm System: It will be placed entering from the patient's left side so that the element that emits and the receiver are on the right hypochondrium of the patient. It is usually necessary to place the arm with a certain degree of angulation with respect to the vertical axis, so that the upper element (emitter) is more cranial than the lower one (receiver) (Fig. 35.3).

Choledochoscope: It is a flexible optical system that allows direct endoluminal exploration of the biliary tract (Figs. 35.4 and 35.5). They are available in 5 and 8 mm thickness, allowing exploration through the cystic or common bile duct, depending on the characteristics of the patient or the situation to be treated. It consists of three parts:

1. Handle, where the control levers are located, that allows the distal end to be articulated. It also contains the connection for the camera that will allow the images to be viewed on a monitor. The handle also has holes called working channels for inserting accessories and to insert saline through a venous perfusion system, to maintain the correct dilation of the biliary tract.
2. Pipeline, through which the fiber optic structures (or wires in case of chip on tip system), movement transmission elements and the work/irrigation channel are located.
3. Tip, which is the distal articulating element that allows visualization, the light emission and image capturing. It also has the output of the working channel.

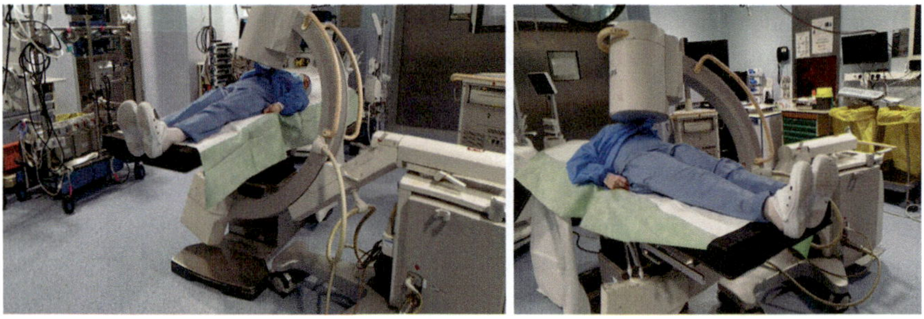

Fig. 35.3 Equipment specific to choledochoscopy

Fig. 35.4 Olympus CHF-290 choledochoscope

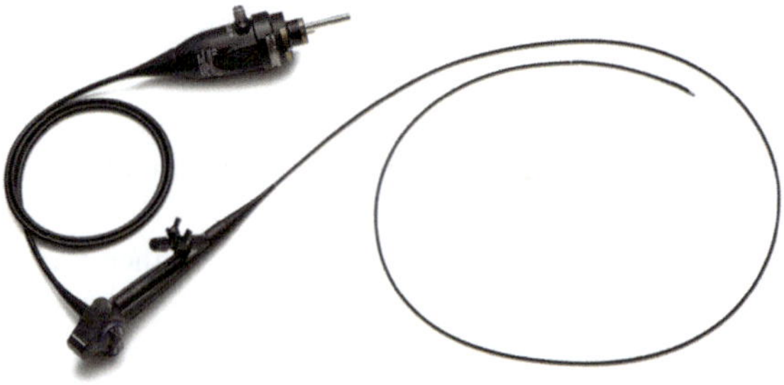

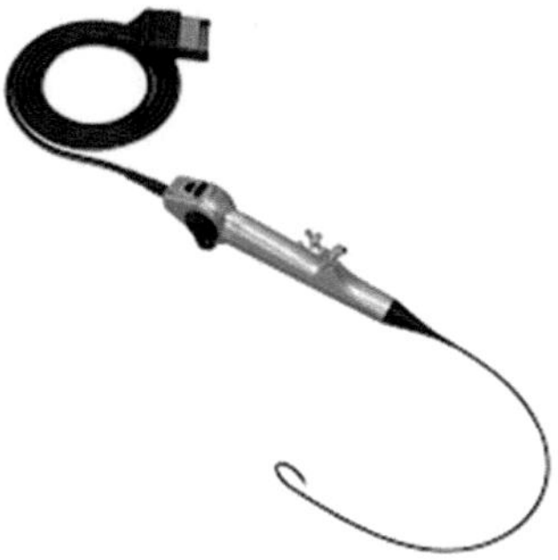

Fig. 35.5 Karl Storz choledochoscope

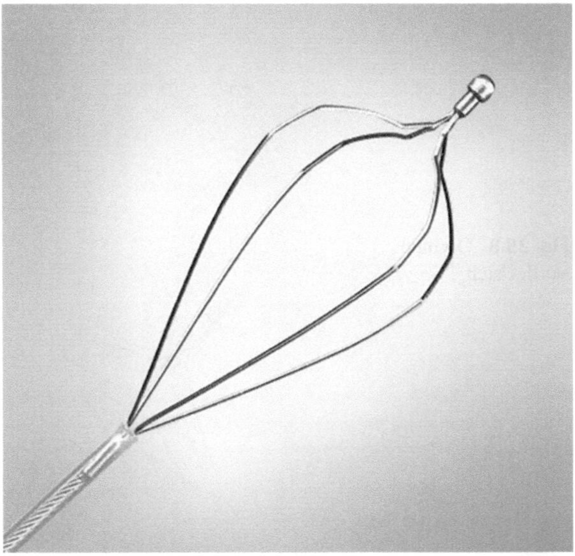

Fig. 35.6 Olympus basket

Dormia baskets of various sizes (Figs. 35.6, 35.7, and 35.8). It is an element based on a braid of metal fibers, usually four, which merge at the distal end, giving the appearance of a basket. The proximal part can be in the form of a plunger or with a gripping system, which allows the wires to be separated at the distal end, forming the basket in which stones can be trapped.

Balloon systems are Fogarty type catheter with a proximal end having an attachment for a syringe (Fig. 35.9). At the distal end, it has a balloon system that can be expanded and collapsed by attaching a syringe at the proximal end. Cather is passed distal to the stones in a collapsed state, and then the balloon is inflated to pull out the stones. In some cases of small lithiasis, it can be used to push it into the duodenum.

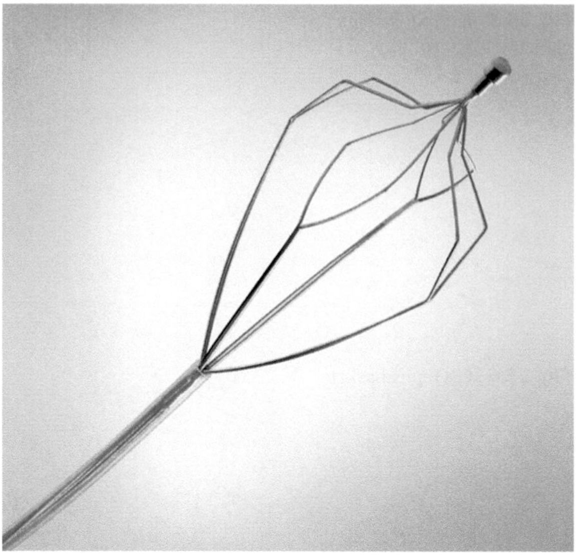

Fig. 35.7 Olympus flower basket

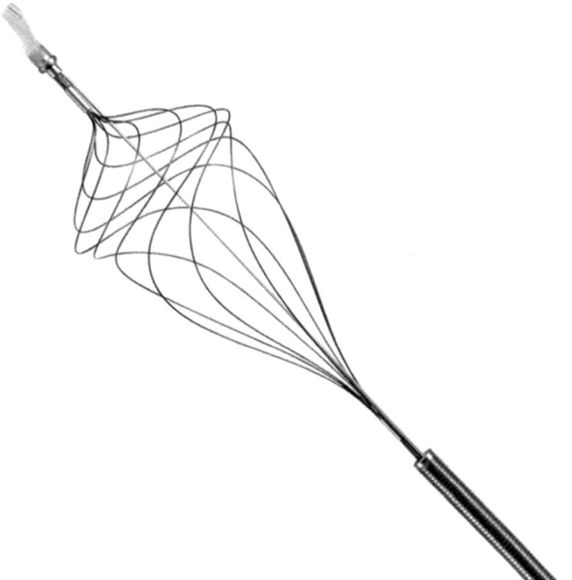

Fig. 35.8 Olympus VorticCatch

Fig. 35.9 Fogarty catheter

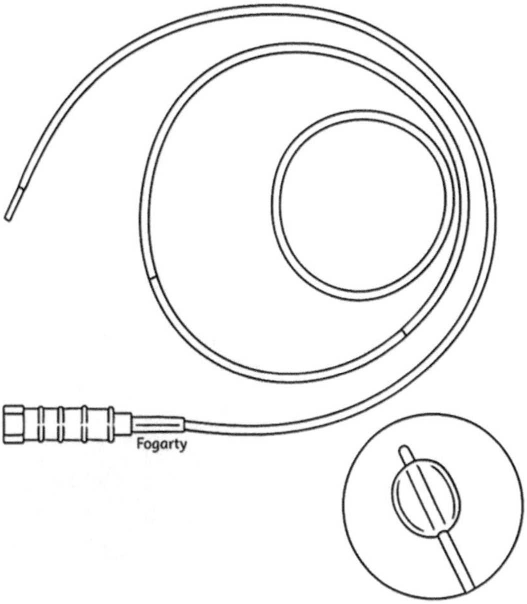

35.3 Tips and Tricks [12, 13]

As with most surgical techniques, there are differences between step-by-step descriptions in books and articles and daily practice with complex cases.

So, it is interesting to keep in mind some tricks that favor the performance of cholangiography and choledochoscopy:

- If using the venipuncture catheter to insert the cholangiography catheter, insert it into the right hypochondrium, with an angle that allows the direction of the cholangiography catheter to be inserted parallel to the cystic duct, favoring thus its intracystic positioning. This option, from the point of view of several authors, is preferable because it allows working with all ports.
- Prior to the introduction of the cholangiography catheter, it is important to break the internal valves of the cystic duct by creating a section and inserting a curved dissector to facilitate a smoother and less difficult insertion of the catheter.
- It is very important to prevent the catheter from leaving the cystic duct, hence the use of Olsen's forceps or placing the titanium clip holding the central part of the distal end of the catheter. The titanium clip serves two purposes: It secures the catheter to the cystic duct, preventing its dislodgement, and it also occludes the walls of the cystic duct to the catheter, preventing contrast leakage. Prior to administering the contrast, asses the catheter permeability with physiological saline.
- To consider that a cholangiography is well done, the complete visualization of the entire biliary tree and the passage of the contrast into the duodenum must be

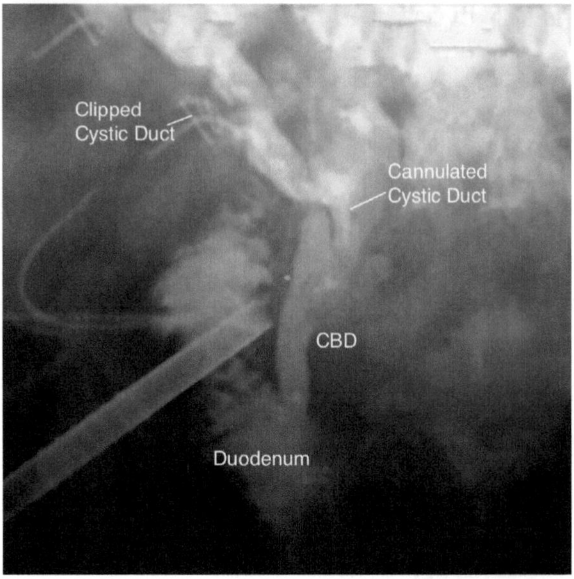

Fig. 35.10 Cholangiogram. (Used with permission from L.E. Machicado) [13]

ensured. In order to ensure correct localization and orientation, the titanium clips can be used as anatomical references and, at the first shot of the C-arm, position a metal element (scissors or artery forceps) on the patient's abdomen, allowing the orientation to be determined on the craniocaudal and right–left axis (Fig. 35.10).

- To facilitate visualization of the biliary tree, traditionally, two radiographs were recommended. The first was taken with the surgical table in Trendelenburg position, injecting approximately 5 cc of contrast through the cholangiography catheter and taking the first radiograph. If the intrahepatic biliary tree is correctly delineated, the position is then changed to anti-Trendelenburg, with the remaining contrast injected (5–15 cc according to the groups), and a second radiograph taken. This second radiograph allows for the detection of the presence of calculi and/or visualization of the contrast passing to the duodenum, or detect bile leaks. With the development of portable radiological fluoroscopy systems, successive images can be obtained without changing plates on the surgical table, making it a safer system in terms of possible surgical site infections.
- Centers that use metal laparoscopy ports must try to align them parallel to the spine, to avoid interference.
- If a lithiasis is detected, the first maneuver may consist of the irrigation of physiological saline under pressure through the same cholangiography catheter. If this is not achieved, the Fogarty can be introduced, and by combining the use of the balloon with irrigation and its withdrawal, the extraction of the stone can be achieved.
- Many teams at the beginning of their experience describe difficulties in obtaining a good visualization of the biliary tract with the choledochoscope, despite having a continuous irrigation of physiological saline through the irrigation channel.

This view can be improved if the saline bag is associated with a pressure applicator, so that the flow is higher and allows better and more continuous dilatation of the bile duct.

- To avoid breaking the fibers of the choledoscope, mainly in the case of the smaller ones, it is important to use forceps with protected metal parts, to reduce the pressure that is transmitted to the end when orienting it toward the incision made in the biliary tract. Ready-made clamps with foam on the ends of the blades can be used, or the metallic clamps can be protected with sterile silicone or plastic elements.
- It is common that the balloon of the Fogarty catheter can rupture with a sudden volume input, it should be checked before the scan the necessary volume, ensure that the balloon is not broken and assess the speed and force of inflation to have them under control at the time of the scan.
- To be able to capture the lithiasis with the Dormia basket, an interesting gesture consists of detecting it with the choledochoscope, going over it with the Dormia closed, opening it, and with circular movements of the Dormia, gradually bringing the lithiasis inside the basket, close by adjusting the threads to the lithiasis and removing it.
- In case of large lithiasis, they can be fractionated with biliary tract exploration forceps. In recent years, several companies have developeddisposable choledoscopy systems with channels suitables for use with laser lithotripsy systems, wich facilitate the destruction of large or difficult-to-move stones.

35.4 Maintenance [14–17]

The choledochoscope is an expensive, fragile, and reusable instrument; you must be very careful with its handling during the examinations and at the time of its cleaning and sterility. According to the World Organization of Gastroenterology and the World Organization of Endoscopy, in their global guidelines, a step-by-step procedure must be followed, the first of which is cleaning by removing macroscopic remains and ensuring that the working channel has been left free, applying saline or pressurized air through it. The second step consists of the removal of the detachable parts (caps, valves, etc.), All the components must be cleaned by hand using the enzymatic soap recommended by the manufacturer at the dilution indicated by the same. Once clean, it must be disinfected, which can be done in an automatic system or manually by use of high-level disinfectants (e.g., glutaraldehyde, ortho-phthalaldehyde, peracetic acid, or water acid electrolyzed) and at the end dry it with pressurized air. Finally, it will be sterilized. It is recommended not to use temperatures higher than 60 °C, the autoclave, hot water, or atmospheric steam, because it can generate alterations to the material that composes it. Theres is the possibility of disposable models, wich, despite having a higher cost, imply a decrease in maintenance costs, with a decrease in the risk of misalignment or incidental breakage.

35.5 Alternatives to Cholangiography and Choledochoscopy

The great alternative that we have today to these more invasive techniques for the study of the biliary tract is the system integrated in many laparoscopy towers for vision with infrared light and detection of indocyanine green. The difficulty of this system is that it requires indocyanine green and optics with the ability to detect infrared light. However, its use is simple; indocyanine green can be injected directly into the gallbladder and promote its passage into the biliary tract, although the effect is more obvious if, at the beginning of anesthetic induction intravenous indocyanine green is injected. The aim is to be able to visualize the biliary tree can reduce the possible injuries of the biliary tract during cholecystectomy, in addition, in expert hands, it is possible to detect absences of uptake that could point to the presence of lithiasis.

Surgeons can use magnetic cholangioresonance and biliopancreatic echoendoscopy to diagnose choledocholithiasis and study the biliary tree if they don't want to use other options. Both are characterized by a high price, in addition the first of them can generate rejection in patients with claustrophobia; with regard to the second, it is very specialist dependent; in expert hands it presents a sensitivity and specificity superior to magnetic resonance studies, but in professionals starting their learning curve the results are not so good. Echoendoscopy has the advantage that if choledocholithiasis is detected, in the same act it can be associated with the therapeutic alternative to choledochoscopy, endoscopic retrograde cholangiopancreatography.

35.6 Safety Considerations [18]

35.6.1 Intraoperative

If we expose ourselves to radiation without protection, a series of harmful effects can occur, ranging from erythema of the exposed areas to hair loss. If the exposure were continued, ulcers could appear. Carcinogenic effects may manifest after years of exposure. Alterations to the germ cells can cause alterations to the offspring.

These effects are determined by the time of exposure and the dose of the same; it is for this reason that it is essential that health personnel who develop their activity with ionizing radiation are exposed in a controlled manner, with protection and with a quantification system of received dosage.

In order to have an image of the dose received, dosimeters have been designed, recommending that all personnel exposed to radiation carry their personal and non-transferable dosimeter, to be able to calculate the radiation received during a given period of time. It is recommended that workers are not exposed to an annual effective dose higher than 50 mSv. Optimize every scan to be shorter and with the lowest dose, exposing only the minimum number of people necessary. In this sense, all personnel not essential for performing the cholangiography should leave the operating theatre at the time of activation of the C-arm, and the personnel who must perform the test, in order to reduce the dose received, must use a padded apron and cervical protector.

35.7 Troubleshooting [12, 13, 19–21]

Despite all precautions, something can always go wrong while performing these procedures. Tables 35.1 and 35.2 can act as a ready reference for such common problems.

Table 35.1 Troubleshooting intraoperative cholangiography (IOC)

Problem	Possible cause	Solution
No contrast flow seen	Catheter malposition or kinking	Reposition the catheter and confirm patency by flushing with saline
Extravasation of contrast	Perforation of the bile duct or high-pressure injection	Stop injection immediately, assess the site, and manage as needed (clip or suture repair)
Poor image quality	Air bubbles in contrast or improper contrast dilution	Remove air from syringe before injection; use appropriate contrast dilution
Reflux of contrast into the gallbladder	Incomplete cystic duct occlusion	Apply a stronger clip or use a bulldog clamp on the cystic duct proximal to the catheter
Overlapping of bowel shadows	Suboptimal patient positioning or excessive bowel gas	Adjust patient position; decompress bowel if possible
Cannulation failure	Spasm or tortuous cystic duct	Use a smaller, more flexible catheter or change the angle of approach
Radiation exposure concerns	Prolonged fluoroscopy time	Plan imaging steps; minimize exposure with intermittent fluoroscopy and proper shielding

Table 35.2 Troubleshooting choledochoscopy

Problem	Possible cause	Solution
Poor visualization	Fogging, inadequate irrigation, or debris	Ensure proper irrigation; warm the scope; flush the working channel
Failure to advance the scope	Stricture, stone, or angulated duct	Use guidewire-assisted entry; consider balloon dilation or stone extraction first
Image blackout or flickering	Loose cable connection or damaged camera head	Check all cable connections; replace or repair equipment as needed
Inability to retrieve stones	Large stone or lack of basket manoeuvrability	Fragment stone with lithotripsy; reposition the scope for better access
Mucosal injury or bleeding	Rough scope manipulation or prolonged contact	Minimize trauma; irrigate and monitor bleeding; stop procedure if persistent
Scope damage	Excessive torquing or improper handling	Follow proper handling protocols; use scope protectors; ensure team training
Loss of orientation	Lack of anatomic landmarks or over-insufflation	Use anatomical cues like duct bifurcation; avoid excessive air insufflation

35.8 Recent Advances and Future Directions

1. *Fluorescence Cholangiography Using Indocyanine Green (ICG)*

This technique uses near-infrared fluorescence imaging after intravenous administration of ICG dye to visualize the biliary tree without contrast injection or radiation. This is now being made available by many laparoscopic cameras manufactures and its availability is increasing. Provides real-time, radiation-free imaging, helps prevent bile duct injury during laparoscopic cholecystectomy, and enhances anatomical orientation. Limitations include limited penetration in obese patients and requires specialized laparoscopic equipment with infrared capabilities.

2. *Digital Choledochoscopy Systems*

Modern digital scopes (e.g., SpyGlass™ DS) offer high-resolution imaging, improved navigation, and integrated therapeutic channels. Advantages include enhanced image clarity, targeted biopsies, lithotripsy compatibility, and ease of use with single-operator systems. This is transforming the approach to intraductal strictures, stone fragmentation, and biliary surveillance.

3. *Enhanced Lithotripsy Techniques*

Electrohydraulic lithotripsy (EHL) and laser lithotripsy (e.g., Holmium:YAG lasers) can now be precisely guided under direct choledochoscopic visualization. This is resulting in minimally invasive management of difficult or impacted stones, reducing the need for open surgery.

4. *3D Reconstruction and Navigation Systems*

Software-assisted 3D mapping of the biliary tree using preoperative CT or MRCP data enhances intraoperative orientation. This is useful in complex biliary anatomy or re-operative settings.

5. *Disposable and Semi-Disposable Choledochoscopes*

These reduce the risk of cross-contamination and maintenance burden, making advanced biliary visualization more accessible.

35.9 Conclusion

Intraoperative cholangiography and choledochoscopy are indispensable tools in the armamentarium of hepatobiliary surgery, aiding in the accurate identification of biliary anatomy and the management of choledocholithiasis. The choice and proper handling of instruments—from cholangiogram catheters, contrast injectors, and fluoroscopy units to flexible or rigid choledochoscopes with appropriate accessories—directly influence procedural success and patient outcomes. Modern technological advancements have made these procedures safer and more efficient, but they require familiarity with equipment, troubleshooting techniques, and vigilance to avoid complications. A structured approach to instrument setup, image acquisition, and intraoperative problem-solving enhances the diagnostic and therapeutic value of these procedures. Ultimately, mastering the tools of cholangiography and choledochoscopy ensures precision in biliary surgery and reinforces the commitment to patient safety and surgical excellence.

References

1. Phillips EH. Routine versus selective intraoperative cholangiography. Am J Surg. 1993;165:505–7.
2. Lorimer JW, Fairfull-Smith RJ. Intraoperative cholangiography is not essential to avoid duct injuries during laparoscopic cholecystectomy. Am J Surg. 1995;169:344–7.
3. del Carmen MAP, Herrera JT, Sánchez CM. Colangiografía transoperatoria selectiva. Factores asociados a coledocolitiasis. Rev Med IMSS. 2003;41(2):159–63.
4. Hoyuela C, Cugat E, Marco C. Opciones actuales para el diagnostico y tratamiento de la coledocolitiasis. Cir Esp. 2000;68:243–53.
5. Valladares LD, Aguirre MEP, Botella AG. Aproximación diagnóstica en la icterícia obstructiva. In: Cirugía AEC, vol. XIV.; 814–815/825–826. 3rd ed. Ed Med Panamericana; 2022.
6. Quintero CJ, Rivas JF, Martínez JL, Osorio VJ, López AD. Exploración laparoscópica de vías biliares con coledocoscopia transoperatoria para manejo de coledocolitiasis: reporte de casos en el HCSAE Pemex del 2008–2013. http://www.medigraphic.com/cirugiaendoscopica.
7. Parrilla, et al. Cirugía AEC. 3rd ed. Editorial Medica Panamericana; 2022.
8. Galloso Cueto Gilberto L, Abel LG, Sergio CC. Instrumental básico y especializado en la colecistectomía video laparoscópica. Rev Med Electrón. [Internet]. 2012 [citado 2023 Mar 18]. 34(1):81–94. http://scielo.sld.cu/scielo.php?script=sci_arttext&pid=S1684-18242012000100008&lng=es.
9. Sánchez-Ismayel A, Rodríguez O, Sánchez R, Benítez G, Bellorín O, Paredes J. Coledocoscopia en la exploración laparoscópica de la via biliar para resolución de coledocolitiasis. Rev Venez Cir. 2007;60:177.
10. Borie F. Colecistectomía y exploración de la vía biliar principal por laparoscopia. In: Tratamiento laparoscópico de la litiasis de la vía biliar principal. https://doi.org/10.1016/S1282-9129(14)69152-2.
11. Quintero CJM, Rivas JF, Martínez JL, Osorio VJC, de Jesús A, López S. Exploración laparoscópica de vías biliares con coledocoscopia transoperatoria para manejo de coledocolitiasis: reporte de casos en el HCSAE Pemex del 2008–2013. Cir Endoscòpica. 2013;14(4):186–91. http://www.medigraphic.com/cirugiaendoscopica.
12. Gupta R, et al. The SAGES manual. Chapter 22. In: Cholangiography. Springer; 2012.
13. Machicato LE. ¿Qué es una colangiografia? Soluciones Quirúrgicas: ¿Qué es una colangiografía intraoperatoria? (doctor-machicado.blogspot.com).
14. del Pilar M, Méndez F, Fernández MJG, Delgado MIC, Oliveros IL, del Robledo Vicente Castellano F. Limpieza y acondicionamiento del material de laparoscopia en cirugía Ocronos. Ocronos. 2021;4(1):58.
15. Criado Álvarez JJ, Peláez Ros B, Fereres CJ. Esterilización en centros sanitarios. Madrid: Ed Fiscam; 2006.
16. Altemeier W. Surgical antiseptics. In: Disinfections, sterilization and preservation, vol. 12. 4th ed. Lippincott Williams & Wilkins; 1991. p. 204–21.
17. Rey J-F, et al. Desinfección de endoscopios-un enfoque sensible a los recursos. WGO/WEO Global Guideline; 2021.
18. Riscos físics ambientals. CFGS.1954.C03/0.08 CFGS – Prevenció de riscos laborals. Generalitat de Catalunya.

19. Navarrete SA, Cantele HE, Leyba JL, Perez Y, Navarrte LS. Colangiografía intraoperatoria por laparoscopia con cateter de Cholangiocath y de teflon. Revista de la Facultad de Medicina. 2000;23(2): Caracas:122–5.
20. Dong ZT, Wu GZ, Luo KL, Li JM. Primary closure after laparoscopic common bile duct exploration verus T-tube. J Surg Res. 2014;189(2):249–54. https://doi.org/10.1016/j.jss.2014.03.055.
21. Yi H, Hong G, Min S, Lee H. Long-term outcome of primary closure after laparoscopic common bile duct exploration combined with choledochoscopy. Surg Laparosc Endosc Percutan Tech. 2015;25(3):250–3. https://doi.org/10.1097/SLE.0000000000000151.

Endostaplers

36

Mohey Elbanna

Surgical staplers are essential surgical tools nowadays, and stapling has become a standard practice. Staplers are used for tissue approximation, tissue sealing, and division. They are convenient, easy to use, time-saving, and provide a consistent tissue approximation if properly used. All surgeons must be aware of the structure and appropriate use of surgical staplers. There are various types of surgical staplers, including staplers for open surgery and staplers for laparoscopic surgery. The staplers apply staples of different open and closed heights. The choice of the stapler depends on the tissue thickness. The outcome of stapling depends on several factors, including tissue properties, thickness, vascularity, the correct stapler height for the tissue thickness, and proper surgical technique.

36.1 History of Stapling

The first stapler was invented in 1908 by Hümer Hültl, a Hungarian surgeon who practiced in Budapest, Hungary. In 1907 the idea occurred to him that a mechanical instrument, which would place rows of metal staples into the wall of a hollow organ before its division may prevent spillage altogether. The instrument was manufactured by Victor Fischer, a businessman and surgical instrument designer. Fischer completed the stapler in the early part of 1908 (Fig. 36.1), in two sizes, one 17 cm long to close the cardia and the other 11 cm long to staple the duodenum. Hültl first used the stapler clinically on 9 May 1908 [1].

Several modifications to the original Fischer–Hültl instrument were made during the following decades. The Hültl–Fischer stapler was later replaced by an easier to

M. Elbanna (✉)
General Surgery, Faculty of Medicine, Ain Shams University, Cairo, Egypt

Faculty of Medicine, Modern University for Technology and Information, Cairo, Egypt

J. S. Ahluwalia (ed.), *User Manual for Minimally Invasive Surgical Equipment*,
https://doi.org/10.1007/978-981-95-9019-3_36

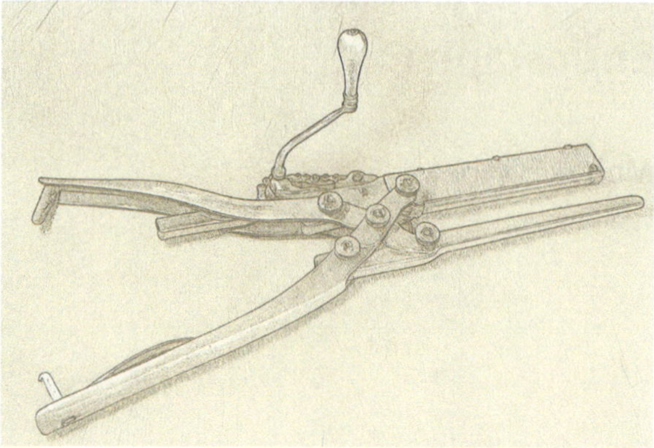

Fig. 36.1 Hültl Stapler

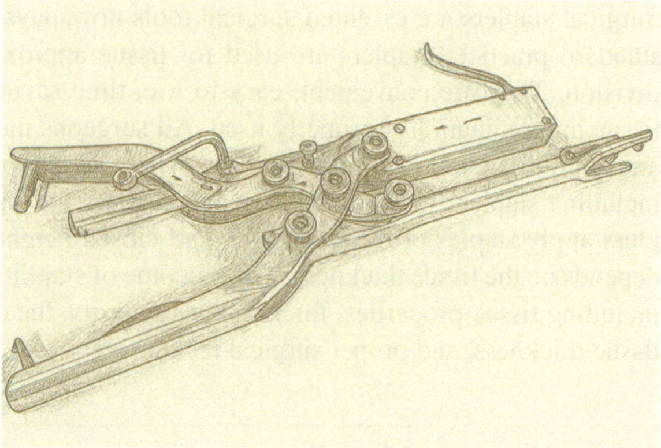

Fig. 36.2 von Petz Stapler

assemble and use stapler developed by another Hungarian surgeon, Alexander von Petz that was introduced in 1921 (Fig. 36.2). During World War II, with its countless injuries, and the need for effective control of hemorrhage, the Soviet engineers succeeded in creating mechanical suturing devices for vascular surgery in 1945. In 1950s, the Soviets designed and manufactured several staplers for GI, Lung, and vascular resections and anastomoses. In 1958, Mark M. Ravitch, Prof. of Surgery at Johns Hopkins University and surgeon-in-chief of Baltimore city hospitals, transferred staplers from the Soviet Union to the USA. A year later, in 1959, Ravitch published an article in the journal "Surgery" describing his experience with surgical staplers for the closure of bronchial stumps [2].

Finally, in 1963, Leon Hirsch, who shared the same spirit of enterprise, supported Ravitch's idea. A year later, he founded United States Surgical Corporation (US Surgical). The modified stapler consisted of just two parts: the stapler itself and an interchangeable cartridge preloaded with staples. The first instrument, named TA (thoraco-abdominal), entered the market in 1967, followed by GIA (gastrointestinal anastomosis) and then other models. The interchangeable cartridges were labeled in different colors (gray, white, blue, gold, and green) to reflect the size of the preloaded staples. Ravitch and his longstanding colleague, Steichen, also developed a stapling course and continued to promote the technique. In the 1970’s, Johnson and Johnson joined the stapling manufacturing business. The 1970’s also witnessed the widespread use of staplers. It is obvious that staplers altered the skills of younger generations of surgeons; many of them now feel uncomfortable with handsewn anastomoses and sometimes challenged by stapler failure [3].

36.2 Types of Endostaplers

Before the advent of endostaplers, some authors classified staplers into five categories: circular, linear, linear cutting, ligating, and skin staplers [4]. Another classification categorizes staplers into circular, linear, curved, and radial. Within each category, several commercial models are available, many of which have their own unique features. They can place staples in a longitudinal, transverse, or oblique manner with respect to the direction of tissue division, with much improved integrity of the staple line. The standard number of staple rows is three rows on each side of the cutting knife [5]. Endostaplers can be classified according to the cutting mechanism into two main types: one with the knife in the reload (e.g., Medtronic) and one with the knife in the stapler (e.g., Ethicon) [6, 7]. In the knife in the reload style, the reload is assembled into the stapler, so that every time we fire, a new blade is used. It places two triple-staggered rows of titanium staples, and simultaneously, the knife divides the tissue in between. In the knife-in-stapler style, the knife is in the stapler itself, and the cartridge is placed in the cartridge magazine.

36.3 Components

Different manufacturers make staplers in different shapes but basic principle, components, and features have a lot in common, and few such variations are described below (Fig. 36.3).

The Signia™ stapler from Medtronic offers latest innovations like fully powered articulation, rotation, and clamping, along with push-button powered firing (Fig. 36.6). It also features adaptive firing, where the firing speed changes automatically based on tissue variability for consistent staple formation. Real-time feedback offers visual and audible feedback to inform decision-making.

Robotic staplers that can be integrated with the robotic surgical system and manipulated by the console surgeon are the latest technological advancement [9].

36.4 Staple Firing

Firing of the staples can be performed manually by pressing the firing trigger or automatically by pressing a button in powered staplers. Most modern staplers bend each staple into a B-shape staple form to secure the tissue in place [10]. Endostaplers

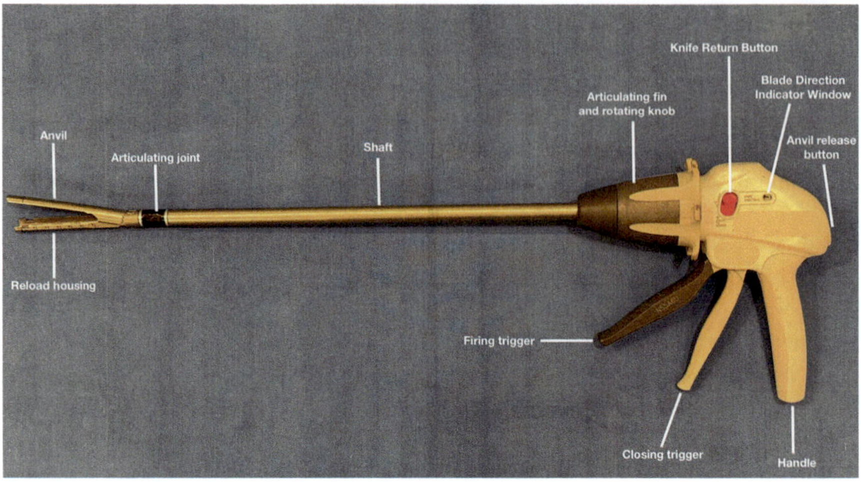

Fig. 36.3 Endostapler with blade built into the device. (1) Handle: Is used to grip the device and adjust its position. (2) Closing Trigger: Is used to close the anvil of the stapler. (3) Firing Trigger: Is used to start stapling once the closing trigger has been pressed to close the stapler and firing trigger lock (if any) has been released. (4) Rotating Knob: Is used to rotate the stapler shaft. (5) Articulation Fin: Is pulled to set the articulating joint free so that the tip can be articulated by pressing it against hard object/tissue. (6) Anvil Release Button: Is used to release the anvil before or after firing. (7) Knife Return Button: Is used if the knife is jammed and cannot be returned after firing. (8) Shaft: Is made in different lengths to suit different kinds of patients. Longer lengths are needed for obese patients. (9) Anvil: Is made of metal and used to push the staples through the tissues into the B form (final shape after firing). (10) Reload Housing: Is the place to insert reload

incorporate a knife for tissue division. Some staplers are equipped with a mechanism for fixation of the device to tissues to improve its stability. By design, the staples precede the knife in the stapler reload. The objective is to place a staple line that is obviously longer than the distance the knife runs to cut between the staple lines [2].

36.5 Optimal Stapling

The aim of stapling is to create a staple line that achieves proper tissue approximation, maintains proper tissue apposition while enabling appropriate homeostasis and tissue perfusion until healing of tissues and anastomoses takes place. Ideal stapling occurs with minimal bleeding, tissue damage, and postoperative leaks. The most important factor in creating an optimal staple line is the formation of well-aligned, well-formed staples, with good vascularization, and without tissue tearing. Optimal stapling is achieved by proper balance between tissue compression and tissue damage, and a balance between tissue perfusion and hemostasis. The tissue thickness and its intrinsic mechanical properties will determine the necessary extent of

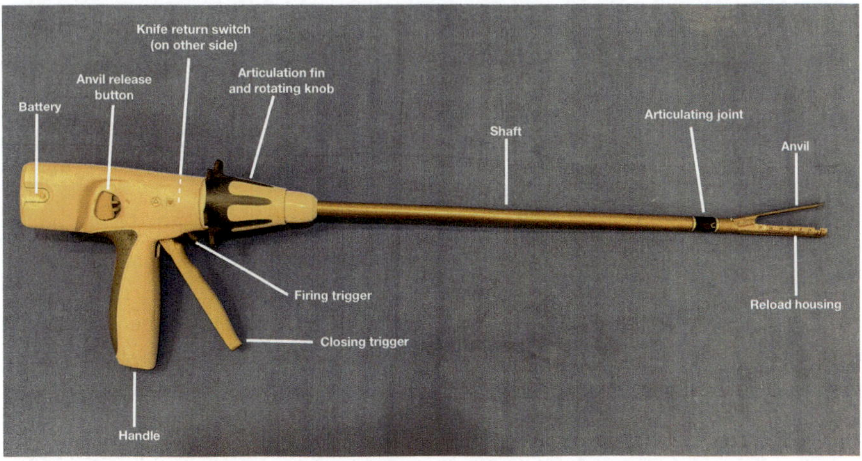

Fig. 36.4 Powered Ethicon endostapler with blade built into the device. (1) Handle: Is used to grip the device and adjust its position. (2) Closing Trigger: Is used to close the anvil of the stapler. (3) Firing Trigger: Is used to start stapling once the closing trigger has been pressed to close the stapler and firing trigger lock (if any) has been released. (4) Rotating Knob: Is used to rotate the stapler shaft. (5) Articulation Fin: Is pulled to set the articulating joint free so that the tip can be articulated by pressing it against a hard object/tissue. (6) Anvil Release Button: Is used to release the anvil before or after firing. (7) Battery: Is used to power the stapler (Fig. 36.4). Should be assembled into the stapler just before use. (8) Knife Return Button: Is used if the knife is jammed and cannot be returned after firing. (9) Shaft: Is made in different lengths to suit different kinds of patients. Longer lengths are needed for obese patients. (10) Anvil: Is made of metal and used to push the staples through the tissues into the B form (final shape after firing). (11) Reload Housing: Is the place to insert reload

compressive force and the adequate length of prefiring compression time. The correct staple height will therefore vary depending on these tissue-specific properties [10].

Tissue apposition and tissue sealing are the intended outcomes of stapling. Understanding how staplers interact with target tissues is key to improving patient outcomes. Different tissues have different thickness and different intrinsic biomechanical properties that determine the ideal compressive force and prefiring compression time for each tissue type. The correct staple height will vary depending on these tissue-specific properties and the tissue pathology. Factors that should be considered by the surgeon include stapler compression, tissue compressibility, staple height, tissue thickness, and tissue type [10].

The best stapler is the one that provides appropriate hemostasis and tissue apposition without significant ischemia or tissue damage. If the closed staple height is too high, tissue apposition may be inadequate and may result in leakage, bleeding, and/or dehiscence. Conversely, if the staple height selected is too low, then ischemia, serosal shearing, or “cheese wiring” may result, potentially leading to leakage or frank necrosis. Staple colors, heights, and dimensions are described in Table 36.1 [10].

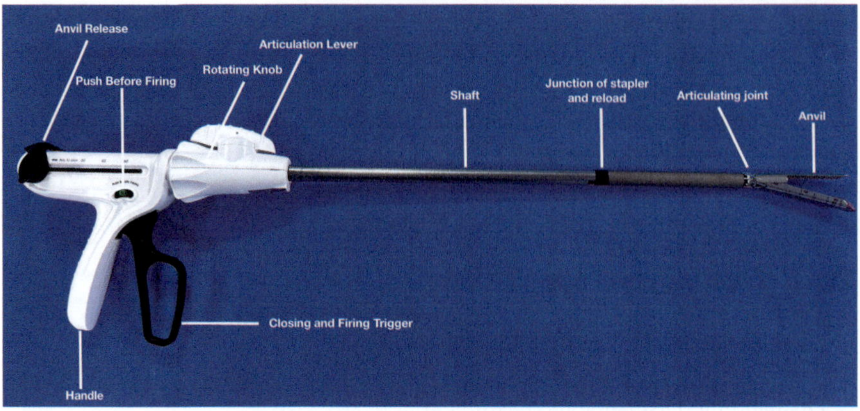

Fig. 36.5 Manual endostapler with blade built into reload. (1) Handle: Is used to grip the device and adjust its position (Fig. 36.5) [8]. (2) Closing and Firing Trigger: Is used to close the anvil of the stapler in the first instance, and after the green button is pushed, it is pressed again to fire the stapler. (3) Push Before Firing Button: Is pressed to engage the trigger to fire the stapler. (4) Rotating Knob: Is used to rotate the stapler shaft. (5) Articulation Lever: Is used to rotate the articulating joint in different directions so that the tip can be articulated as per the need of the situation. (6) Anvil Release: Is used to release the anvil before or after firing by pulling it backwards. (7) Shaft: Is made in different lengths to suit different kinds of patients. Longer lengths are needed for obese patients. (8) Anvil: Is made of metal and used to push the staples through the tissues into the B form (final shape after firing)

When staples close, they attain B-shaped form. Such a form achieves secure closure with resultant appropriate tissue apposition. If the staples close in inappropriate forms, this may result in leakage or bleeding. One must examine the final formation of staple pins after firing.

Tri-staple technology was devised by Covidien in 2010 that is purchased by Medtronic (Norwalk, CT) in 2015. Tri-staple cartridges consist of three rows of staples on each side of the knife; each row has a different staple open and closed height to cover a range of tissue thickness (Table 36.2). The staples increase in height from the inner row to the outer row. They might improve burst pressure strength and reduce the tissue compression stress on the outer staple row [12, 13].

36.6 Tissue Properties

The unique properties of the different types of tissues in the body have a major impact on the choice of the stapler and staple height. Gastrointestinal tissues, like other tissues, have a biphasic nature due to having both liquid and solid properties. Different tissue types have inherently different ratios of liquid and solid components as well as air components. In addition, biochemical properties such as the protein content and metabolic profile are also differentiating factors. Moreover, the extrinsic blood supply will also vary by tissue type and will contribute further to differentiation. The compressive load necessary to form a stable anastomosis will

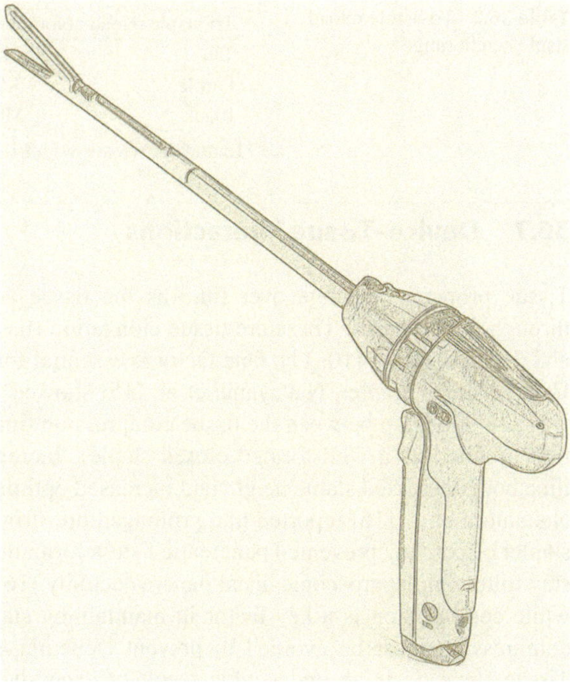

Fig. 36.6 Medtronic Signia stapler

Table 36.1 Dimensions of commonly available staple cartridges

Color	Tissue type	Open staple height	Closed staple height
Gray	Mesentery	2.0 mm	0.75 mm
White	Vascular	2.5 mm	1.0 mm
Blue	Standard	3.5 mm	1.5 mm
Gold	Standard/thick	3.8 mm	1.8 mm
Green	Thick	4.1 mm	2.0 mm

depend on these inherent tissue properties, as well as the current physical condition of the tissues to be joined. Tissue compression is of paramount importance for tissue healing while maintaining adequate perfusion as well as achieving limited ischemia and tissue destruction. Optimal stapling of any tissue requires an adequate tissue compression time to decrease the fluid in the tissue, to allow elongation of the tissue being compressed, smooth firing of the instrument, and consistent staple line formation. These requirements must be balanced against the risk of increased tissue tearing and excessive tensile strength [10, 14].

Table 36.2 Tri-staple reload staple height range

Tri-staple reload color	Range of staple height	Port size
Tan	2 mm–3.5 mm	12 mm
Purple	3.5 mm–4.8 mm	12 mm
Black	More than 4.8 mm	15 mm

Endo GIA reloads with tri-staple technology

36.7 Device–Tissue Interactions

Tissue properties change over time as the tissue is compressed. Tissues pass through three phases. These are tissue elongation (tissue creep), stress relaxation, and tissue shearing [10, 11]. One factor is essential for the three phases: Time [5]. Using a linear stapler, Nakayama et al. [15] showed in stomach tissue that there was a relationship between the tissue compression time and optimal staple formation (defined as a well-formed closed staple). Increasing prefiring compression time both decreased staple height and increased optimal staple formation rate [15]. Nakamura et al. [16] reported that prolonged pre-firing compression with a linear stapler effectively prevented pancreatic fistula formation and reduced the length of stay following laparoscopic distal pancreatectomy [16]. It is important to note that while compression is a key factor in maintaining staple line integrity, excessive compression must be avoided to prevent ischemia and tissue destruction [14]. Tissue shearing is an undesirable result of excessive tissue compression. More recent studies confirm the concept that increased compression is associated with desirable outcomes: lower leak rates, increased intraluminal pressure, improved hemostasis, and minimized wound contraction, potentially leading to decreased stricture rates [17, 18].

The mechanical properties of tissues are also influenced by inherent patient differences, including specific tissue location, accessibility, comorbidities, prior medications/therapy, and the pathological condition of the tissue. Differences in the profile for each patient with these variables not only influence the tissue thickness but also its compressibility. For example, the changes in thickness associated with irradiation may alter the inherent compressibility of the tissue. As the tissue becomes less compressible, an increased amount of pressure needs to be applied by the stapler to the tissue to ensure that the desired closed staple height is obtained [14].

However, all these factors must be considered in the context of perhaps the most relevant variable: The experience and surgical technique of the surgeon [10].

Advances in technology cannot overcome deficiencies in technique, such as indelicate handling of the tissues, tension on anastomoses, ischemic anastomoses, and the attempted salvage of unsatisfactory stapled anastomoses. In such cases, takedown and construction of another anastomosis is the only viable option. Howard analyzed the studies on medical error in surgical stapler use [19]. He concluded that human misuse of the stapler may be the most important risk factor. Surgeon's experience and understanding of the tissue properties, the principles of gastrointestinal anastomosis, and proper stapler use are essential factors for successful stapling [19].

Table 36.3 Types of stapler malfunctions reported (Lucas et al. [20])

Type of surgical malfunction	Number reported	Percentage of total (%)
Malformed staples/staple line	62	32
Staple line nor forming/staples missing	38	20
Sticking/locking/jamming	31	16
Tissue damage/leaks	29	15
Misfire	20	10
Stapler not cutting	6	3
Cartridge not properly loaded	4	2
Stapler broke	5	2.5
Total	195	Cases surveyed

This conclusion was supported by a study performed by Lucas et al. [20]. They surveyed stapler malfunctions and reported the types of stapler malfunctions (Table 36.3) [20]. However, it is noticeable that the most common cause of stapler malfunction or staple malformation is human error or misuse of the stapler [21].

36.8 Troubleshooting

Many unexpected events can happen while using endostaplers, and the following table (Table 36.4) gives an outline to such situations and their solutions.

Table 36.4 Staplers' problems, causes and solution

Problem	Possible cause	Solution
The stapler fails to fire	Improper tissue thickness, device malfunction, or jammed reload	Remove and inspect the stapler, check for a jammed reload, and replace if needed
Partial staple line/ incomplete firing	Poor tissue compression, faulty cartridge, or early firing	Wait for full compression time, reload and refire, use a new stapler if needed
Bleeding from the staple line	Inadequate compression, incorrect staple height	Use correct staple height, ensure full compression before firing
Misfire or mechanical resistance	Stapler jammed, faulty mechanism, or over-thick tissue	Do not force, remove the stapler carefully, and replace with new device
Staple line dehiscence	Tension on tissue, wrong staple height, or misalignment	Reinforce with sutures or clips, revise with a new staple line if required
Device not articulating or opening	Mechanical fault, user error	Check articulation controls; replace the device if faulty
Difficulty inserting through the trocar	Oversized stapler or narrow trocar port	Use the appropriate trocar size or port; consider an alternate access site
Reload not engaging	Misalignment, defective reload, or improper loading	Realign, reload properly and replace reload if damaged
Tissue slippage during firing	Inadequate grasp, poor positioning, or wet tissue	Reposition tissue, dry area, and ensure adequate tissue capture before firing

36.9 Conclusion

Endoscopic staplers have revolutionized the field of minimally invasive surgery by enabling precise, efficient, and hemostatic tissue division and anastomosis. As with any advanced surgical tool, a thorough understanding of its mechanics, appropriate usage, and potential pitfalls is essential to maximize its benefits and minimize complications. Mastery of endostapler techniques not only enhances surgical outcomes but also improves patient safety and recovery times. Continued advancements in stapler technology, coupled with ongoing surgical training and critical intraoperative judgment, will ensure that endostaplers remain an indispensable component of the modern laparoscopic toolkit.

References

1. Robicsek F, Konstantinov I. Hümer Hültl: the father of the surgical stapler. J Med Biogr. 2001;9:16–9.
2. Akopov A, Artioukh D, Molnar T. Surgical staplers: the history of conception and adoption. Ann Thorac Surg. 2021;112:1716–21.
3. Gaidry AD, Tremblay L, Nakayama D, Ignacio RC Jr. The history of surgical staplers: a combination of Hungarian, Russian, and American innovation. Am Surg. 2019;85:563–6.
4. McGuire J, Wright IC, Leverment JN. Surgical staplers: a review. J R Coll Surg Edinb. 1997;42(1):1–9.
5. Baker RS, Foote J, Kemmeter P, et al. The science of stapling and leaks. Obes Surg. 2004;14:1290–8. https://doi.org/10.1381/0960892042583888.
6. Stapling and Laparoscopy: Product Catalogue 2005. Tyco Healthcare. https://www.akinglobal.com.tr/uploads/subdir-141-4/COVIDIEN%20(TYCO%20)-AUTOSUTURE.pdf.
7. Ethicon Product Catalogue 2022. Johnson & Johnson. https://www.jnjmedtech.com/sites/default/files/user_uploaded_assets/html_exports/echelon-plus-stapler/pdf/ECHELON-Stapler-Product-Brochure.pdf.
8. https://qianjingmed.en.made-in-china.com/product/IZMQNoXYMlVK/China-Endoscope-Instrument-Human-Staples-Single-Use-Laparoscopic-Linear-Stapler-for-Cardiothoracic-Surgery.html.
9. Giffen Z, Ezzone A, Ekwenna O. Robotic stapler use: is it safe?-FDA database analysis across multiple surgical specialties. PLoS One. 2021;16(6):e0253548. https://doi.org/10.1371/journal.pone.0253548. PMID: 34166443; PMCID: PMC8224848.
10. Chekan E, Whelan RL. Surgical stapling device-tissue interactions: what surgeons need to know to improve patient outcomes. Med Devices (Auckl). 2014;7:305–18. https://doi.org/10.2147/MDER.S67338. PMID: 25246812; PMCID: PMC4168870.
11. Akiyoshi T, Ueno M, Fukunaga Y, et al. Incidence of and risk factors for anastomotic leakage after laparoscopic anterior resection with intracorporeal rectal transection and double-stapling technique anastomosis for rectal cancer. Am J Surg. 2011;202(3):259–64.
12. Endo GIA. Reloads with tri-staple technology. Technical Brochure. https://www.medtronic.com/content/dam/medtronic-wide/public/united-states/products/surgical-stapling/gia-stapler-with-tristaple-technology-value-analysisbrochure.pdf.
13. Derici S, Atila K, Bora S. The effect of the cartridge used in laparoscopic sleeve gastrectomy on the development of a staple-line leak. Am Surg. 2018;84:1499–503.
14. Collopy BT. Colorectal anastomotic leak rates are measures of technical skill in surgery. ANZ J Surg. 2001;71(9):508–10.
15. Nakayama S, Hasegawa S, Nagayama S, et al. The importance of precompression time for secure stapling with a linear stapler. Surg Endosc. 2011;25(7):2382–6. 31.

16. Nakamura M, Ueda J, Kohno H, et al. Prolonged peri-firing compression with a linear stapler prevents pancreatic fistula in laparoscopic distal pancreatectomy. Surg Endosc. 2011;25(3):867–71.
17. Nakayama S, Hasegawa S, Hida K, Kawada K, Sakai Y. Obtaining secure stapling of a double stapling anastomosis. J Surg Res. 2015;193(2):652–7. https://doi.org/10.1016/j.jss.2014.08.044. Epub 2014 Sep 3.
18. Myers SR, Rothermel WS, Shaffer L. The effect of tissue compression on circular satpler lne failure. Surg Endosc. 2011;25(9):3043–9.
19. Howard JE. Understanding medical error in surgical stapler use: a philosophical and scientific analysis. Honors Undergraduate Theses 797; 2020. https://stars.library.ucf.edu/honorstheses/797.
20. Lucas S. Avoiding surgical stapler misuse - surgical stapler misuse - 2020's #1 health technology hazard. Plymouth Meeting; 2019. Retrieved date from https://www.ecri.org/events/webinar-avoiding-surgical-stapler-misuse-2019/.
21. Miller J. Recommendations to avoid surgical stapler misuse - 2020's #1 health technology hazard. Avoiding surgical stapler misuse - 2020's #1 health technology Hazard. Plymouth meeting; 2019. Retrieved from https://www.ecri.org/events/webinaravoiding-surgical-stapler-misuse-2019/. Myers SR, Rothermel WS Jr, Shaffer L. The effect of tissue compression on circular stapler line failure. Surg Endosc 2011;25(9):3043–9.

37 Gynecology Surgery: Special Instruments

Preeti Jindal, Muskan Mittal, and Mandeep Kaur

The history of laparoscopic gynecology can be traced back to the early twentieth century, when German physician Georg Kelling conducted a rudimentary form of laparoscopy in 1901 [1]. Utilizing a cystoscope, he inspected the abdominal cavity of a canine subject. In 1910, Hans Christian Jacobaeus further advanced this approach, performing laparoscopy on human patients [2]. However, it was during the 1960s that modern laparoscopy in gynecology truly commenced to develop, primarily due to the contributions of Dr. Kurt Semm, a German gynecologist. He introduced several groundbreaking innovations, including automated insufflation devices and electrosurgical instruments, which facilitated the execution of more intricate gynecological procedures laparoscopically [3]. By the 1980s and 1990s, laparoscopy had become a widely accepted and preferred technique in gynecology, revolutionizing the field by offering less invasive alternatives to conventional open surgery.

The majority of the instruments utilized in laparoscopic gynecological surgeries are shared with other abdominal surgeries. However, there are certain instruments that are almost exclusively employed in laparoscopic gynecological surgeries, and these will be the focus of this chapter.

37.1 Uterine Manipulator

Uterine manipulators are specially designed instruments to be inserted from the transvaginal route into the uterine cavity to provide precise control and movement of the uterus during laparoscopic gynecological procedures. This greatly enhances

P. Jindal · M. Mittal
The Touch Clinic, Mohali, India

M. Kaur (✉)
Department of Fertility Services, STAR Hospital, Jalandhar, Punjab, India

J. S. Ahluwalia (ed.), *User Manual for Minimally Invasive Surgical Equipment*,
https://doi.org/10.1007/978-981-95-9019-3_37

visualization during pelvic surgery without the need for additional instruments placed laparoscopically. Since the uterus is not held externally with any instrument, this does not interfere with other laparoscopic instruments and also does not lead to any bleeding intra-abdominally (as compared to uterine manipulation with myoma screw or forceps placed laparoscopically). The various parts of a uterine manipulator are tailored to serve specific functions like movement of the uterus, stability of the instrument and access to the uterine cavity. Uterine manipulators are now available in many different shapes, and some have special functions. Below is a description of the key components that will fit the description of most of such instruments (some of the parts are found in some of the models only) (Fig. 37.1).

37.1.1 Components

1. Handle

   This is the part of the manipulator that the surgeon or assistant holds to control the movements of the uterus once the instrument is in place. It is often ergonomically designed to allow for easy rotation, angulation, and movement. This allows for anteversion, retroversion, lateral, and rotational movements of the uterus during surgery as and when required at different steps in the procedure.

2. Shaft

   This is the elongated and slender portion of the manipulator that extends into the uterine cavity through the cervix. It extends from the handle to the instrument's tip. Its length can vary depending on the model and size of the uterus. It serves as the connection between the external handle and the intrauterine components and may

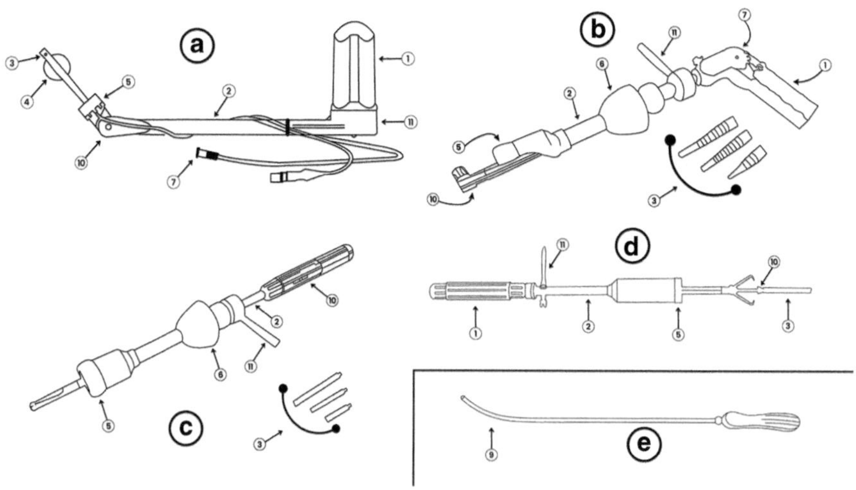

Fig. 37.1 (a–e) different types of uterine manipulators

contain mechanisms to enable controlled movement of the instrument's tip by the handle. Depending on the model, the shaft may be straight or curved to facilitate easier insertion and uterine manipulation.

3. Tip (Intrauterine Portion)
   This portion is inserted into the uterus. Depending on the model, it may be fixed or detachable to confirm the length of the uterine cavity. If it is a fixed length, there may be a mechanism to control the length of the tip that can be inserted into the uterus to prevent inadvertent uterine perforation. The tip of the instrument engages with the uterine cavity to provide direct manipulation of the uterus.

4. Balloon or Inflatable Device
   In certain models (e.g., Vcare and Advincula Delineator), a balloon is available and can be inserted into the uterus and inflated to secure the manipulator in place. This ensures stability and prevents slippage during surgery.

5. Colpotomy Cup (Vaginal Cup)
   This is a cup-shaped structure designed to be positioned at the junction of the cervix and vagina. If constructed from transparent material, it will facilitate visualization of the surrounding tissues and simplify its deployment. The cup serves to delineate the vaginal fornix, ensuring that the incision during colpotomy is safe and precise. Additionally, it protects the surrounding structures, such as the bladder and rectum, during surgical procedures.

6. Cervical Seal or Collar
   This serves as a seal around the manipulator shaft at the level of the cervix, preventing the leakage of pneumoperitoneum gas and intra-abdominal fluids, particularly during and after colpotomy.

7. Dye Injection Port
   Some of the models incorporate a channel integrated into the manipulator, enabling the injection of fluids or dyes into the uterine cavity or fallopian tubes. This technique, known as chromopertubation, facilitates the assessment of the patency of the fallopian tubes.

8. Manipulator Locking Mechanism
   This device secures the handle in a predetermined position once the desired uterine position is attained. Consequently, the uterus remains in place during the critical stages of the procedure, thereby alleviating user fatigue.

9. Uterine Depth Gauge (Sound)
   Certain manipulators possess an integrated or separate uterine sound (or depth gauge) that facilitates the measurement of the depth of the uterine cavity. This data serves as a reference to determine the optimal length of the intrauterine tip, thereby ensuring precise placement and minimizing the risk of uterine perforation.

10. Articulating Joint

This joint enables the manipulator tip to move in various directions (anteversion, retroversion, and lateral movements), thereby providing enhanced control over the position of the uterus. This facilitates optimal positioning during the procedure.

11. External Locking Ring or Adjustable Stop

If an adjustable ring or stopping mechanism is present on the shaft, it assists the operator in adjusting and fixing the depth of the uterine manipulator to prevent over-insertion into the uterine cavity and perforation.

These components collaborate to provide effective uterine manipulation, enhancing the safety and precision of laparoscopic gynecological procedures. Different models and brands may offer variations or additional features tailored to specific surgical requirements. It is advisable to consider a range of models available to surgeons and select the one that best aligns with their expertise and operating style. If a particular model proves suboptimal, it is prudent to transition to another type to ensure enhanced safety and efficiency during procedures. Different models may suit various operators based on their approach to procedures and operating style variations.

37.1.2 Placing a Uterine Manipulator

Utilizing a uterine manipulator necessitates meticulous handling and technique to ensure accurate placement, effective uterine mobilization, and patient safety during laparoscopic gynecological procedures. This comprehensive guide provides a step-by-step protocol for the proper utilization of a uterine manipulator in laparoscopic surgeries, including hysterectomy, myomectomy, and endometriosis excision.

1. Patient Preparation
   - Positioning: The patient is placed in a lithotomy position (legs in stirrups). Proper positioning is essential for optimal access to the pelvic region.
   - Anesthesia: General anesthesia is preferred.
   - Disinfection: The perineum and vaginal canal is made sterile using the standard protocol of the hospital.
2. Cervical Dilation (if Necessary)

If the cervix is constricted, gentle dilation using cervical dilators may be necessary. This procedure facilitates the insertion of the manipulator into the uterine cavity.

3. Assemble the Uterine Manipulator

Depending on the model, the manipulator may require assembly. This entails attaching the colpotomy cup, adjusting the intrauterine tip (if the instrument has multiple sizes of tips, ensure the appropriate one is used), and deflating the balloon if applicable. Verify that the manipulator is configured with the suitable components for the intended surgical procedure (e.g., a colpotomy cup for hysterectomy and a dye injection port for tubal patency testing).

4. Lubrication

Lubricate the intrauterine portion (tip or balloon) of the uterine manipulator with a sterile, water-based lubricant. This facilitates smooth insertion and minimizes the risk of trauma to the cervix or uterus.

5. Insert the Uterine Manipulator
   - Insertion into the Cervix: Gently insert the tip of the uterine manipulator into the cervical canal. Apply steady, gentle pressure to advance the tip into the uterine cavity.
   - Exercise caution when attempting to manipulate the manipulator, as excessive pressure may result in injury or perforation of the uterus.
   - Balloon Inflation (If Applicable): If the manipulator possesses an inflatable balloon, inflate the balloon within the uterus using saline or air to secure the manipulator in position.
6. Position the Colpotomy Cup

If a colpotomy cup (vaginal cup) is part of the setup in a given procedure, it should be positioned at the cervix. The colpotomy cup serves as a visual aid and a guide for the surgeon during the colpotomy incision, assisting in the visualization and delineation of the vaginal fornices during a total laparoscopic hysterectomy.

7. Secure the Manipulator

Adjust the turning mechanism on the manipulator handle to position the uterus in the desired location. Certain manipulators are equipped with a locking mechanism that secures the uterus in place, thereby preventing unintended movement during surgery and reducing strain on the user.

8. Manipulate the Uterus
   - Anteversion and Retroversion: Utilize the handle to tilt the uterus forward (anteversion) or backward (retroversion) in accordance with the surgical imperative.
   - Lateral Movements: Additionally, the uterus can be rotated laterally (side to side) to facilitate improved access to the ovaries, fallopian tubes, or other pelvic structures.
   - Rotation: Certain manipulators facilitate the rotation of the uterus to enhance surgical visibility.
9. Perform the Surgical Procedure
   - Once the uterus is positioned correctly, the laparoscopic surgery is performed. The manipulator enables the surgeon to manipulate the uterus as necessary throughout the procedure, enhancing access to the operative site.
   - For procedures such as hysterectomies, the colpotomy cup serves as a guide, assisting the surgeon in making the colpotomy incision safely and efficiently.
10. Dye Injection (if Required)

If chromopertubation is to be performed, a dye is injected from the port on the manipulator and observed by the surgeon to assess tubal patency.

11. Removal of the Manipulator
    - After completing the surgical procedure, deflate the intrauterine balloon (if applicable).
    - Gently remove the uterine manipulator from the cervix and vaginal canal.
    - Check for any bleeding or trauma to the cervix or vagina upon removal.

37.1.3 Maintenance

Proper care of a uterine manipulator is paramount for ensuring its continued functionality, patient safety, and extended lifespan, particularly for reusable models. Sterilization and meticulous handling are indispensable in preventing infection, equipment damage, or malfunction. The following general guidelines provide a comprehensive framework for the responsible care of uterine manipulators:

1. Disassemble

   Separate the parts, such as the handle, shaft, colpotomy cup, and any balloon components, if the uterine manipulator has such separable parts. Take care of small detachable parts loss during cleaning.

2. Pre-Cleaning (Rinsing)

   Immediately after surgery, rinse the manipulator thoroughly with sterile water or saline to remove blood, tissue, and other bodily fluids. This initial rinse is crucial to prevent the formation of biofilms. Refrain from using chemicals not approved by the manufacturer, as this may compromise the material or integrity of the instrument.

3. Manual Cleaning
   - Soaking: To facilitate the cleaning of the instrument, it is recommended to immerse it in an enzymatic detergent solution. Ensure that the detergent used is specifically approved for surgical instruments. Adhere to the instructions of the manufacturer regarding the concentration and soaking time.
   - Brushing and Scrubbing: Utilize soft, sterile brushes to meticulously clean the internal channels, crevices, and inaccessible areas, including the dye injection ports, balloons, and seals. Exercise caution to avoid damaging delicate components.
4. Ultrasonic Cleaning (optional)
5. Sterilization (For Reusable Devices)

   According to the compatibility of a given uterine manipulator and hospital policy, it may be sterilized using autoclave, ethylene oxide, plasma, etc.

6. Storage

   Store the uterine manipulator in a clean, dry, and sterile environment.

7. Single-Use Disposable Devices

   These devices should be safely disposed of according to the medical waste guidelines of your healthcare facility immediately after use.

8. Routine Maintenance
    - Regular Checks: Conduct routine inspections of all reusable manipulators to ascertain their optimal functionality. This entails verifying the functionality of moving components, locking mechanisms, and internal channels.
    - Professional Servicing: Upon detecting indications of wear or malfunction, promptly dispatch the manipulator for professional servicing or repair. Certain components, such as balloons or seals, may necessitate periodic replacement.

37.1.4 Troubleshooting

If an issue arises during the performance of a gynecological surgery involving the uterine manipulator, it is crucial to comprehend fundamental troubleshooting concepts. Below are prevalent issues that may occur with uterine manipulators, along with the corresponding troubleshooting steps to address them:

1. Difficulty in Insertion of Uterine Manipulator
    - Cervical Stenosis—Gently dilate the cervix using a cervical dilator before attempting insertion again.
    - Insufficient Lubrication—Apply a sterile, water-based lubricant to the manipulator tip to ease the insertion.
    - Improper Sizing of the Intrauterine Tip—Ensure the tip of the manipulator is the appropriate size for the patient's uterine cavity. If it's too large, select a smaller-sized tip or manipulator.
2. Uterine Manipulator Slipping out of the Uterus
    - Inadequate Insertion Depth—Ensure that the manipulator tip is fully inserted into the uterine cavity.
    - Inadequate Tension or Loose Locking Mechanism—Ensure proper tension and tighten the locking mechanism.
    - Deflated or Damaged Intrauterine Balloon—Ensure balloon is properly inflated inside the uterine cavity and rule out any leak or damage.
3. Limited or Restricted Movement of the Uterus
    - Stiffness or Malfunction of Articulating Joints of Manipulator—Clean and lubricate the joints.
    - Improper Positioning of the Manipulator Tip—Ensure the tip is fully inserted into the uterine cavity.
    - Obstruction by Surrounding Organs—Do proper adhesiolysis.
4. Colpotomy Cup Not Positioning Properly

Improper Sizing of the Colpotomy Cup—Ensure proper matching of the cup size to the patient's anatomy.

Misalignment of Cup—Make sure the cup is correctly aligned in the vaginal vault.

5. Balloon Fails to Inflate or Deflate (Balloon-Type Manipulators)
    - Leak or rupture in the balloon—Replace the balloon or the manipulator.
    - Damaged or kinked inflation tubing—Unkink the tube.

6. Difficulty in Dye Injection (During Chromopertubation)
   - Blockage in the dye injection port—Clean with brush or force saline into it with a syringe.
   - Improper connection to the dye syringe—Secure the connection.
   - Incorrect placement of the intrauterine tip—Reposition the tip and make sure it is positioned within the uterine cavity.

37.2 Laparoscopic Myoma Screw

Laparoscopic myomectomy involves the removal of uterine fibroids (myomas), and laparoscopic myoma is used for the manipulation and extraction of fibroids. It is usually available in 5 mm and 10 mm sizes and has a screw-shaped, sharp tip (giving it its name) with a handle at the back (Fig. 37.2).

37.2.1 Components

1. Handle—It is meant for a secure grip by the surgeon or assistant. The handle may be made of plastic or metal.
2. Shaft—This is the area between the handle and the screw-shaped tip. It is made of solid metal without a sheath to give good strength to the instrument, to facilitate the movement and extraction of fibroids.
3. Screw—These are screw-shaped threads meant for securing grip on fibroid. Rotation of the instrument in clock-wise direction advances it into the fibroid due to the screw shape of this part. Rotation in a counter-clockwise direction enables it to come out of fibroid. It may be fixed onto the shaft separately (less desirable as the joint may break) or the whole instrument may be made from a single piece of metal (except the handle).
4. Tip—Sharp tip enables entry of myoma screw into fibroid.

Fig. 37.2 Laparoscopic myoma screw

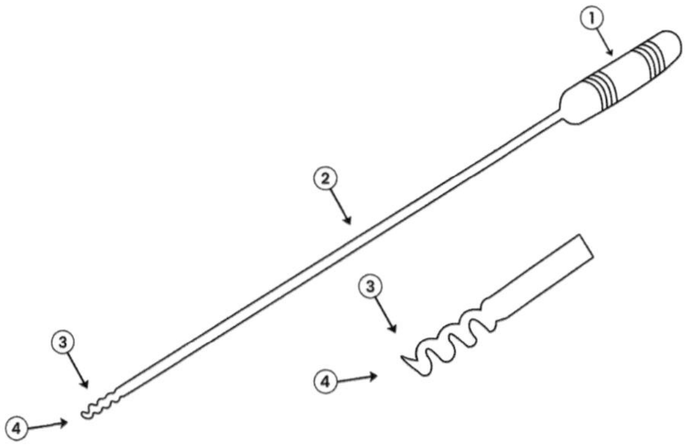

37.2.2 Key Features and Benefits

The laparoscopic myoma screw offers several key features and benefits that contribute to its efficacy and versatility in myomectomy procedures:

1. Secure Tissue Fixation: The corkscrew tip of the myoma screw enables secure fixation of fibroids. Fibroids are hard to hold with other instruments. Screw allows surgeons to manipulate and mobilize them with ease during laparoscopic surgery as compared to other instruments.
2. Minimized Tissue Trauma: Since the screw has a sharp tip, it can be inserted into the fibroid through a small opening in the uterine musculature, and dissection can proceed very close to fibroid minimizing trauma to normal tissue.
3. Enhanced Visualization: As the fibroid gets tightly fixed by the screw, it becomes easy to manipulate the fibroid, making visualization better.
4. Reduced Operative Time: The use of the laparoscopic myoma screw can contribute to shorter operative times by streamlining the fibroid manipulation and extraction process, thereby enhancing surgical efficiency and reducing patient anesthesia exposure.

37.2.3 Maintenance

Immediately after use, clean, scrub, sterilize, and store as per the hospital policy.

37.2.4 Troubleshooting

1. Difficult Insertion into Myoma
   - Blunt Screw Tip: Over time, the tip of myoma screws may become blunt. If possible, it should be sharpened. Otherwise, the instrument should be replaced.
   - Inadequate Pressure: Ensure you are applying consistent pressure while inserting the myoma screw into the fibroid.
   - Fibroid Location: If the fibroid is in a hard-to-reach location, adjust the positioning of the laparoscope and other instruments to get better access.
2. Screw Slipping During Manipulation
   - Loose Insertion: If the screw slips out while pulling or rotating the fibroid, ensure it has been inserted deeply enough. The screw should be rotated sufficiently into the fibroid to create a firm anchor.
   - Wrong Technique: Use a twisting motion to insert and secure the screw rather than pushing directly. This ensures better traction and reduces the chance of slipping.
   - Weak Fibroid Tissue: In cases where the fibroid tissue is soft or fragile, it may tear easily. Try using toothed forceps instead.

3. Instrument Malfunction
   - Inspect for mechanical damage like loose joints, cracks, or bends.
   - Verify that the screw's threads are intact and not compromised. Damaged threads can diminish the screw's grip and impair its ability to secure the fibroid.
   - Use a myoma screw that does not have a joint at the shaft and screw junction, as this joint can break while applying excessive force.
4. Difficulty Removing the Myoma Screw
   - Overpenetration: If the screw is excessively embedded, gently rotate it counterclockwise while extruding it to avoid tissue damage.
   - Grip on Adjacent Tissues: Verify that the screw has not inadvertently grasped adjacent uterine tissue. Reexamine the screw's position under direct visualization prior to removal.

37.3 Vaginal Tube

Many uterine manipulators are equipped with a colpotomy cuff. However, if this component is absent, a standalone vaginal tube may be utilized. In a laparoscopic hysterectomy, it plays a crucial role in facilitating the surgical procedure by aiding in visualization and manipulation of the uterus. It is typically used in conjunction with a uterine manipulator. The vaginal tube is inserted into the vaginal canal and provides several key functions during the surgery (Fig. 37.3).

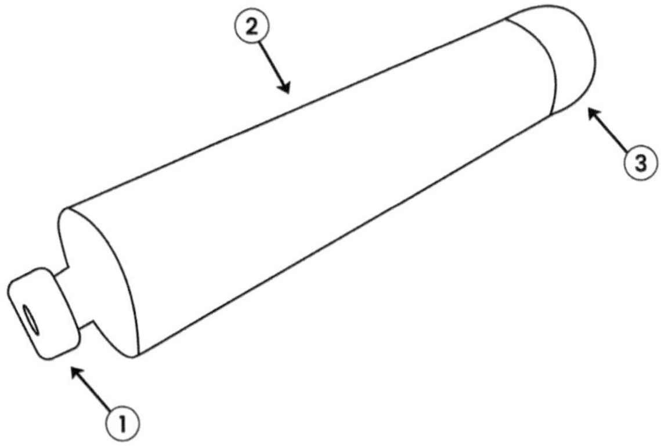

Fig. 37.3 Vaginal tube

37.3.1 Components

1. Seal: This allows passage of the instrument to hold the cervix without leakage of gas. This can of 5 mm or 10 mm size.
2. Shaft: This is a hollow tube that is inserted into the vaginal canal. This keeps the vaginal canal open. This can be of different sizes to ensure a proper fit in the vaginal canal.
3. Cervical Cup (Colpotomy Cup): A round cup that fits snugly around the cervix, used to help define the vaginal fornices during surgery. It serves as a visual guide for the surgeon to perform a safe colpotomy.

37.3.2 Key Functions of the Vaginal Tube

1. Visualization: It helps define the vaginal fornices, giving the surgeon a clear view of where to safely make incisions in the vaginal vault.
2. Manipulation: It allows the uterus to be moved in different directions, providing better access and exposure of the uterine ligaments and blood vessels during dissection.
3. Cervical Stabilization: The vaginal tube stabilizes the cervix and keeps it in place during the laparoscopic procedure, aiding in the precise removal of the uterus without damaging nearby structures.
4. Colpotomy Guide: It serves as a guide for the surgeon when performing the colpotomy.

37.4 Laparoscopic Fallopian Ring Applicator

This is a specialized surgical instrument used in laparoscopic procedures to apply silicone to the fallopian tubes, often during sterilization procedures or in cases where tubal occlusion is needed. Below are the key aspects and functionality of the device (Fig. 37.4):

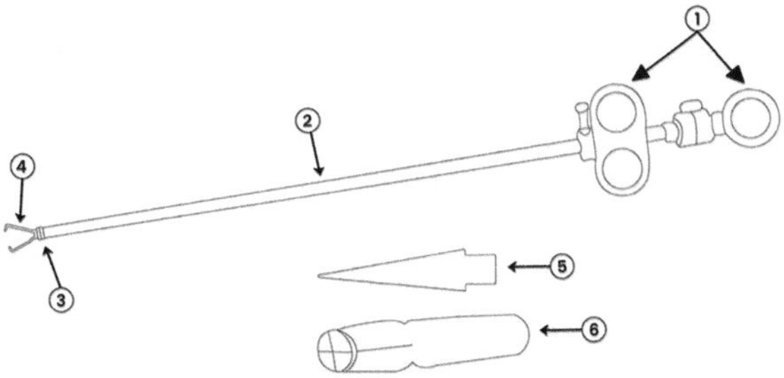

Fig. 37.4 Laparoscopic fallopian ring applicator

37.4.1 Components

1. Handle: The portion of the instrument that the surgeon holds, typically ergonomically designed to provide a secure grip. It may include a trigger mechanism to release the ring onto the fallopian tube.
2. Shaft: A long, narrow tube that extends from the handle to the tip. It usually has a tube inside a tube mechanism for ring deployment.
3. Ring Applicator Tip: The distal end of the instrument, which securely holds and deploys the silicone ring, is designed to fit the ring precisely and release it accurately over the looped portion of the fallopian tube.
4. Jaws: These are used to grasp the tubes.
5. Ring Loader: This component is detachable from the main device and is utilized for installing the stretchable rings onto the device by sequentially dilating them.
6. Ring Pusher: This is used to push the ring loaded onto the ring loader's tip toward the tip of the ring applicator.
7. Rings: Usually made of silicon or plastic, these rings constrict the loop of the fallopian tube, causing permanent blockage.

Ring Deployment: When the fallopian tube is in position, the handle is compressed, which releases the ring and deploys it around a loop of the fallopian tube to occlude it.

Usage: The primary advantages of employing the laparoscopic ring applicator for tubal ligation are its expedited execution and minimal damage to the tubes, as opposed to conventional methods such as cutting or cauterization. This facilitates the possibility of successful recanalization in the event of future need.

37.4.2 Maintenance

- Sterilization: The applicator must be properly sterilized between uses to prevent infection.
- Inspection: Check the applicator for any signs of wear and tear, especially the grasping jaws, which are very delicate, to ensure proper function during surgery.
- Ring Replacement: Ensure that the applicator is loaded with fresh sterilization rings for each procedure, and they are loaded just before the procedure.

37.4.3 Troubleshooting

Troubleshooting a fallopian tube applicator entails identifying and resolving prevalent issues that may occur during its utilization. Below are some typical problems, their potential causes, and recommended solutions:

1. Applicator Fails to Deploy the Ring

   The ring may not deploy due to incorrect loading, insufficient pressure applied to the trigger, or mechanical jamming. To resolve this issue, ensure proper ring loading, apply firm and consistent pressure to the trigger, and inspect for any mechanical jamming. Jamming may be overcome by cleaning and lubricating the instrument.

2. Inconsistent Ring Release

   Worn-out rings or incorrect technique could be the reasons. Replace any damaged rings and ensure proper handling.

3. Unexpected Resistance During Use

   Improper cleaning, lack of lubrication, and damage to the instrument could be the cause. Proper cleaning and lubrication can help overcome this resistance. In case of damage to the instrument, it may require professional repair or replacement.

In conclusion, laparoscopic gynecological surgery instruments have revolutionized the field of minimally invasive surgery. Their design and functionality not only enhance surgical precision but also contribute to improved patient outcomes, including reduced recovery times and minimized postoperative pain. As technology continues to advance, the development of innovative instruments will likely further refine surgical techniques, making procedures safer and more effective. Mastery of these instruments is crucial for gynecologists seeking to provide optimal care, and ongoing education and training will ensure that practitioners remain adept at utilizing these sophisticated tools to their fullest potential.

References

1. Hatzinger M, Badawi JK, Häcker A, Langbein S, Honeck P, Alken P. Georg Kelling (1866–1945): Der Erfinder der modernen Laparoskopie [Georg Kelling (1866–1945): the man who introduced modern laparoscopy into medicine]. Urologe A. 2006;45(7):868–71. German. https://doi.org/10.1007/s00120-006-1068-9.
2. Hatzinger M, Kwon ST, Langbein S, Kamp S, Häcker A, Alken P. Hans Christian Jacobaeus: inventor of human laparoscopy and thoracoscopy. J Endourol. 2006;20(11):848–50. https://doi.org/10.1089/end.2006.20.848.
3. Bhattacharya K. Kurt Semm: A laparoscopic crusader. J Minim Access Surg. 2007;3(1):35–6. https://doi.org/10.4103/0972-9941.30686. PMID: 20668618; PMCID: PMC2910380.

Hysteroscope

38

Mandeep Kaur

Hysteroscopy is the visual examination of the cervix and interior of the uterus with an endoscope. Commander Pantaleoni in 1869 performed the first hysteroscopy on a postmenopausal woman, where he visualized a polyp and did chemical cauterization [1]. The equipment has transformed extensively over the years. A complete understanding of how to assemble the hysteroscope or resectoscope and its irrigation system is essential for smooth and safe surgery. Fluid management systems that maintain adequate and consistent intrauterine pressures are essential for operative procedures.

Monitor, camera, light source, and fluid management system (irrigation system) are discussed in their respective chapters and will not be detailed here.

38.1 Hysteroscope

A hysteroscope is a specialized, thin, telescope-like instrument employed by gynecologists to visualize the interior of the uterus. Both diagnostic and operative procedures pertaining to the uterine cavity can be performed with this, offering direct visualization of the endometrial lining, uterine walls, and the tubal ostia. Typically, an operative hysteroscope has a channel for insertion of an instrument, and this makes it a little larger in diameter as compared to a diagnostic hysteroscope (Fig. 38.1).

M. Kaur (✉)
Department of Fertility Services, STAR Hospital, Jalandhar, Punjab, India

J. S. Ahluwalia (ed.), *User Manual for Minimally Invasive Surgical Equipment*,
https://doi.org/10.1007/978-981-95-9019-3_38

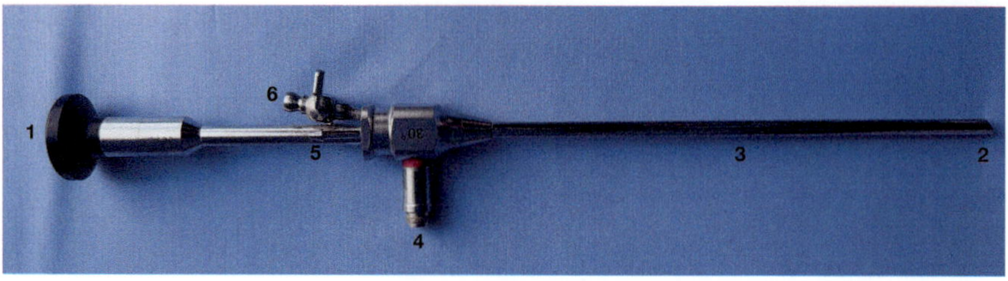

Fig. 38.1 Components of an operative hysteroscope

38.2 Components

1. *Camera Connector*: This end is connected to a camera head to transmit an image to the sensor on the camera head. A chip-on-tip type of hysteroscope will have the proximal end attached to the camera system permanently, as the sensor is on the tip of the scope.
2. *Tip*: This has the far end of the rod lens system, which transmits the image to the eyepiece at the camera end (near end). This also has a distal end of fiber optic system that carries light into the cavity.
3. *Shaft*: This is a long, thin tube that connects the proximal and distal end of hysteroscope. Its length may vary from 25 to 40 cm. The purpose of the shaft is to provide access without the need for incisions.
4. *Light Source Connector*: The fiber optic cable from the external light source is attached here to illuminate the uterine cavity.
5. *Irrigation and Suction Ports*: Channels for the inflow of fluids (such as saline) and the outflow of fluids for suction and visualization purposes.
6. *Instrument Ports*: In operative hysteroscopes, surgical instruments, such as scissors, forceps, or lasers, are introduced through the operative channels.

38.3 Types of Hysteroscopes

There are various types of hysteroscopes depending on their size, design, and intended use. Here's a detailed look at the various types of hysteroscopes:

1. Diagnostic Hysteroscopes

Diagnostic hysteroscopes are typically designed to be thinner, minimizing discomfort, and often avoiding the need for cervical dilation. They are commonly utilized for office-based procedures and straightforward diagnostic examinations. Their diameter can range from 2.7 mm to 4 mm, and the commonly available sizes are 2.7 mm, 3.0 mm, 3.5 mm, and 4.0 mm. These smaller sizes allow easier insertion through the cervix with minimal anesthesia.

2. Operative Hysteroscopes

Operative hysteroscopes are typically larger in size due to the necessity of accommodating surgical instruments employed during procedures such as the

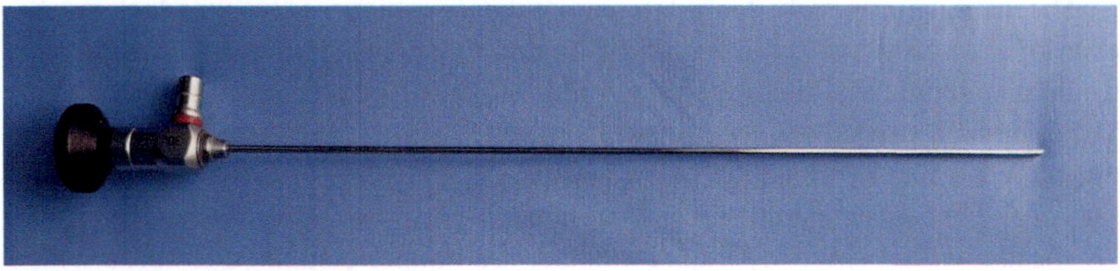

Fig. 38.2 2.9 mm hysteroscope

removal of fibroids, polyps, or adhesions. Their diameter can range from 5 mm to 10 mm. Commonly available sizes are 5.5 mm, 6.0 mm, 8.0 mm, and 10.0 mm. The larger diameter is necessary to allow for additional channels that can house surgical instruments like scissors, lasers, or forceps.

3. Mini Hysteroscopes

   Mini hysteroscopes are specifically designed to minimize discomfort and eliminate the necessity for cervical dilation. They are ideal for use in office-based diagnostic procedures or minor operative interventions, providing a less invasive alternative. Their diameter size can vary from 1.9 mm to 3 mm, and commonly available diameters are 1.9 mm, 2.0 mm, and 2.7 mm. These miniature hysteroscopes are experiencing a surge in popularity due to their capacity to offer a comfortable experience, especially for patients with a narrow cervical canal or those who require multiple procedures (Fig. 38.2).

4. Flexible Hysteroscopes

Flexible Hysteroscopes Generally thinner (ranging from 3 mm to 4 mm) and used for diagnostic purposes in more complex anatomical situations, such as when the uterus is angled. They may have a control system on their head so as to angulate the tip to aid in insertion and visualization.

5. All-in-One Hysteroscopes

   All-in-one will have all the components like scope, irrigation channels, and instrument channel built into a single unit. The advantage is that this arrangement makes is easier to use and saves time during procedure. This may also decrease the overall diameter of the assembly.

38.4 Sheath

The sheaths that cover the telescopes provide protection as well as allow the passage of fluid or gas for distention and instruments for operative procedures. There is usually an inner and outer fenestrated sheath, with space in between them for the passage of the distension media. The inner sheath allows clean fluid into the cavity, while the outer fenestrated sheath helps to evacuate the fluid out of the cavity, thereby making it a continuous flow system. This double channel provides minimal inflow resistance with a slightly higher outflow resistance. This resulting continuous flow increases visibility while maintaining intrauterine pressure and distention.

The instruments may be locked in place either by a rotary or twisting lock mechanism or with a snap-in connection type design. Operating sheaths additionally have single or multiple working (operating) channels incorporated into the inner sheath. The combined outer diameter of newer instruments may be as low as 3.6 mm, and they may not require dilatation of the cervix. The operating channels allow the passage of 3–7 Fr caliber instruments such as scissors, graspers, and electrocautery probes.

Sheaths with a single operating channel are thinner compared to those with a double operating channel, for which the cervix may need dilatation, according to the maximum diameter of the assembled hysteroscope.

38.5 Types of Sheaths

- Diagnostic sheaths: These are typically thinner and simpler in design, as they are primarily used to facilitate diagnostic procedures where no surgical instruments are required (Fig. 38.3). Their diameter typically ranges from 3 to 5 mm to allow easier access through the cervix. They do not have a channel for instrumentation, and may or may not have channels for irrigation.
- Operative Sheaths: Operative sheaths are larger and more complex because they are designed to accommodate surgical instruments, irrigation, and suction during procedures (Fig. 38.4). Their diameter typically ranges from 5 mm to 10 mm.
- Bipolar Sheaths: These sheaths are specially designed for use with bipolar electrosurgical systems, which are used for tissue resection. They have a handle to be used with bipolar energy and resection loops.

38.6 Ancillary Instruments and Working Elements

Several instruments, such as scissors, graspers, forceps, electroprobes, resectoscopes, and laser probes, are now available for operative hysteroscopy, facilitating a wide range of surgical procedures. They range from 3 to 7 Fr in diameter and can be passed through the operating channels in the sheath.

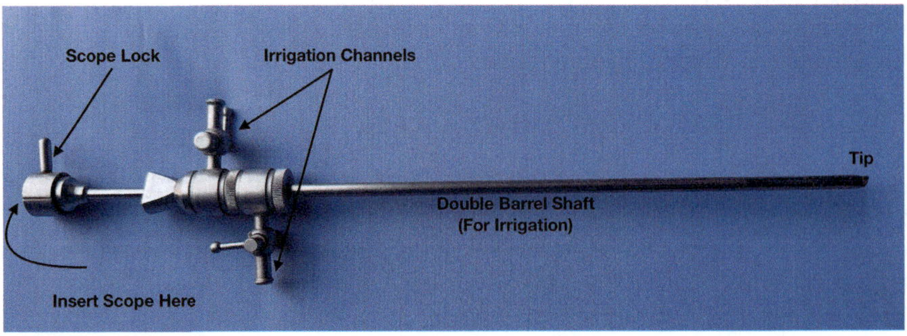

Fig. 38.3 Diagnostic sheath

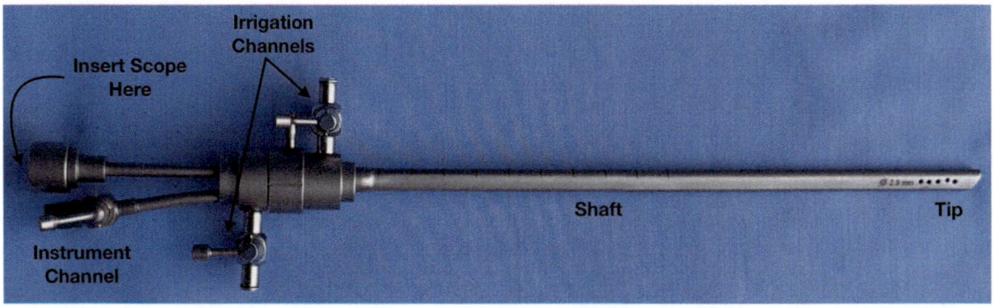

Fig. 38.4 Operative sheath

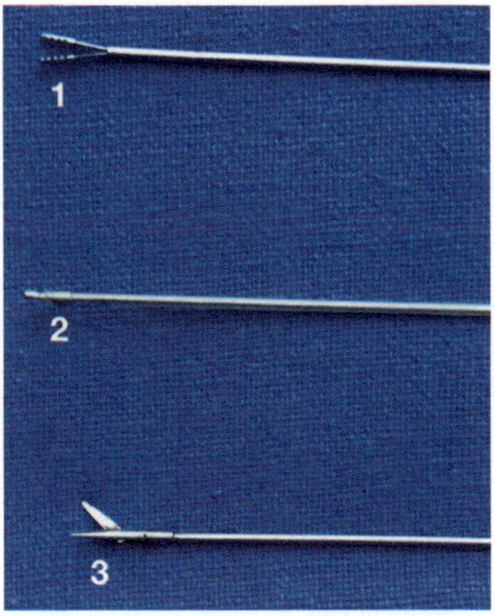

Fig. 38.5 Some ancillary hysteroscopic instruments: 1—Grasper. 2—Monopolar coagulation probe. 3 Mono-polar-scissors

Nonelectrolyte solutions used to distend the uterine cavity, for use of monopolar energy sources, require extreme caution and monitoring to prevent complications such as fluid overload and electrolyte disturbances. Bipolar energy sources allow the use of electrolyte solutions which are comparatively safer (Fig. 38.5).

38.7 Distension Media

A panoramic view of the uterine cavity and the cervical canal needs distension by a transparent medium. Liquid media can be either electrolytes or nonelectrolyte.

An ideal medium should be:

Isotonic—Making it non-hemolytic
Transparent—Allowing ample visualization
Rapidly cleared from the body
Nontoxic
Nonallergic

38.7.1 Electrolyte Solutions

Aqueous electrolyte solutions, such as physiological or 0.45% saline and Ringer's lactate, are usually used for diagnostic hysteroscopy. Operative procedures using mechanical tools, laser, or bipolar current allow the use of such solutions. The presence of electrolytes in the media makes the procedure safer and reduces the risk of hyponatremia in case it is excessively absorbed. It is important to bear in mind that excessive absorption of saline (>1.5–2 L) may still produce pulmonary edema, and caution needs to be exercised.

38.7.2 Nonelectrolyte Solutions

Nonelectrolyte solutions with low viscosity, such as 1.5% glycine solution, 3% sorbitol, and 5% mannitol, and fluids with high viscosity, such as high molecular weight dextran, are used for operative hysteroscopy when monopolar electric current is required, since they are electrolyte-free. The quantity of fluid instilled and recovered should be carefully monitored and calculated in order to estimate the amount of fluid absorbed by the body, so that complications such as hyponatremia and other electrolyte imbalances can be prevented. Usually, the acceptable fluid deficit should not be more than 1000–1500 mL in patients with normal cardiovascular function and not more than 750 mL in patients with compromised cardiovascular function. The deficit crosses the safe limits, the procedure should be terminated and appropriate safety measures be taken immediately.

38.8 Factors Influencing Absorption of Distension Fluid Include

- *Intrauterine Pressure*: This plays a crucial role in fluid absorption into the body. The higher the intrauterine pressure, the greater the degree of absorption. When this pressure surpasses the mean arterial pressure, systemic fluid absorption significantly increases [2]. Moreover, intrauterine pressure exceeding 75 mm Hg leads to an increased volume of fluid passing back along the fallopian tubes and into the peritoneal cavity [3].
- *Mean Arterial Pressure*: The lower the mean arterial pressure, the lower the intrauterine pressure needed to cause fluid to enter the systemic circulation. Therefore, caution is necessary in the elderly and individuals with cardiovascular comorbidities [4].
- *Depth of Myometrial Penetration*: When tissue damage extends into the deeper myometrium, instilled fluid can be rapidly absorbed through open myometrial venous sinuses. The risk of fluid absorption is even higher during myomectomies, where large blood vessels are breached, facilitating the absorption of fluid under pressure.

- *Duration of Surgery*: The longer the procedure, the more time for fluid to accumulate within the body [5].
- *Size of Uterine Cavity*: Larger cavities offer a greater endometrial surface area for fluid absorption. Procedures are also likely to last longer and require more instilled fluid. Achieving adequate intrauterine pressures for proper visualization becomes more challenging.

38.9 Fluid Management System

Uterine walls are thick and in apposition with each other, and therefore a positive pressure is required for their distension, unlike the urinary bladder, which has thin, easily distensible walls. The goal is to use the lowest possible intrauterine pressure, which is around 40–80 mm of Hg in order to achieve adequate visualization of the uterine cavity. As the intrauterine pressure exceeds the mean arterial pressure, the risk of medium absorption increases. Newer devices measure the fluid pressure and the flow rate and allow limiting the intrauterine pressure. Higher filling pressures are associated with higher pain scores in office hysteroscopy, while lower filling pressures may affect the visibility.

Details of such systems are mentioned in a separate chapter on irrigation systems.

38.10 Electrosurgery in Hysteroscopy

Two types of circuits are routinely employed for surgeries. In the monopolar circuit, current passes from the generator to an active electrode and returns from the surgical site through the patient. However, in a bipolar circuit, there is a return electrode adjacent to the active electrode, which facilitates current flow without any major flow of current through the patient. The relative nonconductive nature of the distension media increases impedance, which necessitates a high voltage for initiation. Hence, the electrosurgical units require a higher peak voltage, and the surgeon and assistant should be well versed with the electrosurgical unit settings needed for various operative hysteroscopic procedures.

38.11 Sterilization and Care

After use, the telescope, sheath, and the instruments need to be rinsed, washed, and dried thoroughly with care, especially while cleaning the internal channels. Ancillary instruments are extremely fragile and delicate and therefore require great attention during cleaning. Sterilization of the instruments can be done using overnight gas, ethylene oxide, or hydrogen gas plasma. All microorganisms and spores are destroyed by these methods. Telescopes need to be handled with care, and one should avoid dropping and bending instruments during sterilization.

38.12 Complications

Bleeding Largely, hysteroscopy is a minor procedure that does not lead to major bleeding. However, since the uterus is a well-perfused organ, during operative resection of endometrium and deeper layers, there is a likelihood of opening up of venous sinuses and active arterial bleeders. Typically, bleeding during operative hysteroscopy can be contained by waiting, stopping irrigation, and applying mechanical plugs (gel-foam, surgical, and fibrillar filaments) and pharmacologic antibleeding agents (e.g., tranexamic acid).

Infection Risk increases with prolonged procedures where the scope is introduced and removed multiple times, or there is evidence of cervicitis or vaginitis. It is safer to administrate intraoperative antibiotic and a course of postoperative antibiotics.

Uterine Perforation Hysteroscopy by itself is a procedure that requires appropriate, and focused conduct. Perforation of the uterine wall can happen due to mechanical perforation with the instrument/endoscope, increased irrigation fluid pressure, overzealous attempts for thick biopsy specimen retrieval, enthusiastic attempts to remove a large myoma, and sometimes, going through a wall defect, taking it to be fallopian tube opening.

Fluid Overload Fluid overload manifests in various symptoms, including shortness of breath, confusion, pulmonary edema, and, in severe cases, heart failure or seizures. To prevent fluid overload, meticulous monitoring of fluid intake and output during the procedure is paramount. The utilization of isotonic fluids is advisable when feasible. Early recognition of the early signs and prompt adjustment of fluid management strategies can effectively mitigate this complication.

38.13 Troubleshooting

- Poor distention of the uterine cavity—Make sure there is no leakage of distension media outside the uterus. Do not dilate the cervix more than required to avoid leak from the cervical os. Increase pressure setting, but not beyond the safe upper limit or mean arterial pressure.
- Poor image quality—Make sure lenses are clean. Avoid hysteroscopy during the menstrual phase. Increase the flow rate and open the exit channel to increase the exchange of dirty fluid with fresh fluid.
- No flow or low flow rate of distention media—Make sure there is no vacuum developing inside containers of distention media.
- Excessive air bubbles inside the uterine cavity—Remove air from tubing and sheath before entering the uterine cavity by flushing them with distention fluid.

In conclusion, hysteroscopy has emerged as a pivotal diagnostic and therapeutic modality in the field of gynecology. This minimally invasive approach enables the evaluation and treatment of intrauterine conditions with unparalleled precision. The direct visualization of the uterine cavity facilitates accurate diagnosis and targeted intervention for abnormalities such as polyps, fibroids, and adhesions. The advancements in hysteroscopic techniques have notably enhanced patient outcomes, characterized by accelerated recovery times and reduced incidence of complications compared to conventional methods. As the technology and expertize in hysteroscopy continue to evolve, its role in the management of uterine pathology is poised to expand, solidifying its status as an indispensable procedure in contemporary gynecology.

References

1. Baskett TF, Pantaleoni DC. Hysteroscopy. In: Eponyms and names in obstetrics and gynaecology, vol. 2019. Cambridge University Press; 1869. p. 310.
2. Garry R, Hasham F, Ms K, Mooney P. The effect of pressure on fluid absorption during endometrial ablation. J Gynecol Surg. 1992;8(1):1–10. https://doi.org/10.1089/gyn.1992.8.1.
3. Hasham F, Garry R, Kokri MS, Mooney P. Fluid absorption during laser ablation of the endometrium in the treatment of menorrhagia. Br J Anaesth. 1992;68:151–4. https://doi.org/10.1093/bja/68.2.151.
4. Bennett K, Ohrmundt C, Maloni J. Preventing intravasation in women undergoing hysteroscopic procedures. AORN J. 1996;64(5):792–9. https://doi.org/10.1016/S0001-2092(06)63267-5.
5. Paschopoulos M, Polyzos NP, Lavasidis LG, Vrekoussis T, Dalkalitsis N, Paraskevaidis E. Safety issues of hysteroscopic surgery. Ann N Y Acad Sci. 2006;1092:229–34. https://doi.org/10.1196/annals.1365.019.

Bariatric Surgery: Special Instruments 39

M. Kirubakaran, Jasmeet Singh Ahluwalia, and C. K. Huang

The development in bariatric surgery (BS) has been exceptional during the last few decades, resulting in a dramatic increase in the number of procedures performed worldwide. BS has been proven to induce and maintain durable weight loss as well as improve metabolic disorders compared to intensive medical treatments. The benefit is also seen in reducing cancer incidence as well as cardiovascular risks in patients with obesity, causing a 5-year increase in life expectancy [1]. Advances in minimal invasive techniques have contributed to reduced operative time, reduced length of hospital stays, reduced scarring, and decreased postoperative complications, increasing their popularity. As a result, laparoscopic surgery is the natural choice for most patients and surgeons, regardless of the type of procedure.

The progress in laparoscopic bariatric surgery (LBS) is indeed remarkable, as laparoscopy in morbidly obese patients is technically demanding, and the procedures themselves are more complex. Among the key factors for the vast increase in the number of bariatric procedures performed worldwide is due to the technical improvement of instruments and surgical technology. Key to the success of LBS is the utilization of specialized instruments designed to facilitate safe and effective surgical interventions. The instruments used by Bariatric surgeons will naturally depend on their experience, suitability and preference in using them.

M. Kirubakaran
Department of Metabolic and Bariatric Surgery, China Medical University and Hospital, Taichung, Taiwan

Department of Surgery, Gleneagles Hospital Penang, Georgetown, Malaysia

J. S. Ahluwalia
Department of Bariatric & Minimal Access Surgery, STAR Superspeciality Hospital, Jalandhar, Punjab, India

C. K. Huang (✉)
Department of Metabolic and Bariatric Surgery, China Medical University and Hospital, Taichung, Taiwan

J. S. Ahluwalia (ed.), *User Manual for Minimally Invasive Surgical Equipment*,
https://doi.org/10.1007/978-981-95-9019-3_39

In this chapter, we will discuss the various instruments commonly used in laparoscopic bariatric surgery, highlighting their purpose and unique features.

39.1 Operating Room Table

The operating table (OT) is the foundation of an operating room setup, and the modular structure of the surgical table must allow adaptation to the patient's body size and withstand high loads in various positions. It should also be maneuverable to provide maximum tilt and rotation to allow gravity to shift the abdominal structures, to allow full visualization. Most standard general-purpose operating tables have weight limits of about 225 kg (500 pounds), which are adequate for most of the bariatric procedures. However, super obese patients with weights greater than 225 kg will require a specific OT table that can accommodate them safely in the Trendelenburg/reverse Trendelenburg positions (Fig. 39.1). Bed accessories such as foot boards, side extensions, straps, cushions, and padding are necessary to safely secure the patient to the bed while positioning and preventing injuries (Fig. 39.2).

39.2 Laparoscopic Access Instruments and Pneumoperitoneum

The success of any surgical procedure will depend on a "good beginning". Gaining access into the peritoneal cavity of a morbidly obese patient can indeed be challenging due to excessive abdominal obesity. The options for establishing pneumoperitoneum in these patients include the standard technique of insufflation after insertion of the Veress needle, the open (Hasson technique), the direct trocar insertion, and optical trocar insertion [2].

The *open entry* (*Hasson technique*) is often touted as a safe approach in laparoscopy, but difficult in obese patients, as these patients have a very thick abdominal wall and a thick peritoneum (Fig. 39.3). Advantages of this technique include faster insufflation, the ability to gain access in a hostile abdomen and minimal risk of injury. The open approach is compromised by insufflation leakage, can be more time-consuming and extremely difficult in superobese patients. No evidence

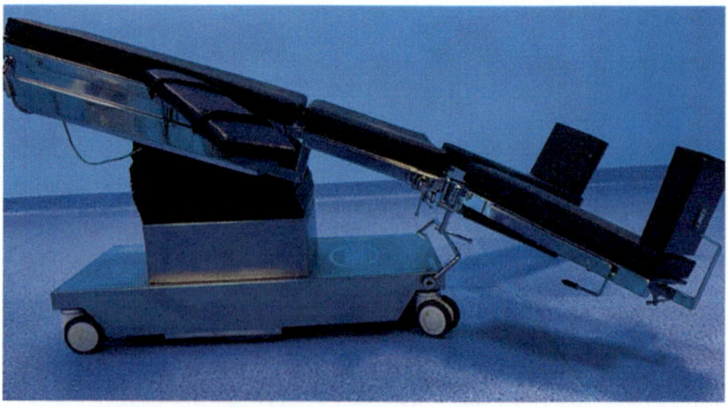

Fig. 39.1 Reverse Trendelenburg position

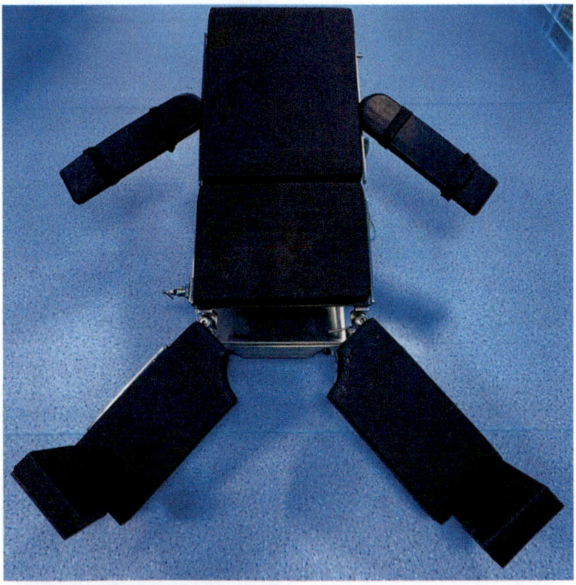

Fig. 39.2 Heavy-weight bearing table with leg split and foot support

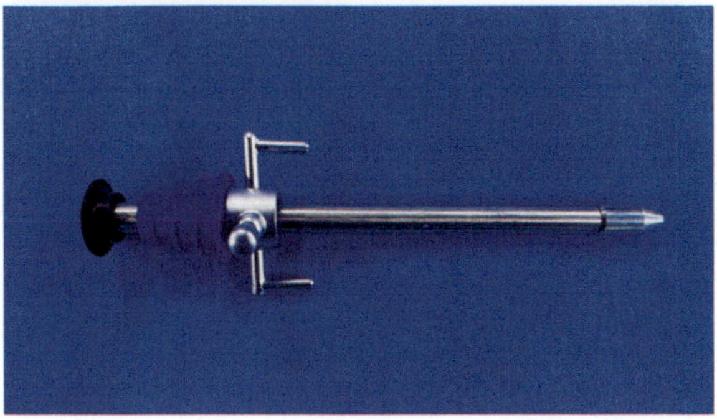

Fig. 39.3 Hassons trocar and cannula

supports that the open entry technique is superior or inferior to the other entry techniques.

The *Veress needle* (Fig. 39.4) and direct trocar insertion are blind techniques and have to be used with caution as they can cause vascular and visceral injuries. Both standard-length Veress needles (both reusable or disposable), ranging from 80 mm to 120 mm and long-length needles of about 150–160 mm, which are preferred in obese patients, are available. The Veress needle diameter is about 2–3 mm and consists of an outer cannula with a beveled needlepoint for cutting through tissues. Inside the cannula is an inner stylet, which is loaded with a spring that "springs forward" in response to the sudden decrease in pressure encountered upon entering the peritoneal cavity. The blunt cannula has a side hole, which enables CO_2 gas to enter the abdominal cavity. The Veress needle should be held like a dart at the time of insertion, and the angle of insertion should vary according to the body mass index (BMI) of the patient, which is about a 45°angle in a nonobese patient to a 90° angle

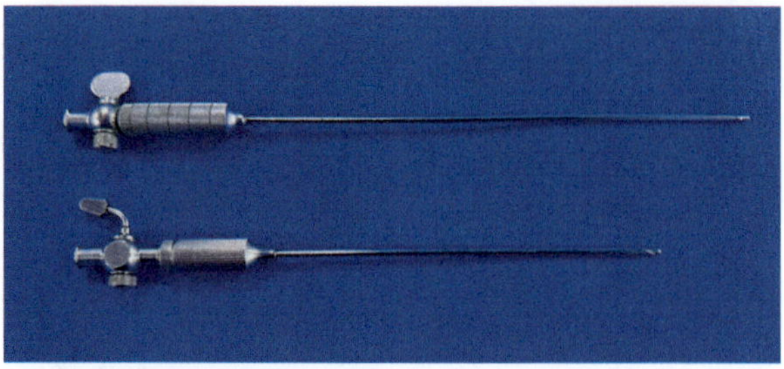

Fig. 39.4 Standard and long-length Veress needles

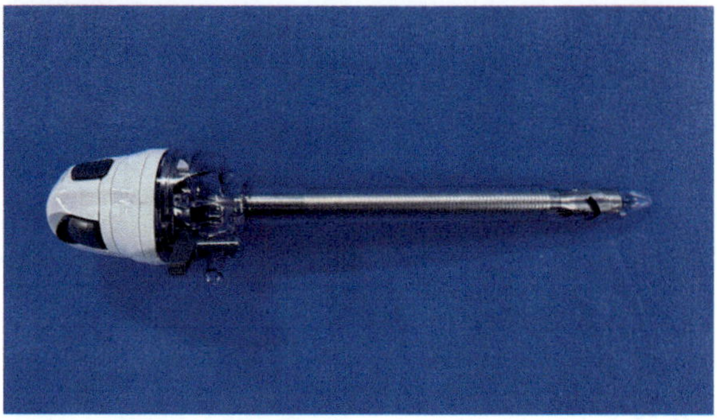

Fig. 39.5 Optical trocars

in an obese patient [3]. Correct positioning can be verified by injecting saline solution, which flows freely without resistance, escape of air from the peritoneal cavity and the water drop test.

Direct trocar insertion is a blind technique that accesses the abdominal cavity without creating pneumoperitoneum. This technique decreases the operating time and is associated with fewer insufflation-related complications such as gas embolism, especially in morbidly obese patients. Direct trocar insertion is not recommended for fellowship surgeons and is not always an easy, safe, and effective technique [4].

An alternative to these blind techniques for access into the abdomen is with an *optical trocar* (Fig. 39.5) under direct view while transecting the abdominal wall layers and with a gentle rotating motion. 0° laparoscope is preferred during optical trocar entry. The optical trocar enters through the layers of the abdominal wall, i.e., subcutaneous fat, anterior rectus sheath, rectus abdominis muscle, posterior rectus sheath, preperitoneal fat, and peritoneum [2].

Sundbom et al. reported on 5470 obese patients in whom pneumo-peritoneum was created using optical trocars. There were six patients (0.11%) who had major vascular injuries (five aortic and one inferior mesenteric artery), implying that central adiposity and the increased distance from the skin to the abdominal cavity is not protective against retroperitoneal injuries [5]. Using the Scandinavian Obesity Surgery Registry to compare Veress needle, optical trocar, and Open Hasson techniques for pneumoperitoneum in 17,446 patients, Sundbaum et al. reported no difference in injury between the Veress needle and optical trocar groups (injury rate for both techniques of 0.08%) with no injuries in the Open Hasson group [6].

Bariatric surgeons should be familiar with all the laparoscopic entry techniques because one approach may not always be feasible, especially in cases of revision surgery. Obese patients must be informed of the risks and complications encountered while gaining access to the abdomen, during laparoscopic bariatric surgery.

39.3 Trocars

Trocars are essential in laparoscopic surgery as they serve as a conduit for instruments to be used in the abdominal cavity. Morbidly obese patients can pose special challenges for abdominal access, secondary to the thickness of the abdominal wall, body habitus, and lack of reliable landmarks.

In addition to being safe and reliable, trocars and cannulas for laparoscopic bariatric surgery should fit snugly to the abdominal wall, allow exchange of instruments of various diameters and be of sufficient length to reach the peritoneal cavity without causing air leaks. Options of standard trocars with 100 mm shafts, ranging from 5 mm to 15 mm are available for most bariatric procedures. Depending on the type of surgery and port positions, there are considerable variations between surgeons and institutions. After establishing initial access into the peritoneal cavity, the other trocars are inserted under direct visualization. Occasionally, extra-long trocars (150 mm shafts) are required in super obese patients or patients with excessively thick abdominal walls (Figs. 39.6 and 39.7).

39.4 Laparoscopes

Obtaining good imaging in morbidly obese patients can be challenging due to the voluminous abdominal cavity, which is expanded with pneumoperitoneum. This requires more illumination compared to nonobese patients. The enlarged viscera due to fatty infiltration and increased tissue adiposity often obscures and reduces the visual field. Inadvertent contact of the laparoscopic lens with the adipose tissue causes soiling of the lens, resulting in poor image quality needing frequent cleaning. In addition, bariatric patients have more lens fogging due to small air leaks at the

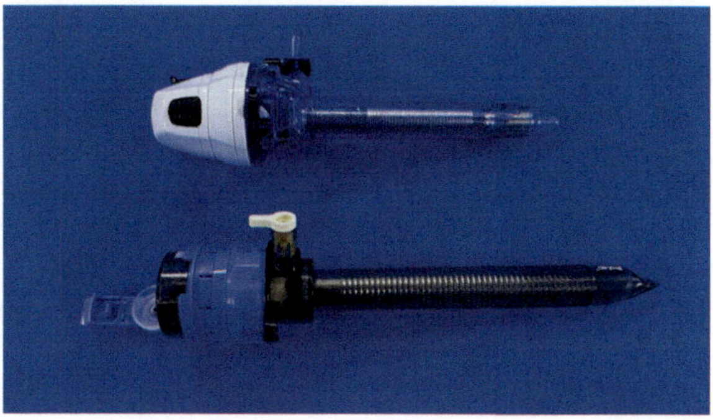

Fig. 39.6 Disposable longer length trocars as compared to standard length

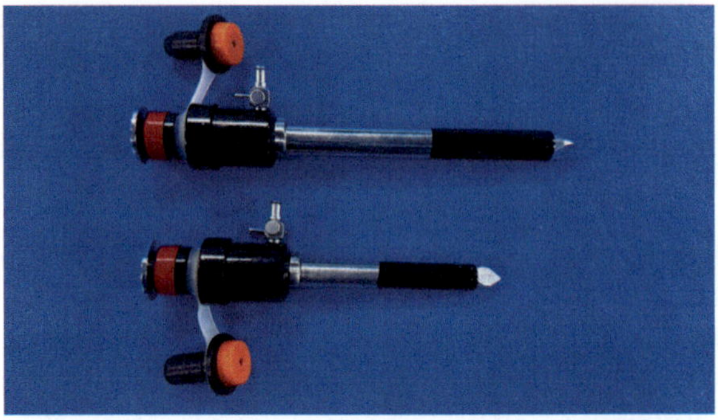

Fig. 39.7 Reusable extra-long trocars with reducers

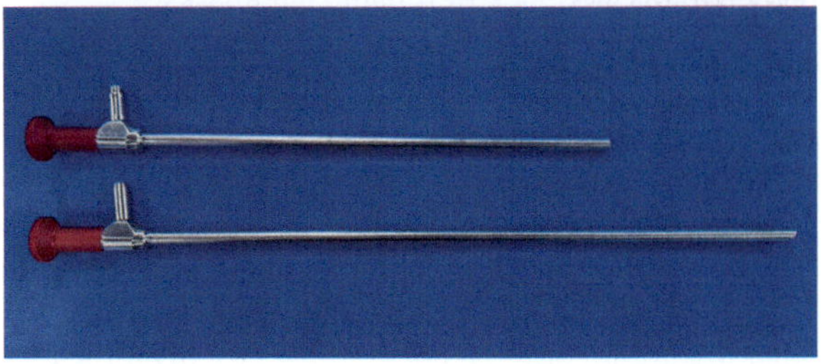

Fig. 39.8 Extra-long telescope as compared to routine telescope

trocar sites as a result of rapid insufflation of relatively cool CO_2 gas. Equipment that minimizes such contacts, prevents, or rapidly corrects lens fogging and quick cleaning of the lens is a necessity.

The laparoscope provides the means of acquiring an image of the abdominal cavity. Laparoscopes are connected to digital imaging systems, allowing visualization on screens and photo or video documentation. "Hopkins" endoscopes consist of a series of quartz rod lenses and fiber bundles surrounding the rod lens for transmission of light. Endoscopes with camera sensors placed on the tip of the endoscope are usually called "chip on the tip" or "video" endoscopes [7]. Recent advances in 3D and 4 K imaging have allowed better visualization of the operative field in minimally invasive surgery. 3D vision overcomes the disadvantage of a traditional 2D laparoscopic system by providing better depth perception, more accuracy with a better surgical field for surgeons, improving hand–eye coordination and reducing errors [8].

Laparoscopes come in various sizes, with a standard length of 32 cm and diameters that range from 3 to 10 mm. The 10 mm diameter is the most commonly used scope and provides the greatest light and visual acuity. However, 5 mm laparoscopes capable of providing images comparable to 10 mm systems are now available in the market. Scopes are angled to various degrees, most commonly from a 0-, 30-, or 45-degree orientation. The angled scopes provide better visibility of the internal structures and areas conventionally blind to a 0° scope, but require more skill in operating them. In bariatric surgery, extra-long laparoscopes (45 cm) are sometimes necessary in superobese patients (Fig. 39.8). As these patients have a large abdominal circumference, excessive abdominal wall thickness together with an expanded abdominal cavity these scopes provide better optimal view and allows for a close-up view of distant sites (e.g., the esophagogastric junction).

39.5 Retracting Instruments

Retraction is another key component in obtaining an excellent field of vision in laparoscopic bariatric surgery. Appropriate retraction of the organs and other structures surrounding the operative area enables easier and precise dissection. In morbidly obese patients, the hypertrophic left lobe of the liver invariably hinders the surgeon's view of the esophagogastric junction and left crus. Appropriate exposure of this region without injuring the liver are key step in bariatric surgery. Several instruments have been developed to facilitate retraction and potentially eliminate the need for an assistant in these surgeries.

39.5.1 Laparoscopic Grasper for Liver Retraction

This classic method for liver retraction utilizes a 5-mm diameter toothed, ratcheted laparoscopic grasper. A 5-mm trocar is introduced in the subxiphoid region. The grasper is introduced through this trocar, passing between the visceral face of the left liver lobe and the stomach and fixing its tooth on the right diaphragmatic crus (Fig. 39.9). Thus, the liver is suspended between the grasper and the abdominal wall, causing a folding of the left liver lobe and exposing the angle of His [9].

39.5.2 Nathanson Liver Retractor

Nathanson liver retractor has been used for decades in laparoscopic surgery and is known to produce a degree of hepatic congestion from vascular compression, resulting in a temporary postoperative rise in liver enzymes. It has also been reported that

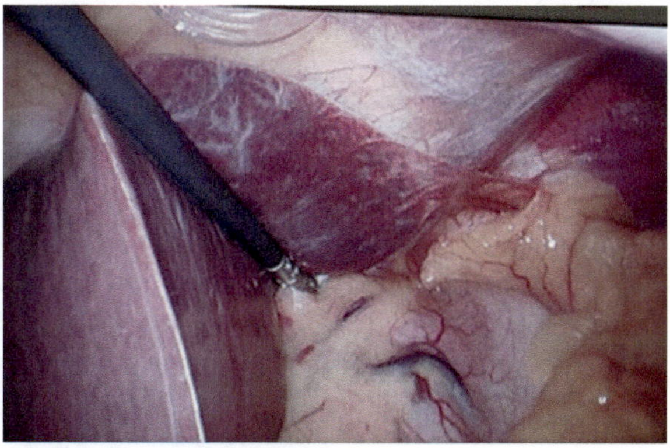

Fig. 39.9 Laparoscopic grasper for liver retraction

NR can cause increased postoperative C-reactive protein (CRP) and increased postoperative pain [10]. It is introduced directly through a subxiphoid incision and does not utilize an extra trocar. The NR is held in position by means of an external holding device, which is attached to the operating table (Fig. 39.10).

39.5.3 Laparoscopic Articulating Liver Retractors

These devices are introduced through a 5- or 10-mm trocar and are strong enough to retract large, heavy livers atraumatically. The tip of the instrument is articulated under direct vision by turning the actuating knob on the handle until the complete shape is formed. Many such retractors in different shapes are available [10] (Fig. 39.11).

39.5.4 Liver Suspension Techniques

Conventional liver retractors are expensive, require additional ports, resulting in pain, and scar formation, in addition to the risk of iatrogenic liver injury during retractor insertion. Furthermore, conventional liver retractors cannot be utilized for single-port surgeries.

To overcome these limitations, Huang et al. developed two simple, rapid, and safe techniques for liver retraction.

(i) V-shaped Liver Suspension Technique (V-LIST)—By using a Penrose drain and laparoscopic stapler. A silicone Penrose drain was inserted into the peritoneal cavity and stapled to the pars condensa of the lesser omentum and parietal peritoneum using a laparoscopic stapler. The left lobe of the liver was retracted by the V-shaped suspension. In their series there were no complications and they reported its potential application in single incision laparoscopic bariatric procedures [11] (Fig. 39.12).
(ii) Another novel liver suspension technique is using an indigenous "T-suspension tape" (TST) made from the fenestrated Teflon tail of a Jackson–Pratt drain and a 2/0 monofilament polypropylene suture (Prolene: straight taper point, ST-70,

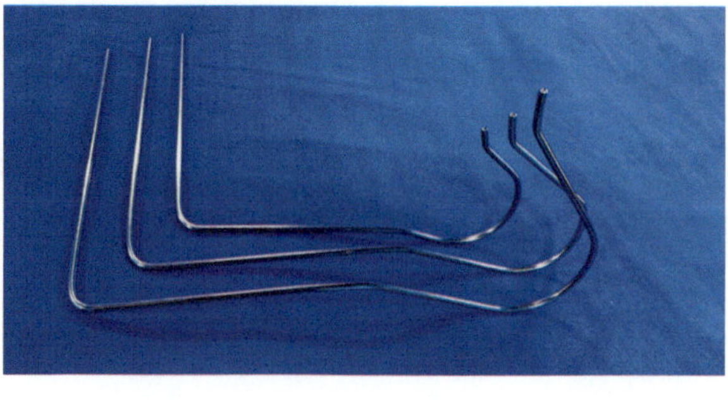

Fig. 39.10 Nathanson liver retraction system with different sizes

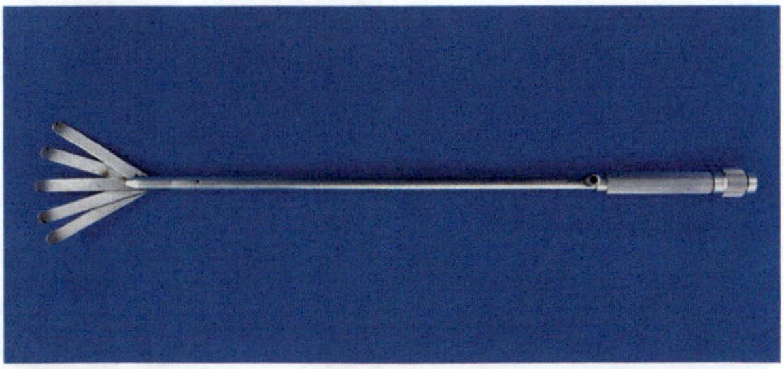

Fig. 39.11 Fan liver retractor

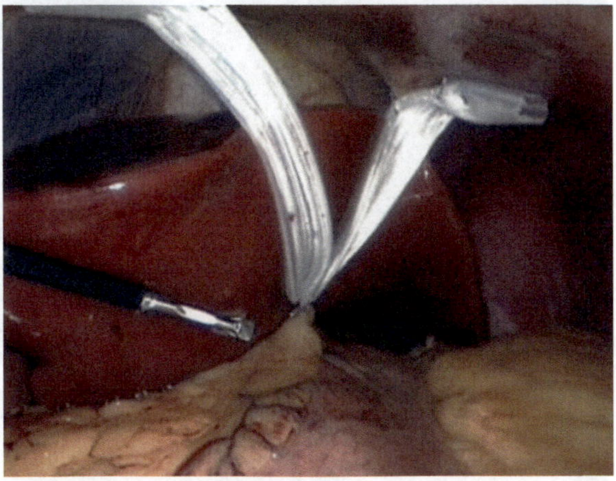

Fig. 39.12 Completed V-shaped suspension of the liver

W8400; Ethicon, Blue Ash, OH) with a long straight needle for liver and gallbladder retraction. The TST was constructed in two steps:

A. A 2–5-cm length of the Teflon tail of the Jackson–Pratt drain was cut off. Smaller lengths are used for gallbladder retraction.
B. The Prolene suture was passed to the midportion of the Teflon tube and secured with multiple passes (three or four) at the center, forming a T-shape with the needle still attached at the end of the suture (Fig. 39.13).

The TST method is a safe, simple, efficient, cost-effective, and feasible technique for retracting the liver, gallbladder, and falciform ligament in laparoscopic bariatric procedures. This novel liver retraction technique is also useful for surgeons embarking on reduced ports as well as single incision bariatric surgery (SILS) [12].

39.6 Hand Instruments for Bariatric Surgery

Key to the success of these surgeries are the hand instruments used by surgeons to perform the necessary tasks. Commonly employed hand instruments in laparoscopic bariatric surgery are dissectors, graspers, scissors, staplers, and energy

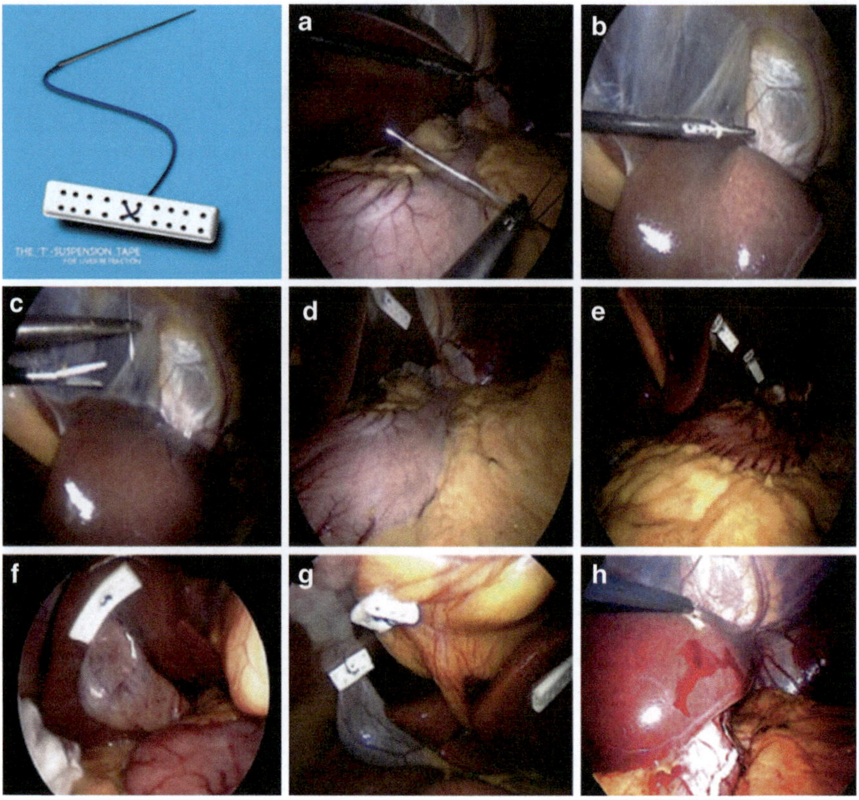

Fig. 39.13 (**a**–**h**) Images showing the design of the "T-suspension tape" by *Huang* et al. for retraction of liver and gallbladder

devices. The proper selection and utilization of these instruments, which are available in reusable and disposable forms, are essential for achieving optimal surgical outcomes.

Most instruments for laparoscopic surgery are available at standard lengths of 32 cm. However, extra-long instruments of about 43 cm—45 cm may be required in laparoscopic bariatric surgery. Several patient factors can determine if extra-long instruments will be required, which include the following:

(a) Body Mass Index (BMI)—Superobese and super–super obese patients will require longinstruments to reach and manipulate structures within the abdominal cavity.
(b) Abdominal Wall Adiposity—Patients with a thicker abdominal wall due to excess subcutaneous fat may need longer instruments to access the surgical area.

(c) Intra-Abdominal Fat Distribution and Large Viscera—Similarly, patients with increased intra-abdominal fat and larger liver or stomach will need longer instruments to perform the surgery.
(d) Abdominal Scarring and Adhesions—Presence of scars and intra-abdominal adhesions may necessitate a variation in the port placements; hence longer instruments may be needed to navigate to the surgical site.
(e) Patient Positioning—Patients may need to change positions from a steep reverse Trendelenburg position to a steep Trendelenburg position in certain conditions. This positioning redistributes the patient's abdominal contents, making it necessary to use longer instruments to maintain maneuverability.

The decision to use extra-long instruments is made by the surgeon based on these individual patient factors, surgical expertize, and preferences. The specific requirements for instrument length may vary based on the surgical technique employed and the patient's unique characteristics.

39.6.1 Grasping Instruments

Graspers are handheld instruments with two opposing jaws used to manipulate tissues during laparoscopic bariatric surgery. These versatile instruments facilitate tissue retraction, dissection, and manipulation. They come in various designs, including straight or curved jaws, in various lengths, fenestrated or non-fenestrated tips, and toothed or atraumatic grasping surfaces. Some graspers feature additional functionalities, such as monopolar or bipolar cautery capabilities, to enable hemostasis during tissue dissection. Graspers enable surgeons to hold and manipulate tissues, perform delicate dissections, and create the necessary working space for the procedure (Figs. 39.14 and 39.15).

39.6.2 Cutting Instruments

Laparoscopic scissors used in bariatric surgery, both standard length and extra-long, are specialized instruments designed to cut, perform sharp dissection, and coagulate

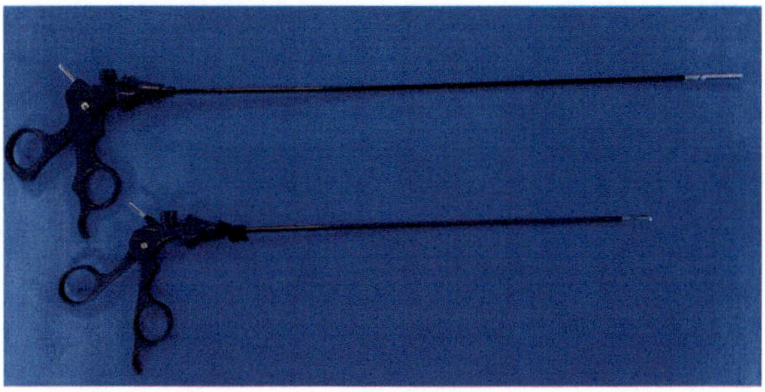

Fig. 39.14 Laparoscopic long vs standard length bowel grasper

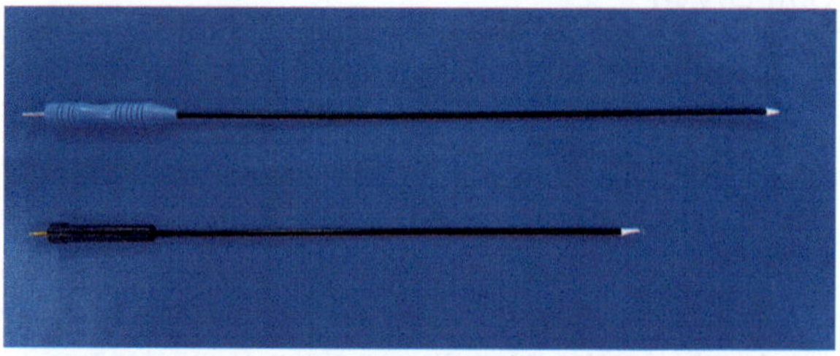

Fig. 39.15 Laparoscopic long vs standard length hook

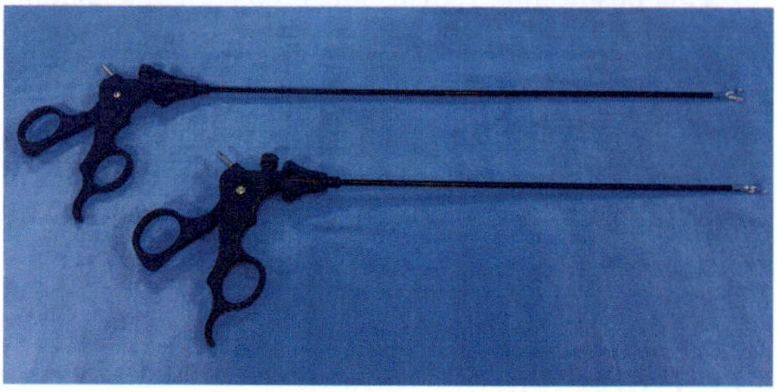

Fig. 39.16 Routine versus longer length laparoscopic scissors

tissues. Scissors used in laparoscopic bariatric surgery are available in different blade configurations, including straight, curved, hook-tip blades, and can be either monopolar or bipolar. Monopolar scissors utilize electrical energy to cut and coagulate tissues, while bipolar scissors pass electrical current only between their tips, allowing for precise coagulation without the need for a return electrode. The choice of scissors depends on the specific surgical task and tissue type being manipulated. Laparoscopic scissors are invaluable for precise tissue dissection and hemostasis during bariatric surgery.

(i) Straight Scissors—Mainly for cutting and dissection.
(ii) Curved Scissors—Preferred by most users, the curvature of the blade allows a better view of the tip.
(iii) Serrated Scissors—Ridges on the blade minimizes tissue or suture slippage.
(iv) Hook Scissors—Encircles the structure before cutting, assuring a firm, and solid grip (Fig. 39.16).

39.6.3 Laparoscopic Suturing Instruments

Suturing is an essential skill in laparoscopic bariatric surgery. It allows for secure tissue approximation, hemostasis of stapler lines or bleeding vessels and creation of anastomosis. Laparoscopic instruments precisely used for suturing include laparoscopic needle holders, suturing devices (endoscopic needle drivers), and extracorporeal suturing (using knot pushers).

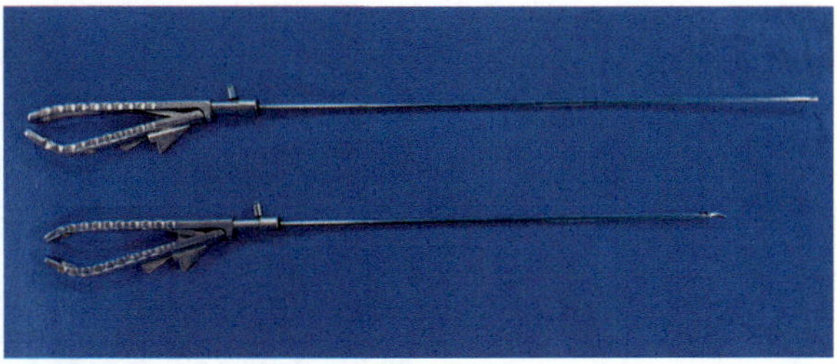

Fig. 39.17 Laparoscopic longer needle holder vs routine length needle holder

(a) Laparoscopic Needle Holders

(i) Curved Needle Holders

Curved needle holders are the most commonly used instruments for suturing in laparoscopic bariatric surgery. Their curved jaws provide the necessary angle to pass the needle through tissue and facilitate precise manipulation.

Examples include the Roeder and Park needle holders.

(ii) Straight needle holders are occasionally used when accessing difficult-to-reach areas or for specific suturing techniques. They offer straight jaw alignment and may provide better maneuverability in certain situations. These instruments are available with different grips depending on surgeon's preference (Fig. 39.17).

(b) Suturing Devices (Endoscopic Needle Drivers)

Endoscopic needle drivers are designed specifically for laparoscopic suturing. They feature long, slender shafts that allow access to deep surgical sited and provide precise control during needle manipulation. "Endo Stitch"™ Suturing Device (Medtronic, USA; Fig. 39.18) is a laparoscopic suturing device with a curved needle that is sharp at both ends. The needle is passed back and forth between the two jaws by activating the forward or backward toggle lever for a grasping device to reload the needle before the next stitch. The ergonomic design allows single handed operation. Suturing in tight spaces, approximating under tension, and obtaining larger tissue bites are not easily performed with these 10-mm devices hence freehand suturing is recommended in these circumstances.

(c) Knot Pushers

They aid in knot tying and securing the suture. They are usually long rods with specially designed tips used to perform extracorporeal knot tying (Fig. 39.19). The knots are thrown outside, utilizing this instrument to push the knot through the cannula and secure it inside.

Laparoscopic suturing instruments play a vital role in laparoscopic bariatric surgery, allowing for precise tissue approximation and anastomoses. The selection of appropriate instruments depends on factors such as surgeon skill and preference, surgical technique, and patient characteristics.

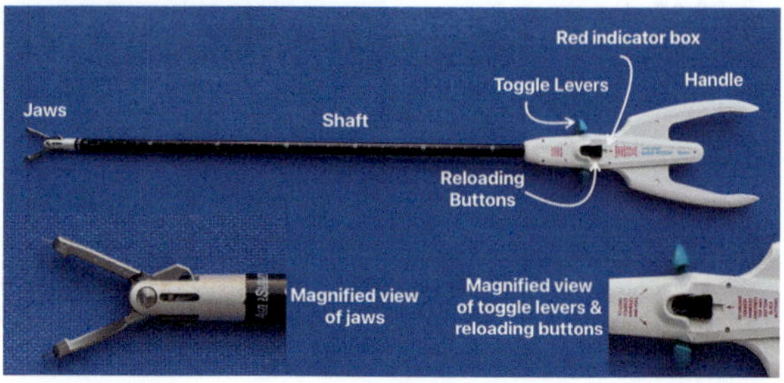

Fig. 39.18 "Endo Stitch"™ suturing device

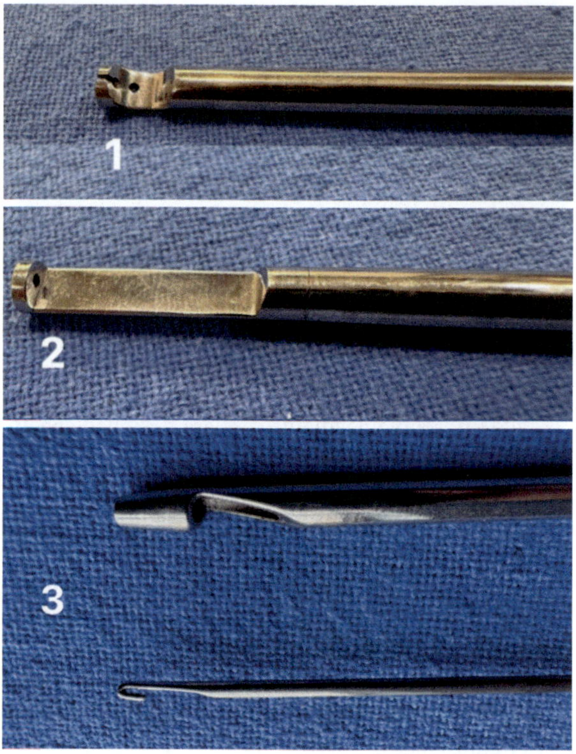

Fig. 39.19 Laparoscopic knot pusher of different styles: 1—Grooved, 2—Closed-loop, and 3—Hooked

39.7 Goldfinger Dissector

The development of innovative surgical instruments has played a significant role in advancing minimally invasive techniques, especially in the field of bariatric surgery. One such instrument is the Goldfinger dissector (GD), which is a handheld instrument designed to assist surgeons in dissection, retraction, and manipulation of tissues during laparoscopic surgery [13].

It consists of a long, slender shaft with a curved or flexible distal tip, and a handle for precise control. The shaft of the GD may or may not be insulated (Fig. 39.20).

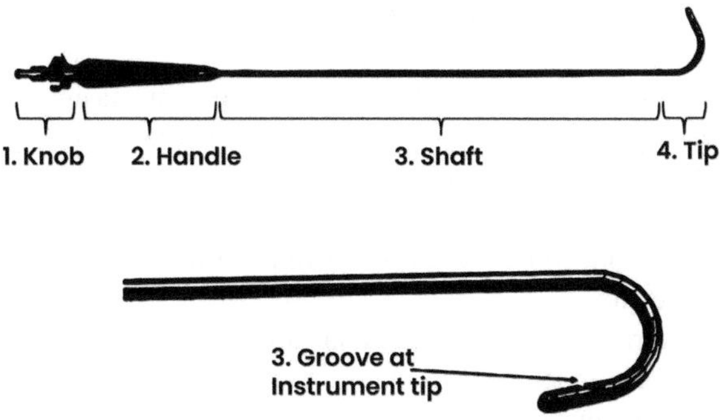

Fig. 39.20 Goldfinger dissector

The GD with its curved or flexible distal tip offers several applications in laparoscopic bariatric surgery, including the following:

(i) Tissue Dissection: The curved or flexible tip aids in the precise dissection of tissues, viscera, adhesions, fat, and vessels, enabling the surgeon to access the operative site and dissect anatomical planes effectively.
(ii) Tissue Retraction: The ratcheting mechanism allows for controlled and secure tissue retraction, reducing the need for additional instruments or assistance, improving visualization and facilitating access to the surgical field.
(iii) Organ Manipulation: The GD can be used to manipulate organs gently, such as the liver or stomach, to expose the surgical site and facilitate the procedure.
(iv) Vessel Dissection and Hemostasis: The dissector's tip can be used to dissect and ligate small blood vessels encountered during the procedure, promoting hemostasis and minimizing bleeding.

The benefits of the GD in laparoscopic bariatric surgery:

(i) Enhanced Precision: The instruments design and maneuverability enable surgeons to perform delicate dissection and manipulation with enhanced precision, reducing the risk of inadvertent tissue injury.
(ii) Improved Visibility: The instrument's ability to retract tissues and organs improves visualization, allowing surgeons to identify important anatomical structures more easily and perform surgery with greater accuracy.
(iii) Reduced Instrument Clutter: The versatile nature of the GD minimizes the need for multiple instruments, reducing instrument exchanges, and optimizing surgical workflow.
(iv) Cost-Effectiveness: The multifunctionality of the GD can potentially reduce the overall instrument cost in laparoscopic bariatric surgery by eliminating the need for additional specialized instruments.

39.8 Energy Devices

Energy devices are utilized to achieve hemostasis, dissect tissues, and seal vessels during laparoscopic bariatric surgery. These devices include monopolar and bipolar electrocautery, ultrasonic dissectors, and advanced energy platforms such as advanced bipolar vessel sealing devices. The appropriate use of energy devices minimizes bleeding, reduces operative time, and enhances the precision of tissue dissection.

Various types of monopolar hooks and spatulas are available, and most scissors have an attachment to connect with the monopolar lead. As usual, standard-sized instruments can be used in most cases, but in superobese patients, extra-long 43 cm–45 cm devices are available. Bipolar devices contain a continuous waveform electrical current between the jaws of the forceps and hence reduce the chances of damage to adjacent tissue. They achieve tissue sealing and hemostasis by thermal coagulation, though they lack the ability to cut.

The surgical evolution of the energy devices used, particularly with ultrasonic energy and advanced bipolar systems, has been the central point in an exponential growth of laparoscopic procedures, including laparoscopic bariatric surgery. Ultrasonic energy device systems convert electrical energy into mechanical energy using frequencies between 23 and 55 kHz. The tissue effects of these devices include mechanical cutting, desiccation, protein coagulation, cavitation, or a combination of these. The tip of the device cuts mechanically with a degree of collateral thermal coagulation used for hemostasis [14].

Advantages of ultrasonic instruments compared to conventional electrosurgery have included improved hemostasis, less thermal damage, combined vessel sealing and tissue dissection capability, and reduced surgical smoke production. Most ultrasonic shears are available at standard lengths of about 37 cm for routine patients and for superobese patients 45 cm length (Fig. 39.21).

LigaSure™ Maryland Jaw (Medtronic, USA) and ENSEAL X1 Curved Jaw Tissue Sealer (EX1; Ethicon, Inc.; Cincinnati, Ohio, USA) are some of the examples of advanced bipolar energy devices that are currently available (Fig. 39.22). Most advanced bipolar devices are capable of sealing vessels up to 7 mm in diameter and have an integrated cutting blade within their jaws to cut the sealed tissue

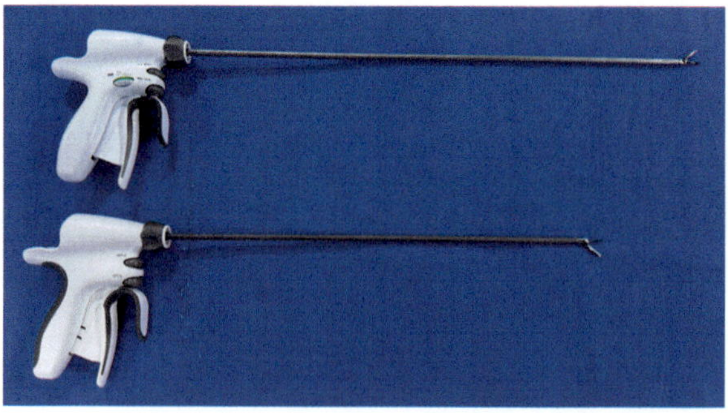

Fig. 39.21 Longer length ultrasonic shears vs routine length

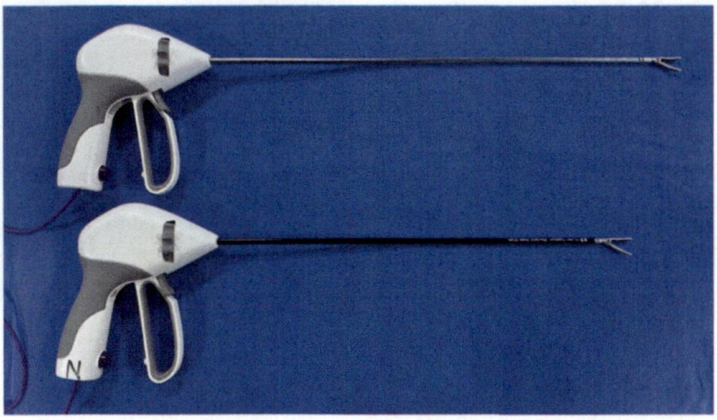

Fig. 39.22 Longer length advanced bipolar device as compared to routine length

once the sealing is complete. Most of such devices are available at the standard 37 mm length and extra-long 44 cm length.

Both ultrasonic energy and advanced bipolar systems are useful in bariatric surgery, and these two advanced power devices are user-friendly and can reduce the surgeon's workload. The choice of the energy device should be based on the familiarity, cost, and preference of the surgeon [14].

39.9 Stapling Devices in Bariatric Surgery

Laparoscopic bariatric surgery has witnessed remarkable advancements in recent years, thanks to innovative surgical instruments that enhance precision, safety, and patient outcomes. One crucial aspect of these procedures is the use of staplers and reloads, which play a pivotal role in dividing tissues and creating secure anastomoses [15]. Linear staplers are used to transect viscera, to divide mesentery and vascular structures, and to create anastomosis. Circular staplers, on the other hand, are primarily used in gastrojejunal anastomosis during laparoscopic roux-en-y-gastric bypass.

Innovation in surgical stapling technology has evolved from manual to power-operated staplers. In contrast with manual staplers, powered staplers use battery power to drive the knife blade and staples, thus eliminating the variable grip force of the surgeon. The choice of a stapler depends on the specific procedure and the surgeon's preference [16].

These stapling devices usually mimic their routine laparoscopic surgery counterparts except for the longer length (Fig. 39.23).

As technology continues to progress, it is likely that further refinements and improvements in the stapling devices will emerge with lower leak rates, better hemostasis, more efficient and safer mechanisms, pushing the boundaries of laparoscopic bariatric surgery even further.

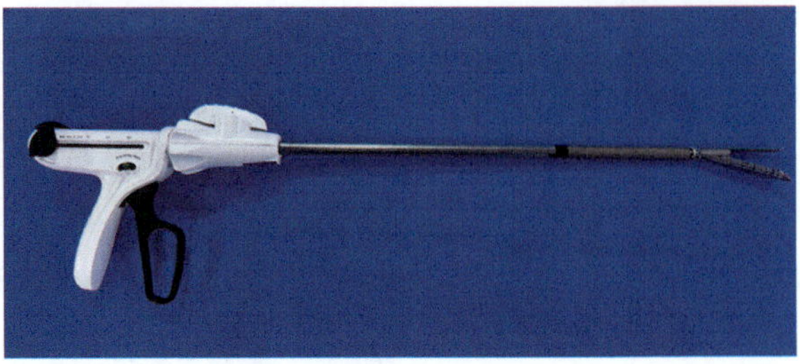

Fig. 39.23 Long length stapling device

39.10 Conclusion

Laparoscopic bariatric surgery involves unique technical challenges for the advanced laparoscopic surgeon. An in-depth knowledge and proper use of a wide array of laparoscopic equipment and instruments greatly help the surgeon and their team perform more advanced and complex laparoscopic bariatric procedures. However, not all of the technology presented in this chapter is necessary to safely complete these operations. As new bariatric procedures are developed and technology improves, bariatric surgeons will have to evolve with the change and keep abreast with the introduction of newer instruments that will hopefully simplify the procedures, adding enhanced efficiency and safety.

References

1. Genser L, Thabut D, Aron-Wisnewsky J. Precision bariatric/metabolic medicine and surgery. J Clin Med. 2023;12(5):1909.
2. Kassir R, Blanc P, Lointier P, Tiffet O, Berger JL, Amor IB, Gugenheim J. Laparoscopic entry techniques in obese patient: veress needle, direct trocar insertion or open entry technique? Obes Surg. 2014;24(12):2193–4.
3. Vilos GA, Ternamian A, Dempster J, et al. Laparoscopic entry: a review of techniques, technologies, and complications. J Obstet Gynaecol Can. 2007;29(5):433–65.
4. Dunne N, Booth MI, Dehn TCB. Establishing pneumoperitoneum: Verres or Hasson? The debate continues. Ann R Coll Surg Engl. 2011;93:22–4.
5. Sundbom M, Hedberg J, Wanhainen A, Ottosson J. Aortic injuries during laparoscopic gastric bypass for morbid obesity in Sweden 2009–2010: a nationwide survey. Surg Obes Relat Dis. 2014;10(2):203–7.
6. Sundbom M, Ottoson J. Trocar injuries in 17,446 laparoscopic gastric bypass: a nationwide survey from the Scandinavian Obesity Surgery Registry. Obes Surg. 2016;26:2127–30.
7. Boese A, Wex C, Croner R, Liehr UB, Wendler JJ, Weigt J, Walles T, Vorwerk U, Lohmann CH, Friebe M, et al. Endoscopic imaging technology today. Diagnostics. 2022;12(5):1262.
8. Momin TD, Wang MF, Zhou Y, et al. Comparison of operative time and sur-geon's subjective assessment in 3D and 2D laparoscopic gastric bypass surgery. Chin J Gen Surg. 2020;29(6):739–44.
9. Babadopulos RFAL, Moura-Jr LG, Fechine V, Rocha MBS, Antunes N, Costa TA, Costa BA, De-Moraes MO. Technique of exposure of the esophagogastric junction obtained by the flexible liver retractor in bariatric surgery: a randomized controlled trial. Arq Bras Cir Dig. 2022;34(4):e1631.

10. Midya S, Ramus J, Hakim A, et al. Comparison of two types of liver retractors in laparoscopic Roux-en-Y gastric bypass for morbid obesity. Obes Surg. 2020;30:233–7.
11. Huang CK, Lo CH, Asim S, Houng JY, Huang SF. A novel technique for liver retraction in laparoscopic bariatric surgery. Obes Surg. 2011;21(5):676–9.
12. Zachariah SK, Tai CM, Chang PC, Se AO, Huang CK. The "T-suspension tape" for liver and gallbladder retraction in bariatric surgery: feasibility, technique, and initial experience. J Laparoendosc Adv Surg Tech A. 2013;23(4):311–5.
13. Talla P, Ekotomati M, O'Leary T, Ben AN. The use of the Goldfinger dissector (GD) in laparoscopic Sacrocolpopexy. Front Med (Lausanne). 2018;5:155.
14. Velotti N, Manigrasso M, Di Lauro K, Vitiello A, Berardi G, Manzolillo D, Anoldo P, Bocchetti A, Milone F, Milone M, De Palma GD, Musella M. Comparison between LigaSure™ and harmonic® in laparoscopic sleeve gastrectomy: a single-center experience on 422 patients. J Obes. 2019;2019:3402137.
15. Clapp B, Schrodt A, Ahmad M, Wicker E, Sharma N, Vivar A, Davis B. Stapler malfunctions in bariatric surgery: an analysis of the MAUDE database. J Soc Laparosc Surg. 2022;26(1):e2021.00074.
16. Rawlins L, Johnson BH, Johnston SS, Elangovanraaj N, Bhandari M, Cohen RV, Rheinwalt KP, Fryrear R, Roy S. Comparative effectiveness assessment of two powered surgical stapling platforms in laparoscopic sleeve gastrectomy: a retrospective matched study. Med Devices (Auckl). 2020;13:195–204.

Urology: Special Instruments 40

Mohammad Talal Abdallah Al-Zubi, Khayry Al-Shami, Manar Al-Shami, and Almu'atasim Khamees

The Greek physician Hippocrates is credited with the earliest written description of an endoscopy. Endoscopy has been practiced for many years in its many crude forms, according to archaeological data. For instance, a three-bladed vaginal speculum was found in the Pompeii ruins, and Roman texts from the first and second centuries describe the value of patient placement, good illumination, and several speculum kinds. The Babylonian Talmud, which was finished around 500 CE, also touches on these devices [1]. Around 1000 CE, or roughly 500 years later, the use of mirrors to reflect light would be added to the ever-expanding collection of endoscopic tools. Later, during the Medieval Ages, more advanced light sources had been added. Yet, there were two significant problems with these early instruments: weak penetration and insufficient illumination. Philipp Bozzini wouldn't solve these problems until the early nineteenth century [2]. In 1806, a German army doctor named Philip Bozzini created the first device to see inside a human body. He gave it the name Lichtleiter. A surgeon may view inside a bodily cavity using the device's flame and angled mirrors. The instrument was designed to see the throat initially, but it was rapidly modified to view the urethra. This served as the impetus for more endoscopic equipment exploration and advancement. In 1878, Maximilian

M. T. A. Al-Zubi (✉)
Department of General Surgery and Anesthesia, Faculty of Medicine, Yarmouk University, Irbid, Jordan
e-mail: Mzubi@yu.edu.jo

K. Al-Shami · M. Al-Shami
Department of Medical Science, Faculty of Medicine, Yarmouk University, Irbid, Jordan
e-mail: 2014899029@alumni.yu.edu.jo

A. Khamees
Department of Medical Science, Faculty of Medicine, Yarmouk University, Irbid, Jordan

Department of General Surgery, Princess Basma Teaching Hospital, Ministry of Health, Irbid, Jordan

J. S. Ahluwalia (ed.), *User Manual for Minimally Invasive Surgical Equipment*,
https://doi.org/10.1007/978-981-95-9019-3_40

Carl-Friedrich Nitze and Joseph Leiter created the first cystoscope that really worked. The tools that urologists use today are the result of continuous research and improvement that started at that time [3]. In this chapter, we will discuss the description, maintenance, and troubleshooting of some of the major urology instruments.

40.1 Cystoscopy

Cystoscopes are available as rigid and flexible devices. They come in a range of sizes that are indicated in French (Fr) gauge. The circumference of a 1 French instrument is 1/3 of a millimeter. When opposed to flexible cystoscopes, rigid cystoscopes employ the Hopkins rod-lens optical system, which has the benefit of offering superior optical clarity. Nevertheless, with the introduction of flexible digital cystoscopes, this is less obvious as they have a camera chip on their tip. Due to the higher irrigant flow rate in the stiff model, visualization is improved as well. Moreover, rigid scopes allow for the employment of a wider range of instruments due to their bigger working channels. The flexible scopes are utilized for routine flexible cystourethroscopy in the office environment since they are lower in size and offer improved patient comfort. In contrast to rigid cystoscopy, which requires the patient to be in the frog-leg or lithotomy position, the flexible endoscope can also be passed with the patient supine. The flexible cystoscope's tip's ability to move makes it possible to more easily scan the bladder and maneuver past obstructions like a protruding bladder neck or a large median prostate lobe [4].

40.1.1 Rigid Cystourethroscopy

- Available in Full HD resolution
- Sapphire glass lens at the proximal and distal ends
- Nitrogen-filled optical system to avoid fogging from the inside
- Three-tube construction for more stability
- Sealing by LASER welding with excellent optical transmission
- Autoclavable

Sets of rigid cystoscopes are made up of an obturator, an optical lens, a bridge, and a sheath, as we can see in Fig. 40.1. Depending on the seller, these settings vary. The tip angles of the optical lenses range from 0 to 120 degrees. 0-degree and 12-degree lenses are commonly used to visualize the urethra, while 30-degree lenses are often used for both diagnostic and therapeutic purposes within the bladder, and 70-degree and 120-degree lenses are used to inspect specific bladder areas.

The bridge joins the sheath and optical lens. Bridges come in many different varieties. The channels on a diagnostic bridge are inoperative. Bridges used in therapeutic situations may have one or two operational channels. In order to simplify ureteral orifice cannulation, specialty bridges called Albarran bridges have a lever that may deflect wires and catheters across the working channel. Patients with high bladder necks or big median prostate lobes may occasionally need this. When trying to cannulate a transplanted ureter or ureters entering the bladder in unusual places,

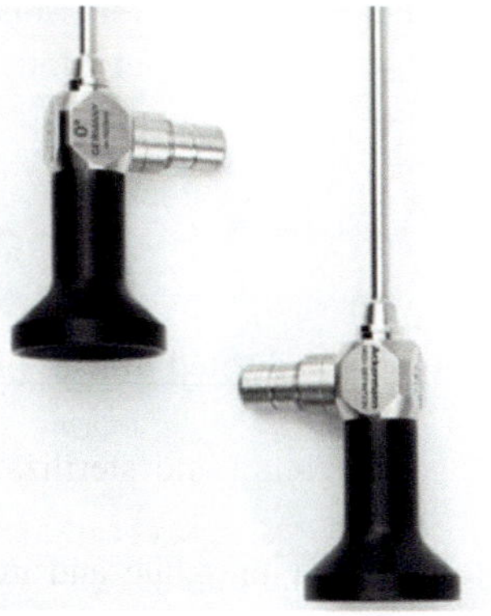

Cysto-Urethroscope sheath including obturator, central valve for use with 4 mm scope	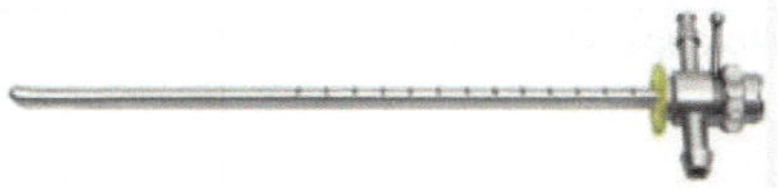
Standard obturator for cysto-urethroscope sheath	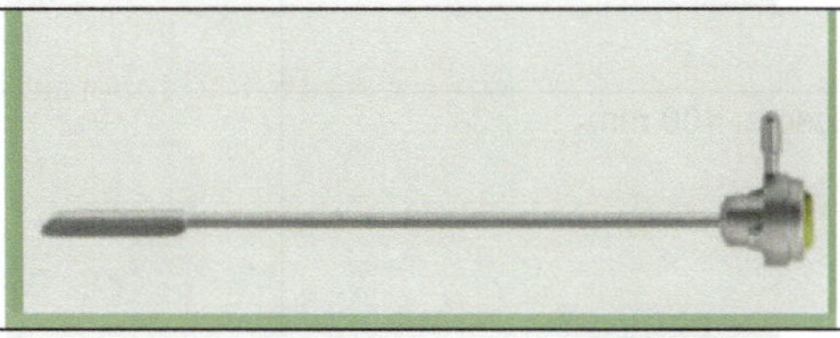
Optical grasping forceps, 4.3 mm, double-action, for 30° scope	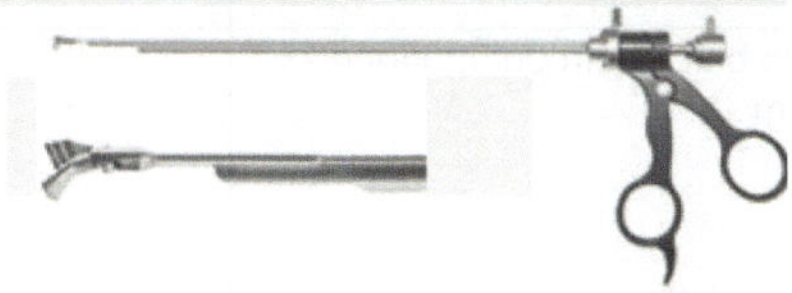
Optical scissors, hook-shaped, double-action.	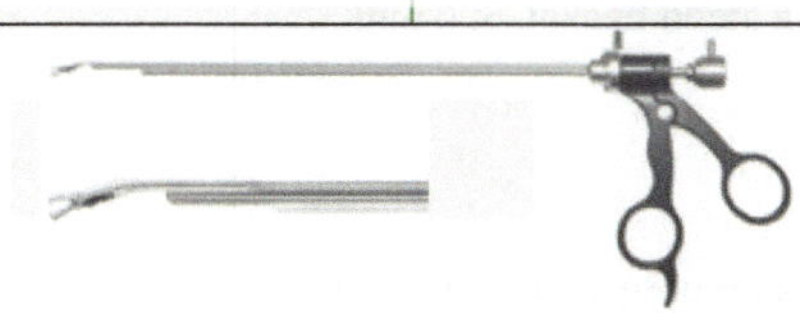
Adapter for optical forceps 32-4066, use with Ackermann resectoscopy outer sheaths.	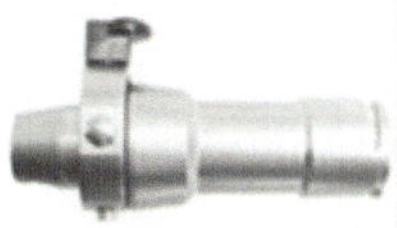

Fig. 40.1 Rigid cystourethroscopy and its additional equipment

Telescope bridge for diagnostics, suitable for 17 -25 Fr. cysto-sheath	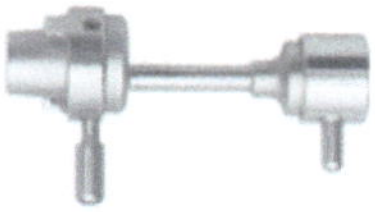
Albarran deflector with 1 instrument channel, lockable, suitable for cysto-sheaths from 17 Fr.	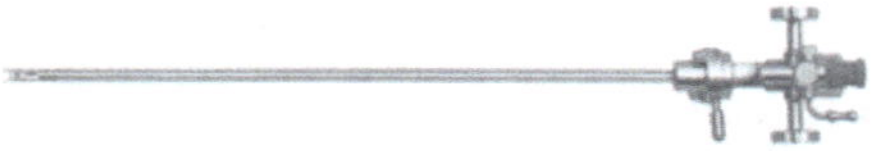
Biopsy forceps, 400 mm	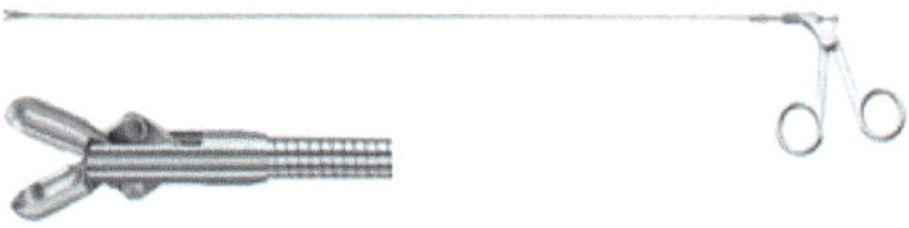
Scissors, 400 mm	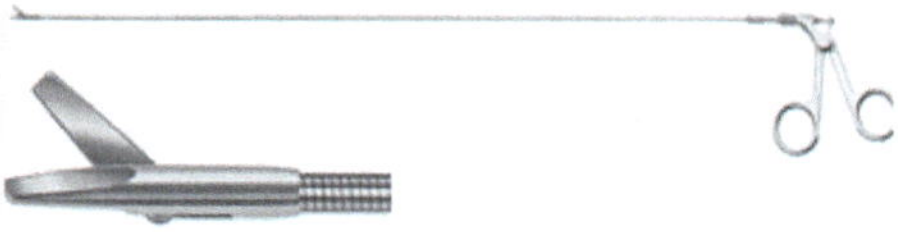
Flexible ball electrode, monopolar, 470 mm	
Dormia stone basket, 600 mm	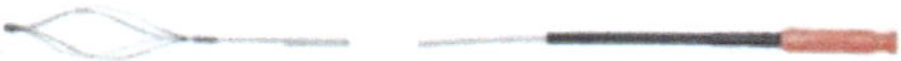
Handle for dormia stone basket	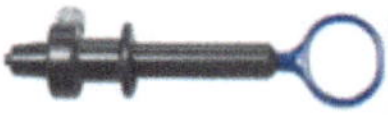

Fig. 40.1 (continued)

it can also be useful. There are many sizes available for the cystourethroscopy sheaths. Sizes for sheaths can range from 15/17 Fr to 25 Fr. For diagnostic cystoscopy, smaller sheaths are desirable since they are less traumatic. For therapeutic operations, bigger sheaths are employed because they provide more irrigation fluid flow and larger instrument working channels. Each sheath features an obturator that blunts the distal end to allow visual assistance-free entry into the bladder.

Flexible Cystoscope	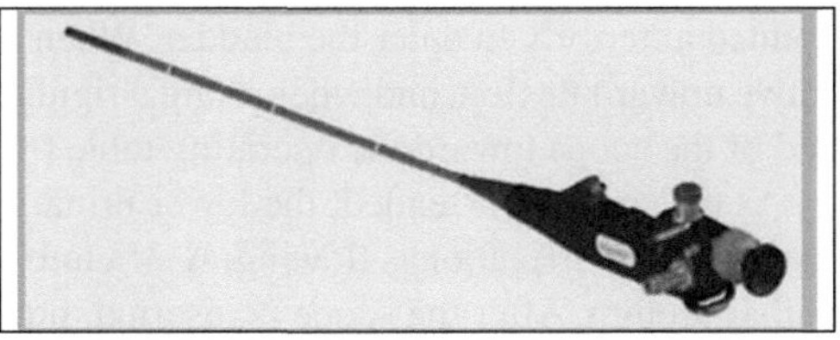

Fig. 40.2 Illustration for flexible cystourethroscopy

40.1.2 Flexible Cystourethroscopy

Flexible cystoscopes typically vary from 14.6 to 16.5 Fr. Dip deflection, field of vision, working channel size, lighting, and optics may vary from model to model (Fig. 40.2). Most versions don't have an offset lens and have a field of vision of about 120 degrees. The direction of tip deflection, which can be either obvious (the same as lever deflection) or paradoxical (opposite direction of lever deflection), spans from 120 to 210 degrees. The same functional route must be used for both the irrigation and the instruments. For instance, passing a flexible grasper through the scope requires stopping the irrigation. To enable the irrigation to be linked while passing instruments, however, adaptors have been created. Several versions provide photodynamic and narrow-band imaging capabilities.

Depending on the circumstance, sterile water or regular saline is employed as an irrigation substance. When utilizing monopolar electrocautery, nonionic irrigants (such as water, glycine, and sorbitol) are necessary. When employing bipolar electrocautery equipment, isotonic irrigating fluids (typical saline/lactated ringers) may be employed. This has the benefit of removing the possibility of electrolyte disruption from systemic uptakes, such as transurethral resection of the prostate (TURP) syndrome. When bladder samples are being obtained for cytologic analysis, sterile water should be utilized.

40.1.3 Technique

The external genitalia are evaluated for any lesions or anatomical anomalies prior to inserting the cystourethroscopy. A sheath obturator can be used to perform a stiff cystourethroscopy insertion on female patients. As the scope is inserted into the bladder, it must be pointed anteriorly. Similar to how a Foley catheter is introduced, a flexible scope can be inserted as well, with the use of active deflection if necessary. To straighten the urethra in males, the penis is stretched to its maximum extent. The penis is grabbed with five fingers of the surgeon's nondominant hand when a stiff scope is passed. The penis is squeezed between the third and fourth fingers of the nondominant hand when a flexible scope is passed, freeing the thumb and index finger to assist in guiding the scope into the urethra. While the scope travels into the anterior urethra, the penis should be positioned between 45 and 90 degrees in relation to the abdominal wall. When the scope has passed the membrane urethra, it is pointed anteriorly to enter the bladder. When using a flexible scope, this is done by active upward flexion, and when using a rigid scope, it is done by lowering the distal end of the scope toward the operating table [4].

As the scope is extended, the lower urinary tract is methodically assessed while the maximum irrigation is flowing. A stricture should be looked for in the penile and bulbar urethra. After the scope is inserted into the membranous urethra, the patient should be urged to unwind. A posterior identification of the verumontanum and utricle is possible once the scope is in the prostatic urethra. It is important to take note of the prostatic urethra's length, the median lobe's size, and whether the bladder neck is blocked. Upon entering the bladder, the mucosa needs to be closely examined. Typically, a rigid cystoscope is used to check as much of the bladder as is visible at first using a 30-degree scope. The ureteral orifices are first identified by looking at the bladder's floor and trigone and noting where and how many there are. Each ureter's efflux should be checked for signs of blood. Checking for bladder stones, trabeculation, bladder diverticula, erythematous patches, or papillary/sessile bladder lesions should be done on the bladder's remaining tissue. The lateral walls can be seen by the surgeon by moving the cystoscope while maintaining a fixed camera position. By retroflecting a rigid scope or utilizing a 70 or 120-degree lens, the dome and posterolateral walls of the bladder are examined. It is best to evacuate the bladder before withdrawing the scope [4].

40.2 Ureteroscope

Ureteroscopies used nowadays might be flexible or semirigid. The most effective application of semirigid ureteroscopes is for distal ureteral procedures. They come in sizes ranging from 7 to 12 Fr, with one or two working channels that are 3 to 6 Fr wide for irrigation and ancillary equipment like baskets, lasers, etc. The semirigid ureteroscopes are usually cheaper, have higher durability, are wider, and have dual working channels. In contrast to the semirigid scopes' angulation range of fewer than 10 degrees, flexible ureteroscopes now have digital video imaging and an angulation range at the tip of up to 275 degrees. This makes it possible for flexible ureteroscopes to enter the kidney and reach the renal pelvis and calyces, especially the lower pole, which has the most tortuosity.

Ureteral access sheaths are a crucial component of flexible ureteroscopy. They can accommodate several ureteroscope insertions into the ureter and kidney without the requirement for a guidewire or the danger of distal ureteral damage from multiple insertions. They are available in diameters ranging from 9 to 16 Fr. The sheaths have two advantages: they prevent repeated damage to the distal ureter and ureteral meatus, and they improve irrigation fluid drainage, allowing for improved vision and reduced intraluminal pressures. Although there is a slight chance that the sheath will result in ureteral wall ischemia, urothelial mucosal tears, and subsequent strictures, as well as ureteral and renal pelvic perforations, these risks are significantly reduced after surgery by the placement of ureteral double pigtail stents, to levels comparable to flexible ureteroscopy without access sheaths [5, 6].

Wire baskets, biopsy forceps, balloon catheters, cold knives, and electrocautery are some of the instruments that can be introduced into the ureteroscope's working channel. In addition to laser fibers, ureteroscopic lithotripsy-specific instruments also include electrohydraulic, pneumatic, and ultrasound probes. Although it is the least efficient choice overall, the ultrasonic probe enables continuous, simultaneous suction with stone ablation to lessen calculi retropulsion. Pneumatic probes must be in direct touch with the stones in order to be successful, and they can only be utilized through stiff and semirigid ureteroscopes. The most adaptable and smallest diameter fibers available are laser fibers (at less than 1 Fr). They range in size from 200 to 360 μm, there are other sizes as well (larger sizes are available for use in the bladder). For usage in the renal pelvis, smaller, more flexible laser fibers are often recommended. Lasers are very efficient for tissue ablation, coagulation, excision, incision, and vaporization in addition to lithotripsy of all forms of stones, especially the holmium:YAG laser [7, 8].

Throughout the past 20 years, the downsizing of scopes and accessories has been one of ureteroscopy's most important technological advancements. The switch from fiber-optic to digital video optical systems is a significant advancement that promotes downsizing. As opposed to fiber-optics with direct-viewing lenses, the digital video optical system employs a charge-coupled device (CCD) camera chip positioned on the tip of the ureteroscope and linked to a monitor display through a single wire. In addition to being smaller than fiber-optic cables, this produces images of superior clarity and has a wider working channel. Even single use such models are also available.

40.2.1 Semirigid Ureteroscopy

- Available in Full HD and HD resolution
- Extra-slim working channel
- Soft tapered sheath allows for easy introduction and atraumatic dilatation
- Semiflexible sheath (Fig. 40.3)

To prevent the angulation required to move into the mid and upper ureters, semirigid ureteroscopy is usually only used on the distal ureter. It may quickly inflict significant harm if not handled carefully when using one. Although utilizing sheaths restricts the scope's potential proximal advancement, it can be advanced into the bladder on its own, over a guidewire, over a brief ureteral access sheath, or even through an empty cystoscope sheath. With difficult urethras, think about advancing the ureteroscope over a guidewire to reduce urethral damage. If the irrigation fluid flow is not lowered and controlled properly, it might push the stone backwards and out of reach while still advancing the scope. To make it easier for semirigid ureteroscopes to enter initially, we prefer to dilate at least the intramural section of the ureter using a dual-lumen catheter or the dilator component of a ureteral access sheath. To make it easier to reintroduce the ureteroscope into the ureter without

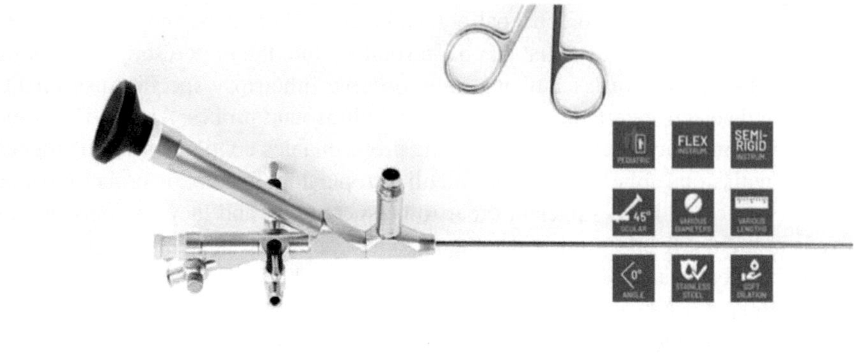

FullHD Standard Uretero-Renoscope, 0°, Ø 6.8 Fr. work. ch., 90° field of view	
Stone grasping forceps, 600 mm	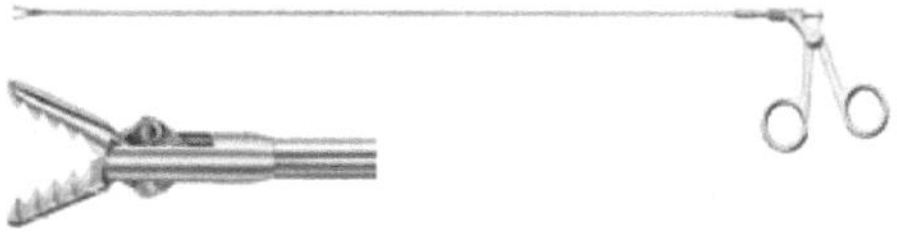
Biopsy spoon, 600 mm	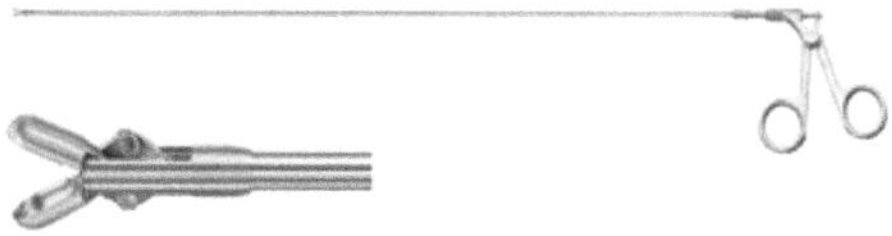
Scissors, 600 mm	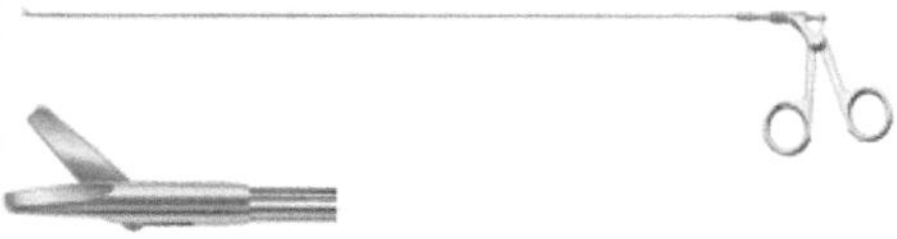
Utero slitting scissors, retrograde cutting, semi-rigid, Ø 4 Fr., 600 mm	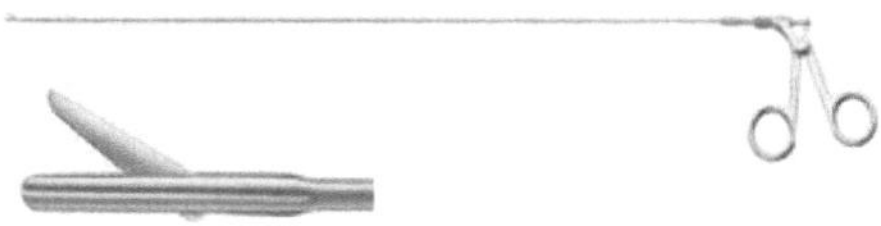
Serrated grasping forceps, teeth interlocks, flexible, Ø 4 Fr., 600 mm	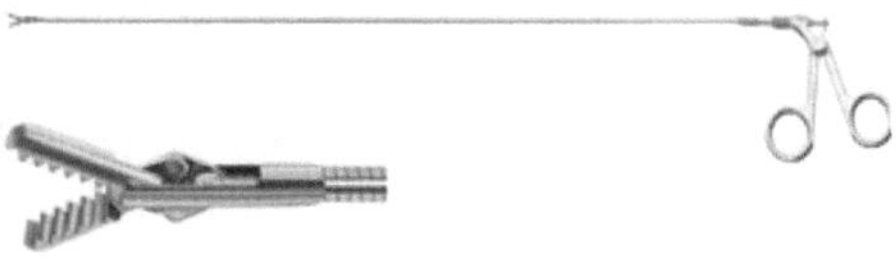

Fig. 40.3 Semirigid ureteroscopy and its additional equipment

Dormia stone basket, Ø 5 Fr., 4 wires, 600 mm	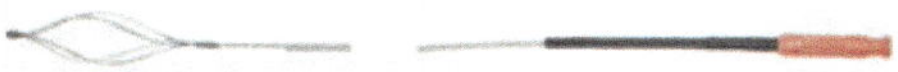
Handle for dormia stone basket, Ø 5 Fr.	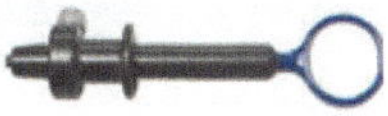
Cleaning brush, 600 mm	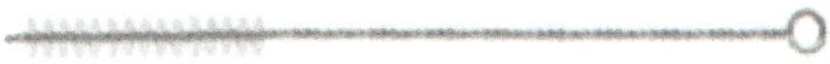
URS adapter	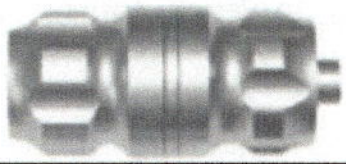
Silicone cap luer lock	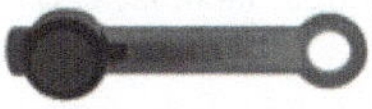

Fig. 40.3 (continued)

having to entirely remove it from the bladder each time, stones that were removed without an access sheath can be placed in the urinary bladder [9].

40.2.2 Flexible Ureteroscopy

Various models are available, and here one is explained for reference.

- Enhanced active dual angular deflection of 275° up and 275° down for maximized versatility
- Memory effect in the sheath for convenient readjustment
- Large viewing angle of 88° for increased visibility
- Total working length of 680 mm with a Ø 1.2 mm working channel (Fig. 40.4)

The "functioning" guidewire, which assisted in "navigating" the ureter, should be withdrawn once the ureteroscope has been introduced into the renal pelvis. A second "safety" guidewire is still in place as a result. The "safety" guidewire's distal end should be kept in its holder or clamped to the drapes so that it won't obstruct the completion of the ureteroscopy. In the "working channel" of the ureteroscope, a small basket (such as a zero-tip basket) or a tiny laser fiber may then be inserted. The ureteroscope should be connected to a standard saline irrigation device, such as

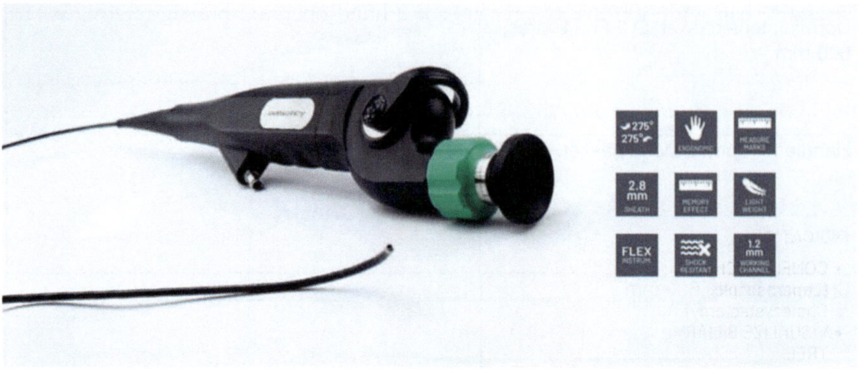

Flexible Uretero-Renoscope, Ø 8.4 Fr. sheath, Ø 3.6 Fr. work. chan., 275° angulation, 60° field of view, 680 mm, includes suction valve, leakage tester and case	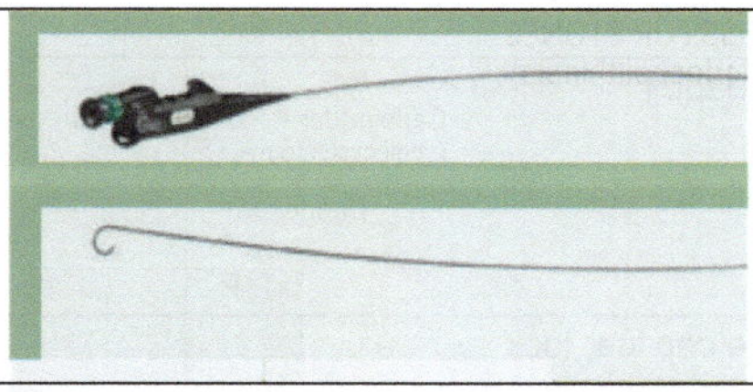
Alligator grasping forceps, flexible, Ø 3 Fr., 120 cm	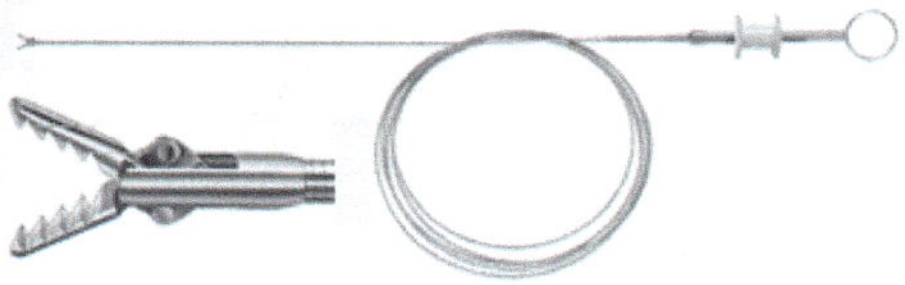
Biopsy forceps, flexible, Ø 3 Fr., 120 cm	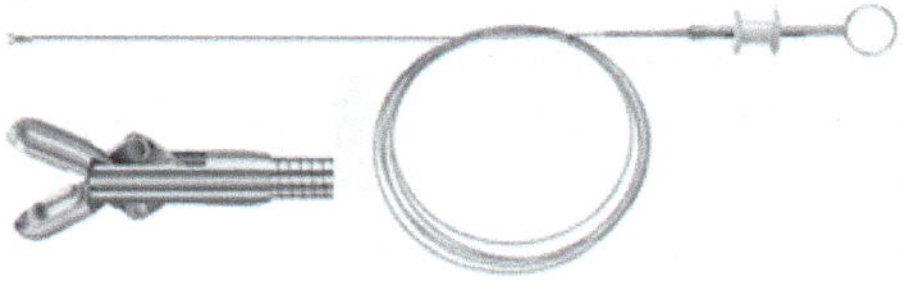
Prong retriever, Ø 1 mm, pointed, flexible, Ø 3 Fr., 120 cm	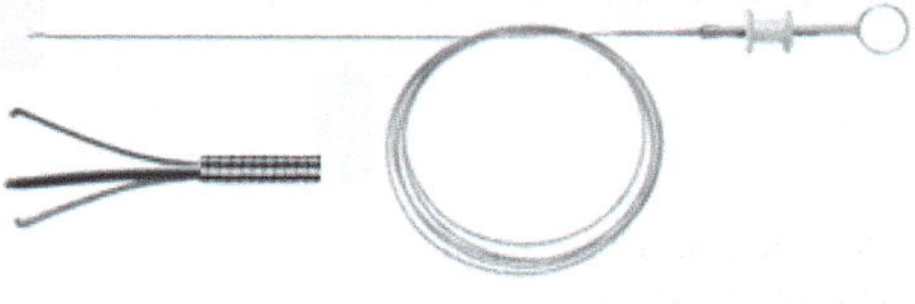
Serrated grasping forceps, flexible, Ø 3 Fr., 120 cm	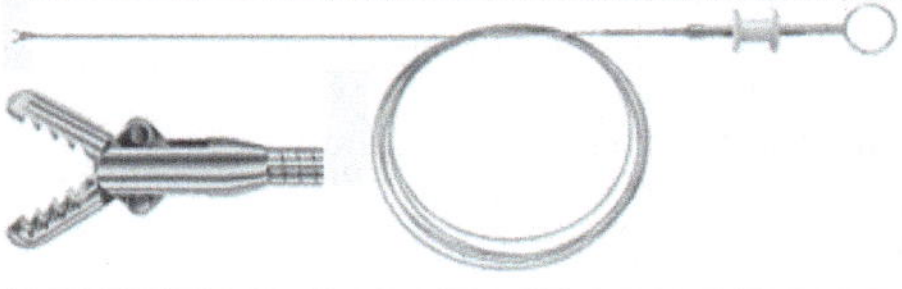
Rat tooth, 2x1 teeth, flexible, Ø 3 Fr., 120 cm	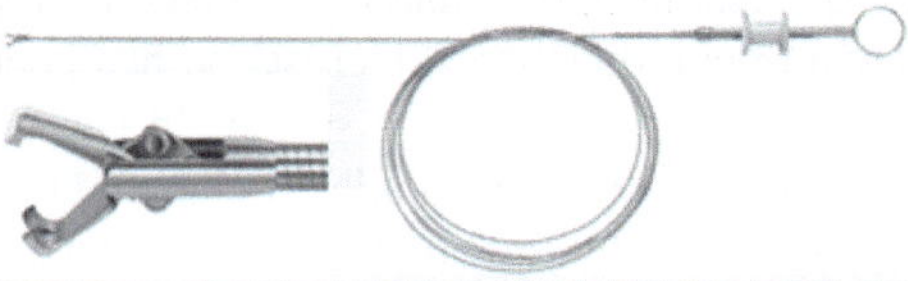

Fig. 40.4 Flexible ureteroscopy and its accessories

a pressure bag with 300 lbs. of pressure or a hand-operated pressure syringe. The irrigation in rigid ureteroscopy is connected to the smaller port since there is frequently a dual-channel. A dual-channel adapter, such as a Tuohy-Borst Y adaptor, should be used if there is only a single channel. As a result, the adjustable diaphragmatic port may still be used for the basket, laser fiber, or guidewire while the irrigation can be coupled to the channel via the offset port. Although there were marginally fewer complications with the pressure bag, most likely because excessively high irrigation pressures were avoided, there was generally no appreciable difference in the rate of complications between the use of a continuous high-pressure irrigation bag versus a hand-operated pressure syringe. While orienting yourself when seeing the renal pelvis, use the safety guidewire as a reference point. A short fluoroscopic picture of the ureteroscope in each calyx will aid in reentry and assist in confirming that the whole calyx has been inspected.

40.2.3 Lasers

The laser may first be tuned to a 5–10 Hz frequency and 5–9 Watts of power for stone fragmentation. Lower power settings with a higher frequency, such as a power level of 0.2 with a frequency of 25–50 Hz, are advised for ureteral stones and stone vaporization. Some lasers have two settings, allowing the surgeon to swiftly switch between one power level and the other. Of course, each laser will need to be adjusted differently, but the basic idea remains the same: whereas lower power and higher frequency settings will maximize vaporization and tend to reduce stone migration, higher power and slower frequency settings tend to enhance stone fragmentation. In contrast to stone fragmentation, laser vaporization works best when the laser fiber is not in close proximity to the object. To melt the stone, simply approach it with the laser fiber up close. The primary drawback of laser stone vaporization is that it takes longer and can reduce the amount of stone that can be used for chemical analysis. In other instances, the core will include a tougher, more resilient stone that may be best handled through stone basket extraction and fragmentation rather than vaporization.

40.2.4 Troubleshooting

For distal ureteral examination and dilatation, some experts propose doing a semi-rigid ureteroscopy immediately prior to all flexible ureteroscopies. It will also aid in the identification of any stones that have unexpectedly moved to the distal ureter. Every ureteroscopy is unique to can present with unforeseen challenges, so always keep a large selection of stents, guidewires, connections, clamps, baskets, and scopes in hand. A "safety" guidewire should be placed in the renal pelvis for access in the event of an unanticipated issue. It must be securely fastened so that it is not unintentionally misplaced, pulled, or removed. Take note of your assistants' abilities and experience. Stiffer guidewires can aid in the implantation of ureteral access sheaths and the progression of double-pigtail stents. They are also less prone to buckle, but they may increase the danger of perforation, so use caution while use them. The dual-lumen catheter is a vital piece of equipment. It can be used as a ureteral dilator, a stone pusher, to inject diluted contrast for retrogrades, to install a second guide wire, or to replace a guide wire. If one kind of guidewire cannot pass through a stricture, impacted stone, or other obstruction, consider another type of guidewire. Hydrophilic wires are often the best choice for this. While doing retrograde pyelograms, combining diluted contrast with lidocaine jelly or simple lubricant increases viscosity while maintaining radio-opacity and helps retain the contrast in the renal pelvis for longer, if desired. To avoid air bubbles, stir the two together slowly and gently. If ureteral strictures are discovered, a double-pigtail stent should be left in place for a few weeks rather than using mechanical or balloon ureteral dilators. To reduce radiation exposure, static, pulsed X-ray images are preferred over live, continuous exposures. It is also advised to use the "Last image hold" option. Understand and operate all of the ureteroscope controls. When the calices and stones are to the left or right, most flexible ureteroscopes will stretch the tip upwards and downwards. Reusable scopes often contain an adjustment that allows the shaft to be moved 90 degrees right or left to ease caliceal inspection and entrance. Disposable ureteroscopes frequently lack this adjustment and must be turned to the left or right by hand as needed, which can be difficult. High-pressure irrigation is one of your most critical and valuable instruments. High flow rates will help with visibility, ureteroscope advancement, and ureteral dilatation, but they may also push the stone closer to the ureter. Excessive pressure can potentially result in a calyceal rupture, which can lead to bacteraemia. Too much flow in the renal pelvis might cause the stone to hop about and travel from calyx to calyx. As a result, in the kidney, just employ the quantity of irrigation flow required for visibility. Higher irrigation flow rates can also be used temporarily to bounce a stone about so that it can be collected by the stone basket. Stone lasering generates a dust cloud. Use the irrigation at the lowest flow rate necessary to keep visibility. When closed, most stone baskets retract (move closer to the ureteroscope). To avoid this, move the stone basket at the same rate as the assistance. This closes the basket around the stone without withdrawing it.

40.3 Resectoscope

The resectoscope is a combination cystoscope and electrosurgical tool that enables direct visual resection of prostate tissue or sick bladder tissue utilizing an electric resection loop. A resectoscope contains a liquid supply, a working channel, a channel for the surgeon to see through, and a handpiece that can spin 360 degrees. Pathological growths are removed with the resectoscope's RF-electrode. The resectoscope must be rotated up to 180 degrees in order to reach sick tissue on the bladder's ventral side (Fig. 40.5).

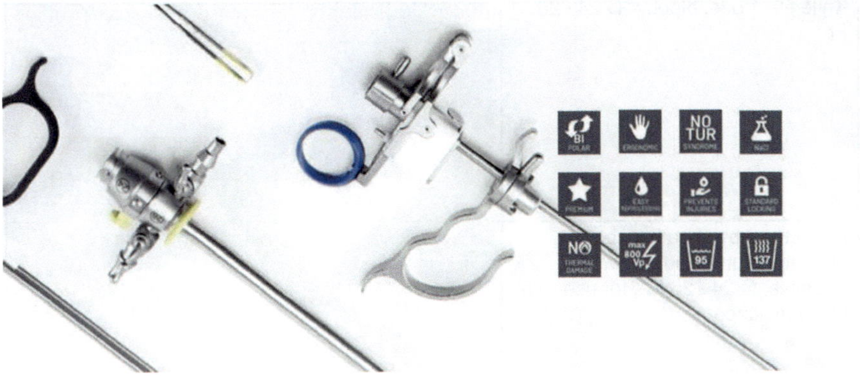

Bipolar working element, closed handle, passive	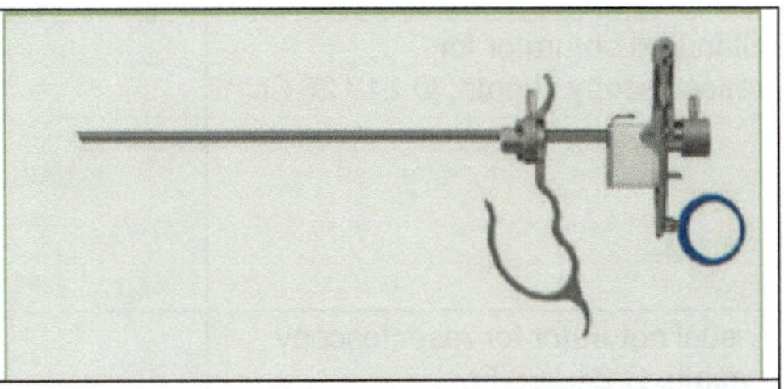
Bipolar working element, closed handle, active	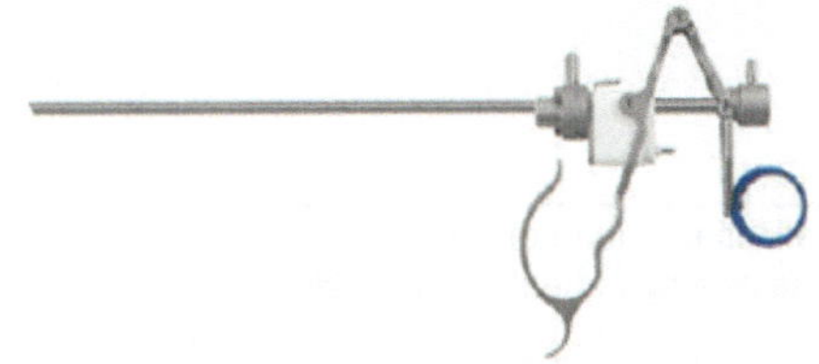
Loop electrode, 90°, bipolar, Ø 24 / 26 Fr.	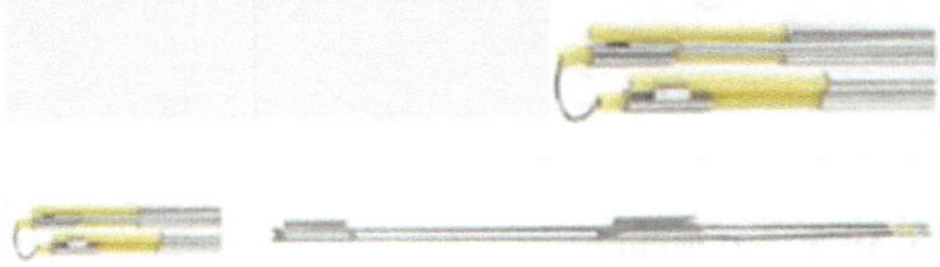
Ball electrode Ø 3 mm, bipolar, Ø 24 / 26 Fr.	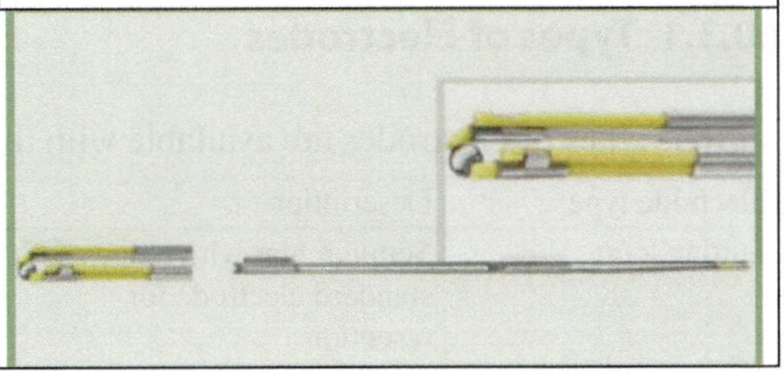

Fig. 40.5 Resectoscope and its additional parts

Knife electrode, bipolar, Ø 24 / 26 Fr.	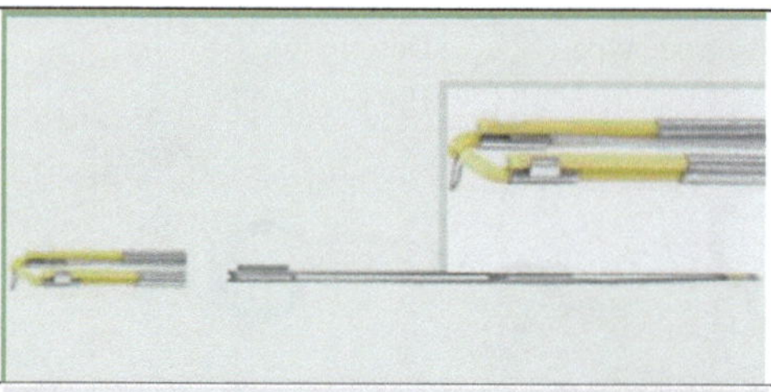
Resectoscopy sheath incl. obturator, continuous-flow, rotatable, Ø 24 / 26 Fr., for use with Ø 4 mm scope	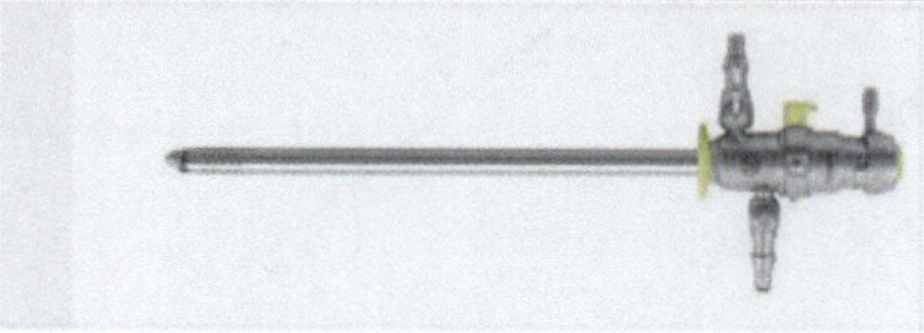
Standard obturator for resectoscopy sheath, Ø 24 / 26 Fr.	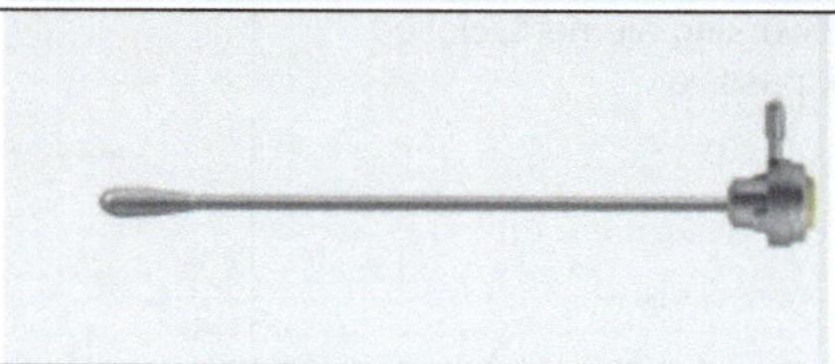
Visual obturator for resectoscopy sheath, Ø 24 / 26 Fr.	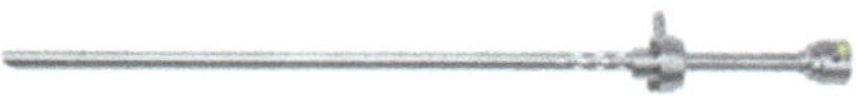
Deflecting obturator for resectoscopy sheath, Ø 24 / 26 Fr.	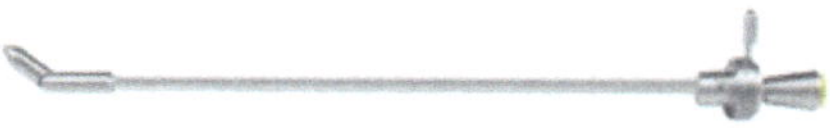

Fig. 40.5 (continued)

40.3.1 Types of Electrodes

Various types of electrodes are available with the resectoscope for various purposes.

Electrode type	Description	Primary uses
Cutting loop	Semicircular wire loop; standard electrode for resection	Resecting enlarged prostate tissue and bladder tumors
Roller ball electrode	Spherical tip electrode for coagulation without cutting	Hemostasis
Collins knife	Thin, needle-like blade	Bladder neck incision Urethrotomy for strictures

(continued)

Electrode type	Description	Primary uses
Hook electrode	Hook-shaped tip	Enucleation of prostate lobes, controlled dissection in difficult anatomy
Button electrode (vaporization button)	Flat, disc-like tip with broad contact surface	Plasma vaporization of prostate tissue. Effective for hemostatic vaporization
Cold knife (mechanical)	Nonelectrical, sharp metal blade	Internal urethrotomy (e.g., for stricture release)—When energy use is contraindicated

40.4 Nephroscope

A nephroscope is a specialized endoscopic instrument used primarily in urology for accessing and visualizing the renal pelvis and calyces during percutaneous nephrolithotomy (PCNL) and other upper urinary tract procedures. It allows diagnosis, stone fragmentation and retrieval, biopsy, and management of upper tract pathology through a percutaneous tract.

Common Sizes
Standard nephroscope: 20 Fr–26 Fr
Mini-nephroscope: 12 Fr–18 Fr
Micro-nephroscope: 4.8 Fr–10 Fr

Clinical Importance
A larger diameter allows the use of bigger instruments and faster fragment removal
Smaller diameter (mini/micro) reduces renal trauma and bleeding

40.4.1 Rigid Nephroscopes

Slim and robust design with Ø 4.8 mm working channel
For use with rigid nephroscopy instruments in 400 or 500 mm length
Available with 45° or 90° angled ocular and 200 mm or 250 mm working length (Fig. 40.6)

The rigid nephroscope is an optical device that enables direct visual control of various treatment operations while allowing inspection of the renal cavitary system. Two versions of nephroscopes have been described: the Wickham model, with the telescope making an angle of 130° with the sheath, and the Amplatz model, with the telescope forming a 90° angle with the sheath. It is made up of the working element and the outer sheath. This houses the optical system and a working channel that is situated in the nephroscope's central axis and enables the insertion of the lithothripter or other working elements (stone forceps, extraction probe, etc). The irrigation

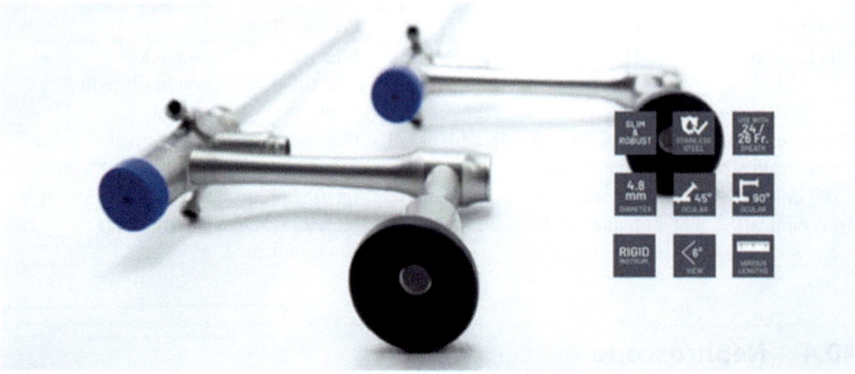

Short Nephroscope, Ø 4.8 mm, 6° viewing angle, 45° ocular	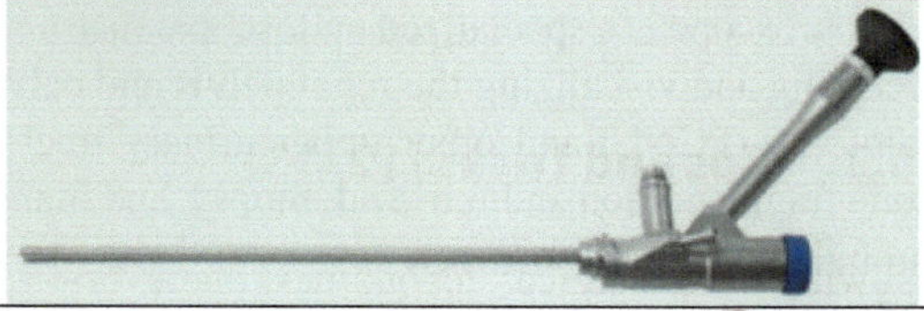
Short Nephroscope, Ø 4.8 mm, 6° viewing angle, 90° ocular	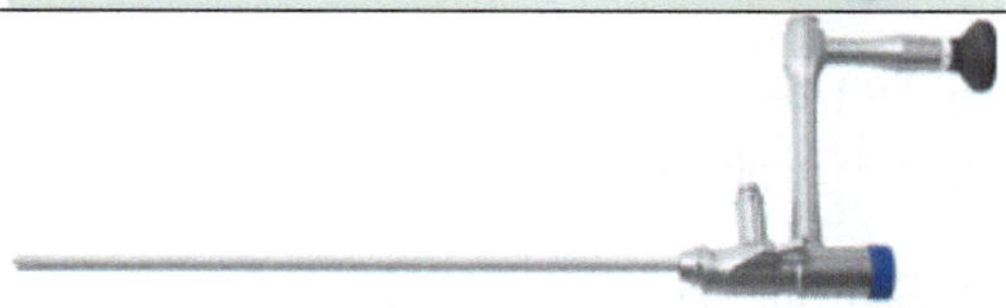
Nephroscopy sheath incl. obturator, 1 stopcock, rotatable	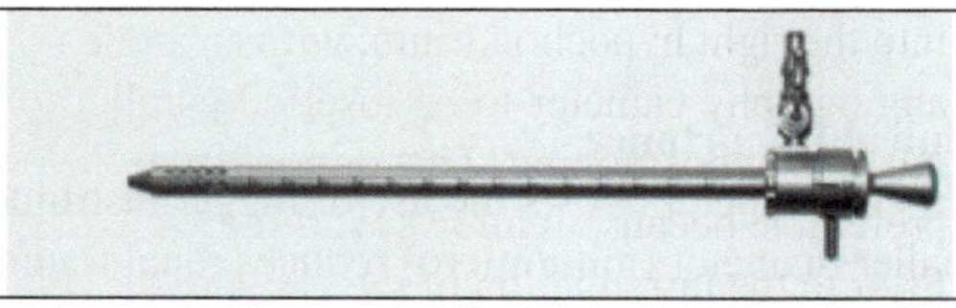
Nephroscopy obturator, cannulated	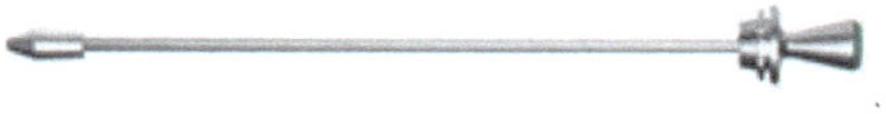
Stone grasping forceps, Ø 3 mm, rigid, ring handle, flushable, 400 mm	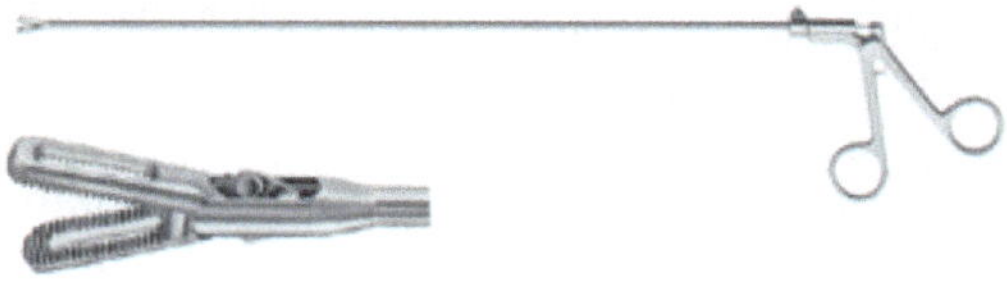

Fig. 40.6 Rigid nephroscope and its equipment

Biopsy spoon, Ø 3 mm, rigid, ring handle, flushable, 400 mm	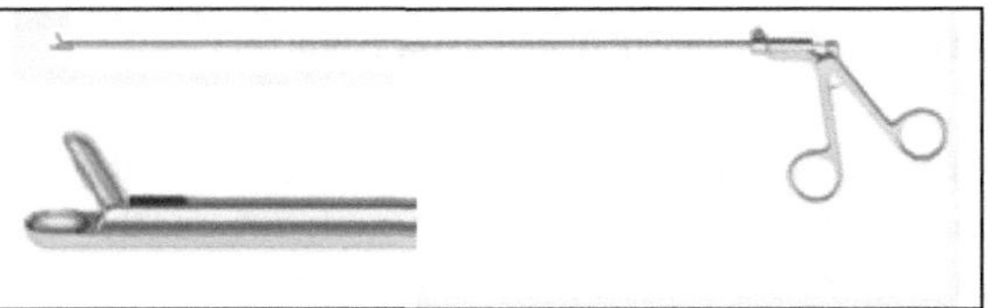
Scissors, Ø 3 mm, rigid, ring handle, flushable, 400 mm	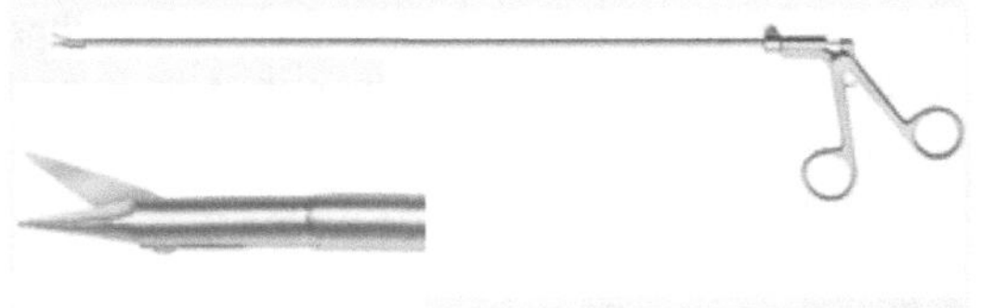
Fenestrated stone grasping forceps, Ø 3 mm, spring handle, 400 mm	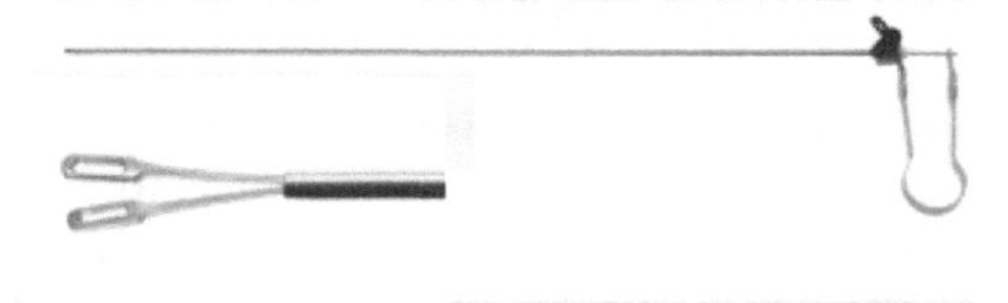
Straight knife, Ø 3 mm, 3-ring handle, 400 mm	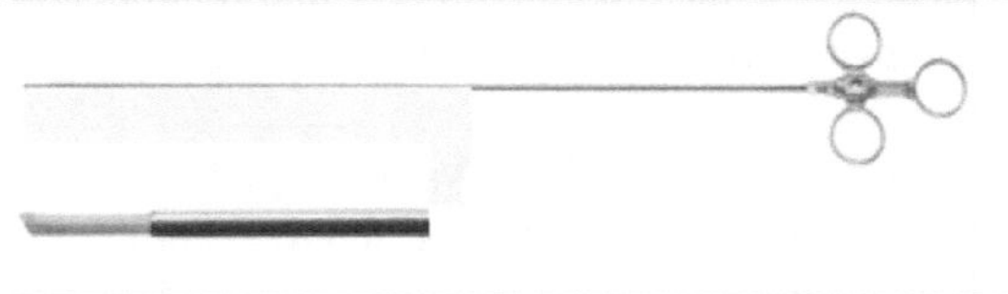
Suction tube, Ø 3 mm, 400 mm	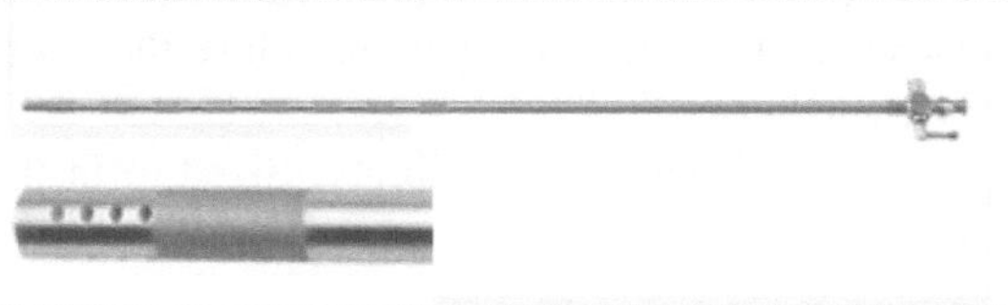

Fig. 40.6 (continued)

fluid's flow is likewise ensured by the same axial channel. The gap between the nephroscope and its sheath is where the fluid exits. The first tool for visualizing the pyelocaliceal system was the rigid nephroscope developed by the Storz firm in 1965. For a very long period, the nephroscope with optical fibers and round lenses was the standard tool for renal percutaneous surgery. Widely used rigid nephroscopes have up to 28 F diameters to enable maximum irrigation and operating channels [10].

The 26 F standard instruments provide excellent visibility and enable the use of a wide range of rigid attachments. Also, continual irrigation through the endoscope provides a sufficient flow to keep the pyelocaliceal system distended throughout the surgery. The evacuation of the washing solution through the Amplatz sheath enables the simple removal of lithotripsy pieces while keeping a clear sight field. Also, the enhanced irrigation flow allows heat created during stone fragmentation to be dissipated. Another significant aspect of this method of irrigation and cleaning fluid evacuation is that a low pressure is maintained in the urinary tracts, lowering the danger of pyelo-renal reflux and, indirectly, fluid absorption and septic dissemination.

40.4.2 Compact Nephroscope

Mini-PCNL (miniperc) is performed using nephroscopes with smaller diameters ranging from 11 F to 18 F. Although not clearly defined, the term "mini-perc" refers to treatments conducted using nephroscopes that are narrower than regular ones. Their usage requires the presence of a lower-caliber functioning channel as well. As compared to normal PCNL, the mini-perc was linked with reduced morbidity (Fig. 40.7).

40.5 Forceps Biopsy

Biopsy forceps are specialized endoscopic instruments used in endourology to obtain tissue samples from the urinary tract for histopathological analysis. They are critical for diagnosing urothelial tumors, inflammatory lesions, strictures, and infections affecting the bladder, ureters, and renal pelvis (Fig. 40.8).

Biopsy forceps consist of the following:

- Flexible or Rigid Shaft: Varies depending on the endoscope being used (rigid cystoscope, ureteroscope, or nephroscope).
- Jaws/Cups: Small, scissor-like cutting edges designed to capture and cut tissue.
- Handle: Mechanism to open and close the jaws, often with a spring-loaded or ratcheted grip.
- Working Channel Compatibility: Sized to fit through the working channels of endoscopic instruments.

Type	Description
Cold cup forceps	Sharp jaws without electrocautery; used for small, clean tissue biopsies
Hot biopsy forceps	Equipped with diathermy for cutting and coagulation; used in vascular lesions
Flexible biopsy forceps	Designed for use through flexible ureteroscopes or flexible cystoscopes
Rigid biopsy forceps	Used with rigid endoscopes (e.g., during TURBT or rigid ureteroscopy)
Fenestrated forceps	Feature holes in the jaws to grip slippery or delicate tissues better

40.5.1 Maintenance

The meticulous maintenance of endourology instruments is paramount to guarantee safety, longevity, and optimal performance. These intricate tools, encompassing scopes and operative instruments, necessitate meticulous handling throughout their use cycle.

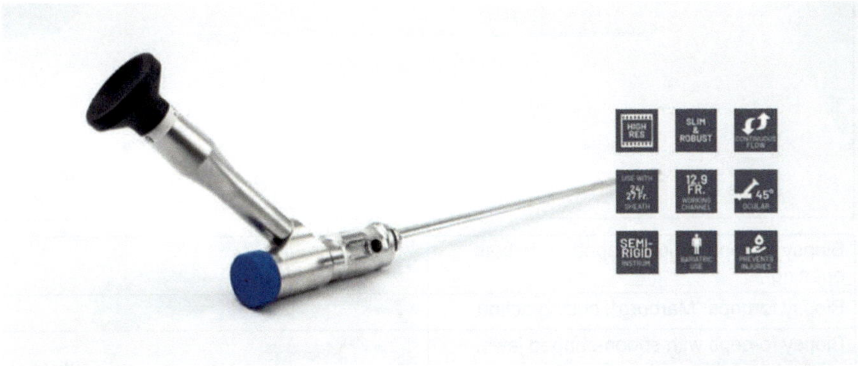

Compact Nephroscope 45°, Ø 18.8 Fr., 12.9 Fr. work. ch., 6° viewing angle, 80° field of view, 220 mm	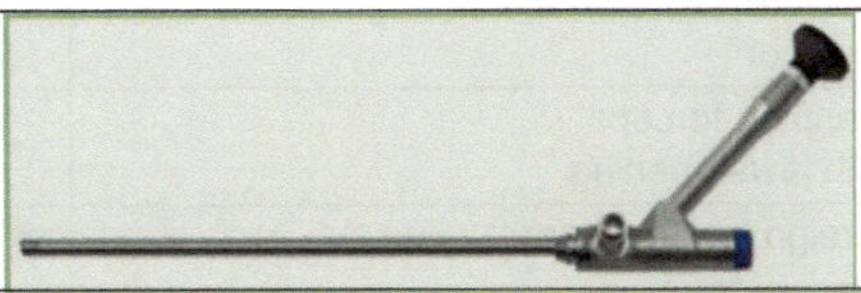
Nephroscopy OP sheath incl. obturator, for use with Amplatz sheath, Ø 24 Fr.	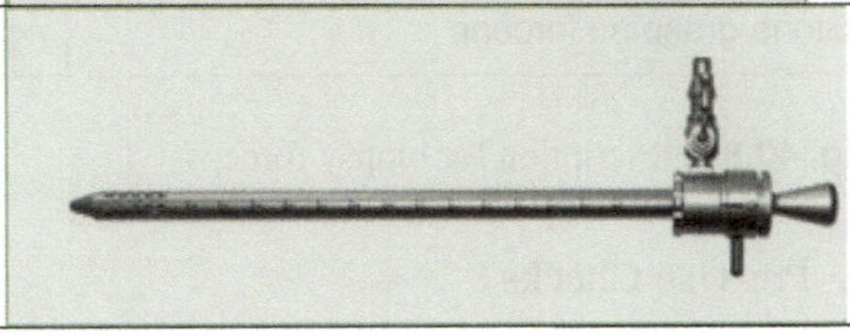
Amplatz sheath, cannulated, Ø 27 Fr.	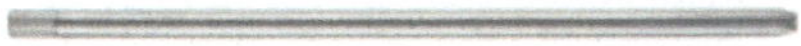
Stone grasping forceps for small stones, Ø 5 Fr., semi-rigid, ring handle, rotatable, 400 mm	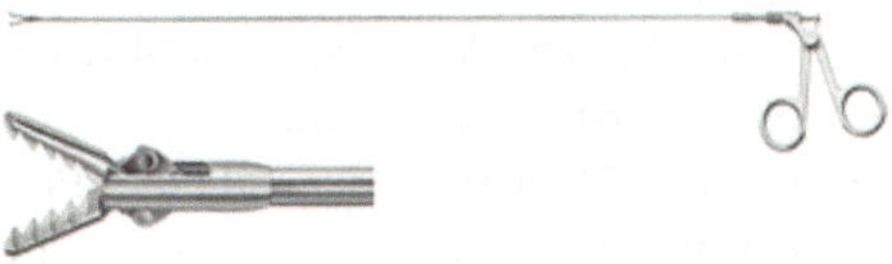
Scissors, Ø 5 Fr., semi-rigid, ring handle, rotatable, 400 mm	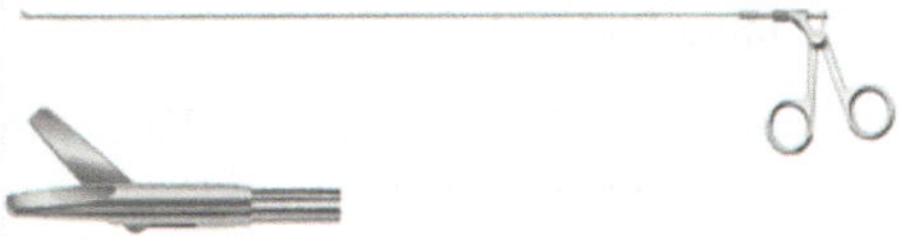
Stone grasping forceps for medium stones, Ø 5 Fr., semi-rigid, ring handle, rotatable, 400 mm	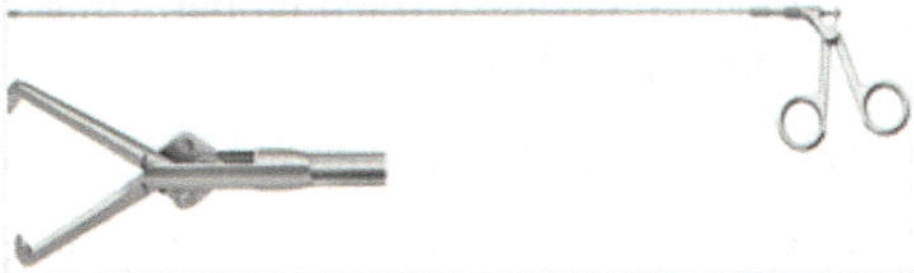
Stone grasping forceps for large stones, Ø 5 Fr., semi-rigid, ring handle, rotatable, 400 mm	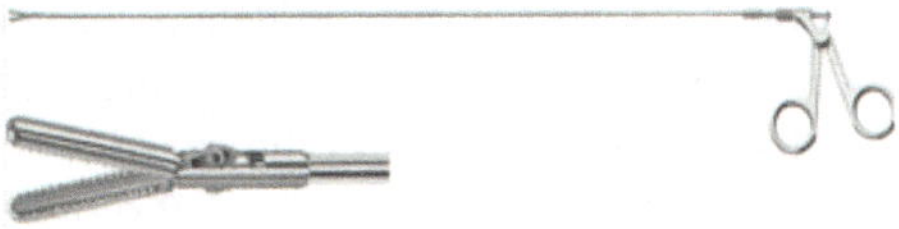

Fig. 40.7 Compact nephroscope and its additional parts

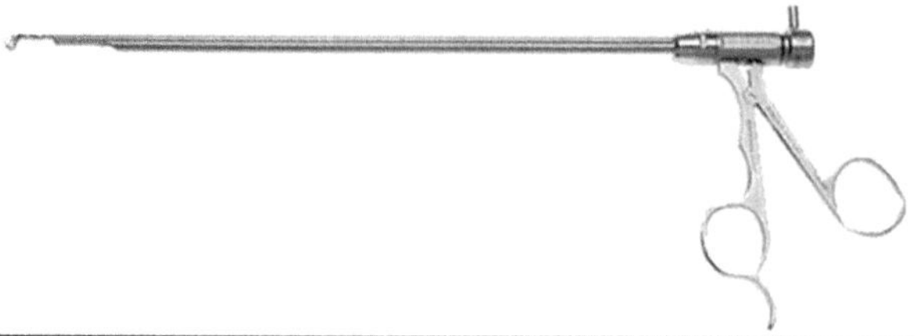

Biopsy forceps spoon shaped jaws, both opening	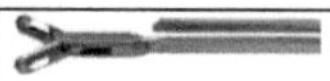
Biopsy forceps "Marburg", cutting action	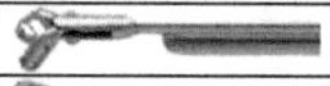
Biopsy forceps with spoon-shaped jaws, retrograde cutting action	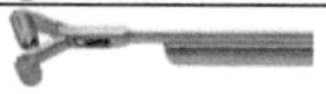
Scissors	
Grasping forceps both jaws opening	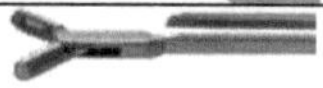
Foreign body forceps	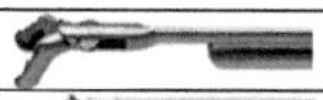
Stone grasping forceps	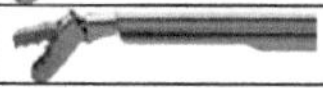

Fig. 40.8 Description for biopsy forceps

1. Pre-Use Checks

    - Inspect for Damage, Bending, or Wear: Thoroughly examine instruments, particularly forceps, baskets, and scopes, for any signs of damage, bending, or wear.
    - Verify Smooth Articulation of Moving Parts: Ensure the seamless articulation of all moving components.
    - Confirm Optical Clarity and Leak-Proofing in Endoscopes: Verify the optical clarity and leak-proofing of endoscopes.

2. Cleaning Protocol

    - Immediate Rinse in Sterile Water: Immediately rinse instruments in sterile water immediately after use to prevent the accumulation of debris.
    - Manual Cleaning with Enzymatic Detergent: Utilize enzymatic detergent for manual cleaning, paying particular attention to working channels using appropriate brushes.

3. Disinfection and Sterilization

    - High-Level Disinfection for Flexible Scopes: Employ high-level disinfection methods, such as glutaraldehyde or peracetic acid, for flexible scopes.
    - Sterilization of Rigid Instruments: Utilize autoclaving techniques, following the manufacturer's specific instructions, to sterilize rigid instruments.
    - Avoid Harsh Chemicals and Prolonged Soaking: Refrain from using harsh chemicals or prolonged soaking, as they can cause damage to optics and seals.

4. Storage

- Dry and Padded Trays: Store instruments in dry, padded trays to prevent mechanical damage.
- Vertical Hanging of Scopes: Whenever feasible, suspend scopes vertically to mitigate angulation strain.
- Labelling and Segregation: Clearly label and segregate delicate components, such as fiber optics or laser fibers.

5. Periodic Maintenance

- Regular Servicing and Calibration: Schedule regular servicing and calibration, particularly for video systems and lasers.
- Proactive Replacement of Worn-Out Parts: Replace worn-out components, including seals and valves, promptly.
- Keep a log of usage and maintenance cycles for each instrument.

40.6 Troubleshooting

Many things can go wrong while performing a minimally invasion urology procedure. The following table outlines some of the common problems.

Problem	Possible cause	Solution
No image or black screen on monitor	Camera cable not connected properly Light source off or faulty Scope lens is dirty or damaged Camera head malfunction	Reconnect the camera and check all connections Ensure the light source is turned on and functioning Clean lens with appropriate solution Try a different camera head or send for repair
Blurry or distorted image	Lens is dirty or fogged Incorrect focus Damaged lens or fiber optics Condensation inside the scope	Clean the lens carefully Adjust focus Inspect for damage, replace if needed Warm the scope before use to prevent fogging
Leakage during procedure (fluid)	Faulty seals or valves Improper connection of inflow/outflow channels Damaged scope or sheath	Inspect seals and valves; replace if worn Recheck all fluid connections Inspect the scope body and sheath for cracks
No irrigation or poor flow	Blocked inflow/outflow channel Kinked tubing Airlock in the system Faulty pump	Flush channels to clear obstruction Straighten tubing Prime system properly Check pump function and settings

(continued)

Problem	Possible cause	Solution
Difficulty inserting scope	Inadequate lubrication Anatomical resistance Incorrect scope size or sheath	Use sterile lubricant generously Reassess patient anatomy Confirm appropriate scope and sheath size
Fogging during use	Temperature difference Inadequate pre-warming Damaged insulation	Warm the scope before use Use antifog solution Inspect and repair insulation if necessary

40.7 Conclusion

Endourology has revolutionized the management of urological disorders by enabling minimally invasive access to the urinary tract. The wide array of instruments—ranging from rigid and flexible endoscopes to precision tools like biopsy forceps, stone retrieval devices, and specialized sheaths—has made procedures safer, more efficient, and patient-friendly. A thorough understanding of these instruments—their structure, function, and compatibility—is essential for any urologist aiming for procedural excellence. Proper selection, handling, and maintenance not only enhance surgical outcomes but also extend the lifespan of the equipment and reduce the risk of complications.

As technology continues to advance, we can expect further miniaturization, improved optics, integration of robotics, and smarter instruments with enhanced therapeutic and diagnostic capabilities. Mastery of current tools, however, remains the foundation on which the future of endourology will be built.

References

1. Davis CJ, Filipi CJ. A history of endoscopic surgery. In: Principles of laparoscopic surgery: basic and advanced techniques. Springer; 1995. p. 3–20.
2. Berci G, Forde KA. History of endoscopy. Surg Endosc. 2000;14(1):5.
3. Ramai D, Zakhia K, Etienne D, Reddy M. Philipp Bozzini (1773–1809): the earliest description of endoscopy. J Med Biogr. 2018;26(2):137–41.
4. Engelsgjerd JS, Deibert CM. Cystoscopy. In: StatPearls [Internet]. StatPearls Publishing; 2021.
5. Kaplan AG, Lipkin ME, Scales CD Jr, Preminger GM. Use of ureteral access sheaths in ureteroscopy. Nat Rev Urol. 2016;13(3):135–40.
6. Delvecchio FC, Auge BK, Brizuela RM, Weizer AZ, Silverstein AD, Lallas CD, et al. Assessment of stricture formation with the ureteral access sheath. Urology. 2003;61(3):518–22.
7. Geavlete P, Multescu R, Geavlete B. Pushing the boundaries of ureteroscopy: current status and future perspectives. Nat Rev Urol. 2014;11(7):373–82.
8. Larizgoitia I, Pons J. A systematic review of the clinical efficacy and effectiveness of the holmium: YAG laser in urology. In: Database of Abstracts of Reviews of Effects (DARE): Quality-assessed Reviews [Internet]. Centre for Reviews and Dissemination; 1999.
9. Giusti G, Proietti S, Rodríguez-Socarrás ME, Saitta G, Bellinzoni P, Gaboardi F. Semirigid ureteroscopy: step by step. J Endourol. 2020;34(S1):S-13–S-6.
10. Mulţescu R, Georgescu D, Geavlete PA, Geavlete B. Equipment and instruments in percutaneous nephrolithotomy. In: Percutaneous surgery of the upper urinary tract. Elsevier; 2016. p. 3–24.

Part IV

Sterilisation

Cleaning of Instruments

41

Merve Tokoçin

The aim of disinfection and sterilization is to ensure that any instrument does not transmit infectious pathogens to patients. Because not all patient care supplies need to be sterilized, healthcare policies should determine the necessity of cleaning, disinfection, or sterilization of a given piece of equipment based on the intended use of the instrument.

41.1 General Principles

Sterilization is a process that destroys or removes all forms of microbial life (including spores) and is provided by physical or chemical methods in healthcare facilities. Disinfection, on the other hand, refers to a process that removes most pathogenic microorganisms except spores [1].

About 50 years ago, Spaulding [2] developed a rational approach to the disinfection and sterilization of patient care supplies and hospital equipment. He thought that the nature of disinfection would be easier to understand if the instruments for patient care were compartmentalized. According to the degree of current risk, he identified three categories—critical, semi-critical, and noncritical [2].

Critical Items—The sterilization of instruments entering sterile tissue or the vascular system is critical because with any contamination, the risk of disease transmission is very high. This category includes surgical instruments, cardiac and urinary catheters, implants and probes used in sterile body cavities. Materials in this category should be purchased sterile, and, if possible, steam sterilization should be provided. If the material is heat sensitive, sterilization can be achieved with ethylene oxide (ETO), hydrogen peroxide gas or chemical agents. Table 41.1 lists several

M. Tokoçin (✉)
Department of General Surgery, University of Health Sciences Istanbul Bagcilar Training and Research Hospital, Istanbul, Turkey

J. S. Ahluwalia (ed.), *User Manual for Minimally Invasive Surgical Equipment*,
https://doi.org/10.1007/978-981-95-9019-3_41

Table 41.1 Methods for disinfection and sterilization of patient care instruments and surfaces [3–5]

Procedure and method	Microbial inactivation level	Process time	Specimen
Sterilization			
High temp Low temp Liquid submersion	Eliminates all microorganisms, including bacterial spores Eliminates all microorganisms, including bacterial spores Eliminates all microorganisms, including bacterial spores	Vapor (~ 40 min) and dry-heat (1–6 h, depending on the temperature) ETO (~15 h) and hydrogen-peroxide (HP) gas (~50 min) Chemical sterilants: A ≥ 2.4% glutaraldehyde (~10 h), 1.12% glutaraldehyde and 1.93% phenol (12 h), 7.35% HP and 0.23% peracetic acid (PA) (3 h), 7.5% HP (6 h), 1.0% HP and 0.08% PA (8 h), and ≥ 0.2% PA (~50 min at 50° C–56° C)	Heat-tolerant critical and semi-critical items Heat-sensitive critical and semi-critical items Heat-sensitive critical and semi-critical items
High-level disinfection *Heat automated* *Liquid submersion* Intermediate-level disinfection Low-level disinfection	Eliminates all microorganisms, without bacterial spores Eliminates all microorganisms, without bacterial spores Eliminates bacteria, mycobacteria, most viruses, and most fungi without bacterial spores Eliminates bacteria, some viruses and fungi without bacterial spores and mycobacteria	Pasteurization (~50 min) Chemical sterilants or high-level disinfectants: A 12% glutaraldehyde (20–45 min), 0.55% OPA (12 min), 1.12% glutaraldehyde and 1.93% phenol (20 min), 7.35% HP and 0.23% PA (15 min), 7.5% HP (30 min), 1.0% HP and 0.08% PA (25 min), and 650–675 ppm chlorine (10 min) EPA-registered disinfectants with tuberculocidal activity, like chlorine-based products or phenolics EPA-registered disinfectants without tuberculocidal activity, chlorine-based products, phenolics and quaternary ammonium solutions or 70%–90% alcohol	Heat-sensitive semi-critical items Heat-sensitive semi-critical items like endoscopes and bronchoscopes Noncritical items (blood pressure cuff) or surfaces (like bed head) with visible blood Noncritical items (blood pressure cuff) or surfaces (like bed head) without visible blood

germicides categorized as chemical sterilants. These may contain ≥2.4% glutaraldehyde formulations, 1.12% glutaraldehyde with 1.93% phenol-phenate, 7.5% stabilized hydrogen-peroxide, 7.35% hydrogen-peroxide with 0.23% peracetic acid, ≥0.2% peracetic acid, and 1.0% hydrogen-peroxide with 0.08% peracetic acid. The specified times are within the range 3–12 h, with the exception of ≥0.2% peracetic acid (sporicidal time of 12 min at 50 °C–56 °C) [6].

Semi-Critical Items—These are instruments that come into contact with mucous membranes or non-intact skin. Anesthesia equipment, endoscopes, laryngoscopes, esophageal manometry probes, and anorectal manometry catheters are included in this category. These medical instruments must be free of all microorganisms (i.e., mycobacteria, fungi, viruses, and bacteria) except for a few bacterial spores. The minimum requirement for semi-critical items is high-level disinfection using chemical disinfectants. It is the complete elimination of all microorganisms in or on the instrument defined by high-level disinfection, except for small numbers of bacterial spores. FDA definition of high-level disinfectants with short-term contact, and they are agents that can kill mycobacterium in a $6 - \log 10$. Cleaning followed by high-level disinfection should remove a sufficient number of pathogens to prevent transmission of infection [7].

As with flexible endoscopes, devices of complex design can be difficult to clean, highly disinfect and sterilize. A detailed cleaning has to precede before any high-level disinfection or sterilization process. Washing endoscopes and flushing channels with sterile water, filtered water, or tap water will prevent side effects associated with the disinfectant retained in the endoscope (e.g., disinfectant-induced colitis).

Glutaraldehyde, hydrogen-peroxide, orthophthalaldehyde (OPA), peracetic-acid with hydrogen-peroxide and chlorine are dependable high-level disinfectants (Table 41.1). These items should be rinsed with water or alcohol as they will come into contact with the respiratory system or GI system mucosa [8]. Alcohol rinsing and air drying significantly reduce the possibility of contamination by eliminating the wet environment that provides the proper environment for bacteria to grow [9]. After rinsing, instruments should be dried and properly stored to protect them from damage and contamination.

Noncritical Items—These items come in contact with intact skin but not in contact with mucous membranes. The risk of transmitting infectious agents to patients has not been documented unless noncritical items come into contact with broken skin and/or mucous membranes. Table 41.1 lists the ones to be used against these items.

Most environmental protection agency (EPA) registered disinfectants have a 10-min suitability label request. However, multiple researchers have also shown the effectiveness of these disinfectants against vegetative bacteria at exposure times of 30–60 s [8–10]. The law requires EPA-registered products to follow all applicable label instructions step-by-step (e.g., use, dilution, shelf life, storage, material compatibility, safe-use, and disposal). If the user chooses a route other than that specified on the label of EPA-registered products, that person assumes responsibility for injuries resulting from off-label use [11]. Mats and reusable cleaning cloths are used regularly to provide low-level disinfection of environmental surfaces. However, because they are often not adequately cleaned and disinfected, the mopping procedure can actually spread heavy microbial contamination throughout the healthcare facility [11].

41.2 Cleaning and Verifying Reusable Medical Instruments

The extreme simplicity of the current scheme can present a major problem today. A new schedule is needed for the inactivation of heat-sensitive or infectious agent species (prions such as Creutzfeldt–Jakob–Patient [CJD]) at the cost of re-care of medical care products that become more complex over time. Therefore, the choice of a disinfection method in some departments remains difficult, even to dictate risk categories for patients.

There is also a dilemma for situations where a semi-critical instrument will come into contact with sterile body tissues. For example, is an upper gastrointestinal endoscope still a semi-critical instrument when used in a patient with esophageal variceal bleeding? All microorganisms, except bacterial spores, must be removed from the endoscope to ensure high-level disinfection. In May 2015, the FDA convened a panel to discuss recent reports and epidemiologic investigations of the transmission of infections associated with the use of duodenoscopes in endoscopic retrograde cholangiopancreatography (ERCP) procedures [12]. This changed from high level disinfection for duodenoscopes to sterilization and modifying the definition of critical items from "objects which enter sterile tissue or the vascular system or through which blood flows should be sterile" to "objects which directly or secondarily (i.e., via a mucous membrane such as duodenoscope) enter normally sterile tissue of the vascular system, should be sterile [13].

Procedures and policies suitable for the cleaning of medical instruments should be issued in cooperation with the manufacturer's instructions and the infection prevention committee of the institution.

The cleaning status of a medical instrument is regulated by:

- Manufacturer's written instructions for use.
- Cleanliness of the instrument surface, and microorganisms to which the instrument is likely to be exposed.
- Design feature of the instrument.
- The type and concentration of the product to be used for cleaning.
- Process, time, and temperature of exposure to the cleaning product.

41.2.1 Pre-Cleaning

Sputum, faces, or coarse dirt such as blood should be cleaned immediately; if it cannot be cleaned, the device should be kept moist by placing a damp towel on it or wetting it with a spray.

For the following processes, the manufacturer's recommendations should always be followed:

- Disassembling—facilitates access of disinfectant and/or sterilizing agent to the device surface.
- Sequencing—Items must be correctly and safely sorted for reasons of incorrect assembly, loss of the instrument, and worker safety.
- Wetting—Prevents dirt from drying on the instrument and makes it easier to clean. A solution with or without enzymes should be selected in accordance with the instructions for use, and this process should not take longer than necessary.

41.2.2 Cleaning

Cleaning is defined as the removal of foreign matter (e.g., organic objects) from the instrument using detergent or enzymatic material together with water. This process is carried out more effectively with manual or mechanical cleaning machines after the coarse dirt is removed from the instruments. It is known that inorganic and organic substances remaining on the surfaces of the tools affect the operability of the tools. Therefore, thorough cleaning is necessary before high-level disinfection and sterilization.

In manual cleaning, the two components should be rubbed together under liquid. An example of scrubbing is rubbing dirty areas with a brush, and this is an old but reliable method. Flowing liquid and pressurized liquids are used to remove dirt and debris from the environment, which helps to remove residues left in the inner channels after brushing. When using the washer disinfector, care must be taken to load the instrument into the cleaner: It must be hinged to ensure adequate contact of the instruments with the detergent solution, the instrument must be fully opened, and the additional apparatus must be completely disassembled. The most common types of mechanical/automatic cleaning include ultrasonic cleaners, washer decontaminators, washer disinfectors, and washer sterilizers.

Ultrasonic cleaning solutions may contain bacterial contamination after cleaning because these solutions are not generally antibacterial. Ultrasonic cleaning largely eliminates bacteria, but with the addition of an effective disinfectant can increase the lethal activity.

Washer sterilizer instruments are modified steam sterilizers that clean by filling the chamber with water and detergent. The instruments are then rinsed and subjected to a brief steam sterilization process. Washer decontaminators/disinfectors work like a dishwasher, using a combination of water circulation and detergent at a certain temperature to remove dirt. Washer disinfectors are devices that can provide adequate cleaning on the surfaces of solid and hollow surgical instruments, thanks to the water flow in the machine and are generally followed by computer control. Therefore, cleaning alone is known to effectively reduce the number of microorganisms on contaminated equipment. In a study, it was determined that the median amount of protein obtained from reprocessed surgical instruments in different hospitals ranged from 8 μg to 91 μg [14]. Compared to nonautomated methods for cleaning reusable accessory devices used for minimally invasive surgery, the automated method was more effective, resulting in >99% reduction in soil parameters [15, 16].

Neutral or near-neutral pH detergent solutions are often preferred for instrument cleaning as they have the best material compatibility profile and good stain removal properties. Enzymes, usually proteases, are sometimes added to neutral pH solutions to assist in cleaning up organic contamination.

Enzymes of this nature attack the proteins that make up most of the common dirt, such as blood. In addition, cleaning solutions may contain lipase and amylase. Enzymatic cleaners should not be considered as disinfectants. Post-cleaning, enzymes must be rinsed from the equipment or adverse reactions may occur.

For the dilution of enzyme-containing solutions, it should be used in contact with the equipment for the period specified in the manufacturer's instructions and manual. Care should be taken when using enzymes in detergent form, as they can cause asthma or other allergic effects. Neutral pH detergent solutions containing enzymes are compatible with metals and other materials used in medical instruments and are the best choice for cleaning sensitive medical instruments, especially flexible endoscopes.

Alkaline-based cleaning agents can be used in the processing of medical devices as they effectively dissolve protein and oil residues; however, they can be corrosive due to their structure. Some data tell us that enzymatic cleaners are more effective at removing microorganisms from surfaces than neutral detergents, but with more recent data, we have not found a difference in cleaning efficiency between enzymatic and alkaline-based cleaners [17]. Cleaning materials must be approved by a team with infection prevention expertize.

During the cleaning process, all of the materials must be immersed in water. For devices that are not suitable for water immersion, aerosol generation should be minimized during cleaning. Lumen devices should be cleaned and rinsed with a brush following the manufacturer's instructions. Meanwhile, the device should be checked for blockage and leakage. Brushing should be done under water, and brushes should be disinfected after each use.

Before mechanical cleaning, it must be ensured that the device to be cleaned is compatible with mechanical cleaning. Ultrasonic washers are highly recommended for semi-critical and critical items. In this way, joints, crevices, lumens, or other hard-to-clean areas can be cleaned. Ultrasonic cleaning solution should be changed at least daily. It should be changed in the presence of visible dirt or more often if necessary. Rubber and polyvinyl chloride (PVC) are not ultrasonically cleaned as they absorb ultrasonic vibration.

Washer disinfectors are highly recommended for cleaning medical equipment suitable for mechanical cleaning, to protect healthcare personnel and to ensure adequate cleaning of the instrument. They remove dirt with water circulation and detergents. Although this practice is not suitable for high-level disinfection, it includes thermal disinfection for low-level disinfection.

To avoid damage to the instrument and also to the patient, rinsing must be done to remove detergent residue. For semi-critical items containing lumen (e.g., endoscopes), the final rinse should be performed with distilled water. Dilution of chemical disinfectants is prevented by drying, thus preventing microbial growth. Instruments can be dried with compressed air, a lint-free cloth or by hand. Instruments with lumen such as flexible endoscopes, 70% isopropyl or alcohol or ethanol can be used to dry the lumen [15, 16, 18] (Table 41.2).

41.2.3 Post Cleaning

After cleaning medical instruments, it is essential to separate them from those that are not clean. The cleaning verification should include a visual that can be understood by someone else [15, 16, 18].

Table 41.2 Summary of advantages and disadvantages of chemical agents used as chemical sterilants [13]

Sterilization method	Advantages	Disadvantages
Per-acetic acid/ hydrogen-peroxide	No activation required	Material compatibility concerns Limited clinical experience Mucosal and respiratory health effects Potential for eye and skin damage
Glutaraldehyde	Many studies about it Not expensive Excellent material compatibility	Respiratory irritation Irritating odor Slow myco-bactericidal activity Coagulates blood/fixes tissue to surfaces Allergic contact dermatitis Limiting employee exposure to ceiling concentration of 0.05 ppm
Hydrogen-peroxide standard)	No activation required Enhance removal of organic matter and organisms No disposal issues No odor Does not coagulate blood/fix tissues to surfaces Inactivates cryptosporidium	Material compatibility concerns Eye damage
Orthophthalaldehyde (OPA)	Fast action No activation required No odor Excellent material compatibility Not coagulated by blood or fixed to surfaces Rapid myco-bactericidal activity	Stains protein gray Expensive Eye-irritation Slowly sporicidal activity Anaphylactic reactions
Per acetic acid (PA)	Standardized cycle Low temperature (50 °C–55 °C) liquid immersion sterilization Environmentally friendly Fully automated Enhance removal of organic material and endotoxin Non-adverse health effects to operators under operating conditions Compatible with materials/ instruments Not coagulate blood/fix tissues to surfaces Sterilant flows through materials/ instruments Rapid sporicidal	Potential material incompatibility Only used for immersible instruments Bioindicator don't suitable for routine monitoring A few instruments can be processed in a cycle Expensive Caused eye or skin damage Not sterile storage AER using 0.2% PA is not FDA cleared as sterilization process

(continued)

Table 41.2 (continued)

Sterilization method	Advantages	Disadvantages
Improved HP (2.0%)	No activation required No odor Nonstaining No special venting requirements Manual/automated applications 12-month shelf-life, 14 days for reuse 8 min at 20 °C claimed	Material compatibility concerns (limited clinical-experience) Organic material resistance concerns (limited data)

41.3 Disinfection

Many disinfectants are used alone or in combination in health institutions. These include alcohols, chlorine and chlorine compounds, formaldehyde, glutaraldehyde, orthophthalaldehyde, hydrogen-peroxide, iodophors, peracetic acid, phenolics and quaternary ammonium compounds, among others. These products are designed for a specific purpose and used in a specific way. Users should carefully read and apply product labels to ensure that the appropriate product is selected for its intended use and applied effectively.

Disinfectants should not be used interchangeably. Inappropriate concentration or selection of disinfectants can lead to increased costs. Because occupational diseases among cleaning personnel have been associated with use of several disinfectants (e.g., formaldehyde, glutaraldehyde, and chlorine), precautions (e.g., gloves and proper ventilation) should be used to minimize exposure (Table 41.3).

Germicide activity against microorganisms is influenced by the internal characteristics of the organism, the properties of the chemical, and environmental factors. By comprehending these factors, current situations are evaluated, and disinfection and sterilization procedures are enhanced in effectiveness [19].

41.4 Sterilization

Medical and surgical devices used in healthcare facilities are generally made of heat-resistant materials, which maintain their stability when exposed to heat and steam during sterilization. However, with the increase in medical devices and instruments made of plastic material since 1950, the requirement for low temperature sterilization has increased. Ethylene oxide gas has been used in heat and humidity-sensitive medical devices and instruments. In the last 20 years, a number of new low temperature sterilization products have been introduced to sterilize medical devices and instruments (hydrogen peroxide gas plasma, peracetic acid immersion, ozone, etc.) [20].

Table 41.3 Summary of advantages and disadvantages of disinfectants [13]

Disinfectant active	Advantages	Disadvantages
Alcohol	Bactericidal, tuberculocidal, fungicidal, and virucidal Fast acting Noncorrosive No staining Used to disinfect small surfaces, such as rubber stoppers on medication vials No toxic residue	Non-sporicidal Affected by organic matter Slow acting against non-enveloped viruses (e.g., norovirus) No detergent/cleaning properties Damages some instruments like hard rubber or deteriorated glue Flammable Evaporates rapidly, making contact time compliance difficult Not recommended to use on large surfaces Outbreaks are ascribed to contaminated alcohol
Sodium hypochlorite	Bactericidal, tuberculocidal, fungicidal, and virucidal Sporicidal Fast acting Inexpensive (in diluted form) Not flammable Unaffected by water hardness Reduces biofilms on surfaces Relatively stable Used as a disinfectant in water treatment EPA registered	Reaction hazard with acids and ammonias Leaves a salt residue Corrosive to metals Unstable when active Affected by organic matter Discolors and stains fabrics A potential hazard is the production of trihalomethane Has an odor Irritating at high concentrations
Improved hydrogen-peroxide	Bactericidal, tuberculocidal, fungicidal, and virucidal Fast efficacy Easy compliance with wet-contact times Safe for workers Benign for the environment Surface compatible Nonstaining EPA registered Not-flammable	More expensive Not sporicidal at low concentrations
Iodophors	Bactericidal, mycobactericidal, and virucidal Not-flammable Used for disinfecting blood culture bottles	Not-sporicidal Shown to degrade silicone catheters Requires prolonged contact to kill fungi Stains surfaces It is an antiseptic rather than disinfectant

(continued)

Table 41.3 (continued)

Disinfectant active	Advantages	Disadvantages
Phenolics	Bactericidal, tuberculocidal, fungicidal, and virucidal Inexpensive in the diluted forms Nonstaining Not-flammable EPA registered	Not-sporicidal Absorbed by porous material Depigmentation of skin is caused by certain phenolics Can cause hyper-bilirubinemia in infants
Ammonium compounds	Bactericidal, fungicidal, and virucidal against enveloped viruses like HIV Good cleaning agents EPA registered Surface compatible Persistent antimicrobial activity Inexpensive in the diluted forms	Not-sporicidal Not tuberculocidal and virucidal against nonenveloped viruses Highwater hardness and cotton/gauze make less-microbicidal Benzalkonium chloride may cause asthma Affected by organic matter Multiple outbreaks ascribed to contaminated benzalkonium chloride
Peracetic-acid/hydrogen-peroxide	Bactericidal, fungicidal, virucidal, and sporicidal like *Clostridium difficile* Active in the presence of organic material Environmentally friendly EPA registered Surface compatible	Lacks stability Potential for material incompatibility, like brass and copper Expensive Odor may be irritating

Sterilization destroys all microorganisms on the surface of an article or in a liquid. While the use of inadequately sterilized critical items represents a high risk of transmitting pathogens, documented transmission of pathogens associated with an inadequately sterilized critical item is exceedingly rare (Table 41.4). This is most likely due to the wide margin of safety associated with sterilization processes used in healthcare facilities. This concept is measured as the probability that each item to be sterilized will be sterile. This possibility is often referred to as the sterility assurance level (SAL) of the product and is defined as the probability of the presence of a single microorganism that may occur on the product surface after sterilization.

Medical equipment that comes into contact with sterile body tissues and fluids is considered a critical item. These items must be sterile when used, as contamination with any microbial contamination can cause disease. These items include surgical instruments, biopsy forceps, and implanted medical instruments. If these products are heat resistant, the recommended sterilization process is steaming sterilization, as this process has the largest margin of safety due to its reliability and lethality [21].

Table 41.4 Summary of advantages and disadvantages of commonly used sterilization technologies [22]

Sterilization method	Advantages	Disadvantages
Steam	Nontoxic to patients, staff, and environment Cycle is easy to control and monitor Rapidly microbicidal Least affected by organic/inorganic soils among sterilization processes listed Rapid cycle time Penetrates medical packaging and device lumens	It is deleterious for heat-sensitive instruments Microsurgical instruments are damaged by repeated exposure It may leave instruments wet and causing them to rust There is potential for burns
Hydrogen-peroxide Gas plasma	Safe for the environment and healthcare personnel Leaves no toxic residuals Cycle time ≥ 28 min, and no aeration necessary Used for heat- and moisture-sensitive items because process temperature < 50 °C Simple to operate, install, and monitor Compatible with most medical devices Only requires an electrical outlet	Cellulose (paper), linens, and liquids cannot be processed Endoscope or medical device restrictions are based on lumen internal diameter and length (see manufacturer's recommendations) It requires synthetic packaging (polypropylene wraps and polyolefin pouches) and a special container tray HP may be toxic at levels >1 ppm TWA
100% ETO	Penetrates packaging materials and device lumens Potential for gas leak and ETO exposure minimized by single-dose cartridge and negative-pressure chamber Simple to operate and monitor Compatible with most medical materials	It requires an aeration time to remove ETO residue ETO is toxic, a carcinogen, and flammable ETO emission is regulated by states, but the catalytic cell removes 99.9% of ETO and converts it to carbon dioxide and water ETO cartridges should be stored in nonflammable liquid storage cabinet It has a lengthy cycle/aeration time
Vaporized hydrogen-peroxide	Safe for the environment and healthcare personnel Leaves no toxic residue; no aeration necessary Cycle time 55 min Used for heat- and moisture-sensitive items (metal and nonmetal devices)	Medical device restrictions are based on lumen internal diameter and length; see manufacturer's recommendations (e.g., stainless steel lumen 1 mm diameter, 125 mm length) It is not used for liquid, linens, powders, or any cellulose materials Requires synthetic packaging (polypropylene) There is limited materials compatibility data There are limited clinical use and comparative microbicidal efficacy data

(continued)

Table 41.4 (continued)

Sterilization method	Advantages	Disadvantages
Hydrogen-peroxide and ozone	Safe for the environment and healthcare personnel Uses dual sterilants, HP, and ozone Does not need aeration because of no toxic by-products Compatible with common medical devices Cycle time 46 min FDA cleared for general instruments, single-channel flexible endoscopes, and rigid and semirigid channeled devices	Endoscope or medical device restrictions are based on lumen internal diameter and length (see manufacturer's recommendations) There are limited clinical uses (limited published data on material compatibility/penetrability/organic material resistance) and limited microbicidal efficacy data It requires synthetic packaging (polypropylene wraps and polyolefin pouches) and a special container tray

References

1. Provincial Infectious Diseases Advisory Committee (PIDC). Best practices for cleaning, disinfection and sterilization of medical equipment/devices. In: All health care settings. 3rd ed. Public Health Ontario; 2016. p. 1–109.
2. Spaulding EH. Chemical disinfection of medical and surgical materials. In: Lawrence C, Block SS, editors. Disinfection, sterilization, and preservation. Philadelphia: Lea & Febiger; 1968. p. 517–31.
3. Centers for Disease Control and Prevention (CDC). Healthcare-associated Infections. Available on: https://www.cdc.gov/hai/data/index.html [Last accessed: 2019, May 20].
4. Ling ML. APSIC guidelines for disinfection and sterilization of instruments in health care facilities. Antimicrob Resist Infect Control. 2018;7:25.
5. William A. Disinfection and sterilization in health care facilities: what clinicians need to know. Clin Infect Dis. 2004;39:702–9.
6. World Health Organization (WHO). Report on the Burden of endemic Health Care-Associated Infection Worldwide. Available on: https://apps.who.int/iris/bitstream/handle/10665/80135/9789241501507_eng.pdf;sequence=1 [Last accessed: 20 May 2019].
7. Centers for Disease Control and Prevention (CDC). Hand hygiene in healthcare settings. Available on: https://www.cdc.gov/handhygiene/ [Last accessed: 20 May 2019].
8. Food and Drug Administration. FDA-cleared sterilants and high level disinfectants with general claims for processing reusable medical and dental devices. Available from: https://www.fda.gov/medicaldevices/deviceregulationandguidance/reprocessingofreusablemedicaldevices/ucm437347.htm. Accessed Jan 2019.
9. Rutala WA, Weber DJ. Reprocessing semicritical items: outbreaks and current issues. Am J Infect Control. 2019;47(Suppl):A79–89.
10. Fields R. Outpatient surgeries outnumber inpatient surgeries at 53M procedures a year. Available from: https://www.beckersasc.com/news-analysis/outpatient-surgeries-outnumber-inpatient-surgeries-at-53m-procedures-a-year.html. Accessed Jan 2019.
11. Centers for Disease Control and Prevention (CDC). Immediate need for healthcare facilities to review procedures for cleaning, disinfecting, and sterilizing reusable medical devices; 2015. Available on: http://emergency.cdc.gov/han/han00382.asp [Last accessed: 20 May 2019].
12. Rutala WA, Weber DJ. ERCP scopes: what can we do to prevent infections? Infect Control Hosp Epidemiol. 2015;36:643–8.

13. William A, Rutala MPH. Disinfection and sterilization in health care facilities: an overview and current issues. Infect Dis Clin N Am. 2016;30(3):609–37.
14. Agüeria DA, Libonatti C, Civit D. Cleaning and disinfection programmes in food establishments: a literature review on verification procedures. J Appl Microbiol. 2021;131(1):23–35.
15. Clausen PA, Frederiksen M. Chemicals inhaled from spray cleaning and disinfection products and their respiratory effects. A comprehensive review. Int J Hyg Environ Health. 2020;229:113592.
16. Rutala WA, Weber DJ. Disinfection, sterilization, and antisepsis: an overview. Am J Infect Control. 2019;47S:A3–9.
17. Mulani MS, Kamble EE, Kumkar SN, et al. Emerging strategies to combat ESKAPE pathogens in the era of antimicrobial resistance: a review. Front Microbiol. 2019;10:539.
18. Protano C, Cammalleri V, Romano Spica V, Valeriani F, Vitali M. Hospital environment as a reservoir for cross transmission: cleaning and disinfection procedures. Ann Ig 2019; 31(5):436–448. M.
19. Modernisation Agency. Ten high impact changes for service improvement and service delivery: a guide for NHS leaders NHS, London. 2004. Available on: https://www.england.nhs.uk/improvement-hub/wp-content/uploads/sites/44/2017/11/10-High-Impact-Changes.pdf [Last accessed: 20 May 2019].
20. Vincenti S, De Waure C, Raponi M, et al. Environmental surveillance of Legionella spp. colonization in the water system of a large academic hospital: analysis of the four–year results on the effectiveness of the chlorine dioxide disinfection method. Sci Total Environ. 2019;657:248–53.
21. Epicentro. Health care-associated infection. Epidemiology. Available on: http://www.epicentro.iss.it/infezioni-correlate/epidemiologia [Last accessed: 20 May 2019].
22. Lautenbach E, Malani PN, Woeltje KF. Practical healthcare epidemiology. 3rd ed. Cambridge University Press; 2018. https://epdf.pub/practical-healthcare-epidemiology-third-edition.html.

Autoclave

42

Irma Cruz Mendoza

To talk about autoclaves and/or sterilizers, it is important first to understand the differences between these two terms. The word sterilizer comes from the Latin word "sterilize," which means "not bearing fruit." An autoclave is used for sterilization. Sterilization refers to the physical, chemical, or gaseous destruction or elimination of all forms of microbial life (including spores) present in inanimate objects.

Autoclaves are primarily used in healthcare facilities, clinical and research laboratories, and public health. Sterilization should be considered as a set of interrelated processes of enormous importance so that health services can be provided within rigorous conditions of asepsis. An autoclave is a thick-walled metal container with a tight seal that allows for working at high pressure. The high pressure enables the water to reach temperatures above its boiling point, and the joint action of temperature and steam produces the coagulation of microorganisms' proteins, including those essential for their life and reproduction, leading to their destruction.

42.1 Operation

Autoclaves work by allowing the entry or generation of water vapor, but restricting its exit, until an internal pressure of 103 kPa is reached, causing the steam to reach a minimum temperature of 121 °C. A typical sterilization time at this temperature and pressure is 20–30 min. Modern autoclaves allow processes at higher temperatures and pressures, with pre-vacuum cycles at 134 °C and 200 kPa for 5 min to sterilize heat-resistant material; they even perform vacuum cycles to accelerate the drying of sterilized material.

Containing fluid at high pressure implies that autoclaves must be solidly manufactured, usually in metal and made completely airtight. However, due to the

I. C. Mendoza (✉)
Department of General Surgery at the Juarez Hospital in Mexico City, Mexico City, Mexico

J. S. Ahluwalia (ed.), *User Manual for Minimally Invasive Surgical Equipment*,
https://doi.org/10.1007/978-981-95-9019-3_42

process involving high-temperature water vapor, certain materials, such as paper and many plastics (except for polypropylene), cannot be sterilized in an autoclave.

Since the material to be sterilized is most likely for clinical use, quality testing methods for the sterilization are required. This means that the pressure and temperature applied will be different for each of the products to be sterilized. Autoclaves are usually equipped with pressure and temperature gauges that allow for verification of the equipment's operation, although additional test methods exist in the market. For example, chemical indicators that change color when a certain temperature is reached, or mechanical indicators that deform under high temperatures and pressure. Through these means, it is possible to sterilize all types of materials except for volatile substances, so caution and knowledge of sterilization processes are required.

42.2 Autoclave Installation

During autoclave installation, several requirements must be met. First, the sterilizer must be placed on a flat and level surface with a minimum bearing capacity that exceed weight of the autoclave. To ensure proper air circulation, free space of at least 10 cm at the sides and 20 cm at the top of the equipment should be left. Another condition is that the sterilizer must be located in a properly ventilated space and not installed near water or heat sources. Finally, it is essential not to cover the air outlet grille of the condenser fan or block the side outlets.

The instructions in the equipment manual must be followed at all times. Place the equipment near a power outlet suitable for the machine's consumption. Level it correctly using the legs or immobilize it using stops, depending on the type of autoclave, to give it stability. Attach a hose to the steam/water outlet and secure the other end to a container or drainage, taking care not to obstruct the passage. Do not install this type of equipment in areas where flammable liquids are stored or in zones of special protection. Connect it to a mains voltage that matches what is indicated on the equipment's nameplate. Do not use the equipment without being connected to a ground outlet. The equipment must have an installation plate indicating the identification number, maximum operating pressure, date of manufacture, inspection level, pressure and date of testing, pressure vessel category and group, and fluid.

42.3 Front Part of the Steam Autoclave

42.3.1 Description of Parts

Different models of autoclaves can have different presentations of parts and controls, but a general description is given below as per Fig. 42.1.

42.3.1.1 Multi-Port Valve

This valve controls the direction and flow of steam into and out of the autoclave chamber.

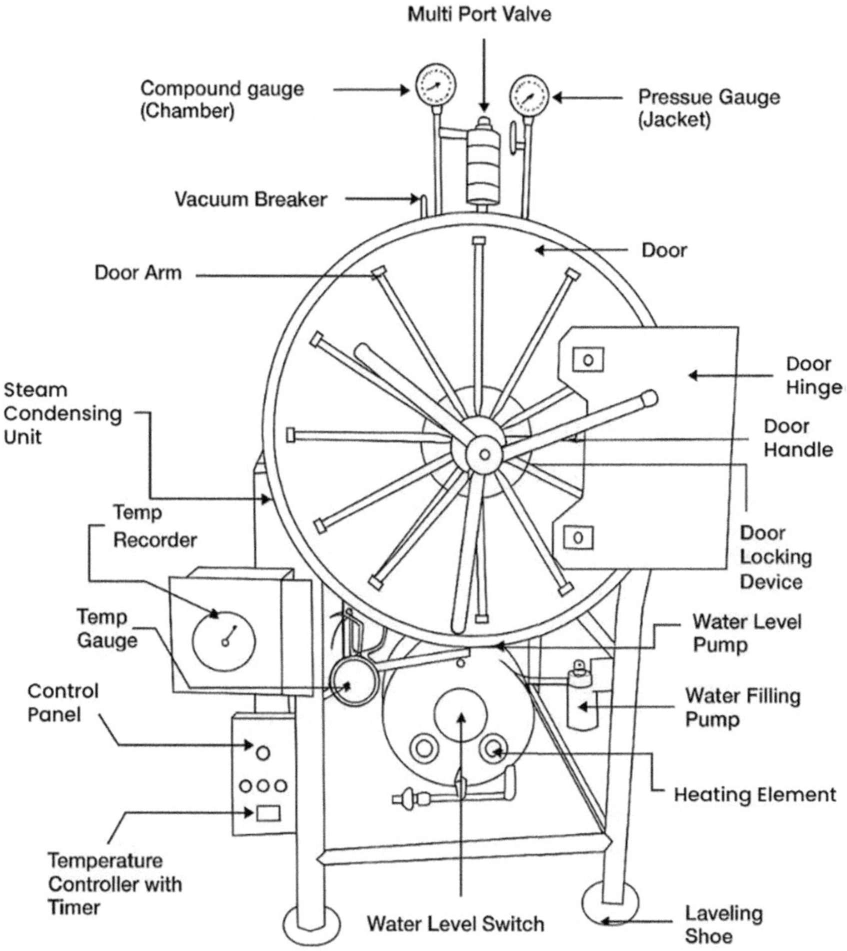

Fig. 42.1 Front of a typical autoclave

42.3.1.2 Compound Gauge (Chamber)

It shows both vacuum and pressure readings inside the main sterilization chamber, ensuring proper operating conditions.

42.3.1.3 Pressure Gauge (Jacket)

Displays the pressure within the jacket space surrounding the main chamber, which helps maintain uniform heat.

42.3.1.4 Vacuum Breaker

Prevents the creation of a vacuum during cooling by allowing air to enter the chamber safely.

42.3.1.5 Door

The main access to the autoclave chamber is where instruments are loaded for sterilization.

42.3.1.6 Door Arm

Supports and enables secure opening and closing of the heavy autoclave door.

42.3.1.7 Door Handle

Used by the operator to open or close the autoclave door manually.

42.3.1.8 Door Hinge

Provides rotational support for the door to swing open or shut.

42.3.1.9 Door Locking Device

A safety mechanism to lock the door during sterilization, preventing accidental opening under pressure.

42.3.1.10 Steam Condensing Unit

Cools and condenses steam after the sterilization cycle, reducing pressure and temperature safely.

42.3.1.11 Temp Recorder

Automatically records the chamber temperature throughout the cycle for documentation and validation.

42.3.1.12 Temp Gauge

A dial-type indicator that shows real-time internal temperature of the autoclave chamber.

42.3.1.13 Control Panel

Contains operational switches, indicators, and status lights used to operate the autoclave.

42.3.1.14 Temperature Controller with Timer

Allows the user to set desired sterilization temperature and duration; ensures precise control.

42.3.1.15 Water Level Pump

Maintains the correct water level within the autoclave for proper steam generation.

42.3.1.16 Water Filling Pump

Supplies water to the autoclave, typically from a reservoir or external supply.

42.3.1.17 Heating Element

Heats the water inside the chamber or jacket to generate the steam required for sterilization.

42.3.1.18 Water Level Switch

A safety sensor that monitors water levels and triggers alerts or auto shutoff if water is too low.

42.3.1.19 Leveling Shoe

Adjustable base feet used to stabilize and level the autoclave on uneven floors.

42.4 Chemical Indicators Used in the Sterilization Process

Indicators were designed to respond to different types of sterilization (Fig. 42.2). Biological indicators are useful for solid and porous instruments and should be placed in each package to allow penetration of the sterilizing agent. They are designed with these indicators to comply with the UNE-ISO 11138 criteria.

Internal Chemical Indicators (Package or Load Control): The best-known internal chemical indicators have been strips printed with different chemical inks; the problem with this type of ink is that interpreting the results is based on a visual color change, and sometimes marginal faults are difficult to distinguish. Chemical integrators cannot be used in place of biological indicators since there is no absolute

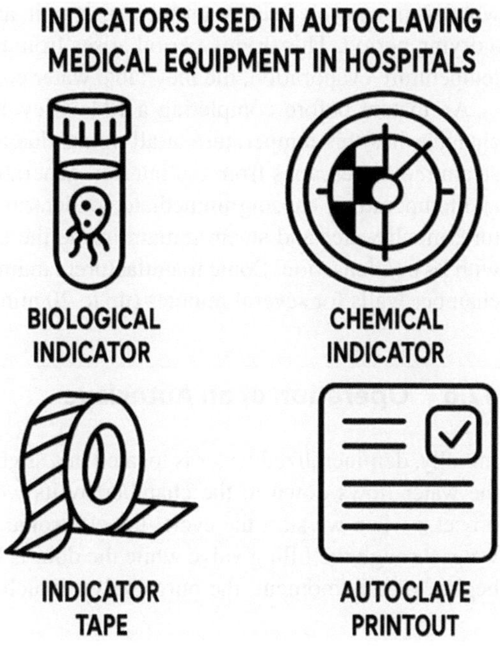

Fig. 42.2 Indicators

agreement between them. These indicators cannot be removed without altering the conditions of sterility, so they are checked at the time of use. If the controls are correct, the autoclave load will be considered correct, and only the affected package will be sterilized again. The chemical indicator should be placed on the part of the package that is considered least accessible to steam penetration.

Another type of autoclave indicator is a biological indicator. These indicators contain a standardized population of resistant bacterial spores, such as Geobacillus stearothermophilus. This bacterium comes in the form of spores in strips or as a suspension in vials. This spore test is used to determine if the sterilization process parameters were sufficient to kill the test microorganisms. This biological indicator is a good test of autoclave success and should be performed regularly. The best practice is to place the biological indicator inside the autoclaved material, preferably in the centre.

42.5 Types of Cycles

The most common cycles that manufacturers incorporate in these machines are:

105 °C cycle, for the disinfection of liquids and delicate objects. Remember that below 120 °C, only disinfection can be discussed, never sterilization. 120 °C cycle, for general sterilization of instruments, gloves, and clinical tissues. 134 °C cycle, for the sterilization of surgical or high-risk material. 143 °C cycle, also called a quick cycle, is mainly used to sterilize instruments that can be used immediately or urgently.

All of these cycles are associated with another cycle called the drying cycle, which is not a cycle itself but rather a part of it, and therefore should be better called a drying period. This drying period arises from the need to eliminate, through mid-temperature evaporation, the inevitable water condensation at the end of the cycle.

An instant before completing a 134 °C cycle, for example, the interior of the chamber has this temperature at all points due to steam. When the cycle ends, the steam rapidly escapes from the interior, generating a very sudden drop in pressure and temperature, causing immediate condensation below 100 °C. At this temperature, much water and steam remain inside the chamber, becoming visibly evident with its condensation. Some manufacturers maintain an elevated temperature of the chamber walls for several minutes (up to 20 min) to evaporate most of this water.

42.6 Operation of an Autoclave

Initially, demineralized water is located in a slightly elevated tank with the goal that the water flows down to the chamber by its weight. Let us assume an automatic process: when we start the cycle, the electronic system allows a certain amount of water through the filling valve while the door is locked. Sequentially, water heating begins. At this moment, the purge valve, which operates thermally, remains open, allowing the hot air to flow through it to the outside. In this way, up to 25% of the interior air can be expelled.

When the water begins to boil at 100 °C, saturated vapor starts forming, gradually leaving the chamber through the aforementioned valve and condensing in the recovery tank. As this entire process is carried out at 1 bar of absolute pressure (0 bar gauge pressure), assuming that is the atmospheric pressure at that moment, as the vapor formed increases, part of the air is also expelled. Once all the water has evaporated, the temperature begins to increase. When it reaches a value above 100 °C, the purge valve (also called the selector) closes, and the pressure gradually starts to rise until it reaches 1 bar on the gauge at a temperature of 120 °C. At this point, the heater begins to reduce its emissions to maintain this pressure. At this moment, the cycle timer starts, which, according to the manufacturer ranges from 8 to 20 min.

Once the cycle is completed, the exit valve opens, allowing the vapor to exit to the recovery tank through a condensation coil. When the pressure reaches an atmospheric level, for some autoclaves, the drying process begins, but for some of them, it is possible to open the door and remove utensils. It is not recommended to rush in opening the chamber since the materials are still very hot, and unwanted condensation is also favored. If a device has a drying phase, it must be completed first.

42.7 Types of Autoclave Sterilization Cycles

Class N Autoclaves The N in this class stands for naked. It is used exclusively for the sterilization of solid products. The sterilized instruments cannot be transported or stored; they must be for immediate use.

Class-B Autoclaves The B in this class stands for big. They sterilize any type of load that can be processed by a large sterilizer: solid, porous, hollow, and all-packed (with single or double layers) materials. They have data processors with mandatory recording of the data.

Class-S Autoclaves The S in this class stands for specific. These sterilizers have cycles defined by the manufacturer, with programs for packed solid, porous, and devices with tubes of specific lengths and diameters. They are devices that usually incorporate a vacuum pump.

42.8 Types of Loads

The types of loads that can be introduced into an autoclave for sterilization are the following:

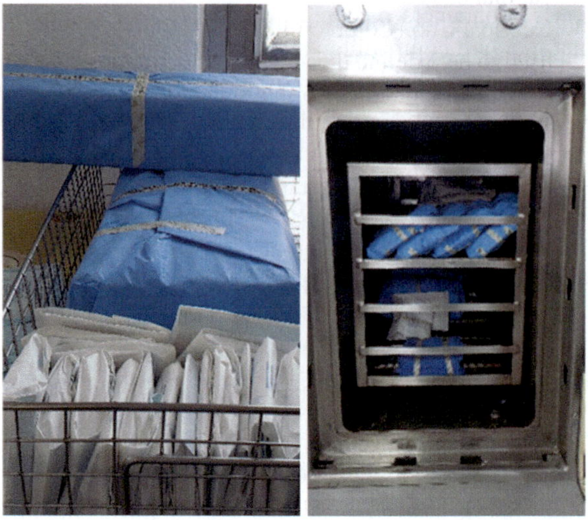

Fig. 42.3 Preparation of load

Solid Load—They are nonporous articles, without slots or fissures, or other features that can obstruct steam penetration into the material. Examples of solid loads are forceps and needle holders.

Porous Load—Material that can absorb fluids, e.g., surgical gowns and gauze.

Type A Hollow Load—An object whose ratio of length of cavity to diameter is greater than 5.

Type B Hollow Load—An object whose ratio of length of cavity to diameter is greater than 1 and less than 5 (Fig. 42.3).

42.9 Special Precautions

Pre-check Before using the autoclave, the interior of the autoclave chamber should be checked in case there is any article left by the last person who used it that might be a danger. Check that the strainer is clean. Check that the door gaskets are not damaged, appear to have no visible defects and are flexible.

Loading Load the autoclave according to the manufacturer's recommendations. Do not overload the autoclave. Do not overload the trays, racks, or baskets and always leaving a space of at least 1 or 2 cm between them.

Use containers prepared to withstand the sterilization temperature and ensure that they are compatible with the autoclave sterilization process. Containers with liquids should be in a heat-resistant plastic tray with about 2.5 cm of water. Containers (bottles, etc.) should not be filled more than 2/3 of their capacity. Keep between 2 and 4 cm of free space between containers. To prevent bottles from exploding during pressurization, the lids of liquid containers should be loosened before loading them into the autoclave. Individual glass parts should be in a heat-resistant plastic tray, on a grate or shelf, never directly on the bottom surface of the autoclave chamber. Check that the autoclave door is completely closed and has a latch in place. Never exceed the maximum pressure of the equipment (as specified in the instruction manual). Also, check before starting the cycle that the correct cycle has been selected for the articles to be sterilized. Do not sterilize or use the autoclave with articles containing corrosive, solvent, volatile, or radioactive materials.

When Opening Do not open the device until the pressure gauge reads zero and the steam valve is open. Use appropriate personal protective equipment (PPE), including thermal contact protection gloves to hold the material if it is at high temperatures, a laboratory coat, eye protection, and closed shoes when opening the autoclave door after a cycle. Use heat-resistant gloves resistant to mechanical hazards if there is a danger of punctures or cuts with sharp/cutting articles.

Once the sterilization cycle is complete, the following considerations must be taken into account, depending on the material to be sterilized:

Solids (instruments). They may lose their temperature quickly by opening the steam valve and emptying the water from the bucket by opening the drain handle slightly.

Liquids (culture media, etc.). Allow them to return to ambient temperature on their own or, as a last resort, open the steam valve slightly. The rapid decompression of liquids causes bottles to break or liquids to spill.

42.10 Periodic Maintenance

Perform equipment maintenance according to the equipment's instructions. Disconnect the power supply before removing the covers. Do not make any modifications to the equipment's wiring. Handling the control element by unqualified personnel can be dangerous. Clean the equipment regularly (preventative maintenance). Clean the drainage filter in the sterilization chamber. Remove any residue collected in it. Clean the sterilization chamber internally, using cleaning agents that do not contain chlorine, as it may corrode stainless steel. Then, wash with plenty of water. Clean the external stainless surfaces with a mild detergent. Eventually, a solvent such as ethylene chloride could be used, taking care to avoid contact with surfaces that have paint coatings, signage, or plastic covers.

Regularly inspect the safety valve and conduct a pressure test. The user should record the test results. Maintain a comprehensive log of all maintenance activities. If an autoclave is found to be malfunctioning, cease its use and prominently display a warning sign to prevent others from misusing it. Inform the manufacturer promptly about the issue and request corrective maintenance. Keep a detailed record of all maintenance performed.

42.11 Troubleshooting

Problem	Possible cause	Troubleshooting/action
The autoclave does not start	Power supply failure Blown fuse	Check power source Replace fuse if needed
Incomplete sterilization	Insufficient temperature/time Overloading	Recheck cycle settings Avoid overloading chamber
Wet packs after the cycle	Improper drying Blocked air vents	Use proper drying cycle Clean air vents
Door not sealing properly	Worn-out gasket Misalignment	Replace gasket Realign door
Pressure is not building up	Leak in chamber Faulty pressure valve	Check for leaks Inspect/replace valve
Unusual noise during operation	Loose components Mechanical failure	Inspect internal components Call for maintenance
Water not heating	Faulty heating element Low water level	Check/replace heating element Refill the water reservoir
Alarm or error codes on display	Sensor failure Software glitch	Refer to the user manual for error codes Restart the system or call the service
Burnt smell or smoke	Electrical short Foreign object inside	Turn off immediately Inspect the chamber and call technician

42.12 Conclusion

Autoclaves play a vital role in maintaining sterility and infection control in hospital environments. Their reliability and efficiency are crucial for ensuring the safety of both patients and healthcare providers. Regular maintenance, proper operation, and prompt troubleshooting of issues are essential to keep autoclaves functioning optimally. As healthcare demands continue to evolve, the integration of advanced monitoring systems and automation will further enhance the reliability of sterilization processes. A well-maintained autoclave is not just a piece of equipment—it is a critical ally in the fight against hospital-acquired infections.

Bibliography

1. https://medical-solutions.com.mx/diferencias-entre-autoclave-y-esterilizador/.
2. Peláez B. Esterilización por gases: óxido de etileno, gas plasma y vapor a baja temperatura y formaldehído. Disponible en: https://elautoclave.files.wordpress.com/2018/04/03-esterilizacisn.pdf.
3. Sociedad de Enfermeras en Pabellones Quirúrgicos y Esterilización. Sistema de esterilización por Plasma de Peróxido de Hidrógeno "Sterrad". Disponible en: http://www.enfermeraspabellonyesterilizacion.cl.
4. Moreno A. Manejo del sistema Sterrad 100S. Disponible en: http://www.hospitalregionaldemalaga.es/LinkClick.aspx?fileticket=m22PqHuC3u0%3D&tabid=459.
5. Herrera W, Montoro J. Eficacia de las intervenciones en esterilización con peróxido de hidrógeno en el aseguramiento de la esterilización del instrumental médico contaminado con priones. Universidad Norbert Wiener; 2018.
6. Muñoz M, Zegarra M. Eficacia del método plasma de peróxido de hidrógeno Sterrad, para optimizar la esterilización de dispositivos médicos termosensibles. Universidad Norbert Wiener; 2018.
7. Dávila G, Reyes A. Eficacia de los dispositivos médicos procesaros en esterilización a baja temperatura con plasma de peróxido de hidrógeno o gas de óxido de etileno. Universidad Norbert Wiener; 2018.
8. https://www.technodomus.com/blog/esterilizacion-2/tecnologia-de-esterilizacion-por-plasma-12.
9. Centers for Disease Control and Prevention (CDC). Guideline for disinfection and sterilization in healthcare facilities. 2008. Ethylene Oxide "Gas" Sterilization. https://www.cdc.gov/infectioncontrol/guidelines/disinfection/sterilization/ethylene-oxide.html. Accedido el 5 de septiembre de 2020.
10. The research was designed and executed by Actionable Research, an independent third-party research firm in conjunction with ChemDAQ™ Inc., a manufacturer of environmental safety monitoring systems. The research sponsor was Advanced Sterilization Products. Todos los datos se recopilaron el equipo de ChemDAQ.

Ethylene Oxide Sterilization

43

Onur Tokoçin

Ethylene oxide (EO) is a flammable-explosive and toxic gas that is odorless and colorless. It is a gas used in the sterilization of instruments sensitive to heat and humidity. Ethylene oxide sterilization is a sterilization process at low temperature (37–55 °C) as compared to the high temperature required in an autoclave.

Ethylene oxide works as a sterilant that reacts with the cell wall and causes irreversible alkalization. It is compatible with many medical materials.

100% ethylene oxide gas or combinations of ethylene oxide with some other gases (HCFC and CO2) can be used. 100% ethylene oxide is flammable and explosive. Since ethylene oxide gas penetrates easily, ventilation is needed at the end of sterilization to remove gas residues on sterile materials.

Before sterilization, the materials must be decontaminated under appropriate conditions, completely disassembled so that the gas can reach all parts of the material to be sterilized, appropriate packaging material must be used, and time, humidity, and temperature must be sufficient.

43.1 Advantages of Ethylene Oxide Sterilization

- All medical equipment and surgical instruments sensitive to heat and humidity can be used.
- Less abrasion on tools.
- Effective against all microorganisms, including spores [except Creutzfeld–Jakob disease (CJD)].
- It penetrates the lumens of packed material and instruments.
- Easy to implement and follow-up.
- Compatible with the majority of medical instruments.

O. Tokoçin (✉)
Department of Emergency Medicine, Arel University Faculty of Medicine, Istanbul, Turkey

J. S. Ahluwalia (ed.), *User Manual for Minimally Invasive Surgical Equipment*,
https://doi.org/10.1007/978-981-95-9019-3_43

- Compatible with sterilization of plastic and lumen instruments.

43.2 Disadvantages of Ethylene Oxide Sterilization

- Sterilization and ventilation time are long.
- Liquids cannot be sterilized.
- Fabric cannot be used as packaging material.
- It is a flammable and explosive gas if not mixed with a flame suppressant.
- May leave toxic residues.
- It is a carcinogen.
- It is expensive.

If ethylene oxide sterilization is to be used, occupational safety and health administration (OHSA) standards should be followed. Within this standard, ethylene oxide levels are also specified for hospital personnel using ethylene oxide as a sterilant and chemical workers using or producing ethylene oxide.

AL "Action Level" Means the concentration of ethylene oxide in air is 0.5 ppm when calculated as an 8-hour time-weighted average.

TWA "Time-Weighted Average" Guarantees that none of the workers will be exposed to ethylene oxide at an airborne concentration of more than 1 particle of ethylene oxide per 1 million airborne particles (1 ppm) when the airborne concentration of ethylene oxide is averaged over an 8-hour time-weighted average.

PEL "Permissible Exposure Limit" Permissible exposure level 1 ppm (8 h TWA).

EL "Excursion Limit" The employer guarantees that no worker will be exposed to more than 5 ppm of ethylene oxide if sampling and averaging over a 15-min period.

43.3 Personal Protection Equipment for Ethylene Oxide

Skin Protection Protective gloves, work apron, boots, or other protective clothing should be worn against the chemical. There should be a safety shower right next to the work area.

Eye/Face Protection Features Chemical-safe goggles. A face shield may also be necessary.

Respirator Have suitable equipment available for use in emergencies such as spills and fires.

43.4 Load Packaging

Proper packaging is crucial to ensure the effectiveness of the sterilization process and maintain the sterility of the items until they are ready to be used. Here are some general guidelines for packing (Fig. 43.1):

1. *Choose Suitable Packaging Material*
   - Use materials that are compatible with ethylene oxide and won't interfere with the sterilization process. Common materials include polyethylene, polypropylene, and Tyvek.
   - Ensure the packaging material allows for the penetration of ethylene oxide and facilitates aeration after sterilization.
2. *Maintain Breathability*
   - Ethylene oxide sterilization requires the penetration of the gas into the packaging to ensure all surfaces of the items are sterilized. Choose packaging materials that allow for breathability.
3. *Proper Sealing*
   - Ensure that the packaging is properly sealed to prevent the entry of contaminants after sterilization. Utilize heat-sealing or other suitable sealing methods based on the packaging material.
4. *Labeling*
   - Clearly label the packaging with necessary information, such as the contents, lot number, expiration date, and sterilization date. Use indelible ink or labels that can withstand the sterilization process.
5. *Documentation*
   - Keep detailed records of the packaging process, including the type of packaging used, the arrangement of items, and any other relevant details. This documentation is essential for quality control and regulatory compliance.

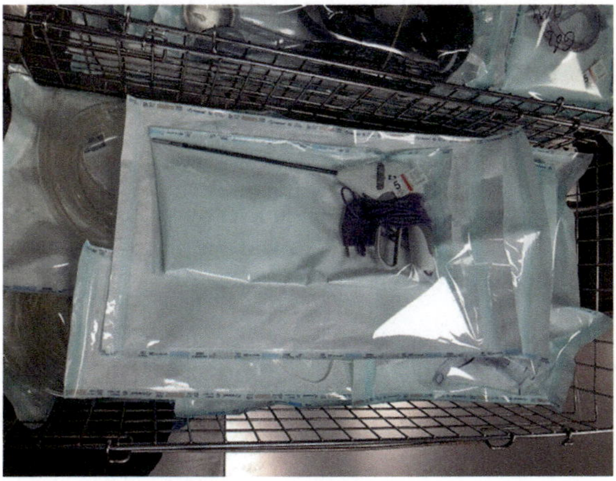

Fig. 43.1 Load packaging

6. *Follow Manufacturer Guidelines*

   - Adhere to the manufacturer's recommendations and guidelines for packaging specific materials or medical devices. Manufacturers often provide instructions on suitable packaging materials and methods.

43.5 Use of the Device for Loading and Unloading

Loading The inner circle of the device is wiped with a damp cloth before each use. If the packages are placed vertically in the basket, they are placed parallel to each other with the plastic sides to the plastic and the paper sides to the paper.

If the packages need to be laid flat, the paper part is placed on the bottom. The chemical and biological indicator package is placed in the center of the load.

Care is taken to ensure that the load in the baskets is not cramped.

Make sure that there is space between the material basket and the sterilizer and that the packages do not touch the inner ring.

Evacuation When the sterilization process is finished and the ventilation process is over, go behind the door of the sterilizer to open it.

Wait for some time (at least 15 minutes) to let any residual gas to evacuate before approaching the load.

The basket is taken out and placed on the table.

The material sterilized with ethylene oxide is transported to the destination with a wheeled trolley.

43.6 Ethylene Oxide Sterilizer Monitoring

It should include physical–mechanical, chemical, and biological controls.

Physical–Mechanical Control Schedule of the program cycle, temperature, pressure, and humidity indicators should be checked at each use.

Chemical Control Multiparameter indicators should be preferred. In each package, a chemical indicator should be placed in the set, and the results should be evaluated before use.

Biological Control The biological indicator agent of choice in ethylene oxide is *Bacillus subtilis* and should be applied every time the device is used (Fig. 43.2).

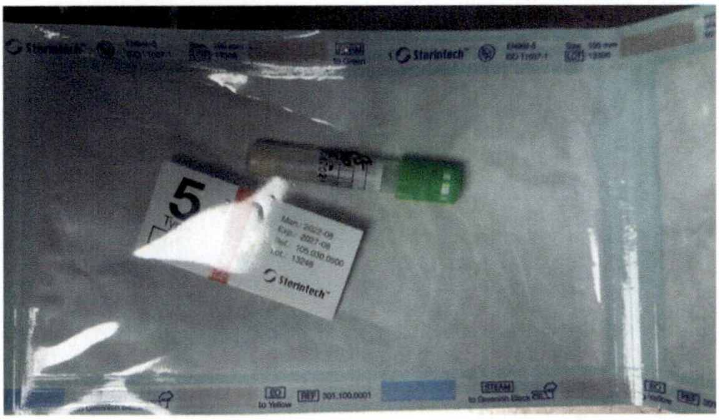

Fig. 43.2 Controls for monitoring sterilization

Documentation Related to Ethylene Oxide Records should be kept on sterilized materials, ethylene oxide workers and monitoring. The hospital management will decide how long the records should be kept.

43.7 Cycle Phases in Ethylene Oxide Sterilization

Most sterilizers follow a structured sequence. Here are the typical cycle steps and sample messages displayed on the touchscreen interface.

1. Preconditioning Phase
   - Purpose: Achieves the required temperature and humidity to prepare for sterilization.
   - Typical message on screen:
   - Phase: Preconditioning.
   - Temp: 55 °C.
   - Humidity: 60%.
   - Time remaining: 30 min.
2. Vacuum Phase
   - Purpose: Removes air to allow better EtO gas penetration.
   - Typical message on screen:
   - Phase: Vacuum.
   - Pressure: minus 60 kilopascals.
   - Pulses: 3 of 3 completed.
3. Gas Injection Phase
   - Purpose: Introduces EtO gas at a defined concentration.
   - Typical message on screen:
   - Phase: Gas injection.
   - EtO concentration: 600 mg/l.
   - Exposure time: 1 h 45 min.

4. Exposure Phase

   - Purpose: Equipment is exposed to EtO gas to achieve sterilization.
   - Typical message on screen:
   - Phase: Exposure.
   - Time remaining: 1 h 15 min.
   - Temp: 55 °C.
   - Humidity: 65%.

5. Evacuation and Aeration Phase

   - Purpose: Removes EtO gas from the chamber and allows safe aeration of equipment.
   - The sterilizer performs a series of vacuum and air pulses.
   - If necessary, equipment may be transferred to a separate aerator.
   - Typical message on screen:
   - Phase: Aeration.
   - Time remaining: 4 h.
   - Temp: 50 °C.

43.8 Unloading

- The cover of the device is never opened before the process is completed.
- Approach the device wearing gloves, protective clothing and an N95 mask.
- The door of the appliance is opened by turning the handle.
- Wait for some time (at least 15 minutes) to let any residual gas escape.
- Baskets are taken out, and materials are brought out of the unit.
- The empty cartridge is removed and disposed of in medical waste.
- The indicator package is taken and inspected.
- The cap of the biological indicator test tube is pressed on while still in the package.
- The biological test is removed from the package, broken with its own apparatus and placed in one of the incubator slots.
- The exposure indicator on each set package and the color change of the chemical indicator in the sterilization bags are checked.

43.9 Toxicology

Studies have shown an increased incidence of cancer in laboratory animals (leukemia, stomach, and brain) and abortions in the human population. Exposure to concentrations of ethylene oxide in air has led to evidence of disruption of genetic material in animals and humans. Hemoglobin alkylation, programmed DNA synthesis, sister chromatid changes, chromosomal aberrations, and functional sperm abnormalities can be observed. Eye contact with the liquid form of ethylene oxide may cause eye irritation, corneal injury, and skin contact may cause severe irritation, frostbite, and blistering. Ingestion may cause gastric irritation and liver damage. Inhalation of ethylene oxide vapors may cause respiratory irritation, lung injury, headache, nausea, vomiting, dyspnea, diarrhea, and cyanosis.

43.10 How to Work Safely with Ethylene Oxide

- Before working with ethylene oxide, it is extremely important that engineering controls are in place, protective material conditions are maintained, and personal hygiene measures are monitored. A combined sterilization/ventilation facility should be used whenever possible.
- Entry to the designated work area must be kept under control.
- Danger warning signs should be posted outside the room.
- Only authorized persons should enter the ethylene oxide area.
- Those entering the ethylene oxide field must have received appropriate training on the hazards and safe handling of ethylene oxide.
- Maintenance and emergency personnel must be informed of the potential hazards. Gas leakage into the work area must be prevented.
- The ethylene oxide device and ventilation cabinets must be in a closed and ventilated area.
- To reduce fire/explosion hazard, cartridges should be stored in a container or storage tank.
- The wheeled trolley used to transport the cylinders should be made of suitable, nonbreakable material.
- All ignition sources (sparks, open flames, and hot surfaces) must be eliminated. Keep away from heat.
- "No smoking" signs should be posted.
- Flammable materials (cardboard, sawdust, etc.) should not be kept in areas where ethylene oxide is used.
- Leaks and ventilation defects should be reported immediately.
- Unprotected persons should avoid contact with material contaminated with ethylene oxide.
- If ethylene oxide is released, wear a suitable respirator immediately and leave the area until the severity of the release is determined.
- In case of leakage or spillage, a contingency action plan and materials should be available to move away from the work area.
- Do not use with incompatible materials such as acids, bases, alcohol, and oxidizing agents.
- The ventilation system in the ethylene oxide work area must use approved, explosion-proof materials and safe electrical systems.
- Consideration should be given to a suitable automatic fire extinguishing system and the provision of leak and fire detection equipment.
- It should be ensured that there are no obstacles to evacuation in corridors and exits.

- Do not weld, cut, join, drill, or do any work that generates heat in empty ethylene oxide tanks, containers, or pipes until you are sure that they have been thoroughly cleaned.
- Before cutting or grounding work in potentially hazardous areas, hard surfaces should be thoroughly wetted to prevent sparking.
- Before intervening in the tanks, they should be checked for leaks.
- During transfer operations, the tanks must be electrically grounded and connected to prevent the buildup of static charges.
- The lid of the tank must not be removed until the tank is safely ready for use.
- Tanks should always be fixed upright to a wall, shelf or other rigid material.
- Tanks should not be intervened with oily hands.
- Tanks should be checked regularly for wear and leakage.
- A suitable pressure regulator must be used.
- Make sure that the material is suitable for the tank pressure and content. The company's recommendations should be followed.
- The precautions in the material safety data sheet (MSDS) must be followed.
- Appropriate emergency supplies should be available for fire and leakage situations.
- The area should be kept clean and well maintained.
- Response equipment should be available.
- Applicable regulations must be complied with.
- An extraordinary action plan to be implemented in case of gas leakage should be kept ready. Drills should be practiced at certain intervals.
- An audible alarm system must be used for the gas level in the ethylene oxide chamber. When the ethylene oxide level exceeds the safety limit, a hand detector should be used in addition to the detection systems that give an audible alarm.

43.11 Maintenance of Ethylene Oxide Sterilizers

Regular maintenance of EtO sterilizers is essential to ensure reliable performance, patient safety, and compliance with regulatory standards. Preventive maintenance should include the following:

- *Routine Inspection*: Check seals, door gaskets, valves, and pressure gauges for wear or damage.
- *Calibration*: Regularly calibrate temperature, humidity, gas concentration, and time controls to maintain sterilization accuracy.
- *Leak Testing*: Perform EtO leak tests frequently to detect and address any gas leakage, ensuring workplace safety.
- *Vacuum Pump and Filters*: Service the vacuum pump and replace filters as recommended by the manufacturer to maintain efficient air evacuation.
- *Sensor Functionality*: Verify and test all sensors (e.g., temperature, humidity, and pressure) for accuracy and responsiveness.

- *Software Updates*: Keep control systems and safety protocols updated as per manufacturer guidance.
- *Documentation*: Maintain a detailed log of all maintenance activities, calibrations, and service interventions for auditing and compliance.

A scheduled maintenance plan, usually semiannual or annual depending on usage, helps prolong equipment life and ensures consistent sterilization efficacy.

43.12 Troubleshooting

Problem	Possible cause	Suggested solution
The sterilizer does not start	Power supply failure or faulty power switch	Check the main power supply, fuses, and switch connections
Cycle aborted mid-process	Door not properly sealed or sensor failure	Ensure the door is fully closed and check the door sensors
Inadequate sterilization	Incorrect temperature, humidity, gas concentration, or exposure time	Verify and recalibrate parameters; check for leaks; ensure load is not overpacked
EtO gas not entering the chamber	Gas cartridge/piping issue or solenoid valve malfunction	Check gas cartridge level, pipeline integrity, and solenoid valve function
Condensation inside the chamber	Poor temperature control or ventilation	Check temperature settings and chamber insulation; improve ventilation
Excessive EtO residue on instruments	Inadequate aeration or improper material selection	Increase aeration time; use only EtO-compatible materials
Alarm sounding repeatedly	Sensor fault or environmental safety breach	Check sensor calibration, EtO leakage; ensure ventilation is adequate
EtO leak detected	Damaged gaskets, seals, or pipe fittings	Replace worn seals and tighten fittings; perform a leak test
Slow vacuum or pressure cycles	Vacuum pump malfunction or filter blockage	Inspect and service the vacuum pump; replace filters
The door will not open after the cycle	Cycle not completed or locking mechanism jammed	Wait for the complete cycle; check the lock mechanism and release override

43.13 Conclusion

Ethylene oxide (EtO) sterilization remains a cornerstone method in hospitals for sterilizing heat- and moisture-sensitive medical devices. Despite its efficacy, the process requires meticulous control of temperature, humidity, gas concentration, and exposure time to ensure sterility without compromising safety. Proper training of personnel, routine equipment maintenance, and adherence to strict safety protocols are crucial to mitigate risks associated with EtO use, including toxicity and flammability. With appropriate handling, EtO sterilization offers a reliable solution for achieving high-level disinfection in modern healthcare settings.

Bibliography

1. ANSI/AAMI ST:79. Comprehensive guide to steam sterilization and sterility assurance in health care facilities. AAMI; 2006.
2. ANSI/AAMI ST41. Ethylene oxide sterilization in health care facilities: safety and effectiveness. AAMI; 2008.
3. Department of Health of the United Kingdom. Health Technical Memorandum 01-01: management and decontamination of surgical instruments: Part B - common elements. NHS England; 2016.
4. Perkins JJ. Growth and death of microorganisms. In: Perkins JJ, editor. Principles and methods of sterilization in health sciences. 2nd ed. Springfield: Charles C Thomas; 1969. p. 56–62.
5. Forsberg K, et al. Quick selection guide to chemical protective clothing. 3rd ed. Van Nostrand Reinhold; 1997.
6. AAMI. Standard for automatic, general-purpose ethylene oxide sterilizers and ethylene oxide sterilant sources intended for use in health care facilities. Arlington: Association for the Advancement of Medical Instrumentation; 1986.
7. ACGIH. TLV® s: threshold limit values and biological exposure indices for 1988–1989. Cincinnati: American Conference of Governmental Industrial Hygienists; 1988.
8. AICHE. Guidelines for hazard evaluation procedures. New York: American Institute of Chemical Engineers; 1985.
9. ASHRAE. ASHRAE handbook: 1985 fundamentals. Atlanta: Society of Heating, Refrigerating and Air-Conditioning Engineers, Inc.; 1985. p. 14.1–14.20.
10. Bollinger NJ, Schutz RH. Niosh guide to industrial respiratory protection. U.S. Department of Health and Human Services, Public Health Service, Centers for Disease Control, National Institute for Occupational Safety and Health, DHHS (niosh) Publication No. 87-116; 1987.
11. Buonicore AJ. In-plant programs to reduce ethylene oxide worker exposure levels. Pharm Eng. 1984;4(4):35–41.
12. CFR. Code of federal regulations. Washington: U.S. Government Printing Office, Office of the Federal Register.
13. Clayton GD, Clayton FE, editors. Patty's industrial hygiene and toxicology, vol. 2a, Toxicology. 3rd ed. New York: Wiley-Interscience; 1978. p. 2186.
14. Federal Register. 48 FR (No. 78): 17297, April 21, 1983. U.S. Department of Labor, 29 CFR, Pan 1910, Occupational exposure to ethylene oxide; proposed rule. Washington: U.S. Government Printing Office, Office of the Federal Register; 1983.
15. Federal Register. 49 FR (No. 122): 25762, June 22, 1984. U.S. Department of Labor, 29 CFR, Part 1910, Occupational exposure to ethylene oxide; final standard. Washington: U.S. Government Printing Office, Office of the Federal Register; 1984.
16. Federal Register. 53 PR (No. 185): 111414–111438, April 6, 1988. U.S. Department of Labor, 29 CFR Part 1910, Occupational exposure to ethylene oxide; final standard. Washington: U.S. Government Printing Office, Office of the Federal Register; 1988.
17. Generoso WD, Cain KT, Hughes LA, Sega GA, Braden PW, Gosslee DG, Shelby MD. Ethylene oxide dose and dose-rate effects in the mouse dominant-lethal test. Environ Mutagen. 1986;8:1–7.
18. Glaser ZR. Special occupational hazard review with control recommendations: use of ethylene oxide as a sterilant in medical facilities. Cincinnati: U.S. Department of Health, Education, and Welfare, Public Health Service, Center for Disease Control, National Institute for Occupational Safety and Health, DHEW (niosh) Publication No. 77-200; 1977.

19. Kercher SL. In-depth survey report: control technology for ethylene oxide sterilization in hospitals at Shriners Hospitals for Crippled Children, Burns Institute Cincinnati Unit, Cincinnati, Ohio, March 18–22, 1985. Cincinnati: U.S. Department of Health and Human Services, Public Health Service, Centers for Disease Control, National Institute for Occupational Safety and Health, DHHS (niosh) Report 1985 (ECTB No. 146-18b), NTIS Publication No. PB-86-123866; 1985.
20. Kercher SL. In-depth survey report: control technology for ethylene oxide sterilization in hospitals at Wooster Community Hospital, Wooster, Ohio. Cincinnati: U.S. Department of Health and Human Services, Public Health Service, Centers for Disease Control, National Institute for Service, Centers for Disease Control, National Institute for Occupational Safety and Health, DHHS (niosh) Report (ECTB No. 146-15b), NTIS Publication No. PB-87-163887; 1985.
21. Kercher SL, Mortimer V. Before and after: an evaluation of engineering controls for ethylene oxide sterilization in hospitals. Appl Ind Hyg. 1987;2(l):7–12.
22. Leidel NA, Busch KA, Lynch JR. Occupational exposure sampling strategy manual. Cincinnati: U.S. Department of Health, Education, and Welfare, Public Health Service, Center for Disease Control, National Institute for Occupational Safety and Health, DHEW (niosh) Publication No. 77-173; 1977.
23. Lynch DW, Lewis TR, Moorman WJ, Burg JR, Groth DH, Khan A, Ackerman LJ, Cockrell BY. Carcinogenic and toxicologic effects of inhaled ethylene oxide and propylene oxide in F344 rats. Toxicol Appl Pharmacol. 1984;76:69–84.
24. Lynch DW, Lewis TR, Moorman WJ, Burg JR, Gulati DK, Kaur P, Sabharwal PS. Sister-chromatid exchanges and chromosome aberrations in lymphocytes from monkeys exposed to ethylene oxide and propylene oxide by inhalation. Toxicol Appl Pharmacol. 1984b;76:85–95.
25. Mortimer V, Kercher SL. In-depth survey report: control technology for ethylene oxide sterilization in hospitals at Bethesda Hospital, Cincinnati, Ohio. Cincinnati: U.S. Department of Health and Human Services, Public Health Service, Centers for Disease Control, National Institute for Occupational Safety and Health, DHHS (niosh) Report (ECTB No. 146-11b), NTIS Publication No. PB-87-164513; 1985.
26. Mortimer V, Kercher SL. In-depth survey report: control technology for ethylene oxide sterilization in hospitals at Bronson Methodist Hospital, Kalamazoo, Michigan. Cincinnati: U.S. Department of Health and Human Services, Public Health Service, Centers for Disease Control, National Institute for Occupational Safety and Health, DHHS (niosh) Report (ECTB No. 146-13b); 1985b.
27. Mortimer VD, Kercher SL. In-depth survey report: modified control technology for ethylene oxide sterilization in hospitals at Community Med Center Hospital, Marion, Ohio. Cincinnati: U.S. Department of Health and Human Services, Public Health Service, Centers for Disease Control, National Institute for Occupational Safety and Health, DHHS (niosh) Report (ECTB No. 146-12c), NTIS Publication No. PB-86-237252; 1986.
28. Mortimer VD, Kercher SL, O'Brien DM. Effective controls for ethylene oxide: a case study. Appl Ind Hyg. 1986;1(1):15–20.
29. niosh. Current Intelligence 35: Ethylene oxide (EtO). Cincinnati: U.S. Department of Health and Human Services, Public Health Service, Centers for Disease Control, National Institute for Occupational Safety and Health, DHHS (niosh) Publication No. 81–130; 1981.
30. niosh. niosh Testimony to the U.S. Department of Labor, Occupational Safety and Health Administration proposed rule: occupational exposure to ethylene oxide. niosh policy statements. Cincinnati: U.S. Department of Health and Human Services, Public Health Service, Centers for Disease Control, National Institute for Occupational Safety and Health; 1983.
31. niosh. niosh manual of analytical methods. Ethylene oxide. Method 1614. Cincinnati: U.S. Department of Health and Human Services, Public Health Service, Centers for Disease Control, National Institute for Occupational Safety and Health; 1987.
32. niosh. niosh manual of analytical methods. Ethylene oxide. Method 3702. Cincinnati: U.S. Department of Health and Human Services, Public Health Service, Centers for Disease Control, National Institute for Occupational Safety and Health; 1987.

33. niosh. niosh respirator decision logic. Cincinnati: U.S. Department of Health and Human Services, Public Health Service, Centers for Disease Control, National Institute for Occupational Safety and Health, DHHS (niosh) Publication No. 87–108; 1987.
34. niosh. Technical report control technology for ethylene oxide sterilization in hospitals. Cincinnati: U.S. Department of Health and Human Services, Public Health Service, Centers for Disease Control, National Institute for Occupational Safety and Health, DHHS (niosh) Publication No. 89–118; 1989.
35. O'Brien DM. In-depth survey report: control technology for ethylene oxide sterilization in hospitals at Euclid General Hospital, Euclid, Ohio. Cincinnati: U.S. Department of Health and Human Services, Public Health Service, Centers for Disease Control, National Institute for Occupational Safety and Health, DHHS (niosh) Report (ECTB No. 146-14b), NTIS Publication No. PB-87-164497; 1985.
36. O'Brien DM. In-depth survey report: control technology for ethylene oxide sterilization in hospitals at St. Francis/St. George Hospital, Cincinnati, Ohio. Cincinnati: U.S. Department of Health and Human Services, Public Health Service, Centers for Disease Control, National Institute for Occupational Safety and Health, DHHS (niosh) Report (ECTB No. 146-17b), NTIS Publication No. PB-86-125200; 1985.
37. Ringenburg VL, Elliott LJ, Morelli-Schroth P, Molina D. Industrial hygiene characterization of ethylene oxide exposures of hospital and nursing home workers. Cincinnati: U.S. Department of Health and Human Services, Public Health Service, Centers for Disease Control, National Institute for Occupational Safety and Health, DHHS (niosh) Report; 1986.
38. Todd WF, Kercher SL, Mortimer VD, O'Brien DM. In-depth survey report: control technology for ethylene oxide sterilization in hospitals at Community Med Center Hospital, Marion, Ohio. Cincinnati: U.S. Department of Health and Human Services, Public Health Service, Centers for Disease Control, National Institute for Occupational Safety and Health, DHHS (niosh) Report (ECTB No. 146-12b), NTIS Publication No. PB-86-116969; 1985.
39. Union Carbide Corporation. Section 8e [Toxic Substances Control Act] report: final report on ethylene oxide two-year inhalation study on rats. Project Report 44-20, Bushy Run Research Center (formerly Carnegie-Mellon Institute of Research), January 28, 1981. Washington: U.S. Environmental Protection Agency, Office of Toxic Substances. Unpublished Report; 1981.
40. World Bank. Techniques for assessing industrial hazards: a manual. Washington: The World Bank, World Bank Technical Paper Number 55; 1988.
41. Zey JN, Mortimer V, Elliott L. Evaluation of ethylene oxide exposures in a hospital sterilization unit. Paper presented at the 1987 All-Ohio Safety and Health Congress and Exhibit, Cleveland, Ohio, April 9, 1987. Cincinnati: U.S. Department of Health and Human Services, Public Health Service, Centers for Disease Control, National Institute for Occupational Safety and Health, DHHS (niosh) Report (ECTB No. 146-12c), ISMS Publication No. PB-86-237252; 1987.

Plasma Sterilization

44

Alpa Morawala and Qurrat Al Ain Atif

Traditional sterilization methods are not always suitable for delicate laparoscopic instruments, leading to the development of advanced sterilization techniques such as plasma sterilization. This chapter explores the technology, advantages, and applications of plasma sterilization in laparoscopic instruments.

44.1 Introduction: Plasma Sterilization for Laparoscopic Instruments

Many laparoscopic instruments are sensitive to high temperatures and moisture, which can limit the choice of sterilization methods. The intricate design of laparoscopic instruments makes it difficult to reach all surfaces with conventional sterilization techniques.

Plasma sterilization is an innovative method used to sterilize medical instruments, including those used in laparoscopic surgery. It uses a low-temperature plasma, typically a combination of hydrogen peroxide and gas, to eliminate microorganisms such as bacteria, viruses, and spores. Plasma sterilization works by creating a unique chemical reaction that disrupts the cellular structure of microorganisms. This mechanism is effective against a wide range of pathogens.

Plasma sterilizers are available globally, and it is imperative to familiarize yourself with their proper usage. Do consult the specific user manual of the sterilizer available at your facility for further understanding. This user manual serves as a comprehensive guide for safe and effective operation of the equipment. It commences with an introduction outlining its purpose, emphasizing its role as a resource for safe and proper usage. The manual highlights a detailed safety measure,

A. Morawala (✉) · Q. A. A. Atif
General Surgery, Barts Health NHS Trust, London, UK
e-mail: A.morawala@nhs.net

J. S. Ahluwalia (ed.), *User Manual for Minimally Invasive Surgical Equipment*,
https://doi.org/10.1007/978-981-95-9019-3_44

including warnings about potential hazards, personal protective equipment (PPE) requirements, and instructions on handling and storing sterilized equipment.

44.2 Equipment Overview (Fig. 44.1)

- Sterilization Chamber: The sterilization chamber is the core of the system where the sterilization process occurs. It houses the instruments to be sterilized. The chamber is typically made of stainless steel or aluminum that are corrosion-resistant and easy to clean. It features secure seals to prevent the escape of gases during the process.
- Vacuum System: The vacuum system is responsible for creating and maintaining the low-pressure environment within the sterilization chamber. A vacuum pump creates the necessary vacuum conditions for plasma sterilization to take place.
- Gas Injection System: This system is responsible for introducing the sterilant gas, often a mixture of hydrogen peroxide and other gases, into the chamber.
- Generator/Power Supply: The generator or power supply produces the plasma used in the sterilization process. Common plasma sources include microwave or radio-frequency generators, which excite the gas to produce plasma.

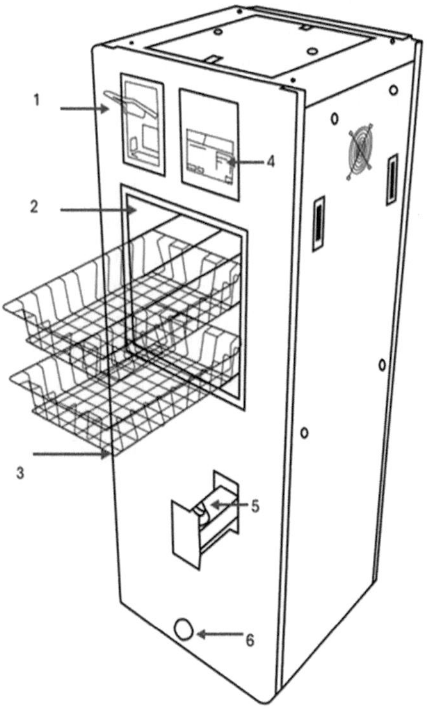

Fig. 44.1 Plasma sterilizer (1) Control system. Thermal printer and USB port for printing cycle information and downloading data. (2) Sterilization chamber/aluminum chamber. (3) Stainless steel drawers for a range of different tools and instruments. (4) Advanced human–machine interface (HMI). (5) Nontoxic H202 sterilizing agent. (6) Vertical sliding door and hands-free opening device

- Control System: The control system manages and monitors the sterilization process, ensuring that parameters are maintained for effective sterilization. Users can select and program sterilization cycles using the control panel.
- Temperature and Pressure Sensors: These sensors monitor temperature and pressure within the chamber, ensuring that conditions remain optimal throughout the sterilization cycle.
- H_2O_2 Vapor Removal System: After the sterilization cycle, a vapor removal system is used to extract residual sterilant gas, ensuring that the sterilized items are safe for handling and use.
- Safety Interlocks and Alarms: These are critical safety features. Interlocks ensure that the system only operates under safe conditions, and alarms notify users of any abnormalities or safety breaches. In case of a safety breach, the system may have an emergency shutdown feature to protect users.
- Advanced Human Interface: The user interface allows operators to select sterilization cycles, monitor the progress, and view critical information. It includes buttons, touchscreens, and displays for user interaction.
- Validation and Compliance Features: These features assist in cycle validation and regulatory compliance.

44.3 System Setup

The setup of a plasma sterilization system is a crucial step to ensure its proper operation and safety. It is essential to follow the equipment manufacturer's specific installation guidelines and recommendations, as different systems may have unique requirements. Regular inspections and maintenance should be performed to ensure that the sterilization system continues to operate safely and efficiently. Ensure that facility's environmental conditions comply with regulatory standards and guidelines for sterilization systems, as set forth by relevant authorities.

44.3.1 Installation

The equipment should be installed in a dedicated, well-ventilated room with sufficient space to accommodate the sterilization system and facilitate access for maintenance. Unlike autoclaves or ethylene oxide-based machines, which often require special piping and connections to water, steam, and for disposal of gas, the plasma sterilizer is usually a "plug-and- play" machine. There are no special drainage or ventilation requirements. It is also worth noting that some plasma sterilizers are built with one-phase electrical supply whereas others are built with three-phase electrical supply. One should provide electric socket accordingly. The installation area should ideally maintain a controlled environment, including temperature and humidity levels that are within the manufacturer's specified range. The installation area should have proper ventilation systems in place. The flooring should be nonporous, easy to clean, and resistant to chemical exposure. Ensure that the equipment is accessible for routine maintenance and service by authorized personnel.

44.3.2 Environmental Requirements

Maintaining specific environmental conditions is critical for the proper operation and effectiveness of a plasma sterilization system. Failure to adhere to these requirements may lead to suboptimal sterilization outcomes or equipment malfunction. For example, the plasma sterilization system typically operates within a specified temperature range. Temperature stability is essential to ensure consistent results. Do not expose the equipment to extreme temperatures that fall outside the specified range, as this can damage system components and affect sterilization efficacy. Some plasma sterilization systems may have specific humidity requirements. Ensure that the relative humidity in the installation area aligns with the manufacturer's recommendations. It is generally advisable to maintain moderate humidity levels. High humidity can lead to condensation within the system, potentially causing damage to electronic components and compromising the sterilization process. Adequate ventilation can help manage humidity. Use environmental monitoring equipment to continuously measure temperature and humidity within the sterilization area.

44.3.3 Ventilation

Even though plasma sterilizers are designed not to emit any harmful by-products, adequate ventilation is essential to manage any potential emissions of sterilant gas during and after the sterilization cycle. The installation area should have effective ventilation systems in place to prevent the buildup of gas concentrations that could pose safety hazards. Implement gas detection and alarm systems to continuously monitor gas levels and promptly notify personnel in the event of gas leaks or emissions. In case of gas leaks or other emergency situations, ensure that the ventilation system can provide rapid gas evacuation and create a safe environment.

44.4 Operating Instructions

44.4.1 Powering On and Off

To safely power on the sterilization equipment, follow these steps:

Ensure the equipment is properly connected to a dedicated power source. Confirm that the emergency shutdown switch is in the "off" position. Switch on the equipment's main power supply using the designated control. Wait for the system to initialize. The user interface may display a start-up sequence or status indicators. Ensure that all safety interlocks are in the correct position to allow equipment operation.

44.4.2 To Power Off the Equipment

Confirm that the sterilization cycle is complete, and the chamber is safe to access. Power down the equipment by using the designated control, typically found on the user interface. Wait for the system to complete the shutdown process. Ensure all indicators show that the equipment is safely powered off.

44.4.3 User Interface

The control panel consist of a touchscreen display, buttons, and indicators. Users can choose sterilization cycles based on the type of equipment and load, and set cycle parameters, including time, temperature, and gas concentration. Users can initiate and terminate sterilization cycles. These display essential information about cycle progress and equipment status. Alert users to any issues, such as safety breaches or cycle abnormalities. It displays messages to help diagnose and address problems.

44.4.4 Selecting Sterilization Cycles

Access the cycle selection feature on the user interface. Choose the appropriate cycle from the available options, considering the load being sterilized. If necessary, adjust parameters like time, temperature, and gas concentration according to the specific requirements. Confirm the selected cycle and parameters before initiating sterilization.

44.4.5 Loading Equipment

Ensure that the sterilization chamber is empty and free of obstructions. Arrange laparoscopic instruments securely within the chamber, avoiding overcrowding. Place instruments in a manner that promotes even gas distribution and effective sterilization. Close and seal the chamber securely according to the manufacturer's guidelines, ensuring all safety interlocks are in place.

44.4.6 Initiating Sterilization Cycles

Once the equipment is loaded and the parameters are set, press the "Start" or "Initiate" button on the user interface. The equipment will initiate the sterilization cycle, which includes vacuum creation, gas injection, plasma generation, and gas removal stages. Follow on-screen prompts and indicators to monitor cycle progress.

44.5 Routine Cleaning and Inspection

Regular cleaning and visual inspections help prevent the accumulation of contaminants and ensure the equipment is in optimal condition. Wipe down the exterior of the equipment with a clean, damp cloth to remove dust and debris. Use a mild, nonabrasive cleaning solution if necessary. Periodically clean the sterilization chamber, focusing on areas where residues may accumulate. Use manufacturer-approved cleaning agents and follow their instructions. Ensure that ventilation components, such as filters or exhaust fans, are free of obstructions and functioning correctly. Conduct visual inspections to identify signs of wear, damage, or corrosion. Pay special attention to gaskets, seals, and electrical connections.

44.6 Preventative Maintenance

Preventative maintenance is essential to maintain equipment performance and safety. Create a maintenance schedule and perform tasks at specified intervals. Calibrate temperature and pressure sensors as recommended by the manufacturer to maintain accuracy. Conduct routine electrical safety checks, including inspections of power cables, plugs, and grounding. Inspect and maintain gas supply components, such as pressure regulators and piping, to ensure proper gas delivery. Regularly test the emergency shutdown system to confirm it functions correctly.

44.7 Replacing Consumables

Replace filters, such as air or gas filters, at recommended intervals to maintain air quality and gas purity. Replace gaskets and seals as needed to maintain chamber integrity and prevent gas leaks. Depending on the system design, components like the RF coils may have a limited lifespan and need replacement per the manufacturer's instructions.

44.8 Troubleshooting

Issue	Possible causes	Troubleshooting steps
Unit not turning on	Electrical faults or power surges Malfunctioning power supply unit	Inspect the power cord and outlet for damage Check internal fuses or circuit breakers Verify correct voltage and current supply
Sterilization cycle failure	Insufficient H_2O_2 Leaks in the chamber Improper loading Inadequate vacuum	Replace H_2O_2 supply Inspect door gasket Arrange instruments optimally Verify vacuum pump operation

(continued)

Issue	Possible causes	Troubleshooting steps
Failure to generate plasma	RF or microwave generator issues Depleted sterilizing agent Chamber contamination	Verify generator Replace H_2O_2 cartridge Clean chamber
Error messages or alarms	Electrical or software malfunction Overheating of components Faulty sensors	Refer to the user manual for error codes Reset the system as per guidelines Clean or realign sensors Contact technical support if unresolved
Slow or incomplete vacuum	Blocked or faulty vacuum pump Leak in the vacuum line or chamber seal	Inspect and clean the vacuum pump Tighten or replace vacuum line connections Check seals and gaskets for leaks
Odor or residue after cycle	Residual hydrogen peroxide Improper aeration phase	Run an additional aeration or drying cycle Ensure the chamber is vented properly and sterilizing agent is used in the correct amount

Formalin Chamber for Laparoscopic Instruments

45

Ferdous Alam and Mukhlesur Rahman Bhuiya

45.1 Introduction

Formalin chamber at ambient temperature is used to sterilize heat sensitive delicate operating instruments like laparoscopes, cystoscopes, air-driven bone saws, electric drills, and wires. It is one of the cheapest and older mode of sterilization. It can provide a high level of disfection (HLD) according to WHO guidelines [2]. Though low temperature steam with formaldehyde (LTSF) has been widely used in health care facilities in Northern Europe for the sterilization of heat-sensitive reusable medical device but formalin chamber is commonly used in rural areas in underdeveloped and developing countries due to low healthcare budget and to reduce health costs.

45.2 Formaldehyde

Formaldehyde comes from the Latin word formica means ant that produces formic acid as a natural defense. It is colorless, toxic, highly soluble in water and commercially available 37%–40% formaldehyde solution with a small amount of stabilizer is called formalin. 10%–12% methanol is added as stabilizer to avoid formaldehyde polymerization. So, a 100% formalin solution is equivalent to 37%–40% formaldehyde. Polymerization of formaldehyde is called paraformaldehyde, which is available in tablet form commercially (Figs. 45.1 and 45.2).

F. Alam (✉)
Department of Surgery, Bangabandhu Sheikh Mujib Medical University, Shahbagh, Dhaka, Bangladesh
e-mail: ferdous697@bsmmu.edu.bd

M. R. Bhuiya
Kumudini Women's Medical College, Mirzapur, Tangail, Bangladesh

J. S. Ahluwalia (ed.), *User Manual for Minimally Invasive Surgical Equipment*,
https://doi.org/10.1007/978-981-95-9019-3_45

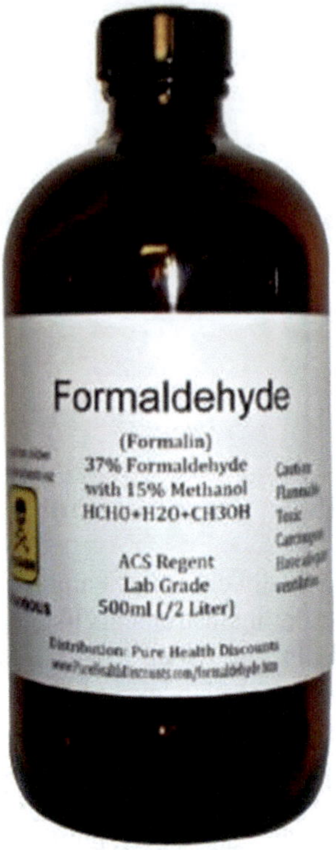

Fig. 45.1 Formalin solution in bottle

$$CH_3OH + \text{HCHO} \rightarrow \text{HCOOH} \rightarrow CO_2 + \text{H}_2\text{O}$$

$$\text{Methanol} + \text{Formaldehyde} \rightarrow \text{Formic acid} \rightarrow \text{Carbon dioxide} + \text{Water}$$

Mechanism of Action: It causes inactivation of microorganisms through the alkylation of the amino and sulfhydryl groups of proteins and of the nitrogenous ring of puric base, resulting alternation in the synthesis of nucleic acids [5].

Spectrum: It has a wide biocidal spectrum (viruses, fungi, TB bacilli, etc.). Its sporicidal action is low at room temperature but acts effectively when it is combined it with heat at temperature of 50–75 °C. This method requires an automated system to avoid and prevent occupational exposure.

Disadvantage: It is extremely irritating to the skin, eyes, nose and respiratory tract. Contacting the product with the conjunctiva can cause permanent injury to the cornea. In very low environmental concentration (between 0.1 to 5 ppm) it can cause irritation to the eye and respiratory tract. In concentrations over 10–20 ppm—It can cause coughing, precordial oppression, tachycardia, and headache. Exposure between 50 and 100 ppm—It can cause pulmonary edema, pneumonia, and death.

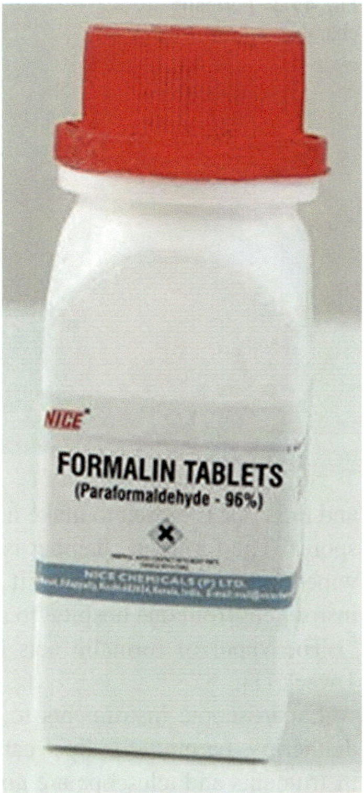

Fig. 45.2 Formalin tablet with container

It has a very pungent odor. It is potentially carcinogenic [3–5]. Occupational exposure precautions should be taken while using it. The permissible exposure limit of formaldehyde is 0.75 ppm in 8 work hours [2].

45.3 Formalin Chamber

Formalin chamber is manufactured with high quality acrylic transparent sheet so that the instruments can be easily viewed. It is lightweight, transparent, corrosion-proof and made from a special grade of polymer with two to three sliding multiple fenestrated trays (Fig. 45.3).

45.4 Procedure of Sterilization in the Formalin Chamber

8–10 formalin (paraformaldehyde) tablets wrapped with moist gauze are placed at the lowermost part of the chamber & sometimes liquid formalin is sprinkled on layers of cotton, and instruments are wrapped in cotton in a sealed box. Heat-sensitive laparoscopic instruments are placed in the upper chamber (as formaldehyde tablet converts to gas within the chamber, which has diffused and effusive characteristics),

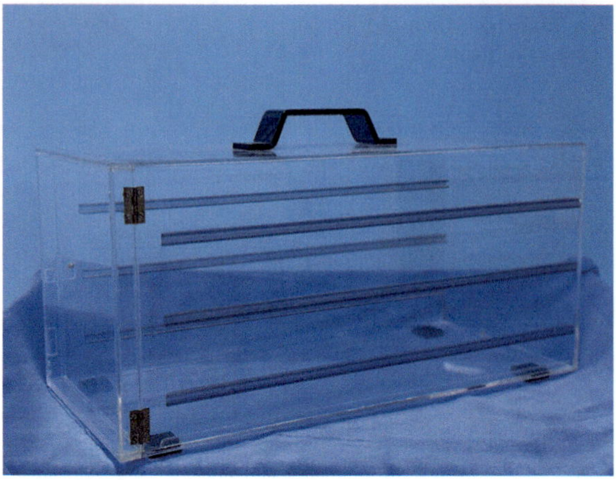

Fig. 45.3 Formalin chamber

and the door is closed to make it air-tight. It takes 12–24 h to be effective in killing spores. The formalin chamber is opened just before surgery, allowing fumes to be wiped out rapidly using fans. It is used by many surgeons to carry their sterilized instrument from one hospital to another.

The vapor of formalin acts for 1 week, and tablets should be changed after 1 week [1].

Laparoscopic instruments to be sterilized are the camera, light cable, tubing, diathermy, harmonic scalpel cable, etc. Rigid metallic trocar, heat-resistant hand instruments and telescope are not recommended as they can be easily sterilized by autoclave and other methods.

In spite of the efficacy of the formalin chamber, it is not recommended now a day as:

1. How many tablets are to be kept is not standardized?
2. How long we have to keep the instruments for exposure is not standardized?
3. What will be the temperature in the chamber is not fixed?
4. How many times can we open the chamber is not standardized?
5. There is a doubt regarding formalin gas leakage from the chamber?
6. Formalin residue can remain on the sterilized goods if the rinsing phase is not 100% efficient. This can be harmful for the patient.
7. Hazards of formalin by itself, as mentioned before.

45.5 Conclusion

At present, formalin tablets are not recommended as they represent a procedure that does not guarantee disinfection or sterilization. Sterilization by low temperature steam with formaldehyde (LTSF) is accepted in countries like the United Kingdom, Germany, Sweden, Denmark, and Norway but not common. In several countries of the world, formaldehyde as a sterilizing agent is discouraged and not approved by FDA.

References

1. Mishra RK. Textbook of practical laparoscopic surgery. 3rd ed. New Delhi: JP Brothers Medical Publishers Ltd; 2013. p. 51–5. ISBN: 978-935025-941-2.
2. Acosta-Gnass SI, Stempliuk VA. Sterilization manual for health centers. Washington, DC: Pan American Health Organization, WHO; 2009. p. 55–95. ISBN: 978-92-75-12926-5.
3. Clark RP. Formaldehyde in pathology departments. J Clin Pathol. 1983;36(8):839–46.
4. Tulis JJ. Formaldehyde gas as a sterilant. In: Briggs Phillips G, Miller WS, editors. Industrial sterilization: international symposium. Durham: Duke University Press; 1973. p. 209–2.
5. Taylor LA, Barbeito MS, Gremillion GG. Paraformaldehyde for surface sterilization and decontamination. Appl Microbiol. 1969;17(4):614–8.

Chemical Sterilization

46

Abd-Elfattah Kalmoush

The elimination of all germs and viruses from an object or product, including all life forms and spore types, is defined as sterilization. Disinfection is a term used to describe a technique that gets rid of most or all harmful germs on inanimate items, with the exception of bacterial spores. Asepsis refers to any actions taken to avoid contaminating instruments or wounds. There are several forms of physical or chemical disinfection and sterilization available. Each one of them must begin by cleaning.

Since we use a variety of laparoscopic devices, some of which are temperature-sensitive, metal, or plastic, there are several techniques that may be used with various instruments [1].

Prior cleaning of an object, organic and inorganic load, type and level of microbiological contamination, concentration and exposure time to germicides, physical characteristics of the object (such as crevices, hinges, and lumens), existence of biofilms, temperature and pH of the disinfection process, and in some cases, relative humidity of the sterilization process (e.g., ethylene oxide) are all elements that can affect the effectiveness of both disinfection and sterilization [2].

46.1 Preparation of Equipment

Instruments must be free of any foreign matter (blood, soil, or anything else), which is typically done using water and another detergent to aid in thorough instrument cleaning. Thus, cleaning is necessary before using any liquid chemical sterilization as well as before using any other sterilizing method. If there is any foreign matter still on the object, liquid disinfectant won't be able to reach the area and the

A.-E. Kalmoush (✉)
General Surgery Department, Faculty of Medicine, Al-Azhar University, Nasr, Cairo, Egypt
e-mail: Abd-ElfattahMorsi.216@azhar.edi.eg

J. S. Ahluwalia (ed.), *User Manual for Minimally Invasive Surgical Equipment*,
https://doi.org/10.1007/978-981-95-9019-3_46

sterilizing procedure won't work properly. Moreover, all equipment should be kept damp until it is cleaned [3].

Friction and fluid under pressure are the two key elements in manual cleaning. Friction is a tried-and-true technique that involves rubbing or scrubbing the stained area with a brush. When brushing is insufficient to remove soil and debris from interior channels, or the design prevents brush passage through a channel, fluid under pressure is utilized [4]. While using a washer-disinfector, caution should be given when loading instruments. Hinged instruments must be fully opened to provide appropriate contact with detergent solutions. Instruments must not be stacked in washers [5].

Due to the fact that these solutions often offer the best material compatibility profile and effective filth removal, neutral or detergent solutions with a pH close to neutral are frequently employed for instrument cleaning. Sometimes neutral pH solutions with proteases added to them help remove organic debris. These formulations' enzymes target proteins, which make up a sizable percentage of typical soil (such as blood, pus). Cleaning solutions may also include amylases and lipases, which are for dissolving starches and fat, respectively. Proteinaceous enzymes can be rendered inactive by a germicide, and enzymatic cleansers do not function as disinfectants. Enzymes must be removed from the equipment, just as with other chemicals, to prevent negative effects on the surgical team and patient [6].

Although in-depth cleaning is essential for high-level disinfection and sterilization, there are no "real-time" tests that can be used in a clinical context to confirm cleanliness. Microorganism identification, chemical detection for organic pollutants, radionuclide tagging, and chemical detection for particular ions can all be used to validate the cleaning procedures in a laboratory testing programme [7, 8].

46.2 Liquid Chemicals

There are indications for sterilizing medical equipment with several liquid chemical sterilants that have received FDA approval. The specified contact times are from 3 to 12 h. With the exception of a few items, the contact duration is determined solely by the requirements to pass the Association of Official Agriculture Chemists (AOAC) Sporicidal Test as a sterilant and not by testing based on simulated usage of devices. In situations where a quicker processing time is needed, such solutions are frequently utilized to achieve a high level of disinfection. Often, a biological indicator cannot be used to monitor chemical liquid sterilants to confirm sterility [9].

While the kinetics for sterilization with liquid sterilants are less well-understood, the survival kinetics of thermal sterilization techniques, such as steam and dry heat, have been thoroughly investigated and defined. According to information found in the literature, sterilization procedures based on liquid chemical sterilants might not generally communicate the same level of sterility guarantee as sterilization accomplished by thermal or physical means. The findings show that the shape of the survival curve might vary based on the liquid sterilant's formulation, chemical make-up, and sterilant's stability, and that the survival curves for liquid sterilants might not display log-linear kinetics. Moreover, the AOAC Sporicidal Test's design does not allow for measurement of the microbiological challenge. As a result, sterilization using liquid chemical sterilants could not guarantee sterility to the same extent as other sterilizing techniques [9].

The accessibility of organisms to sterilants is one of the distinctions between thermal and liquid chemical procedures for the sterilization of equipment. In contrast to liquids, heat can effectively permeate barriers, including biofilms, tissues, and blood, to achieve organism death. Moreover, certain liquid chemical sterilants' viscosity prevents them from reaching microbes on mating surfaces and in tight lumens of devices. The environment in which the device is processed after sterilization with liquid chemical germicides is another drawback. In order to preserve sterility after processing and during storing, devices cannot be wrapped or effectively encapsulated during processing in a liquid chemical sterilant. Moreover, equipment may need to be rinsed with saline after being exposed to the liquid chemical sterilant. Liquid chemical sterilants have intrinsic limits, thus their usage must be limited to reprocessing crucial equipment that are heat-sensitive and incompatible with conventional sterilizing techniques [10, 11].

46.3 Mode of Action

Chemical agent act on microorganism following:

1. Interfering with the enzymatic system
2. Coagulation of protein
3. Disruption of the cell membrane
4. Oxidative damage

Chemical sterilization may be with liquids or gases.

46.4 List of Agents

Liquid
Alcohol
Aldehydes—Formaldehyde and Glutaraldehyde
Phenol
Halogens—Iodine and chlorine
Oxidizing agents—Hydrogen peroxide and peracetic acid
Dyes

Chemical class	Common forms	Mechanism of action	Common uses	Contact time	Benefits	Disadvantages
Alcohols (ethanol and isopropanol)	Solutions (60â€"90%)	Denature proteins and disrupt membranes	Skin antisepsis, small surfaces, and thermometers	15–30 s	Rapid action, no residue, and cheap	Flammable, not sporicidal, and dries skin

(continued)

Chemical class	Common forms	Mechanism of action	Common uses	Contact time	Benefits	Disadvantages
Aldehydes (glutaraldehyde, formaldehyde, and OPA)	Liquid	Alkylates proteins, DNA, and RNA	High-level disinfection of instruments (e.g., endoscopes)	10–30 min (glutaraldehyde); 12 min (OPA)	Sporicidal, effective on all microbes	Toxic fumes, skin/eye irritant, and requires ventilation
Halogens (chlorine and iodine)	Liquids, tablets (e.g., sodium hypochlorite and povidone-iodine)	Oxidize cellular components and denature proteins	Surface disinfection, blood spills, water disinfection, and skin antisepsis	1–10 min (depends on use)	Broad spectrum and inexpensive	Corrosive, inactivated by organic matter, and unstable
Hydrogen peroxide (and peracetic acid)	Liquid, vapor and gas plasma	Oxidative damage to lipids, DNA, and proteins	Surface disinfection, instrument sterilization, and room fumigation	10–30 min	Sporicidal and eco-friendly by-products	Corrosive at high concentrations and eye/skin irritant
Phenolics (e.g., cresols and hexachlorophene)	Liquids and sprays	Disrupt cell walls and precipitate proteins	Environmental cleaning, noncritical items	10–30 min	Stable and residual activity	Toxic if absorbed and not for neonatal use
Quaternary ammonium compounds (QACs)	Liquids, sprays and wipes	Disrupt membranes and denature proteins	Low-level disinfection: Floors, furniture, and walls	10 min	Noncorrosive, pleasant odor	Limited action on spores, TB, and some viruses

46.5 Alcohol

There are different types of alcohol used in sterilization such as isopropanol (70%), propanol (60%), and ethanol (80%).

These alcohols are tuberculocidal, fungicidal, and virucidal but do not kill bacterial spores. They are also fast bactericidal rather than bacteriostatic against vegetative forms of bacteria. The ideal bactericidal concentration is 60%–90% solutions in water (volume/volume), and their cidal action declines significantly below 50% concentration [12].

Alcohol's ability to kill bacteria is most likely attributed to its ability to denaturate proteins. Absolute ethanol is less bactericidal than alcohol and water solutions since proteins denature more rapidly in the presence of water [12].

Alcohols work well against bacteria and fungi, but not so well against viruses. They fail to eradicate bacterial spores. The primary uses of alcohols are for surgical and sanitary hand and skin disinfection due to their quick action and skin compatibility.

Drawbacks: Their effect is not long-lasting (no depot effect), lack of sporicidal action, and they cannot penetrate protein-rich materials [13].

46.6 Formaldehydes

It has a strong antibacterial effect and works against spores. It can be utilized as a liquid or gas.

The Mechanism of Action: By alkylating the amino and sulfhydral groups of proteins and the ring nitrogen atoms of purine bases, formaldehyde inactivates bacteria. It is a multipurpose germicide that works against bacteria, fungi, and viruses. Moreover, spores are destroyed at greater concentrations [13].

Use: It is used to cleanse rooms and preserve antimicrobial specimens.

Paraformaldehyde tablets are being used for the reduction of the bacterial population and the storage of nonwrapped sterilized instruments. For this purpose, 1 tablet/dm3 is needed. The exposure time required for bacterial count reduction is no less than 3 h.

Formaldehydes can cause severe respiratory and skin irritation and have been linked to carcinogenesis, and hence their use is now being restricted in hospitals.

46.7 Glutaraldehyde

It is used as a 2% buffer solution. Although glutaraldehyde aqueous solutions are acidic, they are often not sporicidal under these conditions. The solution doesn't become sporicidal until it is "activated" (made alkaline) to a pH of 7.5–8.5 using alkalinizing chemicals. Since glutaraldehyde molecules polymerize at alkaline pH values, these solutions, once activated, have a shelf life of about 2 weeks.

Mechanism of Action: Sulfhydryl is alkylated, which changes the production of RNA, DNA, and proteins. Extremely poisonous yet less so than formaldehyde against bacteria.

Glutaraldehyde exists in a number of different forms in aqueous solution, such as hemiacetal and aldol ring structures as well as large α-, β-unsaturated polymers containing carbon–carbon double bonds.

A contact time of at least 20 min is needed to have a high level of disinfection. Sterilization requires a 10-h contact time and higher concentration of glutaraldehyde (e.g., Cidex Plus which contains 3.4% gluteraldehyde).

One of the new replacements for glutaraldehyde in high-level liquid disinfection is OPA, o-phthalaldehyde. OPA shares many chemical similarities with glutaraldehyde and has similar toxicity, but the lower vapour pressure reduces the smell and vapor concentrations.

CIDEX OPA is very effective against a wide range of microorganisms, has a near-neutral pH level, and its character is a clear, pale blue liquid with a pH of 7.5. It contains 0.55% ortho-phthalaldehyde in an aqueous base containing buffers, chelating agents, and a corrosion inhibitor. This solution is ready to use right from the bottle and does not require activation or mixing.

The steps to use glutaraldehyde are as follows:

- Wear personal protective equipment.
- Clean the medical instruments prior to dipping them in solution.

- Dip the instruments entirely into the liquid for the desired time as prescribed by the manufacturer.
- Please note that the time for high-level disinfection and sterilization will be different.
- Rinse the instruments properly with sterile water or saline and make sure no glutaraldehyde is left behind.
- Dry the instruments.
- Dispose of used solution as per manufacturer guidelines.

Use: Glutaraldehyde is one of the most frequently employed as a powerful disinfectant for laparoscopic instruments in-between cases due to its short contact time for high-level disinfection. Glutaraldehyde is not corrosive to metals and does not harm rubber, plastics, or instruments with lenses.

Effective against viruses, fungi, and tubercle bacilli [14].

46.8 Phenols

The mechanism of action is bacterial cell membrane damage resulting in lysis.

Types of phenols are commonly used in hospitals and their uses [15]:

Type of phenol	Uses in hospitals
Phenol (carbolic acid)	Used in low concentrations as a disinfectant and antiseptic for surfaces and instruments.
Chloroxylenol	Antiseptic for skin disinfection, handwash formulations, and surgical scrubs.
Hexachlorophene	Used in antimicrobial soaps and preoperative skin preparations (limited use due to toxicity).
Cresols	Disinfecting hospital floors, toilets, and noncritical equipment.
Thymol	Occasionally used in mouthwashes and topical antiseptics due to antifungal and antibacterial properties.
Orthophenylphenol	Surface disinfectant in hospitals; effective against bacteria and fungi.
Triclosan (phenolic derivative)	Found in antibacterial soaps, though use has declined due to resistance concerns.

46.9 Halogens

46.9.1 Iodine

Iodine and iodophors are widely used antiseptic agents in medical practice due to their broad-spectrum antimicrobial activity. Iodine is a potent oxidizing agent that kills bacteria, viruses, fungi, and even some spores by disrupting protein and nucleic acid structure through oxidative damage. However, elemental iodine in its pure form is irritating to the skin and mucosa, stains tissues, and has limited solubility. To overcome these drawbacks, iodophors such as *povidone-iodine* were developed. These are complexes of iodine with a solubilizing carrier (e.g., polyvinylpyrrolidone), which slowly release free iodine, reducing toxicity while maintaining antimicrobial effectiveness. Iodophors are commonly used for *preoperative skin preparation*, *wound cleansing*, *vaginal douching*, and *disinfection of mucous membranes*. They are generally well-tolerated, but caution is advised in individuals with iodine sensitivity or thyroid disorders [16].

46.9.2 Chlorine

Chlorine is a highly reactive, greenish-yellow gas at room temperature, known for its strong oxidizing properties. In medical and healthcare settings, chlorine is most commonly used in the form of *sodium hypochlorite* solutions (commonly referred to as bleach). It is an *effective and broad-spectrum disinfectant*, capable of killing bacteria, viruses, fungi, and even resistant spores at appropriate concentrations. Its action is based on the release of *free chlorine*, which denatures microbial proteins and disrupts essential enzymatic functions. Due to its *low cost and rapid antimicrobial action*, chlorine is widely used for *disinfecting hospital surfaces*, decontaminating *blood and body fluid spills*, sterilizing *laundry* from isolation wards, and even in *emergency water purification*. A typical concentration for general surface disinfection is 0.5%–1%, while a stronger 1:10 dilution of household bleach is recommended for spills involving blood or high-risk fluids. However, chlorine solutions are *corrosive*, can *irritate skin and mucous membranes*, and lose potency rapidly, especially when exposed to light and air, thus requiring *fresh preparation and cautious handling* [15].

46.10 Oxidizing Agents

46.10.1 Hydrogen Peroxide

By generating harmful hydroxyl free radicals, hydrogen peroxide is able to destroy DNA, membrane lipids, and other vital cell constituents. In greater concentrations, it destroys all organisms, including spores [17].

Uses: 3%–6% is used to clean endoscopes and soft lenses.

For plasma sterilization, use 6%–7.5% H2O2.

46.10.2 Peracetic Acid

Mode of Action: Proteins are denatured, cell wall permeability is disrupted, and proteins, enzymes, and other metabolites' sulfhydral and sulphur linkages are oxidized [18].

Microbicidal activity. At a concentration of 100 ppm, peracetic acid inactivates gram-positive and gram-negative bacteria, fungi, and yeasts in about 5 min.

200–500 ppm are needed when organic stuff is present. The dose range for viruses is vast (12–2250 ppm), with 1500–2250 ppm inactivating the poliovirus in yeast extract in 15 min. Bacterial spores in suspension are rendered inactive at 500–10,000 ppm (0.05%–1%) in 15 s to 30 min.

Use: Automated devices use peracetic acid to chemically sterilize medical and surgical devices (such as endoscopes and arthroscopes) [19].

46.11 Dyes

Aniline dye and acridine dye both have mild bactericidal effects but are bacteriostatic at high concentrations.

Gram +ve bacteria are more susceptible to aniline dye than gramme –ve bacteria.

Crystal violet, dazzling green, and malachite green are aniline dyes.

Proflavine, acriflavine, euflavine, and aminacine are acridine dyes.

46.12 Conclusion

Chemical disinfectants and sterilants play a critical role in infection prevention and control within hospital environments. Their selection and application depend on several factors, including the nature of the item or surface to be treated, the level of disinfection required (low, intermediate, or high), and safety considerations for both patients and healthcare workers. Each chemical class has its own advantages and limitations—while some provide rapid and broad-spectrum activity (like alcohols and halogens), others are better suited for sterilizing delicate instruments (such as ethylene oxide and glutaraldehyde). Understanding the mechanism of action, appropriate contact times, and potential hazards associated with each agent ensures effective disinfection while minimizing risks. An informed, evidence-based approach to the use of these agents is essential for maintaining a safe and sterile hospital environment.

References

1. Ratula WA, Weber JA. The healthcare infection control practices advisory committee (HICPAC). Guidelines for disinfection and sterilization in health care facilities. Atlanta: CDC; 2008.
2. Mathur P. Hospital acquired infections prevention and control. 1st ed. Philadelphia: Lippicott Williams & Wilkins; 2010.
3. Alfa MJ, Nemes R, Olson N, Mulaire A. Manual methods are suboptimal compared with automated methods for cleaning of single-use biopsy forceps. Infect Control Hosp Epidemiol. 2006;27:841–6.
4. Loukili NH, Zink E, Grandadam S, Bientz M, Meunier O. Effectiveness of detergent-disinfecting agents on Escherichia coli 54127 biofilm. J Hosp Infect. 2004;57:175–8.

5. Baxter RL, Baxter HC, Campbell GA, et al. Quantitaive analysis of residual protein contamination on reprocessed surgical instruments. J Hosp Infect. 2006;63:439–44.
6. Murdoch H, Taylor D, Dickinson J, et al. Surface decontamination of surgical instruments: an ongoing dilemma. J Hosp Infect. 2006;63:432–8.
7. Dancer SJ. How do we assess hospital cleaning? A proposal for microbiological standards for surface hygiene in hospitals. J Hosp Infect. 2004;56:10–5.
8. Alfa MJ, Nemes R. Manual versus automated methods for cleaning reusable accessory devices used for minimally invasine surgical procedures. J Hosp Infect. 2004;58:50–8.
9. Favero MS. Sterility assurance: concepts for patient safety. In: Rutala WA, editor. Disinfection, sterilization and antisepsis: principles and practices in healthcare facilities. Washington, DC: Association for Professional in Infection Control and Epidemiology; 2001. p. 110–9.
10. Rutal WA, Weber DJ. New developments in reprocessing semicritical items. Am J Infect Control. 2013;41:S60–6. [PubMed] [Google Scholar].
11. Sattar SA, Adegbunrin O, Ramirez J. Combined application of simulated reuse and quantitative carrier test to assess high-level disinfection: experiments with an accelerated hydrogen peroxide-based formulation. Am J Infect Control. 2002;30:449–57.
12. Ali Y, Dolan MJ, Fendler EJ, Larson EL. Alcohols. In: Block SS, editor. disinfection, sterilization, and preservation. Philadelphia: Lippincott Williams & Wilkins; 2001. p. 229–54.
13. Occupational Health and Safety Administration. OSHA fact sheet: formaldehyde: occupational safety and health administration. U.S. Department of Labor; 2002.
14. Scott EM, Gorman SP. Glutaraldehyde. In: Block SS, editor. Disinfection, sterilization, and preservation. Philadelphia: Lippincott Williams & Wilkins; 2001. p. 361–81.
15. Kayser FH, Bienz KA, Eckert J, Zinkernage RM. Medical microbiology principles of sterilization and disinfection. Thieme; 2005. p. 34–42.
16. Rutala WA, Weber DJ. The benefits of surface disinfection. Am J Infect Control. 2004;32:226–31.
17. Dettenkofer M, Wenzler S, Amthor S, Antes G, Motschall E, Daschner FD. Does disinfection of environmental surfaces influence nosocomial infection rates? A systematic review. Am J Infect Control. 2004;32:84–9.
18. Block SS. Peroxygen compounds. In: Block SS, editor. Disinfection, sterilization, and preservation. Philadelphia: Lippincott Williams & Wilkins; 2001. p. 185–204.
19. Malchesky PS. Medical applications of peracetic acid. In: Block SS, editor. Disinfection, sterilization, and preservation. Philadelphia: Lippincott Williams & Wilkins; 2001. p. 979–96.

Part V

Robotic Surgery

Da Vinci System

47

Hany Takla

47.1 Background/Introduction

The da Vinci Surgical System, created by Intuitive Surgical Inc., is widely recognized as the leading platform for robotic-assisted minimally invasive surgery, with over 10,600 systems operating in more than 69 countries [1]. The company was founded in 1995 by Dr. Frederick Moll, Rob Younge, and John Freund and released the first version of the da Vinci system in 1998. FDA approval was granted in 2000 for general surgery applications and in 2001 for urologic and thoracic surgery applications [2].

The da Vinci system is used in general, thoracic, urologic, gynecologic, colorectal, and head and neck surgery applications, with over 17 million operations performed till 2024 [1].

Compared to traditional laparoscopic surgery, the da Vinci system has two significant technological advantages: A three-dimensional endoscope with integrated fluorescence capability and EndoWrist surgical instruments that allow for 7 degrees of freedom of motion at each instrument tip. These features enable improved exposure and manipulation of the operative field [3]. Additional advantages of the da Vinci system will be discussed in relevant sections later in this chapter.

There are currently several da Vinci model systems in use globally, including the da Vinci Si, X, and Xi, DV5 as well as special use-case models such as the single-port access da Vinci SP. For the purpose of this chapter we are only discussing the daVinci Xi platform. Each system uses the same framework of components: a surgeon console, a patient cart, and a vision cart. The patient cart, parked next to the operating table and patient, allows for docking of EndoWrist instruments and the endoscope into any of the four available robotic arms. The surgeon console provides

H. Takla (✉)
Orlando Health Weight Loss and Bariatric Surgery Institute, Orlando Health, Orlando, FL, USA

J. S. Ahluwalia (ed.), *User Manual for Minimally Invasive Surgical Equipment*,
https://doi.org/10.1007/978-981-95-9019-3_47

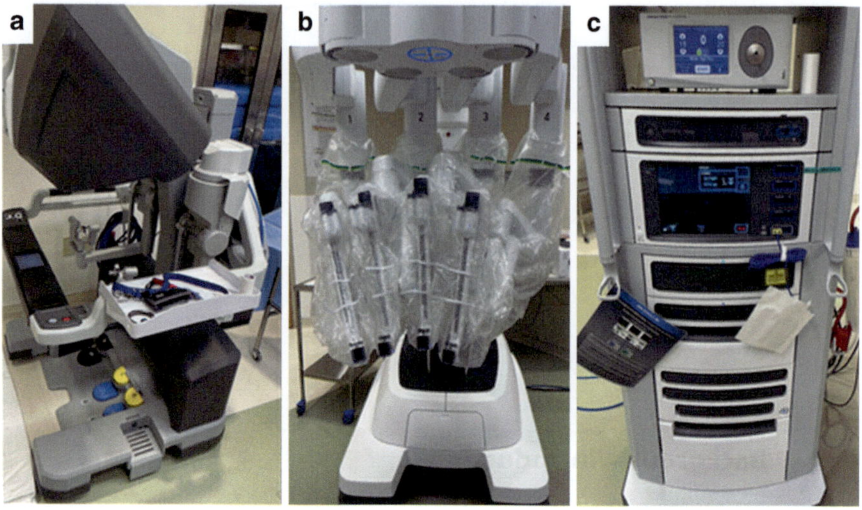

Fig. 47.1 (**a**) Surgeon console; (**b**) Patient cart with sterile covers applied to arms; (**c**) Vision cart housing the electrocautery and image processing systems. Out of frame, an adjustable monitor allows staff at the patient's bedside to view the surgical field

the operating surgeon with a three-dimensional view of the surgical field, and master hand controls allow the surgeon to manipulate both the docked instruments and camera on the patient cart. Finally, the vision tower provides a view of the surgical field to the operating room staff at the patient's bedside and houses the video processing and electrosurgery systems. This chapter will briefly overview each component of the da Vinci Xi model (Fig. 47.1).

47.2 Da Vinci Subsystems: Surgeon Console

The surgeon console is placed away from the sterile field, allowing the surgeon to view the surgical field and manipulate up to three surgical instruments and the endoscope. Major components of the surgical console are labeled in Fig. 47.2. The surgeon console provides several electronic controls to adjust the position of the 3D viewer, armrest, and foot switch panel according to the surgeon's preference. These ergonomic settings can be saved to a user's profile, which may be created using the touchpad on the armrest. In addition to position settings, user profiles will also keep users' camera, sound, microphone, tremor reduction, motion-scaling, and instrument power preferences.

Once the surgeon console is ergonomically fitted to the surgeon, the surgeon can view the operating field by looking through the binocular lenses of the 3D viewer. Because of the incorporation of two cameras in the da Vinci endoscope, separate offset video feeds are transmitted to the left and right lenses of the surgeon console, enabling depth perception. Thus, a three-dimensional view of the operating field is

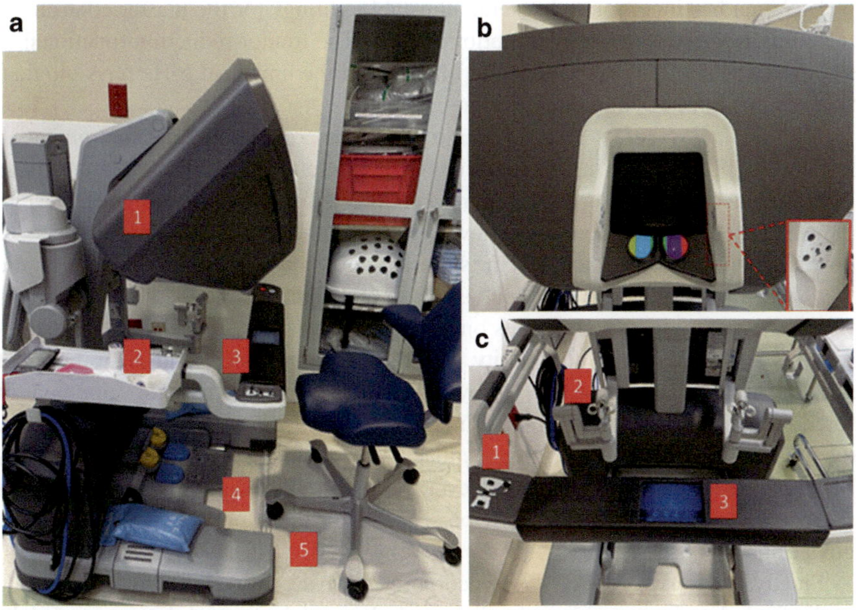

Fig. 47.2 (**a**) Side-view of the surgeon console. (**A-1**) 3D viewer; (**A-2**) Side table; (**A-3**) Armrest; (**A-4**) Footswitch panel; and (**A-5**) Surgeon's chair. Placing a spare towel or blanket underneath the rollers reduces extraneous chair movement. (**b**) Frontal aspect of the 3D viewer. On either side of the surgeon's head are speakers and a microphone, allowing for easy communication between the surgeon and OR staff. (**c**) Armrest and controls; (**C-1**) Ergonomic controls; (**C-2**) Hand controls; and (**C-3**) Touchpad controls

created utilizing two two-dimensional screens. Finally, communication between the surgeon and the other operating room staff is made possible via the placement of a microphone and speakers next to the surgeon's head.

As mentioned previously, the armrest lies beneath the 3D viewer and houses ergonomic controls and a central touchpad. While viewing through the binocular lenses, the surgeon's elbows or forearms should rest comfortably on the armrest to avoid shoulder and upper back fatigue. The surgeon console's power and emergency shutdown controls are also located on the armrest for ease of access.

Beyond the armrest under the 3D viewer are the master controllers floating in an open space bordered by guard rails. The placement of the master controllers relative to the 3D viewing lenses is intended to simulate the natural orientation of the user's eyes and hands. The surgeon can move EndoWrist instruments docked at the patient cart by grasping each controller with their index or middle finger and thumb. "Pinching" the thumb and index finger together will allow for grabbing the tissue with a grasper instrument or cutting the tissue when scissors are docked. Additionally, a clutch mechanism can be engaged on each master controller to allow the surgeon to reposition their hands under the 3D viewer without moving the docked surgical instruments inside the patient.

Da Vinci has incorporated several adjustable settings for the master controllers, including tremor reduction and motion scaling. The tremor reduction functionality stabilizes the surgical instruments by filtering out the universal 6-Hz physiological tremor, thus minimizing unintended movements.

Motion-scaling refers to the relative movement of the surgical instrument in response to the user moving the master controller a set distance. These features have been shown to enhance surgeon accuracy and precision while operating [4]. Despite the utility of these functionalities, however, one of the most challenging aspects of operating with the da Vinci system is the lack of haptic feedback. Without haptic feedback, a surgeon solely relies on visual cues from the operative field to assess the forces exerted by their instruments onto tissues. Developing a gestalt of these cues requires a high degree of familiarity with the da Vinci system and many hours of robotic surgery experience [5–7]. However more recently with the development of force feedback instruments in Da Vinci DV5 system, this issue has largely been overcome. The discussion of force feedback instruments benefits and capabilities is beyond the scope of this chapter however it does provide an additional depth to the surgeon's experience, adding a new perspective for the experienced as well as the novice surgeon.

Finally, the foot plate (Fig. 47.3) incorporates two sets of pedals. On the right side of the foot plate are two pairs of yellow and blue pedals, termed the energy pedals. The rightmost set of energy pedals controls and activates the energy modes of the surgical instrument controlled by the right master controller. Likewise, the left pair of pedals control the energy activation of the instrument controlled by the left master

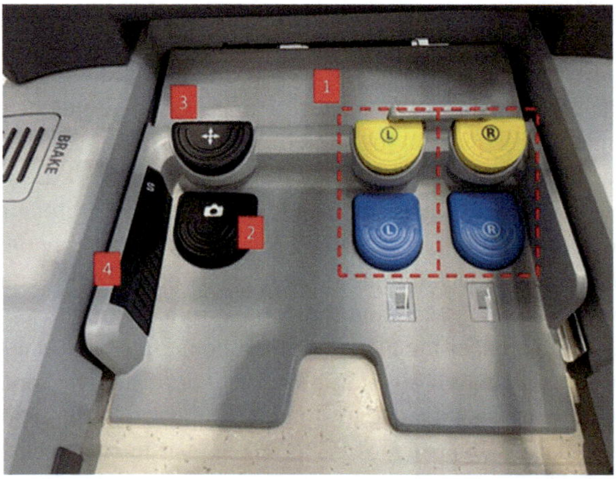

Fig. 47.3 (**1**) Left and right pairs of energy pedals. Blue and yellow pedals initiate the primary and secondary energy modes, respectively, for the corresponding instrument. (**2**) Camera pedal. Allows the surgeon to switch the master controllers from the surgical instruments to the camera. (**3**) Master clutch: Disengages the master controllers. (**4**) Kickplate: Allows the surgeon to switch which arms are being manipulated by the master controllers

controller. The blue and yellow pedals within each pair correspond to the instrument's primary and secondary energy modes, respectively. For example, for grasper EndoWrist instruments, pressing the blue pedal will activate coagulation-mode electrocautery, and pressing the yellow pedal will activate cut-mode electrocautery. However, depending on the instrument being utilized, these functions may change—the daVinci EndoWrist and Sureform stapler instruments uses the blue pedal to first clamp tissue and the yellow pedal to fire the stapler and transect the tissue between the stable lines.

There are three additional pedals on the left side of the foot switch. Pressing and holding the pedal denoted with a camera will allow the master controllers to move the endoscopic camera. Pulling in with the master controllers will instruct the camera to zoom in, and pushing away will cause the camera to zoom out. The button with the four cardinal arrows is the master clutch, allowing the surgeon to completely decouple the master controllers from the surgical instruments, allowing for repositioning of the surgeon and the camera to a more comfortable or advantageous position. Lastly, the left kick-plate pedal allows the surgeon to change which two out of the four arms they are currently controlling with the master controllers.

47.3 Da Vinci Subsystems: Patient Cart

The patient cart is the operative component of the da Vinci system, comprising the instrument and camera arms controlled by the surgeon console. The patient cart is part of the sterile field, and the arms of the patient cart must be sterilely draped prior to the start of the procedure. An integral aspect of the da Vinci system is the incorporation of a remote centre into each of the patient cart arms. This remote center serves as the fulcrum around which the arm of the patient cart moves the docked instrument, resulting in minimal stress on the patient's abdominal wall and less post-procedural pain.Once all instrument cannula is inserted into the patient, the patient cart should be docked at the side of the operating table. The patient cart will recommend a suggested orientation based on the type of the procedure being performed. The boom containing all instrument arms can be rotated over the patient. To ensure proper positioning of the boom and patient cart, the boom emits laser crosshairs, which should, in most cases, be centered on the endoscope camera port.

While the surgeon primarily interacts with the surgeon console, a second assistant must be available at the patient cart to switch instruments and perform other patient-side activities such as specimen collection (Fig. 47.4). Additionally, the arms of the patient cart may collide during the procedure. If this occurs, the assistant can utilize several clutch controls on each arm in order to obtain more clearance.

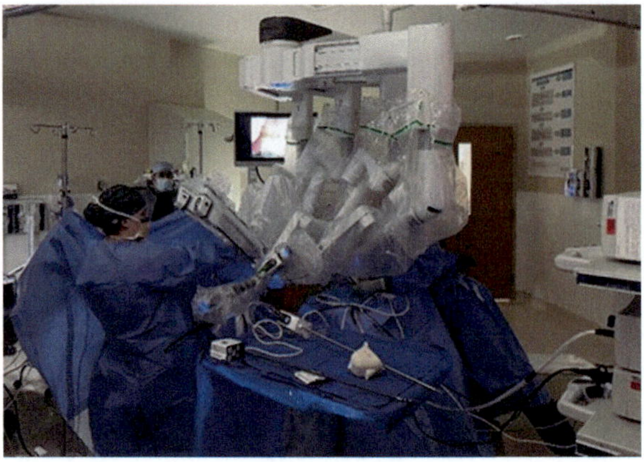

Fig. 47.4 The second assistant, often the scrub technician, performs patient-side activities such as docking the patient cart arms, switching instruments, providing mesh or suture materials for the surgeon, and removing specimens. Again, the assistant can view the operative field using either the vision cart monitor or extra monitors

47.4 Da Vinci Subsystems: Vision Cart

The vision cart (Fig. 47.1c) houses advanced vision and energy technologies and allows the da Vinci's system components to communicate. Atop the tower, there is a large two-dimensional high-definition display in which members of the operative team can view the procedure, and the assistant at the bedside can toggle between the right and left lenses of the robotic camera. The display is a touch screen and allows individuals to draw with their fingers on the monitor. The operating surgeon sitting at the console can see the live drawings made on the monitor while looking into the console. This assists in proctoring procedures and telesteration if needed during the procedure for a novice surgeon or a surgical trainee.

47.5 EndoWrist Instruments

EndoWrist surgical instruments are comprised of the following five components [8] from distal to proximal:

1. The Primary Effector: Located at the tip of the instrument (e.g., cautery hooks, scissors, and graspers).
2. The Wrist: Designed to mimic the range of motion of the human wrist.
3. The Shaft: Provides length to the instrument and allows rotation of the tip.
4. Instrument Housing: Connects the instrument to the patient cart arm.
5. Release Levers: Allows removal of the instrument.

The most crucial factor that distinguishes the EndoWrist instruments from standard laparoscopic surgical instruments is the inclusion of the wrist joint—enabling the tip of the instrument to have seven degrees of freedom. Because of this added mobility, EndoWrist instruments afford a significantly greater degree of control and precision for the operating surgeon. A wide variety of instruments is available for purchase through intuitive surgical. However, it must be noted that each instrument has a maximum usage limit, most often ten procedures. Unfortunately, the da Vinci patient cart will not allow instruments at their usage limit to be used again. Therefore, EndoWrist instruments must be replaced much faster than laparoscopic instruments.

47.6 Simulation and Dual Console Surgery

Similar to laparoscopic surgery, there is a need for surgeons new to the da Vinci system to practice core skills before attempting robotic-assisted procedures. To that end, intuitive has created a robust simulation library, SimNow, for new users to train on the da Vinci system. The SimNow platform is the central learning hub, providing gamified exercises that users can perform on training surgeon consoles. These exercises are then scored, incorporating the user's time to complete the given task, camera/instrument movement efficiency, and any mistakes made during the exercise. These scores are designed to highlight how a user can improve their robotic surgery prowess. The learning curriculum is designed to progress users from simple tasks, such as controlling the camera view, to more complex tasks requiring frequent use of all three instrument arms and endoscope adjustment. Additionally, virtual case exercises, such as laparoscopic cholecystectomy, are available.

In addition to simulation, a unique feature of the da Vinci system is the option to incorporate a second surgeon console in the operating room. Having two surgeon consoles in the operating room allows control of the instruments and endoscopes to be passed from one console to another. Generally, this allows trainees to attempt small parts of a more extensive procedure under the guidance of the senior surgeon, who can retake control of the instruments at any time. Additionally, while one console is able to control the surgical instruments, the user at the other console can create and control a digital pointer/cursor visible to the user at the other console, allowing for in-the-moment teaching opportunities and instruction.

47.7 Conclusion

In conclusion, the Da Vinci surgical system has revolutionized the field of robotic surgery and has had a significant impact on how minimally invasive procedures are performed. The system's ability to provide surgeons with high-definition 3D imaging and a range of motion greater than the human hand has made it a popular choice for many procedures, including prostatectomies, gynecological surgeries, thoracic, bariatric, ENT, hepatobiliary and hernia repair procedures. Patients who undergo surgeries using the Da Vinci system typically experience less pain, reduced scarring, shorter hospital stays, and faster recovery times compared to traditional open surgery.

Despite the many benefits of the Da Vinci system, there are still some limitations and challenges to be overcome. One of the biggest concerns is the high cost of the equipment, which can limit its availability in some hospitals and healthcare facilities [9]. Additionally, the system's dependence on a reliable Internet connection and the potential for technical malfunctions can lead to delays or cancellations of procedures [10]. However, ongoing advancements in technology and continued research is addressing these issues, and we can expect to see even more remarkable outcomes in the years to come. Overall, the Da Vinci surgical system is an exciting development in the field of robotic surgery, and it has already had a significant impact on patient outcomes and the future of surgical care.

References

1. Intuitive Surgical Annual Report 2021; 2022.
2. George EI, Brand TC, LaPorta A, Marescaux J, Satava RM. Origins of Robotic Surgery: From Skepticism to Standard of Care. JSLS. 2018;22(4). https://doi.org/10.4293/JSLS.2018.00039.
3. Schneider A, Feussner H. Mechatronic Support Systems and Robots. Biomedical Engineering in Gastrointestinal Surgery. 2017:387–441. Published online January 1. https://doi.org/10.1016/B978-0-12-803230-5.00010-5.
4. Richter F, Orosco RK, Yip MC. Motion scaling solutions for improved performance in high delay surgical teleoperation. Proc IEEE Int Conf Robot Autom. 2019;1590–5. https://doi.org/10.1109/ICRA.2019.8794085.
5. Reiley CE, Akinbiyi T, Burschka D, Chang DC, Okamura AM, Yuh DD. Effects of visual force feedback on robot-assisted surgical task performance. J Thorac Cardiovasc Surg. 2008;135(1):196–202. https://doi.org/10.1016/J.JTCVS.2007.08.043.
6. Golahmadi AK, Khan DZ, Mylonas GP, Marcus HJ. Tool-tissue forces in surgery: a systematic review. Ann Med Surg (Lond). 2021;65. https://doi.org/10.1016/J.AMSU.2021.102268.
7. Jourdes F, Valentin B, Allard J, Duriez C, Seeliger B. Visual haptic feedback for training of robotic suturing. Front Robot AI. 2022;9. https://doi.org/10.3389/FROBT.2022.800232/FULL.
8. Da Vinci Xi User Manual PN551400-15Rev.B2021.12; 2021.
9. Khorgami Z, Li WT, Jackson TN, Howard CA, Sclabas GM. The cost of robotics: an analysis of the added costs of robotic-assisted versus laparoscopic surgery using the National Inpatient Sample. Surg Endosc. 2019;33(7):2217–21. https://doi.org/10.1007/S00464-018-6507-3.
10. Mehta A, Cheng Ng J, Andrew Awuah W, et al. Embracing robotic surgery in low- and middle-income countries: Potential benefits, challenges, and scope in the future. Ann Med Surg (Lond). 2022;84:104803. https://doi.org/10.1016/J.AMSU.2022.104803.

GPSR Compliance

The European Union's (EU) General Product Safety Regulation (GPSR) is a set of rules that requires consumer products to be safe and our obligations to ensure this.

If you have any concerns about our products, you can contact us on ProductSafety@springernature.com

In case Publisher is established outside the EU, the EU authorized representative is:

Springer Nature Customer Service Center GmbH
Europaplatz 3
69115 Heidelberg, Germany

Batch number: 10889555

Printed by Printforce, the Netherlands